Psychodynamic Diagnostic Manual (PDM)

A collaborative effort of the

American Psychoanalytic Association
International Psychoanalytical Association
Division of Psychoanalysis (39) of the American Psychological Association
American Academy of Psychoanalysis and Dynamic Psychiatry
National Membership Committee on Psychoanalysis in Clinical Social Work

The correct way to cite this book is:

PDM Task Force. (2006). *Psychodynamic Diagnostic Manual*. Silver Spring, MD:
Alliance of Psychoanalytic Organizations

Published by the Alliance of Psychoanalytic Organizations[*]
Psychodynamic Diagnostic Manual (PDM)
10125 Colesville Road, Suite 194
Silver Spring, MD20901
301-789-1660
http://www.pdm1.org

Library of Congress Control Number:2006923050

ISBN 0-9767758-2-4 (paper); 0-9767758-1-6 (cloth)

---

[*]The Alliance of Psychoanalytic Organizations is a program of the Interdisciplinary Council on Developmental and Learning Disorders

Psychodynamic Diagnostic Manual (PDM)

TABLE OF CONTENTS

Outline of the PDM Classification System

PART I—CLASSIFICATION OF ADULT MENTAL HEALTH DISORDERS

Symptom Patterns: The Subjective Experience—S Axis 91

PART III—CONCEPTUAL AND RESEARCH FOUNDATIONS FOR A PSYCHODYNAMICALLY BASED CLASSIFICATION SYSTEM FOR MENTAL HEALTH DISORDERS

Research Foundations

PSYCHODYNAMIC DIAGNOSTIC TASK FORCE

Sponsoring Organizations and Steering Committee

American Psychoanalytic Association
Jon Meyer, MD
President

Ruth S. Fischer, MD
(for Newell Fischer, MD
Past President)

International Psychoanalytical Association
Professor Daniel Widlöcher
Past President

**American Psychological Association
Division of Psychoanalysis (39)**
Jaine L. Darwin, PsyD
Past President

American Academy of Psychoanalysis
Ronald Turco, MD
Past President

**National Membership Committee on
Psychoanalysis in Clinical Social Work**
Barbara Berger, PhD, BCD
Past President

Stuart G. Shanker, DPhil
York University
Toronto, Ontario

Stanley I. Greenspan, MD (Chair)
George Washington University Medical School
Washington, DC

PDM Task Force

Stanley I. Greenspan, MD, Chair

Nancy McWilliams, PhD, Associate Chair   Robert S. Wallerstein, MD, Associate Chair

Adult Mental Health Disorders
Coordinating Committee

Robert S. Wallerstein, MD, (Chair)

Otto Kernberg, MD

Nancy McWilliams, PhD

Herbert Schlesinger, PhD

Jonathan Shedler, PhD

Drew Westen, PhD

Adult Personality Disorders

Nancy McWilliams, PhD (Chair)

Eve Caligor, MD

Abby Herzig, PsyD

Otto Kernberg, MD

Jonathan Shedler, PhD

Drew Westen, PhD

Adult Symptom Patterns

Malkah Notman, MD

Héctor Ferrari, MD

Paul Fink, MD

Abby Herzig, PsyD

Marvin Hurvich, PhD, ABPP

Judy Ann Kaplan, LCSW, BCD

Thomas Kenemore, PhD, LCSW

Edward J. Khantzian, MD

Martha Kirkpatrick, MD

Jodi Licht, PsyD

David G. Phillips, DSW

Stanley I. Greenspan, MD

*Consultants to the Symptom
Patterns Work Group:*
Rachel Barbanel-Fried, PsyD
Edward Dewey, PsyD
Nadine Khoury, PsyD
Rachel Miller, PsyD
Sarah Sarkis, PsyD

Profile of Mental Functioning for Adults and Children

Paul Fink, MD

Bernard Friedberg, MD

Stanley I. Greenspan, MD

Joseph Palombo, MA

Stuart G. Shanker, DPhil

Child and Adolescent Mental Health Disorders

Joseph Palombo, MA (Co-Chair)

Bernard Friedberg, MD (Co-Chair)

Alex Burland, MD (deceased)

Amy Eldridge, PhD

Theodore Fallon, Jr., MD, MPH

Ruth Fischer, MD

Stanley I. Greenspan, MD

Leon Hoffman, MD

Thomas K. Kenemore, PhD,

Paulina Kernberg, MD (deceased)

Stuart G. Shanker, DPhil

Serena Wieder, PhD

Conceptual and Research Foundations

Barbara Berger, PhD, BCD

Sidney J. Blatt, PhD

Reiner Dahlbender, MD, PhD

Peter Fonagy, PhD, FBA

Stanley I. Greenspan, MD

Judy Ann Kaplan, LCSW, BCD

Bertram Karon, PhD

Nancy McWilliams, PhD

David G. Phillips, DSW

Daniel B. Rosenfeld, MA, LCSW BCD

Stuart G. Shanker, DPhil

Jonathan Shedler, PhD

Howard Shevrin, PhD

Robert S. Wallerstein, MD

Joel Weinberger, PhD

Drew Westen, PhD

Daniel Widlöcher, PhD

Consultants

Arnold Cooper, MD

Sherwood Faigen, MA

R. Dennis Shelby, PhD

George Stricker, PhD

PDM Task Force

Barbara Berger, PhD, BCD
Dean of Admissions
Institute for Clinical Social Work
Chicago, Illinois

Sidney J. Blatt, PhD
Professor, Psychiatry and Psychology
Departments of Psychiatry and
Psychology
Yale University
New Haven, Connecticut

Alex Burland, MD (deceased)
Training/Supervising
Psychoanalyst
The Psychoanalytic Center of
Philadelphia
Philadelphia, Pennsylvania

Eve Caligor, MD
Clinical Professor of Psychiatry
Columbia University College of
Physicians and Surgeons
New York, New York

Reiner Dahlbender, MD, PhD
Medical Director, MEDICLIN –
Clinic for Psychosomatic Medicine and
Psychotherapy,
Member of the Medical University of
Hannover/University of Ulm, Hannover/Ulm,
Germany

Amy Eldridge, PhD
Dean
Institute for Clinical Social Work
Chicago, Illinois

Theodore Fallon, Jr., MD, MPH
Psychoanalytic Center of
Philadelphia
Philadelphia, Pennsylvania

Héctor Ferrari, MD
Professor
Department of Mental Health University of
Buenos Aires Medical School
Buenos Aires, Argentina

Paul Fink, MD
Professor of Psychiatry
Temple University School of
Medicine
Philadelphia, Pennsylvania

Ruth Fischer, MD
Clinical Professor of Psychiatry
University of Pennsylvania School of Medicine
Philadelphia, Pennsylvania

Peter Fonagy, PhD, FBA
Freud Memorial Professor of
Psychoanalysis
Sub-Department of Clinical Health
Psychology
University College
London, England

Bernard Friedberg, MD
President
Foundation of the Psychoanalytic
Center of Philadelphia
Voorhees, New Jersey

Stanley I. Greenspan, MD
Clinical Professor of Psychiatry and Pediatrics
George Washington University Medical School
Bethesda, Maryland

Abby Herzig, PsyD
George Washington University
Psychoanalytic Candidate
NYU Psychoanalytic Institute at
NYU Medical Center
New York, New York

Leon Hoffman, MD
Director
Pacella Parent Child Center
New York Psychoanalytic Institute
and Society
New York, New York

Marvin Hurvich, PhD, ABPP
Professor of Psychology
Long Island University
Brooklyn, New York

Judy Ann Kaplan, LCSW, BCD
President
National Membership Committee
on Psychoanalysis in Clinical
Social Work
Practicing Psychoanalyst
New York University
School of Social Work
New York, New York

Thomas K. Kenemore, PhD, LCSW
Institute for Clinical Social Work
Chicago, Illinois

Otto Kernberg, MD
Professor of Psychiatry
Weill Medical College
Cornell University
Westchester, New York

Paulina Kernberg, MD (deceased)
Director of Child and Adolescent Psychiatry
New York Hospital
Cornell Medical Center
Westchester Division
Westchester, New York

Edward J. Khantzian, MD
Clinical Professor of Psychiatry
Harvard Medical School
The Cambridge Hospital and
Tewksbury Hospital
Cambridge, Massachusetts

Martha Kirkpatrick, MD
Clinical Professor
David Geffen School
University of California at Los Angeles
Los Angeles, California

Jodi Licht, PsyD
Postdoctoral Candidate in
Psychoanalysis and Psychotherapy
Adelphi University
Garden City, New York

Nancy McWilliams, PhD
Visiting Professor of Clinical
Psychology
Graduate School of Applied &
Professional Psychology
Rutgers University
Piscataway, New Jersey

Malkah Notman, MD
Clinical Professor of Psychiatry
Harvard University
Cambridge, Massachusetts

Joseph Palombo, MA
Clinical Social Worker
Founding Dean and Faculty Member
Institute for Clinical Social Work
Chicago, Illinois

David G. Phillips, DSW
Supervising and Training Analyst
Psychoanalytic Institute of the Postgraduate
Center for Mental ealth
Adjunct Associate Professor Wurzweiler School
of Social Work
Yeshiva University
New York City, New York

Daniel B. Rosenfeld, MA, LCSW BCD
Illinois Society for Clinical Social Work
Chicago, Illinois

Herbert Schlesinger, PhD
Clinical Professor of Psychology in
Psychiatry
College of Physicians and Surgeons
Columbia University
New York, New York

Stuart G. Shanker, DPhil
Distinguished Research Professor
of Philosophy and Psychology
Director, The Milton and Ethel
Harris Research Initiative
York University
Toronto, Ontario

Jonathan Shedler, PhD
Associate Professor
Graduate School of Professional
Psychology
University of Denver
Denver, Colorado

Howard Shevrin, PhD
Professor of Psychology
Department of Psychiatry
Director
University of Michigan Program of
Research in Neuro-Psychoanalysis
University of Michigan Medical Center
Ann Arbor, Michigan

Robert S. Wallerstein, MD
Emeritus Professor and
Former Chair
Department of Psychiatry
University of California
San Francisco
School of Medicine
San Francisco, California

Joel Weinberger, PhD
Professor
Derner Institute
Adelphi University
Garden City, New York

Drew Westen, PhD
Professor
Department of Psychology and
Department of Psychiatry and
Behavioral Sciences
Emory University
Atlanta, Georgia

Daniel Widlöcher, PhD
Former IPA President
Service of Psychiatry
Hospital of Salpêtrière
Paris, France

Serena Wieder, PhD
Associate Chair
Interdisciplinary Council on
Developmental and Learning
Disorders
Silver Spring, Maryland

Consultants

Arnold Cooper, MD
Stephen P. Tobin and Dr. Arnold M. Cooper
Professor Emeritus
Weill Cornell Medical College
Westchester, New York

Sherwood Faigen, MA
Institute for Clinical Social Work
Chicago, Illinois

R. Dennis Shelby, PhD
Institute for Clinical Social Work
Chicago, Illinois

George Stricker, PhD
Distinguished Research Professor
Adelphi University
Garden City, NY 11530

Acknowledgements

Support provided by the Milton and Ethel Harris Research Institute, York University, Toronto, Canada, and the Interdisciplinary Council on Developmental and Learning Disorders.

The PDM Task Force thanks Jan Tunney for her extraordinary skill in being the hub of communication, coordination, and organization for all the work groups, Jane Mild LaRoque for her excellent editing, Sue Morrisson for her careful editing of the references and work on the manuscript, and Jill Sobieski for all her help in putting the book together. Special thanks to Dottie Jeffries of the American Psychoanalytic Association for her invaluable ongoing guidance on dissemination and public and media communication.

Introduction

OVERVIEW

The *Psychodynamic Diagnostic Manual* (PDM) is a diagnostic framework that attempts to characterize an individual's full range of functioning—the depth as well as the surface of emotional, cognitive, and social patterns. It emphasizes individual variations as well as commonalities. We hope that this framework brings about improvements in the diagnosis and treatment of mental disorders and permits a fuller understanding of the functioning of the mind and brain and their development. The goal of the PDM is to complement the DSM and ICD efforts of the past 30 years in cataloguing symptoms by explicating the broad range of mental functioning.

The PDM is based on current neuroscience, treatment outcome research, and other empirical investigations. Research on brain development and the maturation of mental processes suggests that patterns of emotional, social, and behavioral functioning involve many areas working together rather than in isolation. Outcome studies point to the importance of dealing with the full complexity of emotional and social patterns. Numerous researchers (e.g., Blatt, Auerbach, Zuroff & Shahar, p. 537; Norcross, 2002; Wampold, 2001) have concluded that the nature of the psychotherapeutic relationship, reflecting interconnected aspects of mind and brain operating together in an interpersonal context, predicts outcome more robustly than any specific treatment approach *per se*.

Westen, Novotny, and Thompson-Brenner (2004; p. 691) have presented evidence that treatments that focus on isolated symptoms or behaviors (rather than personality, emotional, and interpersonal patterns) are not effective in sustaining even narrowly defined changes. Shedler and Westen (p. 573), Dahlbender and colleagues (p. 615), and Blatt and colleagues (p. 537) have developed reliable ways to measure complex patterns of personality, emotion, and interpersonal processes that constitute the active ingredients of the psychotherapeutic relationship. Braconnier, Widlöcher, and colleagues discuss the range of problems for which psychodynamic approaches are suitable (p. 403). A number of recent reviews (e.g., Fonagy, p. 765, and Leichsenring, p. 819) demonstrate that in addition to alleviating symptoms, psychodynamically based therapeutic approaches improve overall emotional and social functioning.

The PDM was created though a collaborative effort of the major organizations representing psychoanalytically oriented mental health professionals; namely, the American Psychoanalytic Association, the International Psychoanalytical Association, the Division of Psychoanalysis (39) of the American Psychological Association, the American Academy of Psychoanalysis, and the National Membership Committee on Psychoanalysis in Clinical Social Work. Their presidents formed a steering committee and recommended members to serve on work groups to construct this classification system.

The diagnostic framework formulated by the PDM work groups systematically describes:

- Healthy and disordered personality functioning;
- Individual profiles of mental functioning, including patterns of relating, comprehending and expressing feelings, coping with stress and anxiety, observing one's own emotions and behaviors, and forming moral judgments; and
- Symptom patterns, including differences in each individual's personal, subjective experience of symptoms.

The PDM adds a needed perspective to existing diagnostic systems. In addition to considering symptom patterns described in existing taxonomies, it enables clinicians to describe and categorize personality patterns, related social and emotional capacities, unique mental profiles, and personal experiences of symptoms. It provides a framework for improving comprehensive treatment approaches and understanding both the biological and psychological origins of mental health and illness.

RATIONALE FOR THE PDM

A clinically useful classification of mental health disorders must begin with an understanding of healthy mental processes. Mental health comprises more than simply the absence of symptoms. It involves a person's overall mental functioning, including relationships; emotional depth, range, and regulation; coping capacities; and self-observing abilities. Just as healthy cardiac functioning cannot be defined simply as an absence of chest pain, healthy mental functioning is more than the absence of observable symptoms of psychopathology. It involves the full range of human cognitive, emotional, and behavioral capacities.

Any attempt to describe and classify deficiencies in mental health must therefore take into account limitations or deficits in many different mental capacities, including ones that are not necessarily overt sources of pain. For example, as frightening as anxiety attacks can be, an inability to perceive and respond accurately to the emotional cues of others—a far more subtle and diffuse problem—may constitute a more fundamental difficulty than periodic episodes of unexplained panic. A deficit in reading emotional cues may pervasively compromise relationships and thinking, and may itself be a source of anxiety.

That a comprehensive conceptualization of health is the foundation for describing disorder may seem self-evident, yet the mental health field has not developed its diagnostic procedures accordingly. In the last two decades, there has been an increasing tendency to define mental problems primarily on the basis of observable symptoms, behaviors, and traits, with overall personality functioning and levels of adaptation noted only secondarily. There is increasing evidence, however, that both mental health and psychopathology involve many subtle features of human functioning, including affect tolerance, regulation, and expression; coping strategies and defenses; capacities for understanding self and others; and quality of relationships. Mounting evidence from neuroscience and developmental studies supports the position that mental functioning, whether optimal or compromised, is highly complex. To ignore mental complexity is to ignore the very phenomena of concern. After all, our mental complexity defines our most human qualities.

Over the past 30 years or so, in the hope of developing an adequate empirical basis for diagnosis and treatment, the mental health field has progressively narrowed its perspective, focusing more and more on simple symptom clusters. The whole person has been less visible than the various disorder constructs on which researchers can find agreement. Recent reviews of this effort have raised the possibility that such a strategy was misguided. Ironically, emerging evidence suggests that oversimplifying mental health phenomena in the service of attaining consistency of description (reliability) and capacity to evaluate treatment empirically (validity) may have compromised the laudable goal of a more scientifically sound understanding of mental health and psychopathology. Most problematically, reliability and validity data for many disorders are not as strong as the mental health community had hoped they would be (see Herzig and Licht, p. 663). Allen Frances, Chair of the DSM-IV American Psychiatric Association Task Force, recently acknowledged that the desired reliability, especially among practicing clinicians, has not been obtained (Spiegel, 2005).

Therefore, the laudatory goal of constructing an evidence-based diagnostic system may have led to a tendency to overstep the existing evidence, to make overly narrow observations, and, in the process, to compromise the important goal of classifying mental health and mental health disorders according to their naturally occurring patterns. Only an accurate description of naturally occurring patterns can guide vital research on etiology, developmental pathways, prevention, and treatment. As the history of science attests (and, as recently emphasized by the American Psychological Association in their guidelines defining "evidence"), scientific evidence includes and often begins with sound descriptions, such as case studies.

Insufficient attention to this foundation of scientific knowledge, under the pressure of a narrow definition of what constitutes evidence (in the service of rapid quantification and replication) would tend to repeat rather than ameliorate the problems of current systems. Efforts to complement the current classification system with a fuller description of mental health and mental health disorders must begin with a consensus of "expert opinion" based on astute clinical observations informed by an accurate appraisal of existing and emerging research (see Part III, Conceptual and Research Foundations, p. 383).

In a recent commentary in the *Journal of the American Medical Association*, Paul McHugh (2005) pointed out that medicine has moved beyond simply describing symptoms to categorizing disorders according to the nature of the functional impairment and etiological factors (if known). Contending that the classification of mental health disorders may have gone too far in focusing on describing symptoms (overlapping categories, excessive comorbidities, etc.), thereby compromising efforts to improve our understanding and treatment of psychopathology, he recommended that the classification of mental disorders also reflect the quality and degree of functional impairment and, where possible, etiology.

The mental health field has a long history of describing symptom patterns. As in the development of many fields, this effort began with pioneers who made meticulous observations and discovered common clusters of patient complaints, symptoms, and behaviors. In attempting to make progress in describing naturally occurring patterns, however, much recent research has been a mixed blessing. On the one hand, carefully constructed questionnaires and structured interviews have led to more reliable judgments about symptom patterns and have facilitated research into what belongs in a pattern, including its antecedents and course. On the other hand, fixed definitions (often made by clinical consensus) and incomplete data have impeded the improvement of descriptions of naturally occurring patterns.

A patient may experience a number of symptom patterns. Many such patterns have long been observed to overlap. In the DSM and ICD systems, the use of fixed definitions and strict criteria (e.g., four out of six, not three out of six, items on a diagnostic checklist) forces an artificial separation of conditions that are frequently related. Symptoms that may be etiologically, phenomenologically, or contextually interconnected are described as comorbid conditions, as if these discrete problems coexist more or less accidentally in the same person, much as a sinus infection and a broken toe might coexist. Assumptions about discrete, unrelated, comorbid conditions are rarely justified by compelling data such as clear genetic, biochemical, and neurophysiological distinctions between syndromes. The cut-off criteria for diagnosis are often arbitrary decisions of committees rather than conclusions drawn from the best scientific evidence.

The development of the PDM reflects our concern that mental health professionals may have uncritically and prematurely adopted methods from other sciences instead of developing empirical procedures appropriate to the complexity of the data in our field. The intent of those who moved the DSM and ICD classifications in the direction of specifying discrete, externally observable disorders was to build a stronger foundation for the diagnosis and treatment of psychopathology. This was a worthy project. Now, however, it is time to take a hard look at the phenomena with which mental health professionals regularly deal and to adapt the methods to the phenomena rather than vice versa (see Blatt, et al., p. 537, and Shedler & Westen, p. 573).

The PDM attempts to do this. Because the current terminology for symptoms and their groupings comes from a long and intellectually serious tradition, we employ the descriptions of symptoms and patterns of symptoms used in the currently prevailing taxonomies, the DSM-IV-TR and ICD-10, systems that represent a valuable history of careful observation and description. In the most recent versions of the DSM and ICD systems, however, some of the more subtle features of many basic symptom patterns have been lost. Most notably, despite the fact that it is usually the patient's subjective suffering that brings him or her to treatment, a full description of the patient's internal experience of the symptoms is often absent.

All approaches to assessment and treatment rely at least in part on patients' reports of their thoughts, feelings, and behaviors. (Does the patient feel depressed? anxious? Does the patient hear voices? think about suicide?) Therefore, despite the fact that mental health professionals are inevitably dealing with the elusive world of subjectivity, we require a fuller description of the patient's internal life to do justice to understanding his or her distinctive experience. We are hoping that with more elaborated depictions, we can make more progress on understanding naturally occurring patterns. The rapidly advancing neuroscience field, including genetic studies, can be only as useful as our understanding of the basic patterns of mental health and pathology. We cannot expect our colleagues in genetics to separate the apples and oranges for us. If we do not properly separate them, we shall continue to frustrate the search for underlying biological pathways and common experiential etiologies.

Even in general medicine, instances in which etiological factors are fully understood are rare. Most commonly, we are at the level of functional rather than etiological explanation. Neoplastic disorders, for example, are often thought to be understood etiologically, but we are still searching for the causes of many malignancies, as we attempt to comprehend the relationship between genetic, environmental, and, in some instances, viral and other infectious processes. We are nonetheless able to describe various malignancies in detail in terms of their functional characteristics. Both in general medicine and in mental health, progress in understanding the functional nature of disorders should eventually facilitate a greater understanding of etiological factors. Functional and etiological understanding together provide the fullest basis for diagnosis and treatment.

In general, there is a healthy tension between the goals of capturing the complexity of clinical phenomena (functional understanding) and developing criteria that can be reliably judged and employed in research (descriptive understanding). It is vital to embrace this tension by pursuing a step-wise approach in which complexity and clinical usefulness influence operational definitions and inform research. A scientifically based system begins with accurate recognition and description of complex clinical phenomena and builds gradually toward empirical validation. Reliance on oversimplification and favoring what is measurable over what is meaningful do not operate in the service of good science.

In addition, we are learning that when therapists apply manualized treatments to selected symptom clusters without addressing the complex person who experiences the symptoms and without attending to the therapeutic relationship that supports the treatment, therapeutic results are short-lived and rates of remission are high (Baumann, Hilsenroth, Ackerman, Baity, Smith, Smith, et al., 2001; Hilsenroth, Ackerman, Blagys, Baity, & Mooney, 2003; Stiles, Agnew-Davies, Hardy, Barkham, & Shapiro, 1998; Westen, Novotny, & Thompson-Brenner, 2004). A recent meta-analysis of outcomes of manualized treatments for targeted symptoms found that symptomatic improvement often did not persist and that fundamental psychological capacities involving the depth and range of relationships, feelings, and coping strategies did not show evidence of long-term change. In a number of studies these critical areas were not even measured (Westen, et al., 2004).

At the same time, process-oriented research has demonstrated that essential characteristics of the psychotherapeutic relationship as conceptualized by psychodynamic models (the working alliance, transference phenomena, and stable characteristics of patient and therapist) are more predictive of outcome than any designated treatment approach *per se*. Most dynamically oriented clinicians pay careful attention to the therapeutic relationship, noting interpersonal patterns, feelings, coping strategies, and other indicators of mental processes. Although underresearched for decades, psychodynamically based treatments have been the subject of several recent meta-analyses and reviews that reveal evidence of their efficacy (see Fonagy, p. 765; Hilsenroth, et al., 2003; Leichsenring, p. 819; Leichsenring & Leibing, 2003).

The importance of focusing on an individual's full range of feelings and thoughts (personal experience) in the context of his or her unique history cannot be underestimated. For example, a major collaborative effort involving the CDC in Atlanta and over 17,000 adults at Kaiser Permanente (the Adverse Childhood Experiences Study [ACE]), found that exposure to developmentally undermining emotional experiences in childhood was associated with increased likelihood of both physical and mental health problems as adults. The rates of physical and mental health problems were surprisingly high in relationship to the number of adverse experiences during childhood, ranging from over 200% for selected physical illnesses to over 4,000% for selected mental health disorders. The study also revealed that both the physical and mental health disorders were associated with complex feelings and thoughts employed to deal with the adverse childhood experiences (Anda, Croft, Felitti, Nordenberg, et al., 1999; Dietz, Spitz, Anda, Williamson, et al., 1999; Dube, Anda, Felitti, Chapman, et al., 2001; Felitti, Anda, Nordenbreg, Williamson, et al., 1998; Foege, 1998; Hillis, Anda, Felitti, Nordenberg, & Marchbanks, 2000; Weiss & Wagner, 1998; see also: *http://www.cdc.gov/nccdphp/ace/index.htm*).

Although the psychoanalytic tradition, or depth psychology, has a long history of examining overall human functioning in a searching and comprehensive way, the diagnostic precision and usefulness of psychodynamic approaches have been compromised by at least two problems. First, until fairly recently, in attempts to capture the range and subtlety of human experience, psychoanalytic accounts of mental processes have been expressed in competing theories and metaphors that have, at times, inspired more disagreement and controversy than consensus. Second, there has been difficulty distinguishing between speculative constructs on the one hand, and phenomena that can be observed or reasonably inferred on the other. Where the tradition of descriptive psychiatry has had a tendency to reify "disorder" categories, the psychoanalytic tradition has tended to reify theoretical constructs.

In recent years, however, having developed empirical methods to quantify and analyze complex mental phenomena, depth psychology has been able to offer clear operational criteria for a more comprehensive range of human social and emotional conditions (see Blatt, et al., p. 537; Dahlbender, Rudolf, & the OPD Task Force, p. 615; Lingiardi, Shedler, & Gazzillo, in press; Shedler & Westen, p. 573; Westen, Novotny, & Thompson-Brenner, p. 691). The current challenge is to systematize these advances with a growing body of rich clinical experience in order to provide a widely usable framework for understanding and specifying complex and subtle mental phenomena.

A psychodynamically based system highlights the processes that contribute to emotional and social functioning. Early in its history, psychodynamic theories speculated about etiological factors. As in all fields of medicine, however, clinicians and researchers quickly learned that the etiologies of psychological disorders are more complex than initial observations and theory had suggested. Consequently, psychodynamic models have moved toward functional understanding of psychopathologies, with the expectation that such understanding will eventually lead to the identification of etiological patterns. In light of all this, the PDM addresses the full range of mental functioning.

The PDM uses a multidimensional approach to describe the intricacies of the patient's overall functioning and ways of engaging in the therapeutic process. It begins with a classification of the spectrum of personality patterns and disorders, then offers a "profile of mental functioning" covering in more detail the patient's capacities, and finally considers symptom patterns, with emphasis on the patient's subjective experience.

DIMENSION I: PERSONALITY PATTERNS AND DISORDERS—P AXIS

The PDM classification of personality patterns takes into account two areas: the person's general location on a continuum from healthier to more disordered functioning, and the nature of the characteristic ways the individual organizes mental functioning and engages the world.

This dimension has been placed first in the PDM system because of the accumulating evidence that symptoms or problems cannot be understood, assessed, or treated in the absence of an understanding of the mental life of the person who has the symptoms. For example, a depressed mood may be manifested in markedly different ways in a person who fears relationships and avoids experiencing and expressing most feelings and in an individual who is fully engaged in all of life's relationships and emotions. There is not just one clinical presentation of the artificially isolated phenomenon known as depression.

DIMENSION II: MENTAL FUNCTIONING—M AXIS

The second PDM dimension offers a more detailed description of emotional functioning—the capacities that contribute to an individual's personality and overall level of psychological health or pathology. It takes a more microscopic look at mental life, systematizing such capacities as information processing and self-regulation; the forming and maintaining of relationships; experiencing, organizing, and expressing different levels of affects or emotions; representing, differentiating, and integrating experience; using coping strategies and defenses; observing self and others; and forming internal standards.

DIMENSION III: MANIFEST SYMPTOMS AND CONCERNS—S AXIS

Dimension III begins with the DSM-IV-TR categories and goes on to describe the affective states, cognitive processes, somatic experiences, and relational patterns most often associated clinically with each one. We approach symptom clusters as useful *descriptors*. Unless there is compelling evidence in a particular case for such an assumption, we do not regard them as highly demarcated biopsychosocial phenomena. In other words, we are taking care not to overstep our knowledge base. Thus, Dimension III presents symptom patterns in terms of the patient's *personal experience* of his or her prevailing difficulties. The patient may evidence a few or many patterns, which may or may not be related, and which should be seen in the context of the person's personality and mental functioning. The multidimensional approach depicted in the following sections provides a systematic way to describe patients that is faithful to their complexity and helpful in planning appropriate treatments.

As the title of this manual makes clear, we have looked at mental health disorders from a frankly psychodynamic point of view. Because we consider it impossible to be unbiased or genuinely atheoretical, we have simply tried to be explicit about our biases insofar as we are conscious of them. We hope that our explication of a psychodynamically influenced diagnosis will be useful to therapists trained in other traditions, including biological, cognitive-behavioral, family systems, and humanistic approaches. A more thorough diagnostic formulation has the potential to inform any treatment plan that seeks to take the whole person into account. We also believe that even fondly held ideas must be subject to potential disconfirmation by empirical investigation. Hence, we hope that this manual will be tested and improved in later editions, as empirical researchers continue to investigate our assumptions.

REFERENCES

Anda, R. F., Croft, J. B., Felitti, V. J., Nordenberg, D., Giles, W. H., Williamson, D. F,. et al. (1999). Adverse childhood experiences and smoking during adolescence and adulthood. *Journal of the American Medical Association, 282,* 1359-1364.

Baumann, B. D., Hilsenroth, M. J., Ackerman, S. J., Baity, M. R., Smith, C. L., Smith, S. R., et al. (2001). The capacity for dynamic process scale: An examination of reliability, validity, and relation to therapeutic alliance. *Psychotherapy Research, 11,* 275-294.

Dietz, P. M., Spitz, A. M., Anda, R. F., Williamson, D. F., McMahon, P. M., Santelli, J. S., et al., (1999). Unintended pregnancy among adult women exposed to abuse or household dysfunction during their childhood. *Journal of the American Medical Association, 282,* 1359-1364.

Dube, S. R., Anda, R. F., Felitti, V. J., Chapman, D., Williamson, D. F., & Giles, W. H. (2001). Childhood abuse, household dysfunction and the risk of attempted suicide throughout the life span: Findings from Adverse Childhood Experiences Study. *Journal of the American Medical Association, 286,* 3089-3096.

Felitti, V. J., Anda, R. F., Nordenberg, D., Williamson, D. F., Spitz, A. M., Edwards, V., et al. (1998). The relationship of adult health status to childhood abuse and household dysfunction. *American Journal of Preventive Medicine, 14,* 245-258.

Foege, W. H. (1998). Adverse childhood experiences: A public health perspective (editorial). *American Journal of Preventive Medicine, 14,* 354-355.

Hillis, S. D., Anda, R. F., Felitti, V. J., Nordenberg, D., & Marchbanks, P. A. (2000). Adverse childhood experiences and sexually transmitted diseases in men and women: a retrospective study. *Pediatrics, 106,* E11.

Hilsenroth, M. J., Ackerman, S. J., Blagys, M. D., Baity, M. R., & Mooney, M. A. (2003). Short-term psychodynamic psychotherapy for depression: An examination of statistical, clinically significant, and technique-specific change. *The Journal of Nervous and Mental Disease, 191,* 349-357.

Leichsenring, F., & Leibing, E. (2003). The effectiveness of psychodynamic therapy and cognitive behavior therapy in the treatment of personality disorders: A meta-analysis. *American Journal of Psychiatry, 160,* 1223–1232.

Lingiardi, V., Shedler, J., & Gazzillo, F. (in press). Assessing personality change in psychotherapy with the SWAP-200: A case study. *Journal of Personality Assessment.*

McHugh, P. R. (2005). Striving for coherence: Psychiatry's efforts over classification. *Journal of the American Medical Association, 293,* 2526-2528.

Norcross, J. C. (2002). Empirically supported therapy relationships. In J. C. Norcross (Ed.), *Psychotherapy relationships that work: Therapist contributions and responsiveness to patients* (pp. 3-16). London: Oxford.

Spiegel, A. (2005, January 3). The dictionary of disorder: How one man revolutionized psychiatry. *The New Yorker,* 56-63.

Stiles, W., Agnew-Davies, R., Hardy, G. E., Barkham, M., & Shapiro, D. (1998). Relations of the alliance with psychotherapy outcome: Findings in the second Sheffield Psychotherapy Project. *Journal of Consulting and Clinical Psychology, 66,* 791-802.

Wampold, B. E. (2001). *The great psychotherapy debate: Models, methods and findings.* Mahwah, NJ: Lawrence Erlbaum.

Weiss, J. S. & Wagner, S. H. (1998). What explains the negative consequences of adverse childhood experiences on adult health? Insights from cognitive and neuroscience research (editorial). *American Journal of Preventive Medicine, 14,* 356-360.

Westen, D., Novotny, C. M., & Thompson-Brenner, H. (2004). The empirical status of empirically supported psychotherapies: Assumptions, findings, and reporting in controlled clinical trials. *Psychological Bulletin, 130,* 631-663.

Part I
Classification of Adult Mental Health Disorders

Introduction: Adult Mental Health Disorders

A Psychodynamic Nosology of Mental Health Disorders

This psychoanalytic nosology of mental disorders is orthogonal in purpose and structure to the American Psychiatric Association's Diagnostic and Statistical Manual of Mental Disorders (DSM). It is not intended to replace the DSM, which has its distinct purposes and uses, but rather to supplement it for purposes of psychoanalytic (psychodynamic[1]) case formulation and treatment planning, especially when intensive psychotherapy seems the treatment of choice. It thus relates to DSM categorizations but is distinct from them in a variety of ways.

The DSM is a taxonomy of diseases or disorders of function. Ours is a taxonomy of people. DSM is categorical, assigning individuals to the appropriate diagnostic rubric. Ours, though it operates within broad categories, is dimensional within each heading description, indicating, in each instance, the spectrum covered. For each, we describe a continuum ranging from a description of a predominant character organization operating within a "normal" range of functioning through a neurotic level of functioning, and beyond—in most instances—onto the most severe extremes of borderline functioning. DSM categories are constructed to put symptoms and attributes that people have in common into the same diagnostic compartment. Within our more dimensional categorizations we try to elucidate what makes each individual unique, recognizably different from every other person in the world.

The DSM is built around overtly observable (and therefore, it was hoped, reliable) clusters of symptoms and attributes without any necessary imputations of meaning; in fact, the intent was to be atheoretical, that is, not to tie the phenomena, identified and categorized, to any overarching theory of mental functioning, psychoanalytic or other. Our nosology is explicitly set within a psychoanalytic framework that focuses on the full range and depth of human mental functioning. Therefore, our intent, in the various dimensions that comprise our nosological array, is to ascribe meanings, as best we can discern and formulate them, to the observed and described phenomena; i.e., symptoms, behaviors, traits, affects, attitudes, thoughts, fantasies, and so on. Since DSM categories consist of

---

[1] Some psychologists have differentiated "psychoanalytic" and "psychodynamic," using the former to refer to psychoanalysis as a specific form of intensive therapy, and the latter to refer to any subject matter or therapeutic approach influenced by psychoanalytic theory. We use the two terms more or less interchangeably.

distinct clusters of symptoms and attributes, which frequently overlap in part with the clusters of symptoms and attributes of other DSM categories, an individual's difficulties can then be put into two (or more) illness categories, called comorbidity, implying that the person is suffering from two different illnesses. Our nosology is built, for each individual, on the conception of a single coherent and meaningful character organization, which can, of course, represent, uniquely for that individual, a particular admixture of the defining characteristics of two (or more) character organizations and symptom patterns.

It is these described differences that fit the DSM and our psychoanalytic nosology to different purposes and uses. The DSM is geared to the reliability of its designated categories for research purposes, the comparison of researched populations across different samples, different sites, and different theoretical frameworks within which the researchers operate; for insurance reimbursement purposes, to distinguish between what is and is not covered by the insurance program; for epidemiological purposes; and for selected treatment purposes, for example, to identify what specific medication is indicated for those within a particular diagnostic rubric. Our taxonomy is geared toward one central purpose of individualized case formulation and treatment planning for psychoanalytic (psychodynamic) therapy and other therapies that attempt to address the full range and depth of human cognitive, emotional, and behavioral functioning.

Personality Patterns and Disorders
P Axis

Work Group Members

Nancy McWilliams, PhD, Chair
Flemington, New Jersey

Otto Kernberg, MD
Westchester, New York

Eve Caligor, MD
New York, New York

Jonathan Shedler, PhD
Denver, Colorado

Abby Herzig, PsyD
New York, New York

Drew Westen, PhD
Atlanta, Georgia

Personality Patterns and Disorders
P Axis

INTRODUCTION

To talk usefully about disorders of personality, we must first address the concept of personality itself. Personality is what one *is* rather than what one *has*. It certainly comprises more than one can see by scrutinizing a person's behavior. Irrespective of the specific problems that bring them to treatment, many patients, as they participate in therapy, come to realize that what they are trying to change is tied up with who they are. They need the therapist to comprehend something psychologically systemic about them that helps them understand why they are repeatedly vulnerable to certain kinds of suffering or difficulty. Psychological problems are often complexly intertwined with personality issues, may be the flip side of someone's strong points, and need to be appreciated in the context of the whole person and that person's culture.

A strength of the psychoanalytic tradition is its longstanding scholarly attention to the question of personality and its structure. Understanding individual people and their development can be more important to treating them than understanding specific disorders or mastering specific techniques. Consequently, when psychodynamic therapists conduct a clinical interview, they try first to get a feel for the patient's personality, then to evaluate the person's strengths, weaknesses, and overall functioning, and only then try to understand his or her symptoms in that context. In outcome studies, investigators are starting to pay adequate attention to the importance of differentiating among patients when evaluating treatments (Blatt, in press; Roth & Fonagy, 1996)—an emphasis that has been historically critical to clinicians but notably absent from much prior clinical research.

For purposes of this classification, we are defining "personality" as relatively stable ways of thinking, feeling, behaving, and relating to others. In this context, "thinking" encompasses not only one's belief systems and ways of making sense of self and others, but also one's moral values and ideals. Each of us has a set of individual assumptions by which we try to understand our experience, a set of values and characteristic ways of pursuing what we see as valuable, a personal repertoire of familiar emotions and typical ways of handling them, and some characteristic patterns of behaving, especially in our personal relationships. Some of these processes are conscious and some are unconscious and automatic (or, in the parlance of cognitive neuroscience, implicit).

The ways in which we habitually try to accommodate to the exigencies of life and to reduce anxiety, grief, and threats to self-esteem are important aspects of personality. People differ in the ways they adapt to circumstance and defend against threat, and they differ in their abilities to integrate these special efforts seamlessly into the conduct of everyday behavior so that the special efforts do not show as such. Depending on their cultural surround and a myriad of other factors, some patterns will be more adaptive than others. When our particular habitual ways of thinking, feeling, acting, and being with others contribute to our living satisfying lives, enjoying mutually satisfying relationships, and pursuing socially useful goals, there is no problem. If they repeatedly cause pain to ourselves or to others, or become preoccupying or conspicuous, they may constitute a personality "disorder."

At the healthy end of the spectrum of personality, at least as it has been construed by theorists in Western cultures, are people who can engage in satisfying relationships, can experience a relatively full range of age-expected feelings and thoughts, can function relatively flexibly when stressed by external forces or internal conflict, have a clear sense of personal identity, are well adapted to their life circumstances, and neither experience significant distress nor impose it on others. By flexibility, we mean that they can look at a problem from several different angles and adopt one of several possible ways of coping with it. At the more disturbed end are people who respond to stress in rigidly inflexible ways (by relying on only one or two coping strategies, for example, irrespective of the situation), and/or who have marked deficits in sense of identity, relations with others, reality testing, adaptation to stress, moral functioning, or affective range, recognition, expression, and regulation.

As there are an infinite number of lenses through which types and disorders of personality can be viewed, clinical observers, theorists, and researchers have suggested many different ways to conceptualize them.[1] For example, there is a vast literature in personality psychology on the "big five" factors of extraversion, neuroticism, openness to experience, agreeableness, and conscientiousness

---

[1] Among earlier theorists of personality, Karl Abraham, Alfred Adler, Otto Fenichel, Sigmund Freud, Erich Fromm, Karen Horney, Melanie Klein, Emil Kraepelin, Otto Rank, Wilhelm Reich, Herbert Rosenthal, and Harry Stack Sullivan have been particularly influential. More recent writers and researchers include Salman Akhtar, Michael Basch, Gertrude and Reuben Blanck, Jack Block, Norman Cameron, Erik Erikson, John Gedo, Lawrence Hedges, Althea Horner, Stephen Johnson, Lawrence Josephs, Otto Kernberg, Heinz Kohut, Jane Loevinger, Dan McAdams, Theodore Millon, Fred Pine, David Shapiro, Jefferson Singer, Lorna Smith-Benjamin, John Steiner, Michael Stone, and Veikko Tahka, among others.

Relevant researchers include Mary Ainsworth and other students of John Bowlby on attachment, Beatrice Beebe and Frank Lachmann on affect and attachment, Leo Bellak on ego strength, Sidney Blatt on object relations, Jack Block and Phoebe Cramer on ego control, resilience, and defenses, Louis Diguer and his colleagues on self and object representations, Robert Emde on emotional development, Peter Fonagy and Mary Target on attachment and mentalization, Stanley Greenspan on ego development, Michael Lewis in cognitive and affective development, Mardi Horowitz on conscious and unconscious mental processes, Rainer Krause on affect, Jane Loevinger on ego development, Doris Silverman on early development, Colin Trevarthan on representation, Edward Tronick on infancy, and Goerge Vaillant on defenses, among many others.

(Costa & Widiger, 2002; McCrea & Costa, 2003; Singer, 2005), but studies of the relationship between these presumably biotemperamental inclinations and personality disorder categories are still in the early stages. In this document, we have drawn on an extensive empirical and clinical literature to derive the best classification that the available evidence supports, but the nature of the subject matter is so complex, and the literature so incomplete, that our synthesis is of necessity both provisional and, though reasonable, somewhat arbitrary.

In the following, we describe the most clinically familiar personality disorders in terms of the cognitive, affective, relational, and defensive functioning associated with each. When empirical studies are available on a topic, we cite (where they exist) representative, well-designed, and recent research findings. When we refer to clinical experience, we cite writings from as far back as many decades ago, on the assumption that astute clinical description is not limited to the contemporary literature. In recent editions of the DSM, some personality disorders and clinically noted syndromes have been omitted because they have stimulated little empirical research (for example, although depressive personality disorders are common, they were excluded from DSM-III and subsequent editions, putatively on the basis of a lack of research—see Hirschfeld, 1991; Kernberg, 1984). Rather than omitting under-researched disorders, we prefer to include those on which there is extensive clinical agreement, in the hope that research will follow that will augment and improve our formulations.

DIFFERENTIAL DIAGNOSIS OF PERSONALITY DISORDERS AS A CLASS

Every human being has a personality. When someone's personality is so rigid or so marked by deficit that he or she has persistent problems in living, we may call it a personality disorder. In fact, there is no hard-and-fast dividing line between personality type and personality disorder—human functioning falls on a continuum. The term "disorder" is a linguistic convenience for clinicians and theorists denoting a condition that merits treatment. It is important to recognize that individuals with well functioning, stable personalities have many features of the pathological personality types depicted here. One can have, for example, an obsessive personality without having an obsessive personality *disorder*.

In diagnosing personality disorder, an essential criterion is the report of the patient and/or knowledgeable others that the patient's psychology has caused significant distress to self or others, is of longstanding duration, and is so much a part of the patient's consistent experience that he or she cannot remember, or easily imagine, being different. Many personality-disordered individuals come for treatment at the urging of others—friends, relatives, or authorities who are alarmed by their disturbed behavior, behavior that the person either discounts or is able to ignore. Others come on their own, seeking therapy not for their personality but for some more specific distress: anxiety, depression, eating disorders, somatic symptoms, addictions, phobias, self-harm, obsessions, compulsions, and relationship problems, among others.

In addition to differentiating "personality disorder" from personality *per se*, it is critical to differentiate personality disorders from symptom syndromes, the direct effects of injury to the brain, and psychoses. Ritualized behavior, for example, may indicate a single obsessive-compulsive problem, or constitute evidence of a pervasive obsessive-compulsive personality disorder, or express a psychotic delusion, or be the result of brain damage. A manic psychosis may express itself as a state of rage that is easily misunderstood as an affect-regulation problem associated with borderline personality organization. An individual suffering a schizophrenic break in response to a separation may be misdiagnosed as having a borderline psychology in which extreme "abandonment depression" (Masterson, 1976) has been evoked—and vice versa: individuals with borderline personality organization are often misunderstood as schizophrenic when they seek help in the context of severe and disorganizing upset about separation.

Finally, it is essential to evaluate whether what appears to be a personality disorder is a response to chronic stress. For example, a man who has emigrated to a society whose language he does not speak may appear paranoid, dependent, or otherwise disturbed in his personality functioning although no such disturbance was visible before his emigration. Any of us can look borderline or even psychotic if under sufficient strain. Hence, it is not possible to diagnose a personality disorder accurately without attention to other possibilities that explain the patient's behavior, the context of that behavior, and the question of whether it represents long-term functioning rather than a more acute state.

LEVEL OF PERSONALITY ORGANIZATION (SEVERITY OF PERSONALITY DISORDER)

By the end of the 19th century, psychiatric classification distinguished between two general types of problems: (1) neurosis, a term that may refer to either minor or major psychopathology in which the capacity to assess reality is not compromised, and (2) psychosis, which involves serious impairments in reality-testing. In the decades since this categorical distinction became conventional, as clinicians became increasingly aware that many people suffer not from an isolated symptom but from issues that pervade their lives in a more total way, they began to distinguish also between neurotic *symptoms* and neurotic *character*, or personality disorder. Some noted that while neurotic individuals are notable for their own suffering, personality-disordered individuals tend to cause others to suffer.

Throughout the 20th century, as therapists compared notes on their experiences with personality-disordered patients, they began describing individuals who seemed too disturbed to be labeled neurotic, and yet too anchored in reality to be considered psychotic. Slowly, a "borderline" group was identified (Frosch, 1964; Knight, 1953; Main, 1957). The concept of a disorder of personality on the border between the psychoses and neuroses was subsequently subjected to empirical research (e.g., Grinker, Werble & Drye, 1968; Gunderson & Singer, 1975) and theoretical elaboration (e.g., Adler, 1985; Hartocollis, 1977; Kernberg, 1975, 1983, 1984; Masterson, 1972, 1976; Stone, 1980, 1986).

Patients in the borderline area often fared badly in the kinds of treatment that usually help neurotic individuals, especially as they would unexpectedly develop intense, problematic, and often rapidly shifting attitudes toward their therapists. Clinicians observed that although they did not show psychotic tendencies outside the therapy, some would develop what appeared to be an intractable "psychotic transference," (i.e., they would experience the therapist as omnipotently good or malevolently bad or as *exactly* like a person from their past, and they could not be persuaded that this impression was not fully warranted).

As Wallerstein notes in Part III, there slowly evolved a consensus among psychoanalytic clinicians that people with diagnosable personality disorders exist on a continuum of severity, from a relatively healthy to a very disturbed level of personality structure. This continuum is conventionally, if arbitrarily, divided into healthy, neurotic, and borderline ranges of personality organization, the borderline range extending from the border of neurotic character organization to the border of psychotic conditions. It is critical to note that the term "borderline," when used by psychoanalytic clinicians to denote a level of severity, has a different meaning from the same term as used in the DSM, in which only one type of borderline organization (the more histrionic, dramatic manifestation of this level of severity) is labeled Borderline Personality Disorder. The DSM conceptualization adopted as its diagnostic criteria most of the descriptors used by John Gunderson (e.g., 1984), who had defined the term operationally for research purposes. Our use is much broader and is more consistent with the clinical experience that accounts for how the term came into wide professional use.

Extensive research using the Rorschach and other psychological tests (e.g., Blatt & Auerbach, 1988) has identified three different general kinds of borderline patients: (1) an anaclitic type (affectively labile, intensely dependent—roughly congruent with the DSM-IV Borderline Personality Disorder) and (2) an introjective type (over-ideational, characterized by social isolation and withdrawal, more likely to receive the DSM diagnosis of paranoid, schizoid, or obsessive personality disorder), both of whom show the "stable instability" (Schmideberg, 1959) of borderline personality organization; and (3) borderline schizophrenics, who are impaired in perceiving fundamental boundaries and are at risk of psychotic decompensation.[2]

Although personality is determined by many factors and is not reducible to a simple Freudian notion of "fixation" or "arrest" at a particular early phase, there is a maturational assumption associated with the dimension of severity. In other words, the severity dimension assumes that for individuals to acquire psychological maturity and achieve satisfying ways of living, they must develop certain vital capacities. We presume that these developmental attainments were compromised in people with personality disorders. This assumption grew out of clinical experience informed by psychoanalytic theory and has subsequently been supported by considerable empirical research.

As suggested by the findings of Clarkin, Kernberg and their colleagues (e.g., Clarkin, Foelsch, Levy, Hull, Delaney & Kernberg, 2001; Clarkin, Levy, Lenzenweger & Kernberg, 2004) and Greenspan and his colleagues (Greenspan, 1989; Greenspan & Shanker, 2004) we recommend evaluating where an individual's personality lies on the dimension of severity by assessing the following capacities. Traditional psychoanalytic terms for these capacities are in parentheses:

- To view self and others in complex, stable, and accurate ways (identity);

- To maintain intimate, stable, and satisfying relationships (object relations);

- To experience in self and perceive in others the full range of age-expected affects (affect tolerance);

- To regulate impulses and affects in ways that foster adaptation and satisfaction, with flexibility in using defenses or coping strategies (affect regulation);

- To function according to a consistent and mature moral sensibility (superego integration, ideal self-concept, ego ideal);

- To appreciate, if not necessarily to conform to, conventional notions of what is realistic (reality testing);

- To respond to stress resourcefully and to recover from painful events without undue difficulty (ego strength and resilience).

---

[2] The anaclitic-introjective or relatedness versus self-definition dimension is a deep-structure tension that individuals tend to resolve in one direction or the other. It overlaps conceptually with the dimension of extroverted/extrotensive-introverted/introtensive and many other similar polarities; e.g., Bakan's (1966) communion-agency, Beck's (1983) sociotropic-autonomous, McAdams's (1988) relationship-independence, and Spiegel & Spiegel's (1978) Nietzsche-inspired Dionysian-Apollonian. It has been found to discriminate between patients at all levels of psychological health, and to have vital implications for the understanding and treatment of depression, personality disorders, and other psychopathologies (Blatt, 2004; Morse, Robins, & Gittes-Fox, 2002; Ouimette, Klein, Anderson, Riso, & Lizardi, 1994). For example, there is emerging research evidence that supportive-expressive therapies work better with anaclitic patients, at least initially, whereas interpretive psychoanalytic treatment is preferable for introjective ones (Blatt, in press, and p. 537; Vermote, 2005).

At the healthier level of personality organization, a person has all these capacities. The ability to laugh at oneself, for example, involves several of them. At the neurotic level, most of them exist to a significant degree, though one or two areas (e.g., broad experience of affects, satisfaction in relationships) may be problematic. Individuals whose personality is organized at the neurotic level tend to be reasonably articulate about the ways in which their functioning is limited by their psychology, whereas for persons in the borderline range, such problems must often be inferred on the basis of careful interviewing and possible psychological testing.

In individuals with personalities in the borderline range, the first five abilities are seriously limited, and, especially in people with narcissistic and psychopathic (antisocial) personalities, the sixth may be compromised. Despite these deficits, individuals in the borderline area have little or no damage in the seventh area, the ability to appreciate conventional notions of reality. The most disturbed patients with borderline organization, however, may have transient problems with reality testing, particularly when reacting to relatively disturbing events, in the context of highly charged relationships, including psychotherapy.

A less global, more discriminating way of assessing level of individual mental health is via the Profile of Mental Functioning described in the next section. At this point, we note that despite our diagnostic tendency to locate a person's center of psychological gravity at one point on the continuum from severely borderline to healthy, many people have elements that might be respectively considered healthy, neurotic, and borderline.

Healthy Personalities (Absence of Personality Disorder)

Psychopathology expresses the interaction of stressors and individual psychology. Some people who become symptomatic when stressed have overall healthy personality functioning, as assessed above. They may have certain favored ways of coping, but they have enough flexibility to accommodate adequately to challenging realities. We all have a style or flavor or type of personality, or a stable mixture of types. The fact that one has, for example, a consistently pessimistic outlook is not a sufficient criterion for diagnosing depressive personality disorder. It is clinically valuable, however, to understand the general personality of a patient, *whether or not a personality disorder exists.*

Neurotic-Level Personality Disorders

Notwithstanding having all of the above capacities in more or less sufficient degree, individuals with personality disorders in the neurotic range are notable for their relative rigidity (Shapiro, 1965, 1981, 1989, 2000). That is, they tend to respond to certain stresses with a limited range of defenses and coping mechanisms. Common disorders at this end of the severity continuum are depressive or depressive-masochistic personality disorder, hysterical personality disorder, and obsessive and/or compulsive personality disorder. The pattern of suffering of individuals in these groups tends to be restricted to a specific area, such as gender and sexuality for the hysterical person, control issues for the obsessive-compulsive person, and loss, rejection, or self-criticism for the depressive individual.

The maladaptive defensive patterns of individuals in the neurotic range may also be limited to the area of their particular difficulty. For example, in contrast to patients with borderline levels of personality disturbance who use defenses that tend to distort reality more globally, the rigid or problematic defenses of neurotic-level patients are more likely to concern one area: problems with authority, for example, rather than problems in all relationships. Outside their areas of difficulty, persons at the neurotic level may have a good work history, maintain satisfactory relations with others, tolerate dysphoric affect without getting sick (somatizing) or taking impulsive and ill-considered actions, and be able and ready to cooperate in psychotherapy.

Neurotic-level patients often have some perspective on their recurrent difficulties and can imagine how they would like to change. Frequently, they come to treatment after having developed a plausible idea about the sources of their problems, and they usually form an adequate working alliance with the clinician. Therapists tend to react to them comfortably, with a natural sense of respect and sympathy and the reasonable expectation of a collaborative therapeutic partnership.

Borderline-Level Personality Disorders

In contrast, persons with borderline personality organization tend to have recurrent relational difficulties, an incapacity for emotional intimacy, problems with work, periods of marked depression and anxiety, and vulnerability to substance abuse and other addictive behaviors such as gambling, shoplifting, binge eating, sexual compulsion, and addictions to video games or the Internet. They are also at greater risk for self-harm via reckless behavior, including self-mutilation, sexual risk-taking, the acquisition of inordinate debt, and similar self-destructive activities.

On the introversion-extroversion dimension, a major dimension noted in personality research (John & Srivastava, 1999), extroverted borderline patients have been much more extensively discussed than introverted ones. There are, however, "quiet borderlines" (Sherwood & Cohen, 1995)—for example, individuals with schizoid, inhibited, or depressive psychologies who do not behave in the dramatically self-destructive ways described in the DSM but who suffer chronic despair, feel little pleasure in love and work, and have serious problems with their sense of identity, relationships, affect tolerance and regulation, resilience, and moral consistency. Common disorders at this end of the severity continuum include paranoid, psychopathic, narcissistic, sadistic, sadomasochistic, hypomanic, somatizing, and dissociative personality disorders.

Clinicians whose descriptions of patients were studied by the Shedler-Westen Assessment Procedure (SWAP), a method for quantifying subtle and sophisticated clinical observations and inferences (Westen & Shedler, 1999a, 1999b, 2000), have emphasized the affect- and impulse-regulation problems of individuals with borderline personality organization. They comment on the extremity and rawness of their clients' emotions and also on their excessive use of defenses that some theorists and researchers (e.g., Kernberg, 1984; Laughlin, 1979; Perry & Cooper, 1989; Vaillant, Bond, & Vaillant, 1986) have labeled "primitive" or "immature"—that is, defenses that are more distorting than those most frequently used by neurotic-level people.

The most commonly noted of such defenses are *splitting* and *projective identification*. Splitting is the tendency to see self and others in moralized, all-good and all-bad categories; i.e., in unrealistically positive ways (as saints, heroes, or rescuers) or in unrealistically negative ways (as hateful villains or abusers), or in both, in oscillating fashion. Projective identification involves failing to recognize troubling aspects of one's own personality, but feeling absolutely certain that another person (e.g., the therapist) has those undesirable qualities and treating that person accordingly—eventually evoking from the other person the attitudes that have been projected with such conviction.[3]

In contrast to the benign "physicianly" attitude that patients with neurotic-level personality disorders tend to elicit in therapists and interviewers, patients at the borderline end of the continuum evoke strong feelings that clinicians may have to struggle to manage or contain. Often these are negative feelings, such as hostility, fear, confusion, helplessness, or boredom; however, powerful rescue fantasies and wishes to cure the patient by love are also common. Patients with severe personality disorders tend to evoke strong tendencies in the therapist to act, not just "sit there." To put it more bluntly, clinicians may find themselves wanting to kill these patients, or else to cross professional boundaries to "save" them.

---

[3] Other defenses noted as characteristic of persons in the borderline range include *denial* (blandly disregarding things that are disturbing, as if they did not exist), *withdrawal* into fantasy, indiscriminate forms of *introjection* (sometimes called "introjective identification," or wholesale taking on of someone else's characteristics, attitudes, values, and even mannerisms), *omnipotent control* (treating another as an extension of oneself, with little recognition that the other person is a separate human being with independent needs, desires, and preferences), primitive *idealization* (seeing another as all-good and larger than life, as a small child might see an admired adult), and primitive *devaluation* (seeing another as completely worthless, with no redeeming qualities whatever). Vaillant's research (1994) adds hypochondriacal concerns, acting out, and passive aggression to the list of psychologically costly defenses that may signal a more severe personality disorder. (The division of defenses into "primitive" or "immature" versus "more mature" or "higher-order" is controversial and not well anchored in developmental research but has become conventional in the literature on the more severe personality disorders.)

Patients at the most disturbed end of the borderline range, especially in periods of intense reactivity, may confuse the therapist into regarding them as psychotic. Some patients who have never had a diagnosed psychotic illness may nonetheless have transient psychotic features such as concrete or over-generalized thinking, pervasive and severe annihilation anxiety, and the unshakable conviction that their own attributions about someone are correct, regardless of anything the other person may say or do. People with the most severe personality disorders may impute their own thoughts and feelings to others, become convinced of the rightness of their most erroneous perceptions, and be ready to act on the basis of such convictions. An example of a person at this end of the borderline continuum would be a man who stalks his love object in the conviction that this person "really" loves him despite all protestations to the contrary. Other patients with severely borderline psychologies report "hearing voices" but—unlike truly psychotic individuals—tend to identify such voices as internal rather than external, and often as recognizable (the voice of an angry parent, for example).

Although some theorists have posited a psychotic level of personality organization, we feel that this formulation may create a confusion of terminology between such illnesses as schizophrenia (or borderline schizophrenia as described by Blatt & Auerbach, 1988) and the personality disorders described here. There is considerable clinical writing endorsing such a hypothesis but as yet little research supporting it, with the arguable exception of some cross-cultural and clinical investigations into psychotic states in histrionic personalities (Hirsch & Hollender, 1969; Hollender & Hirsch, 1964; Langness, 1967; Richman & White, 1970, Wallerstein, 1967; Zetzel, 1968) that are clearly neither schizophrenia nor psychotic mood disorders. There are numerous anecdotal and autobiographical accounts of individuals without severe mania, depression, or schizophrenia, who, under stress, have had brief psychotic episodes, or whose reality testing fails in certain areas, but whether this can be interpreted as a psychotic-level personality organization is uncertain. The diagnostic picture is complicated by the fact that some people who become psychotic have had a preexisting personality disorder. Typically, after receiving medication that reduces their psychotic symptoms, such individuals then manifest a diagnosable disorder of personality.

IMPLICATIONS OF THE SEVERITY DIMENSION FOR PSYCHOTHERAPY

Experienced therapists behave with important differences in emphasis, level of activity, explicitness of boundary-setting, frequency of sessions, and other features of technique, depending on their evaluation of a patient's location on the severity dimension. Sometimes this adaptation to the individual patient is intuitive, and sometimes it reflects the therapist's training to the effect that there is a continuum from exploratory to supportive treatment that correlates roughly with the level-of-organization dimension.

There follow a few inferences that are commonly drawn from an assessment of the severity of a patient's character pathology. We offer them with several caveats. First, we note that they are very general recommendations for which many exceptions exist. They are not "rules" in any sense. Second, many patients have some capacities in the neurotic range while also showing specific deficits more typical of borderline organization. And some people fall more or less between the neurotic and borderline groups, which, because they are designated ranges on a continuum, do not have clearly demarcated boundaries. Third, as many clinical writers have noted, even psychologically healthy individuals can look borderline when they are seriously misunderstood. Finally, idiosyncratic aspects of a given patient may obviate the common clinical wisdom about the implications of severity levels.

Patients at the neurotic-to-healthy end of the continuum are helped by conventional psychoanalytic exploratory therapy and psychoanalysis.[4] For those who have a personality disorder, psychoanalysis and intensive psychodynamic therapy are the treatments of choice. (Brief treatments may help with a presenting problem, but they have little effect on personality structure.) The therapist can ordinarily expect to develop a reliable working alliance rather quickly and to feel a sense of partnership with the self-observing capacity of the patient. Regressive responses to treatment tend to be contained within the therapy hour; the patient may become aware of powerful and primitive feelings toward the therapist, but at the end of the session, he or she can usually retrieve a mature sensibility.

Transferences of less disturbed patients exist in the context of the patient's capacity to see that certain reactions to the therapist *are* transferences. Thus, they are usually addressable by the clinician without risking intolerable damage to the patient's self-esteem. For example, an obsessional woman experiences her therapist *as if* he or she were her mother; when the therapist points out such reactions, she feels more interested than hurt. Countertransference with higher-functioning people tends to be mild and usually is experienced by the therapist as more interesting than emotionally disruptive. Because less disturbed patients generally have adequate tolerance of anxiety and ambiguity, open-ended exploration tends to facilitate the sense of discovery, mastery, and progress in such individuals, supporting their sense of agency and counteracting their chagrin about whatever they discover. Investigation of historical antecedents of their current feelings and behavior usually contributes to motivation to change.

---

[4] Because they tend to be cooperative, motivated, curious, and able to tolerate anxiety and other painful affects, they are also good candidates for most types (humanistic, gestalt, cognitive-behavioral, etc.) and modalities (individual, couple, family, group) of treatment.

Patients in the borderline range need therapeutic relationships that take into account their extreme anxiety, intense reactivity, potential for disorganizing regression, lack of self- and object constancy, and the profound fears that coexist with their deep needs for attachment. Borderline patients are helped by clear limits and structure, and they usually need to look at and hear from the clinician so that they can develop a sense of the therapist as a "real person" (hence, both the psychoanalytic couch and long silences are ordinarily contraindicated). Although patients with borderline psychologies suffer painfully and may thus evoke from clinicians an inclination to respond to their neediness with increased availability and special adaptations to their pain, efforts by therapists to extend themselves or make exceptions to an established frame (e.g., to offer unusually long or frequent sessions, or to schedule appointments at times outside the therapist's normal work periods, or to be available at any hour for emergencies) may induce unmanageable regressions and painful levels of emotional disorganization in them.

Whatever the treatment frame (in terms of session frequency, cost, length, etc.) adopted by the two parties, the therapist should maintain it consistently and help the patient express negative feelings about its limitations. Specific contractual agreements about self-destructive acts may be necessary, in which the ongoing treatment relationship is contingent on the patient's keeping self-harming behaviors under control. At the same time, the therapist must be capable of genuine devotion, over a long period of time. Borderline patients may be exquisitely sensitive to shifts in the affective tone of the therapist and may become easily terrified that they will be criticized, rejected, and abandoned. Their most disturbing symptoms may come back at times of separation from the therapist and, ironically, during treatment crises caused by their beginning to change for the better and to feel trust and hope in the therapeutic relationship.

Transferences in borderline patients tend to be intense and impossible for the patient to see as transferential (i.e., despite the absence of psychosis in the patient, the transference involves distortion of psychotic proportions). For example, a man regards his therapist as alternately a saint and a monster. When the therapist suggests that he is reacting as if the therapist had qualities like those of his mother, he may exclaim, "Yes, it's just my luck to have gotten a therapist exactly like her!" Often, the borderline patient's nonverbal behavior and the therapist's countertransference reactions give more useful information than the patient's verbalizations. Investigation of historical antecedents of the current behavior of a patient in the borderline range may not facilitate change; in fact, it may be used to rationalize not changing (e.g., "How could I possibly be different, given my background?!"). Thus, treatment should generally focus on the here-and-now, especially the ways in which the patient experiences the therapist. Therapies that are helpful to borderline patients tend to be active, structured, and affectively expressive. Because patients with borderline personality organization know they provoke strong reactions in other people, therapists who try to appear completely neutral and unreactive can be experienced as insincere or dangerously out of touch.

Toward the psychotic end of the borderline continuum, supportive therapy is usually the treatment of choice. Clinicians may need to be explicitly educative, to explain to the patient their understanding of his or her problems, and to be particularly careful not to contribute to any anxieties that are avoidable. They should identify the patient's strengths and build on them rather than encouraging an open, uncovering attitude that may terrify a fragile person. They may need to monitor medication compliance and find ways of reinforcing basic self-care. Their overall therapeutic stance needs to be authoritative enough that the patient feels safe in the care of someone competent, who will not be destroyed by the patient's psychopathology. At the same time, the clinician must convey exquisite respect and a deeply egalitarian attitude, so that the patient's humiliation about his or her symptoms (or even about simply being a patient and needing help) is minimized.

TYPES OF PERSONALITY DISORDERS

There are many different ways to distinguish psychologically between one person and another. All of them are, of course, oversimplifications. Any therapist who gets to know a particular patient intimately finds that over time, that person no longer seems to fit neatly into a category; the person's individuality eventually becomes more impressive than his or her conformity with an abstraction. Nevertheless, especially for purposes of treatment planning and for the therapist's sense of how to proceed in the early phases of therapy, it is clinically useful to consider which personality type or types most closely correspond to the psychology of one's patient.

Mental health professionals have several typologies to choose from. As previously noted, we have developed this taxonomy of personality disorders on the basis of both clinical reports and empirical research. Given that both clinical inference and empirical investigation are affected by the categories and assumptions that observers bring to their work, and given that sociocultural differences also affect our understanding of personality difference and disorder, we note that the categorization we offer may be incomplete, that individuals may have combinations of these syndromes, and that some of the following disorders are more adaptive or less adaptive depending on the person's sociocultural milieu.

In many empirical critiques of the DSM Personality Disorders section, writers have lamented the fact that when a patient meets the criteria for one personality disorder, he or she often meets the criteria for one or more others. This problem is an artifact of the DSM preference to treat personality types as discrete, mutually exclusive entities rather than complex and inevitably overlapping combinations. Because all personality disorders involve self-defeating behavior—otherwise they would not be considered disorders—they all have masochistic aspects by definition. Similarly, because all personality structures are characterized by a strategy for supporting self-esteem, they all have narcissistic functions. At different points in treatment, varying aspects of a patient's personality come into sharp focus. Such facts do not negate the value of understanding broad differences among individuals.

In the following list, those personality disorders characterized by habitual reliance on less effective and more costly ways of defending tend to exist, not surprisingly, predominantly in the borderline range (another reason that a given patient may meet the DSM criteria for more than one personality disorder—in this case Borderline Personality Disorder and another personality diagnosis). For example, individuals with psychopathic (antisocial) personality disorder, whose habitual defensive operations include omnipotent control, projection, denial, and splitting (Meloy, 1995) typically have borderline personality organization; projective tests show many to be close to the border with the psychoses (Gacano & Meloy, 1994). Those personality disorders that involve rigid use of more effective defenses (e.g., people with obsessive-compulsive personality disorder who rely on intellectualization and people with hysterical personality disorder who overuse repression) exist predominantly in the neurotic range.

Although many questions remain, which require research to settle, about the growing evidence that early attachment styles generally persist throughout the lifespan, some connections between personality disorders and early attachment styles have been suggested (e.g., Fonagy, Gergely, Jurist, & Target, 2002; Levy & Blatt, 1999; West & Keller, 1994). When Bradley, Heim, and Westen (2005) factor-analyzed clinical descriptions of the relational patterns of a diverse group of patients toward their therapists, four of the five factors that emerged matched descriptions of attachment styles found by researchers who study infants (e.g., Ainsworth, Blehar, Waters, & Wall, 1978).[5]

Clinical experience and research findings (e.g., Silberschatz, 2005; Weiss, 1993; Weiss, Sampson, & the Mount Zion Psychotherapy Research Group, 1986) suggest that particular unconscious beliefs accompany the various types of personality. These beliefs can produce behaviors that may appear inconsistent, but

---

[5] In terms of the language in which we have framed the proposed typology, some interesting hypotheses can be considered. In people without personality disorders, early attachment may have been secure. In neurotic-level personality disorders generally, early attachment may have been secure or may have had some anxious, ambivalent, and avoidant aspects. In individuals with a borderline psychology, attachment is likely to have been disorganized/disoriented (Fonagy, Target, Gergeley, Allen, & Bateman, 2003; Sperling, Sharp, & Fishler, 1991). In chronically anxious, phobic, passive-aggressive, dependent, and counterdependent people, attachment is likely to have been insecure in the anxious direction (Trull, Widiger, & Frances, 1987). In those with dissociative personality disorders, histories marked by disorganized-traumatic attachment may be more common. In sadistic and psychopathic individuals, there seems to have been a more or less complete failure of attachment.

may amount to contrasting ways of expressing the same central issue. For example, an obsessive-compulsive woman, unconsciously preoccupied with the issue of control of aggression, may be either compulsively prompt or regularly late, fastidiously neat in most areas yet improbably messy in some, ingratiatingly compliant or oppositionally stubborn, depending on how, at the moment, she tries to solve the problem of feeling controlled by others. A man with hysterical personality disorder, unconsciously preoccupied with sexuality and gender and their relationship to power, may be either promiscuous or inhibited or both (e.g., highly seductive, but unresponsive or unsatisfied in actual sexual involvements because of unconscious fear of his partner's imagined power). A paranoid person may alternate between feeling tempted to attack others and being terrified of attack by others. *Traits* (e.g., neatness, sexual expressiveness, provocativeness, in the above examples) often coexist with their seeming opposites. Personality distinctions, thus, have more to do with differences in underlying themes, schemas, or conflicts than with differences in traits, which may represent particular expressions of unconscious preoccupations. In recent editions of the DSM, personality disorders are generally described by observable traits. This may not be consistent with current clinical observations and research.

In describing each of the following personality disorders, we begin with some descriptive and conceptual information, including possible etiology in instances in which there is reasonable clinical and/or empirical consensus on the topic. Where we have data to this effect, we locate the personality type on Blatt's self-definition versus relatedness (introjective-anaclitic) continuum, a dimension of psychological make-up that has been shown to have important implications for therapy. Given the frequency with which personality-disordered individuals express themselves via behavior that induces strong affect, we also mention the characteristic emotional reactions of therapists when relating to patients with the various personality disorders (i.e., the usual countertransferences evoked by the kind of patient in question). Finally, for each personality disorder we note general implications for psychotherapy. We have tried to represent the various conditions more organically than as a list of traits, given that seemingly opposing traits serving the same purpose can coexist within the same personality type. At the end of each section, we summarize schematically the temperamental, thematic, affective, cognitive, and defensive patterns that define the personality type in question.[6]

---

[6] We emphasize again that these "types" are prototypes that no individual patient may match precisely, and that the range of personalities one observes in clinical settings is probably not a representative sample of personalities at large. Other than in section headings, we do not refer to diagnostic entities in capital letters (e.g., patients with Borderline Personality Disorder"), and we avoid acronyms (e.g., "patients with BPD"). People whose personalities are problematic do not have something comparable to a disease, nor does a personality completely define who they are. By avoiding capitalization and initials, we are also trying to resist a tendency that has crept into the mental health field, under the influence of pharmaceutical and insurance companies, to reify complex syndromes, implying that they exist as discernible "things" rather than as interrelated patterns of cognition, emotion, and behavior that are frequently seen in clinical practice.

P101. Schizoid Personality Disorders
P102. Paranoid Personality Disorders
P103. Psychopathic (Antisocial) Personality Disorders P103.1 Passive/Parasitic P103.2 Aggressive
P104. Narcissistic Personality Disorders P104.1 Arrogant/Entitled P104.2 Depressed/Depleted
P105. Sadistic and Sadomasochistic Personality Disorders 105.1 Intermediate Manifestation: Sadomasochistic Personality Disorder
P106. Masochistic (Self-Defeating) Personality Disorders P106.1 Moral Masochistic P106.2 Relational Masochistic
P107. Depressive Personality Disorders P107.1 Introjective P107.2 Anaclitic P107.3 Converse Manifestation: Hypomanic Personality Disorder
P108. Somatizing Personality Disorders
P109. Dependent Personality Disorders P109.1 Passive-Aggressive Versions of Dependent Personality Disorders P109.2 Converse Manifestation: Counterdependent Personality Disorders
P110. Phobic (Avoidant) Personality Disorders P110.1 Converse Manifestation: Counterphobic Personality Disorder
P111. Anxious Personality Disorders
P112. Obsessive-Compulsive Personality Disorders P112.1 Obsessive P112.2 Compulsive
P113. Hysterical (Histrionic) Personality Disorders P113.1 Inhibited P113.2 Demonstrative or Flamboyant
P114. Dissociative Personality Disorders (Dissociative Identity Disorder/ Multiple Personality Disorder)
P115. Mixed/Other

P101. Schizoid Personality Disorders

Individuals with schizoid personalities exist on a range from high-functioning to deeply disturbed. They are highly sensitive and reactive to interpersonal stimulation, to which they tend to respond with defensive withdrawal. They easily feel in danger of being engulfed, enmeshed, controlled, intruded upon, and traumatized, dangers that they associate with becoming involved with other people. On the anaclitic-introjective dimension, they are firmly at the pole of introjection and self-definition. They may appear notably detached, or they may behave in a minimally socially appropriate way while privately attending more to their inner world than to the surrounding world of human beings. Some schizoid individuals withdraw physically into hermit-like reclusiveness; others retreat in more psychological ways, to the fantasy life in their minds.

Although seriously schizoid individuals may appear to be indifferent to social acceptance or rejection, to the extent of having quirky characteristics that serve to put others off, this putative indifference may have more to do with establishing a tolerable level of space between themselves and others than with ignorance of social expectations. The DSM distinguishes between schizoid and schizotypal personalities, indicating that the latter is characterized by cognitive or perceptual distortions and marked eccentricity or oddness. Research has not demonstrated that schizoid and schizotypal personalities are qualitatively different; schizotypy, or the combination of quirky qualities with rather magical thinking, seems to be a trait rather than a type of personality, one that can be associated with schizoid personality and also some other personality types (Shedler & Westen, 2004).

Schizoid individuals are often characterized as loners and tend to be more comfortable by themselves than with other people. At the same time, they may feel a deep yearning for closeness and have elaborate fantasies about emotional and sexual intimacy (Doidge, 2001; Guntrip, 1969; Seinfeld, 1991). They can be startlingly aware of features of their inner life that tend to be unconscious in individuals with other kinds of personality, and they consequently may be perplexed when they find that others seem to be unaware of aspects of themselves that to the schizoid person seem obvious. Contrary to appearances, clinical experience does not support the notion that some schizoid people are completely content in their isolation; in psychotherapy, even extremely withdrawn schizoid individuals have eventually revealed a longing for intimacy, and this observation has been borne out by empirical research (Shedler & Westen, 2004).

Nor does clinical literature support the DSM contention that schizoid individuals rarely experience strong emotions (Shedler & Westen, 2004, p. 638). Rather, they often feel pain at a level so excruciating as to require their defensive detachment in order to endure it. They do well in psychotherapies that both allow emotional intimacy and respect their need for sufficient interpersonal space. They may communicate their concerns most intimately and comfortably via metaphor and emotionally meaningful references to literature, music, and the arts.

- **Contributing constitutional-maturational patterns**: Highly sensitive, shy, easily overstimulated
- **Central tension/preoccupation**: Fear of closeness/longing for closeness
- **Central affects**: General emotional pain when overstimulated, affects so powerful they feel they must suppress them
- **Characteristic pathogenic belief about self**: Dependency and love are dangerous
- **Characteristic pathogenic belief about others**: The social world is impinging, dangerously engulfing
- **Central ways of defending**: Withdrawal, both physically and into fantasy and idiosyncratic preoccupations

P102. Paranoid Personality Disorders

Paranoid personality disorders may be considered as among the more severe personality disorders, found at the borderline level of organization, though it is possible that higher-functioning paranoid individuals exist, but are not often seen clinically (given the paranoid person's problem with trust, he or she has to be suffering greatly to seek help). Paranoid psychology is characterized by unbearable affects, impulses, and ideas that are disavowed and attributed to others, and are then viewed with fear and/or outrage. Paranoid psychologies are on the introjective, self-definition end of the continuum from relatedness to self-definition.

Projected feelings may include hostility, as in the common paranoid conviction that one is being persecuted by hostile others; dependency, as in the sense of being deliberately rendered humiliatingly dependent by others; and attraction, as in the belief that others have sexual designs on the self or the people to whom one is attached (for example, in the common phenomenon of paranoid jealousy or the syndrome of erotomania). Other painful affects such as hatred, envy, shame, contempt, disgust, and fear may also be disowned and projected. Although this disorder is described in somewhat one-dimensional ways in the DSM, persons with paranoid personality disorder have complex subjective experiences.

Because pathologically paranoid individuals tend to have histories marked by felt shame and humiliation (Meissner, 1978), they expect to be humiliated by others and may attack first in order to spare themselves the agony of waiting for the "other shoe to drop," the inevitable attack from outside. Their expectation of mistreatment creates the suspiciousness and hypervigilance for which they are noted, attitudes that sadly tend to evoke the humiliating responses that they fear. Their personality is defensively organized around the theme of power, either the persecutory power of others or the megalomanic power of the self.

Paranoid patients tend to have trouble conceiving that thoughts are different from actions, a belief possibly encouraged because in their formative years, they were criticized or humiliated for attitudes rather than behavior. Some clinical reports suggest that they have experienced a parent as seductive or manipulative and are consequently alert to the danger of being exploited in a seductive way by the therapist and others. They exist in an anxious conflict between feeling panicky when alone (afraid that they will be damaged by an unexpected attack and/or afraid that their destructive fantasies will damage or already have damaged others) and anxious in relationship (afraid that they will be used and destroyed by the agenda of the other).

Therapeutic experience attests to the rigidity of the pathologically paranoid person (Shapiro, 1981). A therapist's countertransference may include strong feelings that mirror those that the paranoid person disowns and projects, such as becoming afraid when a patient expresses only the angry aspects of his or her emotional reaction and shows no sense of personal vulnerability or fear.

The clinical literature emphasizes the importance of maintaining a patient, matter-of-factly respectful attitude, the communication of a sense of strength (lest paranoid patients worry unconsciously that their negative affects could destroy the therapist), a willingness to respond with factual information when the paranoid patient raises questions (lest the patient feel evaded or toyed with), and attending to the patient's private conviction that aggression, dependency, and sexual desire—and the verbal expressions of any of these strivings—are inherently dangerous. It is best not to be too warm and solicitous, as such attitudes may stimulate a terror of regression and consequent elaborate suspicions about why the therapist is "really" being so nice.

- **Contributing constitutional-maturational patterns**: Possibly irritable/aggressive
- **Central tension/preoccupation**: Attacking/being attacked by humiliating others
- **Central affects**: Fear, rage, shame, contempt
- **Characteristic pathogenic belief about self**: Hatred, aggression and dependency are dangerous
- **Characteristic pathogenic belief about others**: The world is full of potential attackers and users
- **Central ways of defending**: Projection, projective identification, denial, reaction formation

P103. Psychopathic (Antisocial) Personality Disorders

In this classification, we have a preference for the earlier term "psychopathic" (Cleckley, 1941; Hare, 1991; Henderson, 1939; Meloy, 1988, 1995) over the more contemporary "antisocial."[7] Many people with this personality disorder are not obviously anti-social—that is, they are not in observable conflict with social norms, and conversely, many people who meet DSM and ICD criteria for antisocial personality are not characterologically psychopathic. Some individuals with psychopathic personality disorder are able to pursue their agendas in contexts of social approval and even admiration (e.g., when a psychopathic person is an intelligence agent). In some occupations, psychopathic behavior is rewarded. Although many psychopathic individuals run into trouble with authorities, some are quite effective at evading accountability for the damage they do to others.

Individuals with psychopathic personality disorder are found throughout the borderline range of severity (Gacano & Meloy, 1994). Their characteristic orientation is toward expressing power for its own sake. They are much more preoccupied with self-definition than with relationship. They take pleasure in duping others and subjecting them to manipulation (Bursten, 1973). Deutsch's (1955) concept of "the imposter" fits within the psychopathic realm. Although the stereotype of antisocial personality involves aggression and violence, clinical observation over many decades (beginning with Henderson, 1939) has differentiated between an aggressive version of psychopathic personality disorder and a passive-parasitic type of psychopath, who use different means of accomplishing exploitative ends. These subtypes may be regarded as more introjective and anaclitic, respectively, within the context of a notably non-anaclitic type of psychology. The introjective processes operating in an aggressive psychopath may constitute an identification with a violent or abusive caregiver.

Psychopathic people feel anxiety as such less frequently or intensely than non-psychopathic individuals (Ogloff & Wong, 1990). There is empirical evidence (Raine, Venables, & Williams, 1990) that many people with this personality disorder have a higher-than-normal physiological threshold for stimulation and therefore seek it addictively. Pathologically psychopathic individuals are notable in lacking the moral center of gravity that, in people of other personality types, tames the striving for power and directs it toward socially valuable ends.

---

[7] Though not with the meaning that the term had in classical German nosology, in which "psychopathy" was a synonym for character pathology. Phenomena that are inherently disturbing tend to be renamed periodically, as the professional community tries to coin morally neutral language and avoid the pejorative tone that can creep into labels for psychopathology. Thus, "psychopathy" replaced the older term, "moral insanity," and later was differentiated from "sociopathy," which originally meant an antisocial psychology without the chilling psychopathic core noted by Cleckley (1941). But "sociopath" and "psychopath" quickly came to be used by many as synonyms.

Psychopathic individuals may be charming and even charismatic, and may read others' emotional states with great accuracy. They may be hyperacute to their surroundings. Their own emotional life, however, tends to be impoverished, and their expressed affect often is insincere and intended to manipulate. Their emotional connection to others is minimal; they typically lose interest in people they see as no longer useful to them. They lack the capacity to describe their own emotional reactions with any depth or nuance and they frequently somatize. Their indifference to the feelings and needs of others, including their characteristic lack of remorse after damaging other people, probably reflects a grave disorder of early attachment. Neglect, abuse, addiction, and/or chaotic undependability in caregivers, or a profoundly bad fit between the child's temperament and that of the responsible adults, may have made a secure attachment impossible.

Treatment in which the therapist persistently tries to reach out sympathetically comes to grief with psychopathic patients, who believe that love and kindness are illusory, and who consequently devalue those who manifest these qualities. It is possible to have a therapeutic influence on many psychopathic individuals, however, if the therapist conveys a powerful presence, behaves with scrupulous integrity, and accepts that what motivates the patient has more to do with what behaviors make him or her look powerful than with other evaluative criteria. The prospects for therapeutic influence are better if the psychopathic person has reached mid-life or later and has consequently experienced a decline in physical power and encountered limits to omnipotent strivings.

- **Contributing constitutional-maturational patterns**: Possible aggressiveness, high threshold for emotional stimulation
- **Central tension/preoccupation**: Manipulating/being manipulated
- **Central affects**: Rage, envy
- **Characteristic pathogenic belief about self**: I can make anything happen
- **Characteristic pathogenic belief about others**: Everyone is selfish, manipulative, dishonorable
- **Central ways of defending**: Reaching for omnipotent control
- **Subtypes:**

P103.1 Passive/Parasitic

Henderson's (1939) more dependent, less aggressive, relatively non-violent manipulator, the "con artist" type

P103.2 Aggressive

Henderson's (1939) more explosive or actively predatory and often violent offender

P104. Narcissistic Personality Disorders

Narcissistic personality disorders exist along a continuum of severity, from the border with neurotic personality disorders to the more severely disturbed levels. Toward the neurotic end of the severity spectrum, narcissistic individuals may be socially appropriate, personally successful, charming and, although somewhat deficient in the capacity for intimacy, reasonably well adapted to their family circumstances, work, and interests. In contrast, people with narcissistic personalities who are organized at the most pathological level, whether or not they are personally successful, suffer from frank identity diffusion, lack a consistent sense of inner-directed morality, and may behave in highly destructive ways. Kernberg (1984) has described such patients as suffused with "malignant narcissism" (that is, narcissism blended with sadistic aggression), considering them closely related to those with psychopathic personality disorder.

The characteristic subjective experience of narcissistic individuals is a sense of inner emptiness and meaninglessness that requires recurrent infusions of external confirmation of their importance and value. Classical depictions of the "as-if personality" (Deutsch, 1942) probably belong in the general area of pathological narcissism. When the narcissistic individual succeeds in extracting such confirmation in the form of status, admiration, wealth, and success, he or she feels an internal elation, often behaves in a grandiose manner, and treats others (especially those perceived to be of lower status) with contempt. When the environment fails to provide such evidence, narcissistic individuals typically feel depressed, shamed, and envious of those who succeed in attaining the supplies that they lack. Their lack of pleasure in either work or love can be painful to witness.

The DSM depiction of the narcissistic personality disorder describes the more arrogant version of this kind of psychopathology (Reich, 1933). It omits consideration of the many persons therapists see who appear overtly diffident and often less successful, who are internally preoccupied with grandiose fantasies (Akhtar, 1989; Cooper & Ronningstam, 1992; Gabbard, 1989; Hunt, 1995; McWilliams, 1994; Rosenfeld, 1987). Less overtly arrogant patients may demand that the therapist teach them how to be "normal" or popular, or complain that they want what more fortunate people have. These subtypes correspond roughly to more introjective and more anaclitic versions of narcissism.

Narcissistic individuals frequently have hypochondriacal preoccupations and tend to somatize. The clinical literature suggests that having experienced early attachment to others as unrewarding and full of hidden agendas (Miller, 1975), people who become markedly narcissistic may have responded by divesting themselves of meaningful emotional investment in others and becoming preoccupied instead with their bodily integrity.

Individuals with narcissistic personality disorder spend considerable energy evaluating their status relative to that of other people. They tend to defend their wounded self-esteem through a combination of idealizing and devaluing others. When they idealize someone, they feel more special or important by virtue of their association with him or her. When they devalue someone, they feel superior. Therapists who work with such individuals tend to feel unreasonably idealized, unreasonably devalued, or simply disregarded. Effects on the therapist may include boredom, mild irritation, impatience, and the feeling that one is invisible.

The clinical literature on narcissistic personality disorder includes diverse speculations about etiology and consequently diverse treatment recommendations, ranging from an emphasis on empathic attunement and exploration of the therapist's inevitable empathic failures (e.g., Kohut, 1971, 1977) to a focus on the systematic exposure of defenses against shame, envy, and normal dependency (e.g., Kernberg, 1975). Like persons whose character structure is more psychopathic, narcissistic patients may be easier to help in therapy if they have reached mid-life or later, when their narcissistic investments in beauty, fame, wealth, and power have been disappointed and when they may have run into realistic limits on their grandiosity.

- **Contributing constitutional-maturational patterns**: No clear data
- **Central tension/preoccupation**: Inflation/deflation of self-esteem
- **Central affects**: Shame, contempt, envy
- **Characteristic pathogenic belief about self**: I need to be perfect to feel okay
- **Characteristic pathogenic belief about others**: Others enjoy riches, beauty, power, and fame; the more I have of those, the better I will feel
- **Central ways of defending**: Idealization, devaluation
- **Subtypes**:

P104.1 Arrogant/Entitled

Reich's (1933) "phallic narcissistic character," Gabbard's (1989) "oblivious narcissist," Rosenfeld's (1987) "thick-skinned narcissist," Akhtar's (1989) "overt narcissist," also described by Cooper & Ronningstam (1992). Behaves with overt sense of entitlement, devalues most other people, strikes observers as vain and manipulative or charismatic and commanding.

P104.2 Depressed/Depleted

Gabbard's (1989) "hypervigilant narcissist," Rosenfeld's (1987) "thin-skinned narcissist," Akhtar's (1989) "covert" narcissist, or the "shy narcissist" of Cooper &

Ronningstam (1992). Behaves ingratiatingly, seeks people to idealize, is easily wounded, and feels chronic envy of others seen as in a superior position.

P105. Sadistic and Sadomasochistic Personality Disorders

Sadistic personality disorder is characteristically borderline and is organized around the theme of domination. Internally, the sadistic person may experience deadness and affective sterility that are relieved by inflicting pain and humiliation, in fantasy and often in reality. The diagnosis of Sadistic Personality Disorder was listed as a provisional category in DSM-III-TR but disappeared in DSM-IV; yet, as Meloy (1997, p. 631) has observed, "burning the map does not eliminate the territory." The reasons for the removal of this syndrome from the DSM are not clear, but may include concern that there is a close relationship between sadistic and antisocial psychologies. The authors of DSM-IV may have felt there is insufficient reliability or validity in a diagnosis that overlaps significantly with another category. But despite the fact that sadism and psychopathy are highly correlated (Holt, Meloy, & Strack, 1999), they are not identical. Not all psychopathic people are notably sadistic, nor are all sadistic people psychopathic.

Except for studies of criminal sexual sadism, there has been very little empirical research on sadistic personality disorders. Millon (1996) offers one of the few comprehensive accounts in the literature. Because sadistic individuals rarely come voluntarily to therapy, they are seen mainly in forensic settings, where clinicians confront numerous patients whose overriding motivation involves controlling, subjugating, and forcing pain and humiliation on others. Despite the paucity of professional description, however, sadistic personality disorder is readily recognizable. Meloy (1997) cites the wife-batterer who smiles broadly and shamelessly while recounting his abuse and the child "who does not angrily kick a pet, but instead tortures animals with detached pleasure" (p. 632). In the search for total control over another, a project Fromm (1973, p. 323) called the turning of "impotence into omnipotence," the sadistic person always chooses as a target those who are subordinate, weaker, comparatively powerless (Shapiro, 1981).

Only a fraction of those who abuse others are characterologically sadistic. While many people strike out when they feel provoked or attacked, sadistic people tend to inflict their tortures with a dispassionate calm (probably originally a defense against being overwhelmed by rage). Thus, forensic scientists distinguish between affective (catathymic) and predatory violence (e.g., Serin, 1991). The hallmark of sadistic personality disorder is the emotional detachment or guiltless enthusiasm with which the individual pursues domination and control. This detachment, which may include the systematic, step-by-step preparation of a sadistic scenario, has the effect (and probably expresses the intent) of dehumanizing the object of sadism. Although it is likely that all individuals with sadistic personality disorder are sadistic in their preferred expressions of sexuality, many people whose sexual fantasies and/or enactments involve sadistic themes are not sadistic generally or in their nonsexual behavior. They thus cannot be considered to have the personality disorder.

Professionals interviewing a sadistic individual typically report feelings of visceral disturbance, vague uneasiness, intimidation, "creepiness." Meloy (1997) mentions goose bumps, the feeling of one's hair standing on end, and other atavistic reactions to a predator/prey situation. Because sadistic individuals are mendacious (Stone, 1993) and may enjoy tormenting the interviewer by lying or withholding verbal descriptions of their sadistic preoccupations, such counter-transferences may be a prime indication of the underlying sadism. Therapists should always take seriously disturbing reactions of this sort as indicating the need for more thorough diagnostic testing and a treatment plan that takes into account the patient's possible dangerousness.

We know of no reports of successful psychotherapy for characterological sadism. Stone (1993), who has carefully analyzed biographical accounts of murderers, considers all the sadistic individuals he has studied to be beyond the reach of therapy. The attachment disorder manifested by treating other living beings as objects to be toyed with rather than subjects to be respected may preclude developing the capacity for therapeutic alliance. In addition, the pleasure in sadistic acts, especially orgiastic pleasure in sexual sadism, may be so reinforcing that efforts to extinguish or reduce the sadistic pattern are doomed to failure. Still, accurate diagnosis of characterological sadism has significant implications for making recommendations to judicial officers, reducing opportunities for harm, helping people affected by a sadistic person, and allocating resources realistically.

- **Contributing constitutional-maturational patterns**: Unknown
- **Central tension/preoccupation**: Suffering indignity/inflicting such suffering
- **Central affects**: Hatred, contempt, pleasure (sadistic glee)
- **Characteristic pathogenic belief about self**: I am entitled to hurt and humiliate others
- **Characteristic pathogenic belief about others**: Others exist as objects for my domination
- **Central ways of defending**: Detachment, omnipotent control, reversal, enactment
- **Subtypes**:

P105.1 Intermediate Manifestation: Sadomasochistic Personality Disorders

Some individuals alternate between sadistic and masochistic attitudes and behaviors (Kernberg, 1988). Patients with this psychology are much more emotionally alive and capable of attachment than those with primary psychopathic, narcissistic, or sadistic personality structures. Their relationships, however, are intense and explosive. Sometimes they let themselves be dominated to an extreme extent, and sometimes they viciously attack the person to whom they previously capitulated. They tend to see themselves as victims of others' aggression whose only choices are to surrender their will entirely or to fight back belligerently. The "help-rejecting complainer" described by Frank and his colleagues (Frank, Margolin, Nash, Stone, Varon, & Ascher, 1952) is one version of this psychology. In psychotherapy, such patients tend to alternate between attacking the therapist and feeling insulted and demeaned by him or her. Because sadomasochistic personality disorder is found at the borderline level of severity, treatment considerations include those for borderline patients generally.

P106. Masochistic (Self-Defeating) Personality Disorders

Individuals with a masochistic personality disorder find themselves repetitively suffering. To others, they appear to keep putting themselves in harm's way. Like "sadism" (named for the Marquis de Sade), the term "masochism" (for Leopold von Sacher-Masoch) originally denoted a sexual psychology in which orgasm is achieved via pain or humiliation. By analogy, the terms became applied to personalities in which some valued experience (e.g., self-esteem, closeness) has become intrinsically associated with necessary suffering. Many prefer the term "self-defeating," which avoids sexual overtones (people with masochistic personalities are not necessarily masochistic in their sexual behavior) and is less associated with "blaming" the victims of abuse for their mistreatment (Herman, 1992).

Self-defeating individuals often strike interviewers as simply depressive, but eventually their masochistic patterns become evident. One indication of characterological masochism noted by many clinicians (but not yet researched) is that psychological and pharmaceutical measures that typically relieve depression tend to be ineffective with masochistic patients. Many self-defeating individuals repeatedly complain to practitioners, sometimes with a faint smile, that their latest intervention has failed. Because depressive and masochistic psychologies share several central dynamics (sensitivity to rejection and loss, inferiority feelings, unconscious guilt, inhibition of conscious anger at others), many people may be regarded as encompassing both. Such patients are aptly diagnosed with a depressive-masochistic personality (Kernberg, 1984; Laughlin, 1956; Westen & Shedler, 1999b), a configuration usually found at the neurotic level of severity. Kernberg (1988) uses this term for persons with neurotic-level depressive and self-defeating dynamics who use faulty ways of processing grief and sadness, have excessive but disavowed dependency needs, and make unreasonably critical demands on themselves.

The more an apparently depressive patient seems aggrieved rather than sad and self-critical, the more masochistic traits may be assumed to predominate. Self-defeating patients typically enter psychotherapy seeking sympathy for their misfortunes and may seem more invested in demonstrating the magnitude of the injustices they have suffered than in resolving their problems. This attitude characterizes people once labeled "moral masochists" (Freud, 1924; Reik, 1941), whose suffering expresses unconscious guilt and who subtly convey a sense of moral superiority through pain or through seemingly altruistic submission to others. Such individuals are clearly on the introjective pole of Blatt's continuum (Blatt & Bers, 1993; Blatt, 2004). Some people who act self-destructively on the heels of every success or victory fit in this group. Cooper (1988) has argued that the narcissistic function of characterological masochism is so inseparable from the self-defeating behaviors that identify masochistic personality disorder that the concept of a "narcissistic-masochistic character" is warranted.

Another version of self-defeating personality structure, one more likely to be at a borderline level of personality organization, is a more relational masochistic pattern located closer to the anaclitic pole (Berliner, 1958; Menaker, 1953). The behavior of some individuals suggests an unconscious belief that attachment requires suffering; that is, that others are there for them only if they are not doing well. Patients who self-mutilate, binge on substances, or become sexually involved with strangers whenever the therapist is on vacation exemplify a borderline level of a masochistic way of revenging themselves (not necessarily consciously) on the absent therapist.

Clinicians working with characterologically masochistic patients initially may feel a strong sympathy for them, which sometimes evokes their own masochistic tendencies (e.g., seeing the patient at inconvenient hours, lowering the fee drastically), but they soon find themselves feeling irritated and even sadistic. A therapist's warm acceptance in response to hearing the patient's troubles (an attitude that is usually vitally helpful to depressive patients) may, by reinforcing in self-defeating people the conviction that it is their suffering that brings connection, unwittingly invite increasing self-destructiveness rather than growth toward self-care. Hence, masochistic patients must eventually be tactfully confronted about their own contributions to their recurrent difficulties, and clinicians confronting them must be prepared to tolerate their resulting anxiety and anger.

- **Contributing constitutional-maturational patterns**: None known
- **Central tension/preoccupation**: Suffering/losing relationship or self-esteem
- **Central affects**: Sadness, anger, guilt
- **Characteristic pathogenic belief about self**: By manifestly suffering, I can demonstrate my moral superiority and/or maintain my attachments
- **Characteristic pathogenic belief about others**: People pay attention only when one is in trouble
- **Central ways of defending**: Introjection, introjective identification, turning against the self, moralizing
- **Subtypes**:

P106.1 Moral Masochistic

Self-esteem depends on suffering; unconscious guilt disallows experiences of satisfaction and success (cf. Reik, 1941).

P106.2 Relational Masochistic

Relationship is unconsciously believed to be dependent on one's suffering or victimization. Existence outside of one's current relationship, however abusive it may be, may seem unimaginable (cf. Menaker, 1953).

P107. Depressive Personality Disorders

Research has established the existence of two different versions of symptomatic depression: the introjective (previously called melancholic), characterized by guilt, self-criticism, and perfectionism, and the anaclitic, characterized by shame, high reactivity to loss and rejection, and vague feelings of inadequacy and emptiness (Blatt & Bers, 1993, Blatt, 2004). When introjective depressive dynamics pervade the personality, the appropriate diagnosis is depressive personality disorder. When more anaclitic dynamics do so, the clinician should also consider the diagnosis of either dependent or narcissistic personality disorder, based on the level of the person's capacity for relationship.

According to the empirical studies of Shedler and Westen (2004), depressive personality (presumably encompassing both introjective and anaclitic versions) is the most common type of personality structure encountered clinically. Individuals with a pathologically depressive personality suffer chronic dysphoric affect, including a disposition to feel guilty and/or ashamed. In DSM-III, III-R and IV, this personality type was omitted in a decision to place all dysphoric phenomena under "Mood Disorders." But many characterologically depressive people have never had a significant episode of clinical depression, and therefore are not diagnosable with a mood disorder. Moreover, clinical experience suggests that many individuals whose overt depressive symptoms are successfully ameliorated by antidepressant medication continue to have problematic characterological depressive features that can be influenced positively by psychotherapy. Hence, we think the diagnosis of depressive personality disorder should be preserved.

Individuals with a depressive personality should be differentiated from those with major depressive illness (although it is possible to have the illness as well as the personality disorder). In the former, the clinician is struck by repetitive personality themes that intensify under stress. In the latter, one is more impressed by both the vegetative symptoms (psychomotor retardation, change in appetite, sleep disturbances, decreased sexual desire or pleasure) and the intensity of dysphoric affect. Whereas antidepressant and/or mood stabilizing medications may alleviate much of the suffering in depressive illness, they tend to have little effect on the more chronic dysphoria of characterologically depressive individuals, and they are particularly ineffective in ameliorating the self-punitive attitude of those with the introjective version of the personality disorder.

Introjectively depressive individuals look inward to find the explanation for painful experiences. (The same phenomenon has been described by cognitive psychologist researchers under the rubric of "attributional styles" [e.g., Peterson & Seligman, 1984]). When mistreated, rejected, or abandoned, they tend to believe they are somehow at fault. This belief may be a residue of the familiar tendency of children in difficult family situations to deny that their caregivers are negligent, abusive, or fragile (ideas that are too frightening), but instead to attribute their suffering to their own badness—something they can try to change. Thus, introjectively inclined depressive people work hard to be "good" but rarely succeed to their own satisfaction. They are more preoccupied with issues of self-worth than with issues of relationship.

Anaclitically depressive individuals are notable for their distress and disorganization in the face of experiences of loss and separation. Their psychologies are organized around themes of relationship, affection, trust, intimacy, warmth, and similar issues. They feel empty, incomplete, lonely, helpless, and weak rather than morally perfectionistic and excessively self-critical. They often complain of existential despair, the feeling that life is empty and meaningless.

Individuals with depressive personality disorders tend to strike therapists as likable, even admirable. They are usually "nice" people. It is vital when treating depressive patients of the introjective type to elicit their negative feelings, especially their hostility and criticism, because they typically idealize the therapist, try to be good patients, and interpret the therapist's noncritical acceptance as evidence that the therapist has not yet noticed how bad they really are. It is also important that they see how they persist in believing that their badness is the cause of whatever difficulties and losses they encounter (Sampson, 1992).

Blatt (e.g., 1998), in reporting his extensive analysis of the Treatment for Depression Collaborative Research Program sponsored by the National Institute of Mental Health, found that brief treatment for introjectively depressive patients, whether pharmacological or psychological, is relatively ineffectual, whereas anaclitically depressed patients may respond positively to short-term interventions. For depressive personality disorders as opposed to depressive symptoms, long-term, intensive therapy is the treatment of choice for both anaclitically and introjectively oriented patients. Blatt's data suggest that interpretation and insight are pivotal to therapeutic progress with introjective patients, while the experience of a reliable relationship seems more central to the improvement of anaclitic ones.

- **Contributing constitutional-maturational patterns**: Possible genetic predisposition to depression
- **Central tension/preoccupation**: Goodness/badness or aloneness/relatedness of self
- **Central affects**: Sadness, guilt, shame
- **Characteristic pathogenic belief about self**: There is something essentially bad or incomplete about me
- **Characteristic pathogenic belief about others**: People who really get to know me will reject me
- **Central ways of defending**: Introjection, reversal, idealization of others, devaluation of self
- **Subtypes:**

P107.1 Introjective

Concerned with self-definition, self-worth, self-critical thoughts

P107.2 Anaclitic

Concerned with relatedness, trust, preservation of attachments

P107.3 Converse Manifestation: Hypomanic Personality Disorder

A much less common personality disorder is found in individuals with powerful depressive dynamics that are obscured by denial (Klein's [1935] "manic defense"), producing a relatively stable state of mood inflation, lack of guilt, and an irrationally positive estimation of the self. Such individuals may have remarkable energy, wit, and charm, but their relations with others are superficial because of their unconscious fear of becoming attached (i.e., deep attachment raises the threat of traumatic loss). Although they might be properly called "counterdepressive," they have historically been seen as characterologically hypomanic (Akhtar, 1992). The use of the same term should not lead us to confuse hypomanic personality disorder (defined by a characterological defense that can be amenable to psychotherapy) with the mood disorder of hypomania (a biologically implicated condition that is appropriately treated pharmacologically). The personality disorder can be distinguished from a manic or hypomanic episode by the relative subtlety, duration, and consistency of the sense of energy, movement, and self-inflation.

Therapists tend to find hypomanic patients initially quite captivating, but they may soon feel confused, overstimulated, irritatingly "entertained," and distanced. Hypomanic individuals are highly resistant to psychotherapy; in fact, they are hard to keep in treatment at all because of their tendency to leave relationships in which they are tempted to attach. They become unconsciously terrified of being abandoned and master that fear by abandoning the other. Unlike people with depressive personality organization, individuals with hypomanic personality disorder are found predominantly in the borderline range and are thus subject to sudden and overwhelming reactions that are hard to contain.

Many therapists, after diagnosing a hypomanic personality disorder, call to the patient's attention the lifetime pattern of abrupt flight that usually pervades the history of a hypomanic individual. They then try to preempt a similar flight from therapy by negotiating an agreement that the person will keep coming for a given number of sessions after any abrupt, unilateral decision by the patient to stop treatment.

- **Contributing constitutional-maturational patterns**: Possibly high energy
- **Central tension/preoccupation**: Overriding grief/succumbing to grief
- **Central affects**: Elation, rage; unconscious sadness and grief
- **Characteristic pathogenic belief about self**: If I stop running and get close to someone, I'll be traumatically abandoned, so I'll leave first
- **Characteristic pathogenic belief about others**: Others can be charmed into not seeing the qualities that make people inevitably reject me
- **Central ways of defending**: Denial (the "manic defense" [Klein, 1935]), idealization of self, devaluation of others

P108. Somatizing Personality Disorders

Given our rapidly increasing knowledge about the brain, the hormonal systems, the nervous systems, and other mental-physiological processes, scientists and theorists have become acutely aware of the artificiality of the traditional

Cartesian distinction between mind and body. Hence, many analytic writers use the term "psyche-soma" when commenting about a person's psychology. It is hard to write about "somatizing" individuals—those in whom painful self-experiences tend to be expressed in bodily states—without suggesting some background notion of a mind-body split, but readers should understand that this difficulty reflects the limitations of language more than a philosophical prejudice in the direction of nineteenth-century beliefs that the mind should "control" the body. Because the human immune system can be compromised by depression and anxiety, episodes of many somatic illnesses may be triggered or exacerbated by psychological elements. Psychosomatic problems (physical illnesses in which emotional factors play a major role) afflict many people from time to time. But some individuals seem to suffer one ailment after another that is not fully explained by a known medical condition or toxin. Vague complaints, shifting pains, gastrointestinal problems, sexual difficulties, and unexplained "spells" are typical. There is a substantial literature attesting to the prevalence of somatization in individuals with little control over their circumstances (Kirmayer, 1984) and in cultures in which the verbal expression of emotion is discouraged (Kazarian & Evans, 2001).

DSM-IV-TR, offering a number of criteria without sufficient research support (four pain symptoms, two gastrointestinal symptoms, one sexual symptom and one pseudoneurological symptom), categorizes this clinical picture as "somatization disorder." By stipulating that the complaints must have begun before age 30, it suggests, however, that this condition is less an "Axis I" syndrome than a personality disorder, a lifelong experience of physical suffering that implicates the characterological defense of somatization. In other words, whereas one person reacts to stress with repression, projection, or intellectualization, another gets sick.

There is scant empirical literature on characterological somatization. Investigation of the psychological aspects of a person's chronic and medically confounding bodily complaints is complicated by the likelihood that some individuals diagnosed as defensive somatizers have an undiagnosed physical illness that explains their somatic preoccupations. The writer Laura Hillenbrand (2003), for example, has documented her long and exasperating experience with physicians who treated her as a characterological somatizer until she was accurately diagnosed with chronic fatigue syndrome. Similar stories abound from people with long-undiagnosed Lyme disease. It is clinically hard to tell whether the self-involved, complaining style common among those with inexplicable, intractable ailments represents preexisting personality characteristics or the psychological consequences of chronic physical discomfort (MacKinnon & Michels, 1971).

Notwithstanding this problem, clinical experience suggests the existence of a personality disorder characterized by the habitual tendency to express dysphoria by somatizing (McDougall, 1989). This psychology is typically found in the bor-derline range; somatizers' bodily preoccupations can verge on somatic delusion. Somatizing patients may present a confusing combination of hypochondriacal preoccupations, diagnosable physical illness known to be stress related, and bod-ily symptoms that express ideas and affects too painful to put into words (con-version reactions). Usually the somatizer consults a psychotherapist reluctantly and in desperation, at the urging of a series of exasperated medical specialists. Frequently, the patient is "sent" to therapy by a doctor or relatives and conse-quently arrives in a resentful, defensive state of mind. Addiction to prescribed pain medications is a common complication.

Although there is some overlap between the two kinds of suffering, somatiz-ing personality disorder should be differentiated from the syndrome of hypo-chondriasis, a more severe condition characterized by excessive concern with the body, exaggerated fears of physical illness, a low threshold of physical discom-fort, rituals related to bodily preoccupations, and an overall substitution of a rela-tionship with the body for meaningful, in-depth relationships with other individuals. In intensive psychotherapy, hypochondriacal patients may become paranoid when the therapist tries to explore transference reactions. Hypochon-driacal patients do not necessarily have the alexithymia described in the next par-agraph.

Somatizing patients are notable for their "alexithymia" (Sifneos, 1973; McDougall, 1989), the inability to express emotions verbally. Although the con-nection between somatization and difficulty putting feelings into words has not been well researched, clinicians have reported this observation frequently, and it is also inferable from research with toddlers and young children. Greenspan (e.g., 1992), for example, found that children who cannot verbalize feelings tend either to act out or to somatize. The French psychoanalysts Marty and M'Uzan (1963) first described somatizers as using "la pensée opératoire" or "operational think-ing," meaning that they were strikingly devoid of fantasy, incapable of symbolic expression, and invested more in "things" than in products of the imagination. Their preoccupations tend to be concrete and repetitive.

Presumably, the early caregivers of somatizing patients did not foster a capac-ity to represent feelings, leaving their bodies to convey what their minds could not (cf. Van der Kolk, 1994). Their alexithymia makes talk therapy difficult but also vital for their improvement. They may have once received some secondary gain from the sick role, but the pain they suffer is real and debilitating, and in adulthood, there is very little that is advantageous about their psychology. Some-times their investment in maintaining a legally disabled status militates against their capacity to improve symptomatically. Their sense of self tends to be fragile, unentitled, and powerless.

Chronic somatizers often report that they feel repeatedly *unheard*—no doubt partly because listeners tune out defensively as their efforts to help are frustrated, but possibly also because of early experiences with caregivers who failed to respond to their communications. With professionals, they may act both helpless and oppositional. The unvoiced hatred that interviewers often feel from somatizing patients may result from their repeated experience of being treated as an annoying complainer and given the message, "It's all in your head." In addition, their internal working model of relatedness may require them to be ill as a condition of being cared about by someone important to them.

Common countertransferences to somatizing patients include a sense of futility, impatience, and irritation. A sense of boredom and inner deadness are also not uncommon in the therapist. Treatment of individuals with this personality structure is difficult and requires patience with their inarticulateness and negativity. Empathic acknowledgment that their suffering is real is critical; otherwise, somatizers may feel accused of malingering. Because any movement toward emotional expression is stressful for them, they frequently become ill and cancel appointments just when a therapist begins to see progress. Central to their improvement is the therapist's tactful encouragement to feel, name, and accept their emotional states.

- **Contributing constitutional-maturational patterns**: Possible physical fragility, early sickliness, some clinical reports of early physical and/or sexual abuse

- **Central tension/preoccupation**: Integrity/fragmentation of bodily self

- **Central affects**: Global distress; inferred rage; alexithymia prevents acknowledgment of emotion

- **Characteristic pathogenic belief about self**: I am fragile, vulnerable, in danger of dying

- **Characteristic pathogenic belief about others**: Others are powerful, healthy, and indifferent

- **Central ways of defending**: Somatization, regression

P109. Dependent Personality Disorders

Individuals with a dependent personality disorder are found anywhere in the range from neurotic through borderline levels of organization. Their psychology is by definition anaclitic as opposed to introjective. The categories of "inadequate" and "infantile" personality in earlier taxonomies connote roughly the same construct. Individuals with characterological dependency define themselves mainly in relation to others and seek security and satisfaction predominantly in interpersonal contexts (e.g., "I am Tom's wife, and I'm okay when things are okay with him"). Psychological symptoms may appear when something goes wrong in a primary relationship. At the neurotic level, dependent people may seek treatment in mid-life or later, after a bereavement or divorce. In some cultures, a dependent personality structure is adaptive, but in Western cultures where independent thinking and individual accomplishment are rewarded, a dependent orientation can be problematic. Even more than other qualities that may characterize a personality disorder, dependency must be evaluated with sensitivity to cultural and subcultural contexts.

Bornstein (1993, 2005) has done the only comprehensive empirical examination of pathological dependency known to us. His findings suggest that it may arise from any or all of the following: overprotective and/or authoritarian parenting, gender role socialization, and cultural attitudes about achievement versus relatedness. Participants in his studies demonstrated "relationship-facilitating self-presentation strategies" such as ingratiation, supplication, exemplification, self-promotion, and intimidation. Although popular prejudice assumes that female patients are more likely than males to be pathologically dependent, Bornstein notes that women may simply be more willing to acknowledge dependency.

Individuals with a dependent personality disorder feel ineffectual when left to themselves and tend to regard others as powerful and effective. Organizing their lives with a view to maintaining nurturing and supportive relationships in which they are submissive, they may feel contented when they have successfully developed such a relationship and acutely distressed when they have not. Emotional preoccupations include performance anxiety and fears of criticism and abandonment (Bornstein, 1993). In therapy, which they may enter readily, they are compliant to a fault. They tend to idealize the therapist, ask for advice, and seek reassurances that they are a "good patient." In an attempt to become special, they may try to "read" the therapist and meet his or her assumed needs. Some insist, even after being informed about professional boundaries, on offering favors and bringing gifts.

The therapist's countertransference is typically benign at first, then increasingly characterized by a sense of burden. Dependent patients may devise unconscious tests to see whether the clinician supports their weak strivings toward autonomy or basks in the patient's invitation to serve as expert and advisor. It is important that the therapist resists seduction into the role of omniscient authority, encourages the patient toward autonomous functioning, and contains the anxieties that arise in the process. Although therapists of patients with dependent personality disorders report being tempted to collude in avoiding negative affect, if they accept the patient's anger and other more aggressive feelings, they may facilitate the patient's sense of agency and acceptance of pride in accomplishment.

- **Contributing constitutional-maturational patterns**: Possible placidity, sociophilia

- **Central tension/preoccupation**: Keeping/losing relationship
- **Central affects**: Pleasure when securely attached; sadness and fear when alone
- **Characteristic pathogenic belief about self**: I am inadequate, needy, impotent
- **Characteristic pathogenic belief about others**: Others are powerful and I need their care
- **Central ways of defending**: Regression, reversal, avoidance
- **Subtypes**:

P109.1 Passive-Aggressive Versions of Dependent Personality Disorder

There does not appear to be sufficient evidence to document that passive-aggressive patterns should be classified as a personality disorder. Because a tendency to punish others indirectly is a feature of several personality disorders at the borderline level (most notably paranoid, masochistic, and especially dependent), it is arguable that passive-aggressivity is better construed as a trait than as a type of personality organization. We recognize, however, a clinically familiar pattern of hostile dependency that may be conceptualized as a variant of dependent personality disorder.

Unlike the straightforward presentation of characterological dependency in uncomplicated dependent personality disorder, dependent individuals with notable hostility resent being tied to another and yet cannot separate psychologically. Aggression that would normally fuel autonomous strivings may be expressed obliquely, in an effort to vent negative affect and "get even" without threatening attachment. Passive-aggressive individuals define themselves by reference to others, but with a negative valence (e.g., "I'm the husband of that bitch"). Like paranoid patients, they attack to preempt expected attack by others, but they do so indirectly. Like masochistic patients, they expect mistreatment, but they fight back, albeit insidiously. They have core narcissistic concerns but are more interpersonally engaged than characterologically narcissistic people. Because they locate themselves in opposition to others' agendas, it is hard for them to conceive of and to pursue their own goals. A main task of therapy is to increase their sense of identity and capacity to accept themselves as agents rather than just respondents and reactors.

It is therapeutically challenging to connect with a person who reaches out with aggression or responds aggressively to others' efforts to attach. The therapist needs a sense of humor as counterpoise to the feelings of irritation and impatience the patient is likely to evoke. Negative feelings emerge quickly in treatment, and power struggles are a risk to avoid. Sometimes stunningly naive about the hostility they exude, passive-aggressive patients need help naming their negative feelings and differentiating verbal from behavioral expressions of anger. To avoid feeding into their oppositionalism, therapists should not seem to be overinvested in their progress. Instead, clinicians need to take their provocations and inconsistencies in stride, keeping the therapy focused on the price the patient pays for passive-aggressive acts.

- **Contributing constitutional-maturational patterns**: Not known; possibly irritable, aggressive
- **Central tension/preoccupation**: Tolerating mistreatment/getting revenge
- **Central affects**: Anger, resentment, pleasure in hostile enactments
- **Characteristic pathogenic belief about self**: The only route to dignity is to sabotage the achievements of others
- **Characteristic pathogenic belief about others**: Other people all want me to conform to their rules
- **Central ways of defending**: Projection (of negativity on to others), externalization, rationalization, denial

P109.2 Converse Manifestation: Counterdependent Personality Disorder:

Bornstein (1993) describes a continuum from maladaptive dependency (submissiveness) through healthy interdependency (connectedness) to inflexible independence (unconnected detachment). Some individuals at the inflexibly independent end of that spectrum have powerful dependent longings that they keep out of awareness via denial and reaction formation. They thus have what amounts to a dependent personality disorder masked by pseudo-independence. In their relationships, they define themselves as the one on whom others depend, and they pride themselves on being able to take care of themselves.

Counterdependent individuals may look askance at expressions of need and may regard evidence of emotional vulnerability in themselves or others with scorn. Often they have some secret area of dependency—on a substance, a partner, a mentor, an ideology; some have a tendency toward illness or injury that gives them a "legitimate" reason to be cared for by others.

Pathologically counterdependent individuals seldom seek psychotherapy but may be pushed into it by partners who feel starved for genuine emotional intimacy. In treatment, they need help to accept their dependent wishes as a natural part of being human before they can develop a healthy balance between connectedness and separateness. Therapists who tolerate their defensive protestations about their independence long enough to develop a therapeutic alliance report that when the counterdependent defenses are given up, a period of mourning for early and unmet dependent needs then ensues, followed by more genuine autonomy.

- **Contributing constitutional-maturational patterns**: Unknown; possibly more aggressive than overtly dependent people
- **Central tension/preoccupation**: Demonstrating lack of dependence; i.e., shameful dependence
- **Central affects**: Contempt, denial of "weaker" emotions (fear, sadness, envy, longing)
- **Characteristic pathogenic belief about self**: I don't need anyone
- **Characteristic pathogenic belief about others**: Others depend on me and require me to be "strong"
- **Central ways of defending**: Denial, reversal, enactment

P110. Phobic (Avoidant) Personality Disorders

As with passive-aggressive personality disorder, we are uncertain whether avoidant personality disorder, or what the psychoanalytic literature has usually termed phobic personality disorder, is a syndrome coordinate with the personality disorders described here. The research of Shedler and Westen (2004) suggests that while clinicians recognize some patients as dominated by specific fears that they handle by avoidance, many seem to consider them as having a variant of a depressive or dependant personality organization, with more fear in the clinical picture.

Many people who enter therapy for one phobic pattern eventually disclose that they have multiple phobias and an overall phobic outlook. The central dynamic in avoidant psychologies is dealing with anxiety by attaching it to specific feared situations that are then assiduously avoided. Characterologically phobic people want to believe that as long as they keep away from particular dangers, they are safe in general. They tend to feel small, inadequate, and threatened when by themselves, and they deal with these feelings by trying to elicit protection from those to whom they impute greater power. Thus, their psychology seems to be organized around anaclitic themes. Just as they avoid certain external phenomena, they may fear their own affect and avoid knowing about their internal emotional states.

In therapy, phobic patients connect in a submissive, anxious way, asking for relief. Often they arrive with addictions to anti-anxiety drugs prescribed by doctors who have responded to their subtle pressures to be magically rescued. Their characterological avoidance may be supported by secondary gains, such as regular home visits by well-meaning friends who try to relieve them of anxiety about going out. In therapy, they have difficulty taking responsibility for their part of the work and may attempt to extract advice and reassurance from the therapist, whose evoked response may oscillate between frustrated withholding and a temptation to patronize or infantilize them (MacKinnon & Michels, 1971).

Like alexithymic individuals, phobic patients need to be encouraged to experience, name, and express their emotions. They may be verbally as well as behaviorally avoidant, changing the subject when anything disturbing enters their consciousness. When they make sweeping proclamations of danger, they should be pressed for details ("And then what would happen?") and asked for specific fantasies. Once there is a secure therapeutic alliance, they should be urged to face the situations they fear. With some patients it is possible to do this informally, while with others, a systematic exposure therapy should be considered. Phobic patients can be expected to have some depressive reactions as they renounce magical wishes for the gratification of their dependency and find themselves being less fearful and avoidant.

- **Contributing constitutional-maturational patterns**: Possible anxious or timid disposition
- **Central tension/preoccupation**: Safety/danger relative to specific objects
- **Central affects**: Fear
- **Characteristic pathogenic belief about self**: I am safe if I avoid certain specific dangers
- **Characteristic pathogenic belief about others**: More powerful people can magically keep me safe
- **Central ways of defending**: Symbolization, displacement, projection, rationalization, avoidance
- **Subtypes:**

P110.1 Converse Manifestation: Counterphobic Personality Disorders

As is the case with hypomanic and counterdependent psychologies, some individuals with counterphobic personalities are psychologically organized around defenses against their fears. People who seek out dangerous situations, those who thrive on risk, and those with a reputation for an unnerving calm in the face of peril may be considered to be in this group, if their tendency to put themselves in jeopardy is so compelling and driven that they cannot resist hazardous opportunities to demonstrate their fearlessness. As in individuals with a straightforwardly phobic personality structure, one can discern some magical thinking behind the activity of counterphobic individuals, most strikingly the internal conviction that they are safe no matter what danger they court.

Although pathologically counterphobic people are unlikely to seek psychotherapy for their personality disorder, they may come for symptomatic problems such as depression or obsessive-compulsive disorder. Treating them for psychological problems can be difficult because of their need to deny ordinary anxieties and their tendency to present themselves with a bravado that makes talking about any feelings difficult. Countertransference reactions may include anxiety about their risk-taking, as well as irritation with their fantasies of omnipotence.

- **Contributing constitutional-maturational pattern**: Unknown
- **Central tension/preoccupation**: Safety/danger
- **Central affects**: Contempt, denial of fear
- **Characteristic pathogenic belief about self**: I can face anything without fear
- **Characteristic pathogenic belief about others**: Others frighten easily and admire my bravery
- **Central ways of defending**: Denial, reaction formation, projection

P111. Anxious Personality Disorders

Many individuals currently diagnosed with Generalized Anxiety Disorder are better understood as having a personality disorder in which anxiety is the psychologically organizing experience. Although the anxious personality disorder is not included in most nosologies, we regard this omission as unfortunate. Characterological anxiety is found in the neurotic through borderline ranges. Toward the border with psychosis, individuals with anxiety-driven psychologies become so filled with dread that defenses such as projection and denial become central to their functioning. In such instances, the diagnosis of paranoid personality disorder may be more appropriate.

In many cases, patients with an anxious personality structure appear at first to be either hysterical (hence the old diagnosis of anxiety hysteria) or obsessional, depending on how they attempt to deal with their pervasive sense of fear. Unlike individuals with either hysterical or obsessive-compulsive personality disorders, however, they are chronically aware of their anxiety because their efforts at defense fail to keep their apprehensiveness out of consciousness. Unlike phobic patients, whose anxieties attach to specific objects or situations, characterologically anxious individuals experience a "free-floating," global sense of anxiety, often with no idea of what frightens them.

Signal anxiety (affective cues that a particular situation has previously been dangerous), moral anxiety (dread of violating one's core values), separation anxiety (fear of loss of an object of attachment), and annihilation anxiety (terror of fragmentation and loss of the sense of self—cf. Kohut's [1977] "disintegration anxiety") may *all* be discernible in patients with anxious personality disorder, in contrast to people in whom one of these tends to predominate. In general, the more severe the level of organization of the anxious person, the more likely it is that annihilation anxiety dominates the clinical picture (Hurvich, 2003). The proximal source of characterological anxiety lies in affective dysregulation (Schore, 2003) and failure to have developed coping strategies or defenses that mitigate normal developmental fears. Individuals with anxious personality disorder typically report having had a primary caregiver who, because of the caregiver's own anxiety, could not adequately comfort them or convey a sense of security or support a sense of agency.

Countertransference with chronically anxious patients may include a responsive anxiety, including a degree of annihilation anxiety severe enough to make the therapist feel overwhelmed, and hence impelled to do something that promises relief to the patient. Although therapists naturally wish to ease the anxious person's suffering as fast as possible, anxiolytic medications for people with this personality disorder should be prescribed with caution because of the risk of addiction. The therapist should evince an attitude of confidence in the patient's own capacities to tolerate and reduce anxiety. It is also important to preserve the therapeutic context by trying to formulate the patient's affective experience and give words to previously inchoate states of feeling (Stern, 1997). Systematic relaxation training, education in meditative disciplines, and cognitive-behavioral techniques to promote anxiety reduction are helpful adjuncts to the process of understanding, naming, and mastering previously unformulated emotional states.

- **Contributing constitutional-maturational patterns**: Anxious or timid temperament
- **Central tension/preoccupation**: Safety/danger
- **Central affects**: Fear
- **Characteristic pathogenic belief about self**: I am in constant danger from forces unknown
- **Characteristic pathogenic belief about others**: Others are sources of either danger or protection
- **Central ways of defending**: Failure of defenses against anxiety; inchoate anxieties may mask more upsetting specific anxieties that are kept out of consciousness

P112. Obsessive-Compulsive Personality Disorders

Obsessions and compulsions are relatively common symptoms, but in Western cultures, many clinicians believe that the neurotic-level syndrome of obsessive-compulsive personality disorder is becoming more subtle or rarer. The obsessive defenses of isolation of affect and intellectualization are common, especially among more cerebral and perfectionistic individuals. But as child-rearing has become less authoritarian, fewer people may struggle with the issues of personal control and moral rectitude central to the obsessive-compulsive character. Because obsessive and compulsive traits can accompany other kinds of personality (especially narcissistic and introjective depressive psychologies), diagnosis of obsessive-compulsive personality disorder requires an understanding of the internal experience, not just the behavior, of the patient.

Central to an obsessive-compulsive psychology is a reluctance to feel emotions associated with being "out of control." This attitude may originate in early dyadic struggles. Freud (1913) related the stubborn, punctilious, and hoarding tendencies of the obsessive-compulsive adult to battles over toilet training, but a controlling parent may also have set up power struggles around eating, sexuality, and general obedience. Obsessive-compulsive individuals, evocatively described by Reich (1933) as "living machines," seem to have identified themselves with caregivers who expected them to be more grown-up than was possible at the time. They regard expressions of subjectivity and affect as "immature," they overvalue rationality, and they suffer humiliation when they feel they have acted childishly. Only when an emotion is logically or morally "justified"—e.g., righteous anger—do they find it acceptable. Although they are generally more preoccupied with issues of self-definition than issues of relationship, there is an anaclitic version of obsessive-compulsive dynamics, exemplified by the compulsive people-pleaser who lives in horror of offending anyone by inappropriate behavior.

Psychoanalytic clinical experience and research (Fisher & Greenberg, 1985; Salzman, 1980; Shapiro, 1965) suggest that obsessive-compulsive people fear that their impulses, especially their aggressive urges, will get out of control. Most obsessive thoughts and compulsive actions involve efforts to undo or counteract impulses toward destructiveness, greed, and messiness. Because guilt over unacceptable wishes is severe, the conscience of the pathologically obsessive-compulsive person is famously rigid and punitive. Self-criticism is harsh; such individuals hold themselves as well as others to a standard close to perfection. They follow rules literally, get lost in details, and have trouble making decisions because they want to make the perfect one. They are scrupulous to a fault but because of all they suppress, they have trouble relaxing, joking, and being fully intimate.

Although obsessive and compulsive qualities tend to go together because they express similar unconscious fantasies, some people have an obsessive personality with little compulsivity while others have a compulsive personality with little obsessionality. Obsessive people are chronically "in their head": thinking, reasoning, judging, and doubting. Compulsive people are chronically "doing and undoing": cleaning, collecting, perfecting.

In therapy, individuals with obsessive and/or compulsive personalities try hard to be cooperative but resist the therapist's efforts to explore their affective world. They may become subtly negativistic, expressing unconscious opposition by coming late, forgetting to pay, and prefacing responses to the therapist's comments with "Yes, but . . . " To the clinician, the relationship may feel like a power struggle. As the patient insists on tendentious argument rather than emotional expression and engagement, the therapist may become impatient and exasperated.

Both cognitive-behavioral and pharmaceutical interventions may help pathologically obsessive-compulsive patients with specific problems, but improving their self-esteem and enriching their emotional life require considerable time with someone willing to help them explore and express those aspects of their personality that they otherwise spend inordinate energy trying to subdue. Given the introjective nature of obsessive-compulsive psychology, psychotherapies that attempt to facilitate insight into the patient's problems are most likely to be helpful.

- **Contributing constitutional-maturational patterns**: Possible irritability, orderliness
- **Central tension/preoccupation**: Submission to/rebellion against controlling authority
- **Central affects**: Anger, guilt, shame, fear
- **Characteristic pathogenic belief about self**: My aggression is dangerous and must be controlled
- **Characteristic pathogenic belief about others**: Others try to exert control, which I must resist
- **Central ways of defending**: Isolation of affect, reaction formation, intellectualizing, moralizing, undoing
- **Subtypes**:

P112.1 Obsessive

Ruminative, cerebral; self-esteem depends on *thinking*, on intellectual achievements

P112.2 Compulsive

Busy, meticulous, perfectionistic; self-esteem depends on doing, on practical achievements

P113. Hysterical (Histrionic) Personality Disorders

Patients with hysterical personality disorder are preoccupied with issues of gender, sexuality, and power. They may come across as flamboyant and attention-seeking, as in the DSM description, or they may strike the interviewer as curiously naïve, conventional, and inhibited. Unconsciously, they tend to regard themselves as weak, defective, and devalued on the basis of their gender, and see individuals of the opposite sex as powerful, exciting, frightening, and enviable (Horowitz, 1991). Before DSM-III applied the term "histrionic" to patients with unconscious gender preoccupations, most psychoanalytic practitioners used the term "hysterical" for neurotically organized individuals with these dynamics, and the term "histrionic" or "hysteroid" for those in the borderline range. The DSM diagnosis of Borderline Personality Disorder is essentially a description of a histrionic person at the borderline level of severity (cf. Zetzel, 1968).

Clinical experience suggests that heterosexual individuals who grow up disappointed by the same-sex parent and overstimulated by the opposite-sex parent may become hysterically organized. Thus, hysterical women tend to describe their mothers as depressed or overburdened and their fathers as larger than life. The opposite-sex parent may have been seductive or sexually inappropriate, sometimes to the point of molestation. In gay and lesbian children with hysterical dynamics, the same-sex parent is often reported as powerful, problematic, or frightening. Unlike transgendered individuals, the hysterical or histrionic person accepts his or her biological gender, but feels that it confers significant disadvantages.

Hysterical and histrionic individuals may seek power via seductiveness ("pseudo-hypersexuality") toward persons of the overvalued gender. Sexual intimacy, however, is a source of significant conflict because of unconscious shame about one's gendered body and fears of being damaged by the more powerful other. Some people with hysterical psychologies are sexually avoidant or unresponsive, while others flaunt their sexuality in an exhibitionistic way, in an effort to counteract unconscious shame and fear. In terms of general personality style, some people with hysterical dynamics resemble the self-dramatizing DSM depiction, while others are inhibited and reserved. Cultural factors may encourage the predominance of one type or the other; for example, hysterical people in Western societies are more likely to dramatize, while those in cultures that try to control the sexuality of people of their gender are apt to be inhibited.

Like schizoid individuals, hysterical patients fear overstimulation, but from inside rather than from outside, and thus view their own feelings and desires with anxiety. The dread of being overwhelmed by affect may be expressed in a self-dramatizing style of speaking, as if emotion is being unconsciously derided by being exaggerated. Cognitive style may be impressionistic (Shapiro, 1965), as the hysterical person prefers not to look too closely at details for fear of seeing too much and being overwhelmed. Medically inexplicable physical symptoms expressing dissociated conflicts (conversion) may be present. Behavior, especially sexual behavior, may be impulsive or driven yet regarded by the hysterical person as curiously unrelated to identifiable internal states. Like narcissistic individuals, hysterical patients may compete for attention that reassures them of their value, but their exhibitionistic and excessively competitive qualities are limited to the realm of sexuality and gender. Outside that arena they are capable of warm and stable attachments.

Therapists' initial responses to neurotic-level hysterical patients tend to be positive. Later, clinicians may feel that attitudes related to their own gender are being evoked. Therapists whose gender is devalued by the patient may feel slightly demeaned, while those whose gender is overvalued may feel narcissistically inflated. At the borderline level, histrionic patients evoke exasperation and apprehension in the therapist, as their intense unconscious anxiety impels them to act out rather than talk. With a therapist of the gender they see as powerful, they may be flagrantly seductive.

Because the psychology of hysterically and histrionically organized patients is so centrally anaclitic, it tends to be the relational aspects of psychotherapy that help them the most. At the same time, because hysterical individuals need to balance their anaclitic orientation with an increase in self-definition, they may respond well to interpretive aspects of treatment. Traditional psychoanalytic therapies that encourage the patient's gradual, self-paced exploration of thoughts and feelings are likely to be helpful to hysterically organized individuals in the neurotic range, whereas treatment of those at the borderline level requires more deliberate handling of boundary issues, confrontation about destructive enactments, and explicit psychoeducation.

- **Contributing constitutional-maturational patterns**: Possibly sensitivity, sociophilia
- **Central tension/preoccupation**: Power and sexuality in own gender/other gender
- **Central affects**: Fear, shame, guilt (over competition)
- **Characteristic pathogenic belief about self**: My gender makes me weak, castrated, vulnerable
- **Characteristic pathogenic belief about others**: People of my own gender are of little value; people of the other gender are powerful, exciting, potentially exploitative and damaging
- **Central ways of defending**: Repression, regression, conversion, sexualizing, acting out
- **Subtypes**:

P113.1 Inhibited

More common in highly structured, moralistic cultures and subcultures, this manifestation of hysterical personality is characterized by emotional reserve, sexual naïveté, inexperience and inhibition, conversion symptoms and somatization.

P113.2 Demonstrative or Flamboyant

More common in liberal and chaotic cultures and subcultures, this manifestation is characterized by a tendency toward repeated crises and dramatizations, seductiveness, and sexual impulsiveness. Problems with achieving a full sexual response are common.

P114. Dissociative Personality Disorder (Dissociative Identity Disorder/Multiple Personality Disorder)

What we label dissociative personality disorder is roughly identical with the DSM-IV-TR diagnosis of Dissociative Identity Disorder. Although the DSM-IV-TR places this condition with other dissociative syndromes (under the general rubric of anxiety disorder) rather than in its section on personality disorders, dissociative identity disorder is a dissociative syndrome that dominates an individual's personality. When dissociative defenses are relied upon as a person's primary and habitual response to stress and negative affect, dissociation becomes characterological in the same way that any other defense can become locked into personality (Brenner, 2001; Bromberg, 1998/2001). When someone is repeatedly traumatized (abused to such an extent that the abuse constitutes torture) during early childhood and has the constitutional capacity to go into trance, or grows up in a family in which dissociation is adaptive, with little opportunity to process traumatic experiences in words and with feeling, the basis for a dissociative personality disorder exists (Kluft, 1985).

While the phenomenon that for many decades was called multiple personality disorder has evoked psychiatric interest for well over a century, its sometimes dramatic manifestations have spawned many controversies about incidence, etiology, relationship to other conditions, and treatment. In some decades, dissociative individuals have been virtually ignored by the mental health community, whereas during others, especially those marked by war and other catastrophes that draw attention to trauma, they have elicited passionate interest. Currently, professionals are divided as to whether individuals with dissociative personality disorder constitute a significant mental health population or whether they are "created" by credulous therapists who unwittingly encourage dissociative reactions in suggestible people.

Our reading of the evidence is that dissociative personality disorder is not rare (see, e.g., Brenner, 2001; Bromberg, 1998/2001). The traumatic history that engenders this condition, usually involving abuse by a primary caregiver, creates in its victims a disposition to placate authorities, including therapists, from whom grave mistreatment is unconsciously feared. Thus, clinicians who convey skepticism about amnesia and altered states of consciousness unwittingly discourage dissociative patients from revealing the dissociative symptoms from which they suffer. Practitioners with the polar opposite attitude, a fascination with the drama of identity shifts and intrusive memories, may unwittingly encourage patients with dissociative defenses to dissociate more and more. Thus, dissociation may be either iatrogenically suppressed and underdiagnosed or iatrogenically provoked.

This disorder exists in the neurotic through the borderline ranges and may involve temporary dissociative reactions with psychotic features. Behavior, affect, bodily experience, or knowledge and memory can be dissociated (Braun, 1988). Patients who dissociate may feel troubled by parts of the body or self they experience as alien or by aspects of personality they experience as "alter." Amnesia for certain states of mind, often described by the patient as "losing time," is a prime indicator of dissociative personality disorder. With this psychology goes an oscillating doubt about which experiences can be trusted and which are confabulated, an uncertainty that may be felt by both patient and therapist. Individuals with this personality disorder may experience profound hopelessness about developing any sense of continuity of self states and feel repeatedly blindsided by shifts in consciousness that they cannot explain.

Dissociative individuals may induce confusion and a sense of futility in the therapist, especially during the early diagnostic process, when attempts to take a history elicit vague, disjointed narratives (Davies & Frawley, 1993). Once they have revealed their history of trauma, dissociative patients may inspire powerful sympathetic wishes to save and rescue. Given the patient's underlying fear of abuse, it is critical that treatment proceed slowly, with consistent attention to maintaining the therapeutic alliance and scrupulous preservation of boundaries. Premature efforts to accomplish the emotional processing or "abreaction" of early trauma risk overwhelming and retraumatizing the dissociative person. Eventually, however, cognitive, emotional, behavioral, and somatic aspects of experience that have been dissociated need to be addressed and reintegrated, at a pace controlled by the client.

- **Contributing constitutional-maturational patterns**: Constitutional capacity for self-hypnosis; early, severe, and repeated physical and/or sexual trauma
- **Central tension/preoccupation**: Acknowledging trauma/disavowing trauma
- **Central affects**: Fear, rage
- **Characteristic pathogenic belief about self**: I am small, weak, and vulnerable to recurring trauma
- **Characteristic pathogenic belief about others**: Others are perpetrators, exploiters, or rescuers
- **Central ways of defending**: Dissociation

P115. Mixed/Other

This category is included to cover individuals with combinations of personality types (e.g., phobic-hysterical or paranoid-schizoid) as well as individuals with unusual personal themes, defenses, affect patterns, and orienting beliefs that do not correspond to the more common constellations depicted in this section.

REFERENCES

Adler, G. (1985). *Borderline psychopathology and its treatment.* New York: Jason Aronson.

Akhtar, S. (1989). Narcissistic personality disorder: Descriptive features and differential diagnosis. *Psychiatric Clinics of North America, 12,* 505-529.

Akhtar, S. (1992). *Broken structures: Severe personality disorders and their treatment.* Northvale, NJ: Jason Aronson.

Ainsworth, M. D. S., Blehar, M. C., Waters, E., & Wall, S. (1978). *Patterns of attachment: A psychological study of the Strange Situation.* Hillsdale, NJ: Erlbaum.

Bakan, D. (1966). *The duality of human existence: Isolation and communion in western man.* Boston: Beacon Press.

Beck, A. T. (1983). Cognitive therapy of depression: New perspectives. In P. J. Clayton & J. E. Barrett (Eds.), *Treatment of depression: Old controversies and new approaches* (pp. 265-290). New York: Raven.

Berliner, B. (1958). The role of object relations in moral masochism. *Psychoanalytic Quarterly, 27,* 38-56.

Blatt, S. J. (1998). Contributions of psychoanalysis to the understanding and treatment of depression. *Journal of the American Psychoanalytic Association, 46,* 722-752.

Blatt, S. J. (2004). *Experiences of depression: Theoretical, clinical and research perspectives.* Washington, DC: American Psychological Association.

Blatt, S. J. (in press). A fundamental polarity in psychoanalysis: Implications for personality development, psychopathology, and the therapeutic process. *Psychoanalytic Inquiry.*

Blatt, S. J., & Auerbach, J. S. (1988). Differential cognitive disturbances in three types of "borderline" patients. *Journal of Personality Disorders, 2(3),* 198-211.

Blatt, S. J., & Bers, S. A. (1993). The sense of self in depression: A psychodynamic perspective. In Segal, Z. V. & Blatt, S. J. (Eds.) (1993). *The self in emotional distress. Cognitive and psychodynamic perspectives.* New York: Guilford Press.

Bornstein, R. F. (1993). *The dependent personality.* New York: Guilford Press.

Bornstein, R. F. (2005). *The dependent patient: A practitioner's guide.* Washington, DC: American Psychological Association.

Bradley, R., Heim, A., & Westen, D. (2005). Transference phenomena in the psychotherapy of personality disorders: An empirical investigation. *British Journal of Psychiatry, 186,* 342-349.

Braun, B. G. (1988). The BASK (behavior, affect, sensation, knowledge) model of dissociation. *Dissociation: Progress in the Dissociative Disorders, 1:* 4-23.

Brenner, I. (2001). *Dissociation of trauma: Theory, phenomenology, and technique.* New York: International Universities Press.

Bromberg, P. M. (1998/2001). *Standing in the spaces: Essays on clinical process, trauma, and dissociation.* Hillsdale, NJ: Analytic Press.

Bursten, B. (1973). *The manipulator: A psychoanalytic view.* New Haven: Yale University Press.

Clarkin, J. F., Foelsch, P. A., Levy, K. N., Hull, J. W., Delaney, J. C., & Kernberg, O. F. (2001). The development of a psychodynamic treatment for patients with borderline personality disorder: A preliminary study of behavioral change. *Journal of Personality Disorders, 15,* 487-495.

Clarkin, J. F., Levy, K. N., Lenzenweger, M., & Kernberg, O. F. (2004). The Personality Disorders Institute / Borderline Personality Research Foundation randomized control trial for borderline personality disorder: Rationale, methods, and patient characteristics. *Journal of Personality Disorders, 18,* 51-72.

Cleckley, H. (1941). *The mask of sanity: An attempt to clarify some issues about the so-called psychopathic personality.* St. Louis: Mosby.

Cooper, A. (1988). The narcissistic-masochistic character. In R. A. Glick & D. I. Meyers (Eds.), *Masochism: Current psychological perspectives* (pp. 117-138). Hillsdale, NJ: Analytic Press.

Cooper, A., & Ronningstam, E. (1992). In A. Tasman & M. Riba (Eds.), *American Psychiatric Press review of psychiatry: Vol. 2* (pp. 80-97). Washington, DC: American Psychiatric Press.

Costa, P. T., Jr., & Widiger, T. A. (Eds.) (2002). *Personality disorders and the five-factor model of personality* (2nd ed.). Washington, DC: American Psychological Association.

Davies, J. M., & Frawley, M. G. (1993). *Treating the adult survivor of childhood sexual abuse: A psychoanalytic perspective.* New York: Basic Books.

Deutsch, H. (1942). Some forms of emotional disturbance and their relationship to schizophrenia. *Psychoanalytic Quarterly, 11,* 301-321.

Deutsch, H. (1955). The imposter: Contributions to ego psychology of a type of psychopath. In *Neurosis and character types: Clinical psychoanalytic studies* (pp. 319-338). New York: International Universities Press.

Doidge, N. (2001). Diagnosing The English Patient: Schizoid fantasies of being skinless and being buried alive. *Journal of the American Psychoanalytic Association, 49,* 279-309.

Fisher, S., & Greenberg, R. P. (1985). *The scientific credibility of Freud's theories and therapy.* New York: Columbia University Press.

Fonagy, P., Gergely, G., Jurist, E. L., & Target, M. (2002). *Affect regulation, mentalization, and the development of the self.* New York: Other Press.

Fonagy, P., Target, M., Gergely, G., Allen, J. G., & Bateman, A. W. (2003). The developmental roots of borderline personality disorder in early attachment relationships: A theory and some evidence. *Psychoanalytic Inquiry, 23,* 412-459.

Frank, J. D., Margolin, J., Nash, H. T., Stone, A. R., Varon, E., & Ascher, E. (1952). Two behavior patterns in therapeutic groups and their apparent motivation. *Human Relations, 5,* 289-317.

Freud, S. (1913). The disposition to obsessional neurosis. *Standard Edition, 12,* 311-326.

Freud, S. (1924). The economic problem of masochism. *Standard Edition, 19,* 159-170.

Fromm, E. (1973). *The anatomy of human destructiveness.* New York: Fawcett.

Frosch, J. (1964). The psychotic character: Clinical psychiatric considerations. *Psychiatric Quarterly, 38,* 91-96.

Gabbard, G. O. (1989). Two subtypes of narcissistic personality disorder. *Bulletin of the Menninger Clinic, 53,* 527-532.

Gacano, C., & Meloy, J. R. (1994). *Rorschach assessment of aggressive and psychopathic personalities.* Hillsdale, NJ: Lawrence Erlbaum.

Greenspan, S. I. (1989). *The development of the ego: Implications for personality theory, psychopathology, and the psychotherapeutic process.* Madison, CT: International Universities Press.

Greenspan, S. I. (1992). *Infancy and early childhood: The practice of clinical assessment and intervention with emotional and developmental challenges.* Madison, CT: International Universities Press.

Greenspan, S. I., & Shanker, S. (2004). *The first idea: How symbols, language, and intelligence evolve from primates to humans.* Reading, MA: Perseus Books.

Grinker, R. R., Werble, B., & Drye, R. C. (1968). *The borderline syndrome: A behavioral study of ego functions*. New York: Basic Books.

Gunderson, J. G. (1984). *Borderline personality disorder*. Washington, DC: American Psychiatric Press.

Gunderson, J. G., & Singer, M. T. (1975). Defining borderline patients: An overview. *American Journal of Psychiatry, 133,* 1-10.

Guntrip, H. (1969). *Schizoid phenomena, object relations and the self.* New York: International Universities Press.

Hare, R. (1991). *The Hare psychopathy checklist: Revised manual.* Toronto: Multi-Health Systems.

Hartocollis, P. (Ed.) (1977). *Borderline personality disorders: The concept, the syndrome, the patient.* New York: International Universities Press.

Henderson, D. K. (1939). *Psychopathic states.* London: Chapman & Hall.

Herman, J. L. (1992). *Trauma and recovery: The aftermath of violence–from domestic abuse to political terror.* New York: Basic Books.

Hillenbrand, L. (2003, July 7). A sudden illness. *New Yorker.*

Hirsch, S. J., & Hollender, M. H. (1969). Hysterical psychoses: Clarification of the concept. *American Journal of Psychiatry, 125,* 909.

Hirschfeld, R. M. A. (1991). Depressive illness: Diagnostic issues. *Bulletin of the Menninger Clinic, 55,* 144–155.

Hollender, M. H., & Hirsch, S. J. (1964). Hysterical psychosis. *American Journal of Psychiatry, 120,* 1066–1074.

Holt, S., Meloy, J. R., & Strack, S. (1999). *Journal of American Academic Psychiatry and the Law, 27,* 23-32.

Horowitz, M. J. (Ed.) (1991). *Hysterical personality style and the histrionic personality disorder.* Northvale, NJ: Jason Aronson.

Hunt, W. (1995). The diffident narcissist: A character-type illustrated in *The Beast in the Jungle* by Henry James. *International Journal of Psychoanalysis, 76,* 1257-1267.

Hurvich, M. (2003). The place of annihilation anxiety in psychoanalytic theory. *Journal of the American Psychoanalytic Association, 51,* 579-616.

John, O. P., & Srivastava, S. (1999). The Big Five trait taxonomy: History, measurement, and theoretical perspectives. In L. A. Pervin & O. P. John (Eds.), *Handbook of personality: Theory and research* (2nd ed., pp. 102-138). New York: Guilford Press.

Kazarian, S. S., & Evans, D. R. (Eds.) (2001). *Handbook of cultural health psychology.* Philadelphia: Elsevier Science and Technology Books.

Kernberg, O. F. (1975). *Borderline conditions and pathological narcissism.* New York: Jason Aronson.

Kernberg, O. F. (1983). Object relations theory and character analysis. *Journal of the American Psychoanalytic Association, 31S,* 247-271.

Kernberg, O. F. (1984). *Severe personality disorders: Psychotherapeutic strategies.* New Haven: Yale University Press.

Kernberg, O. F. (1988). Clinical dimensions of masochism. *Journal of the American Psychoanalytic Association, 36,* 1005-1029.

Kirmayer, L. (1984). Culture, affect, and somatization. *Transcultural Psychiatric Research Review, 21,* 160–169.

Klein, M. (1935). A contribution to the psychogenesis of manic-depressive states. In R. Money-Kyrle (Ed.), *The writings of Melanie Klein: Vol. 1. Love, guilt and reparation and other works, 1921-1945* (pp. 262-289). New York, Free Press, 1975.

Kluft, R. (Ed.) (1985). *Childhood antecedents of multiple personality.* Washington, DC: American Psychiatric Press.

Knight, R. (1953). Borderline states in psychoanalytic psychiatry and psychology. *Bulletin of the Menninger Clinic, 17*, 1-12.

Kohut, H. (1971). *The analysis of the self: A systematic approach to the psychoanalytic treatment of the narcissistic personality disorders.* New York: International Universities Press.

Kohut, H. (1977). *The restoration of the self.* New York: International Universities Press.

Langness, L. L. (1967). Hysterical psychosis: The cross-cultural evidence. *American Journal of Psychiatry, 124*, 143-151.

Laughlin, H. P. (1956). *The neuroses in clinical practice* (pp. 394-406). Philadelphia: Saunders.

Laughlin, H. P. (1979). *The ego and its defenses* (2nd ed.). New York: Jason Aronson.

Levy, K., & Blatt, S. J. (1999). Attachment theory and psychoanalysis. *Psychoanalytic Inquiry, 19*, 541-575.

MacKinnon, R. A., & Michels, R. (1971), *The psychiatric interview in clinical practice.* Philadelphia: Saunders.

Main, T. F. (1957). The ailment. *British Journal of Medical Psychology, 30*, 129-145.

Marty, P., & M'Uzan, M. de (1963). La pensée operatoire. *Revue Française de Psychoanalyse, 27 (Suppl.)*, 345–356.

Masterson, J. F. (1972). *Treatment of the borderline adolescent: A developmental approach.* New York: Wiley-Interscience.

Masterson, J. F. (1976). *Psychotherapy of the borderline adult: A developmental approach.* New York: Brunner/Mazel.

McAdams, (1988). *Power, intimacy, and the life story: Personological inquiries into identity.* New York: Guilford Press.

McCrae, R. R., & Costa, P. T., Jr. (2003). *Personality in adulthood: A five-factor theory perspective* (2nd ed.). New York: Guilford Press.

McDougall, J. (1989). *Theaters of the body: A psychoanalytic approach to psychosomatic illness.* New York: Norton.

McWilliams, N. (1994). *Psychoanalytic diagnosis: Understanding personality structure in the clinical process.* New York: Guilford Press.

Meissner, W. W. (1978). *The paranoid process.* New York: Jason Aronson.

Meloy, J. R. (1988). *The psychopathic mind: Origins, dynamics, and treatment.* Northvale, NJ: Jason Aronson.

Meloy, J. R. (1995). Antisocial personality disorder. In G. O. Gabbard (Ed.), *Treatments of psychiatric disorders: Vol. 2* (pp. 2273-2290). Washington, DC: American Psychiatric Press.

Meloy, J. R. (1997). The psychology of wickedness: Psychopathy and sadism. *Psychiatric Annals, 27*, 630-633.

Menaker, E. (1953). Masochism: A defense reaction of the ego. *Psychoanalytic Quarterly, 22*, 205-220.

Miller, A. (1975). *Prisoners of childhood: The drama of the gifted child and the search for the true self.* New York: Basic Books.

Millon, T. (1996). *Disorders of personality: DSM IV and beyond.* New York: Wiley.

Morse, J. Q., Robins, C. J., & Gittes-Fox, M. (2002). Sociotropy, autonomy, and personality disorder criteria in psychiatric patients. *Journal of Personality Disorders, 16*, 549-560.

Ogloff, J., & Wong, S. (1990). Electrodermal and cardiovascular evidence of a coping response in psychopaths. *Criminal Justice and Behavior, 17*, 231-245.

Ouimette, P. C., Klein, D. N., Anderson, R., Riso, L. P., & Lizardi, H. (1994). Relationship of sociotropy/autonomy and dependency/self-criticism to DSM-III-R personality disorders. *Journal of Abnormal Psychology, 103*, 743-749.

Perry, J. C., & Cooper, S. H. (1989). An empirical study of defense mechanisms. *Archives of General Psychiatry, 46*, 444-452.

Peterson, C., & Seligman, M. E. (1984). Causal explanations as a risk factor for depression: Theory and evidence. *Psychological Review, 91,* 347-374.

Raine, A., Venables, P., & Williams, M. (1990). Relationships between central and autonomic measures of arousal at age 15 and criminality at age 24. *Archives of General Psychiatry, 47,* 1003-1007.

Reich, W. (1933). *Character analysis.* New York: Farrar, Straus, & Giroux.

Reik, T. (1941). *Masochism in modern man.* New York: Farrar, Straus.

Richman, J., & White, H. (1970). A family view of hysterical psychosis. *American Journal of Psychiatry, 127,* 280-285.

Rosenfeld, H. (1987). Afterthought: Changing theories and changing techniques in psychoanalysis. In *Impasse and interpretation: Therapeutic and anti-therapeutic factors in the psychoanalytic treatment of psychotic, borderline, and neurotic patients* (pp. 265-279). London: Tavistock.

Roth, A., & Fonagy, P. (1996). *What works for whom? A critical review of psychotherapy research.* New York: Guilford Press.

Salzman, L. (1980). *Treatment of the obsessive personality.* New York: Jason Aronson.

Sampson, H. (1992). The role of "real" experience in psychopathology and treatment. *Psychoanalytic Dialogues, 2,* 509-528.

Schmideberg, M. (1959). The borderline patient. In S. Arieti (Ed.), *American handbook of psychiatry* (vol. 1, pp. 398-416). New York: Basic Books.

Schore, A. N. (2003). *Affect dysregulation and disorders of the self.* New York: Norton.

Seinfeld, J. (1991). *The empty core: An object relations approach to psychotherapy of the schizoid personality.* Northvale, NJ: Jason Aronson.

Serin, R. (1991). Psychopathy and violence in criminals. *Journal of Interpersonal Violence, 6,* 423-431.

Shapiro, D. (1965). *Neurotic styles.* New York: Basic Books.

Shapiro, D. (1981). *Autonomy and rigid character.* New York: Basic Books.

Shapiro, D. (1989). *Psychotherapy of neurotic character.* New York: Basic Books.

Shapiro, D. (2000). Dynamics of character: Self-regulation in psychopathology. New York: Basic Books.

Shedler, J., & Westen, D. (2004). Refining personality disorder diagnosis: Integrating science and practice. *American Journal of Psychiatry, 161,* 1350-1365.

Sherwood, V. R., & Cohen, C. P. (1995). *Psychotherapy of the quiet borderline patient: The as-if personality revisited.* Northvale, NJ: Jason Aronson.

Sifneos, P. (1973). The prevalence of "alexithymia" characteristics in psychosomatic patients. *Psychotherapy and Psychosomatics, 22,* 255-262.

Silberschatz, G. (2005). *Transformative relationships: The control-mastery theory of psychotherapy.* New York: Routledge.

Singer, J. A. (2005). *Personality and psychotherapy: Treating the whole person.* New York: Guilford Press.

Sperling, M. B., Sharp, J. L., & Fishler, P. H. (1991). On the nature of attachment in a borderline population: A preliminary investigation. *Psychological Reports, 68,* 543-546.

Spiegel, H., & Spiegel, D. (1978). *Trance and treatment: Clinical uses of hypnosis.* New York: Basic Books.

Stern, D. B. (1997). *Unformulated experience: From dissociation to imagination in psychoanalysis.* Hillside, NJ: Analytic Press.

Stone, M. H. (1980). *The borderline syndromes: Constitution, personality, and adaptation.* New York: McGraw-Hill.

Stone, M. H. (Ed.) (1986). *Essential papers on borderline disorders: One hundred years at the border.* New York: New York University Press.

Stone, M. H. (1993). *Abnormalities of personality: Within and beyond the realm of treatment.* New York: Norton.

Trull, T. J., Widiger, T. A., & Frances, A. (1987). Covariation of criteria sets for avoidant, schizoid, and dependent personality disorders. *American Journal of Psychiatry, 144,* 767-771.

Vaillant, G. E. (1994). Ego mechanisms of defense and personality psychopathology. *Journal of Abnormal Psychology, 103,* 44-50.

Vaillant, G. E., Bond, M., & Vaillant, C. O. (1986). An empirically validated hierarchy of defense mechanisms. *Archives of General Psychiatry, 42,* 597-601.

Van der Kolk, B. A. (1994). The body keeps the score: Memory and the evolving psychobiology of posttraumatic stress. *Harvard Review of Psychiatry, 1,* 253-265.

Vermote, R. (2005). *Touching inner change: Psychoanalytically informed hospitalization-based treatment of personality disorders: A process-outcome study.* Unpublished doctoral dissertation. Katholieke Universiteit Leuven, Belgium.

Wallerstein, R. S. (1967). Reconstruction and mastery in the transference psychosis. *Journal of the American Psychoanalytic Association, 15,* 551-583.

Weiss, J. (1993). *How psychotherapy works: Process and technique.* New York: Guilford Press.

Weiss, J., Sampson, H., & the Mt. Zion Psychotherapy Research Group (1986). *The psychoanalytic process: Theory, clinical observation, and empirical research.* New York: Guilford Press.

West, M., & Keller, A. (1994). Psychotherapy strategies for insecure attachment in personality disorders. In M. B. Sperling & W. H. Berman (Eds.), *Attachment in adults: Clinical and developmental perspectives* (pp. 313–330). New York: Guilford Press.

Westen, D., & Shedler, J. (1999a). Revising and assessing Axis II: Part 1: Developing a clinically and empirically valid assessment method. *American Journal of Psychiatry, 156,* 258-272.

Westen, D., & Shedler, J. (1999b). Revising and assessing Axis II: Part 2. Toward an empirically based and clinically useful classification of personality disorders. *American Journal of Psychiatry, 156,* 273-285.

Westen, D., & Shedler, J. (2000). A prototype matching approach to personality disorders: Towards DSM-V. *Journal of Personality Disorders, 14,* 109-126.

Zetzel, E. (1968). The so-called good hysteric. *International Journal of Psycho-Analysis, 49,* 256-260.

Profile of Mental Functioning
M Axis

WORK GROUP MEMBERS

Paul Fink, MD
Philadelphia, Pennsylvania

Stanley I. Greenspan, MD
Bethesda, Maryland

Bernard Friedberg, MD
Voorhees, New Jersey

Joseph Palombo, MA
Chicago, Illinois

Stuart G. Shanker, DPhil
Toronto, Ontario, Canada

Profile of Mental Functioning
M Axis

The following describes categories of basic mental functions that we believe help clinicians to capture the complexity and individuality of the patient. For each category, we have provided illustrations that exemplify different levels of healthy-to-impaired functioning. These descriptions are not intended to be used for ratings; we offer them to amplify what might be considered in each category.

The descriptions cover a variety of areas of mental functioning. While no profile can hope to capture the full richness of mental life, the following attempts to highlight a number of crucial areas. The first category on *capacity for regulation, attention, and learning* underlines fundamental processes that enable human beings to attend to and learn from their experiences. The second category concerns the *capacity for relationships and intimacy (including depth, range, and consistency)*. The third category, the *quality of internal experience (level of confidence and self-regard)*, attempts to capture the level of confidence and self-regard that characterizes an individual's relationship to others and the larger world. The fourth category delineates the basic nature of the individual's *capacity for affective experience, expression, and communication*, and that person's ability to express the full range of pre-representational and representational patterns of affects. The fifth category, *defensive patterns and capacities*, highlights the way the individual attempts to cope with and alter wishes, affect, and other experiences, and the degree to which he or she distorts experience in the process.

The sixth category, the *capacity to form internal representations*, concerns the individual's capacity to symbolize affectively meaningful experience (i.e., to organize experience in a mental, rather than somatic or behavioral form). This capacity to represent or mentalize enables the individual to use ideas to experience, describe, and express internal life. The seventh category, the *capacity for differentiation and integration*, involves the individual's ability to build logical bridges between internal representations (i.e., to separate fantasy from reality and to construct connections between internal representations of wishes, affects, self and object relationships, and the past, present, and future). The next category, *self-observing capacities (psychological mindedness)*, concerns the individual's ability to observe his or her own internal life. This category is an extension of the capacity for differentiation and integration but is a significant enough advance to warrant its own description. The last category involves the *capacity to construct or use internal standards and ideals (sense of morality)*. An outgrowth of other mental functions and an integration of a number of them, the capacity to formulate internal values and ideals reflects a consideration of one's self in the context of current and future experiences.

Mental functions include very basic capacities that do not depend on verbal exchanges, such as engaging in relationships and using gestures to express and respond to affects (i.e., the affects are not represented, symbolized, or mentalized), as well as capacities that we usually communicate verbally, such as self-observation.

By necessity, some of these categories overlap. Each one, however, highlights an important feature of mental functioning that cannot quite be described by the others. Nor can critical human features be accounted for without reference to these or similar constructs. We emphasize again that the following profile of mental functioning is simply an attempt to systematize the richness of human emotional experience. Any such attempt is inevitably an approximation of infinitely complex processes.

There is a growing body of research demonstrating that it is possible to measure these components of mental functioning as well as others. Examples of important systematic efforts include:[1]

- **Scales of Psychological Capacities (SPC)**—From the Menninger Psychotherapy Research Project, PRPII, 17 scales designed to create a profile of personality functioning, which would reflect changes in underlying personality organization, i.e., structural changes in the ego (DeWitt, Hartley, Rosenberg, Zilberg, & Wallerstein, 1991; Wallerstein, 1988; Zilberg, Wallerstein, DeWitt, Hartley, & Rosenberg, 1991)

- **Karolinska Psychodynamic Profile (KAPP)**—Created in Sweden, 17 scales of personality attributes (Weinryb, Rossel, & Asberg, 1991)

- **Operationalized Psychodynamic Diagnosis (OPD)**—Created by German researchers. (Dahlbender, Rudolf, & OPD Task Force, p. 615)

- **Structured Interview of Personality Organization (STIPO)**—Created by the Kernberg-Clarkin group at Cornell, covering 94 areas of inquiry, divided into six overall domains of personality functioning (Clarkin, Caligor, Stern, & Kernberg, 2004; Stern, Clarkin, Caligor & Kernberg, 2005)

- **McGlashan Semistructured Interview (MSI)**—Similar to the STIPO, covering 32 areas of personality functioning (Miller, McGlashan, Rosen, Cadenhead, Cannon, Ventura, et al., 2004)

- **Analytic Process Scales (APS)**—Created by Waldron and his group in New York, designed as a process measure to assess the contributions of the analyst, of the patient, and of the interactional characteristics of their relationship (Waldron, Scharf, Crouse, Firestein, Burton, & Hurst, 2004; Waldron, Scharf, Hurst, Firestein, & Burton, 2004)

---

[1]Wallerstein describes the more recent of these approaches in greater depth in this volume's section on research (p. 511).

- **Psychotherapy Process Q-Set (PPQS)**—A Q-sort providing for the description and classification of treatment processes and as an outcome measure of personality change (Jones, 2000)

- **Shedler-Westen Assessment Procedure (SWAP)**—Also a Q-sort geared to assessment of overall personality functioning (Shedler & Westen, p. 573)

- **Object Relations Inventory (ORI)**—Created by Blatt and his colleagues at Yale, organized as a measure of personality structure, into two separate scales of personality organization (Blatt, & Auerbach, 2001; Blatt, Auerbach, & Levy, 1997; Blatt, Chevron, Quinlan, Schaffer, & Wein, 1988; Blatt, Stayner, Auerbach, & Behrends, 1996; Diamond, Blatt, Stayner, & Kaslow, 1991)

- **Ego Function Assessment (EFA)** - Created by Leopold Bellak and his collaborators under a grant from the National Institute of Mental Health. Measures twelve aspects of ego strength (Bellak & Goldsmith, 1984; Bellak & Hurvich, 1969; Bellak, Hurvich & Crawford, 1970; Bellak, Hurvich & Gediman, 1973)

Capacity for Regulation, Attention, and Learning

Consider constitutional and maturational contributions, including:
- Auditory processing and language
- Visual-spatial processing
- Motor planning and sequencing
- Sensory modulation

and related capacities for:
- Executive functioning
- Memory (working, declarative, and non-declarative)
- Attention
- Overall intelligence
- Processing affective and social cues

Illustrative Descriptions of the Range and Adequacy of Functioning
- Focused, organized, and able to learn most of the time, even under stress
- Focused, organized, calm, and able to learn except when over- or understimulated (e.g., noisy, active, or very dull setting); challenged to use a vulnerable skill (e.g., a person with weak fine motor skills is asked to write rapidly); or ill, anxious, or under stress.
- Only when very interested, motivated, or captivated can attend, be calm, and learn for short periods and to a limited degree (i.e., has problems with language, motor, or visual-spatial processing).
- Attention is fleeting (a few seconds here or there) and/or is very active, agitated, or mostly self-absorbed, and/or lethargic or passive. Learning capacity is severely limited due to multiple "processing" difficulties.

Related studies include: Bucci, 1985; Greenspan, 1989; Greenspan & Shanker, 2004; Hartmann, 1965; McGaugh, 2003; Nagera 2001; Schore, 1994.

Capacity for Relationships and Intimacy
(Including Depth, Range, and Consistency)

Illustrative Descriptions of the Range and Adequacy of Functioning

- Deep, emotionally rich capacity for intimacy, caring, and empathy, even when feelings are strong or under stress in a variety of expectable contexts.
- Intimacy, caring, and empathy are present but disrupted by strong emotions and wishes such as anger or separation anxiety (e.g., person withdraws or acts out).
- Superficial and need-oriented, lacking intimacy and empathy.
- Indifferent to others or aloof and withdrawn.

Related studies include: Bell 2001; Blatt & Auerbach, 2001; Blatt, Auerbach, & Levy, 1997; Blatt, Chevron, Quinlan, Schaffer, & Wein, 1988; Blatt, Stayner, Auerbach, & Behrends, 1996; Dahlbender, Rudolf, et al., p. 615; DeWitt, Hartley, Rosenberg, Zilberg, & Wallerstein, 1991; Diamond, Blatt, Stayner, & Kaslow, 1991; Kantrowitz, Katz, Paolitto, Sashin, & Solomon, 1987a; Levy 2001; Miller 1998; Meissner 2000a; Waldron, Scharf, Crouse, Firestein, Burton, & Hurst, D, 2004; Waldron, Scharf, Hurst, Firestein, & Burton, 2004; Wallerstein, 1988; Wallerstein, Robbins, Sargent, & Luborsky, 1956; Weinryb, Rossel, & Asberg, 1991; Zilberg, Wallerstein, DeWitt, Hartley, & Rosenberg, 1991.

Quality of Internal Experience
(Level of Confidence and Self-Regard)

Illustrative Descriptions of the Range and Adequacy of Functioning

- Sense of well-being, vitality, and realistic self-esteem. Present even when under stress.
- Sense of well-being, vitality, and realistic self-esteem. Disrupted by strong emotions or stress, but with eventual recovery of feelings of well-being.
- Feelings of depletion, emptiness, and incompleteness, along with self-involvement unless experiences are nearly "perfect." Self-esteem is vulnerable.
- Depletion, emptiness, incompleteness and self-involvement dominate.

Related studies include: Krystal, 1974, 1975; Meissner 2005a; Meissner 2005b.

Affective Experience, Expression, and Communication

Note: The following descriptions combine the individual's capacity to experience, comprehend, and express affects. Some individuals are relatively stronger or weaker in either affect comprehension or affective expression. Similarly, individuals differ in the way they express or comprehend affects though gestures, such as facial expressions or voice tone, as well as with words. These unique patterns should be captured in the narrative characterizing the individual.

Illustrative Descriptions of the Range and Adequacy of Functioning

- Most of the time uses a wide range of subtle emotions and wishes in a purposeful manner, even under stress. Reads and responds to most emotional signals flexibly and accurately even when under stress (e.g., comprehends safety vs. danger, approval vs. disapproval, acceptance vs. rejection, respect vs. humiliation, partial anger, etc.).

- Often purposeful and organized, but not with a full range of emotional expressions (e.g., seeks out others for closeness and warmth with appropriate glances, body posture, and the like, but becomes chaotic, fragmented, or aimless when very angry). Often accurately reads and responds to a range of emotional signals, except in certain circumstances involving selected emotions and wishes, very strong emotions and wishes, or stress.

- Some need-oriented, purposeful islands of behavior and emotional expressions. No cohesive larger integrated emotional patterns. In selected relationships can read basic intentions of others (such as acceptance or rejection), but unable to read subtle cues (e.g., respect, pride, or partial anger).

- Mostly aimless, fragmented, unpurposeful emotional expressions (e.g., no purposeful grins, smiles, or reaching out with body posture for warmth or closeness). Distorts the intents of others (e.g., misreads cues and therefore feels suspicious, mistreated, unloved, angry, etc.).

Related studies include: Bates, 2000; Blum & Schneider, 2000; Boesky, 2000; Bucci, 2000; Coen, 2000; Corona & Levinson, 2000; De Folch & Kavka, 2000; Green, 1999; Hernández, 1999; Jappe & Lebe, 2000; Kantrowitz, Paolitto, Sashin, Solomon, & Katz, 1986; Mariotti, 2000.

Defensive Patterns and Capacities

Illustrative Descriptions of the Range and Adequacy of Functioning

- Demonstrates an optimal capacity to experience a broad range of thoughts, affects, and relationships and handles stresses with minimal use of defenses that suppress or alter feelings and ideas. Tends to use defenses and coping strategies that support flexibility and healthy emotional functioning, including sublimations, altruism, humor, etc.
- Makes use of defenses to keep potentially threatening ideas, feelings, memories, wishes, or fears out of awareness, without significant distortion of experiences. May use defenses, such as intellectualization and rationalization, and, to a limited degree repression, reaction formation, and displacement.
- Makes extensive use of defenses that distort experience and/or limit the experience of relationships in order to deal with internal and external stressors and to keep feelings and thoughts out of awareness. Uses defenses such as disavowal, denial, projection, splitting, and acting out.
- Demonstrates a generalized failure of defensive regulation leading to a pronounced break with reality through the use of delusional projection and psychotic distortion.

Related studies include: Clarkin, Caligor, Stern, & Kernberg, 2004; Cramer, 1999; DeWitt, Hartley, et al., 1991; Meissner, 2000a; Meissner, 2000b; Meissner, 2000c; Meissner, 2000d; Miller, 1998; Safyer & Hauser, 1995; Schlessinger & Robbins, 1975; Stern, Clarkin, Caligor, & Kernberg, 2005; Wallerstein, 1988, 2001; Weinryb, Rossel, & Asberg, 1991; Zilberg, Wallerstein, DeWitt, Hartley, & Rosenberg, 1991.

Capacity to Form Internal Representations

Illustrative Descriptions of the Range and Adequacy of Functioning

- Uses internal representations to experience a sense of self and others and to express the full range of emotions, wishes. Able to use internal representations to regulate impulses and behavior.

- Uses internal representations to experience a sense of self and others and to express a range of emotions, wishes, except when experiencing selected conflicts or difficult emotions and wishes. Able to use internal representations to inhibit impulses.

- Uses representations or ideas in a concrete way to convey desire for action or to get basic needs met. Does not elaborate on a feeling in its own right (e.g., "I want to hit but can't because someone is watching" rather than "I feel mad"). Often puts wishes and feelings into action (i.e., impulsive behavior) or into somatic states ("my stomach hurts").

- Unable to use internal representations to experience a sense of self and others or to elaborate wishes and feelings (e.g., acts out or demands excessive physical closeness when needy).

Related studies include: Arnold, Farber, & Geller, 2004; Blatt & Auerbach, 2001; Blatt, Auerbach, Levy, 1997; Blatt, Chevron, Quinlan, Schaffer, & Wein, 1988; Blatt, Stayner, Auerbach, & Behrends, 1996; Clarkin, Caligor, Stern, & Kernberg, 2004; Cooper, 2005; DeWitt, Hartley, et al., 1991; Diamond, Blatt, Stayner, & Kaslow, 1991; Meissner, 2000e; Mikulincer & Shaver, 2005; Moretti, 1999; Stern, Clarkin, Caligor, & Kernberg, 2005; Symons, 2004; Szecsody, Varvin, Amadei, Stoker, Beenen, Klockars, et al., 1997; Wallerstein, 1988, 2001; Weinryb, Rossel, & Asberg, 1991; Zilberg, Wallerstein, DeWitt, Hartley, & Rosenberg, 1991.

Capacity for Differentiation and Integration

Illustrative Descriptions of the Range and Adequacy of Functioning

- Is able to connect internal experiences of self and non-self; self and others; fantasy and reality; past, present, and future; and a range of wishes, emotions, and feeling states. Can separate and comprehend differences in these patterns of internal experiences.

- Is able to differentiate and integrate experience, but with some constriction. Strong emotions, wishes, and selected specific emotions, wishes, or stresses can lead to the temporary fragmentation or polarization (all-or-nothing extremes) of internal experience.

- The capacities for differentiation and integration are limited to just a few emotional realms (e.g., very superficial relationships). Challenges outside these limited areas often lead to the fragmentation or polarization (all-or-nothing extremes) of internal experience.

- Internal experience is fragmented most of the time. For example, unable to make emotionally meaningful differentiations of experiences of self and non-self, past and present, or different wishes and feelings.

Related studies include: Blatt & Auerbach, 2001; Blatt, Auerbach, Levy, 1997; Blatt, Chevron, Quinlan, Schaffer, & Wein, 1988; Blatt, Stayner, Auerbach, & Behrends, 1996; Clarkin, Caligor, Stern, & Kernberg, 2004; DeWitt, Hartley, et al., 1991; Diamond, Blatt, Stayner, & Kaslow, 1991; Kantrowitz, Katz, Paolitto, Sashin, & Solomon, 1987b; Sandell, Blomberg, Lazar, Carlsson, Broberg, & Schubert, 2000; Stern, Clarkin, Caligor, & Kernberg, 2005; Wallerstein, 1988, 2001; Weinryb, Rossel, & Asberg, 1991; Zilberg, Wallerstein, DeWitt, Hartley, et al., 1991.

Self-Observing Capacity (Psychological-Mindedness)

Illustrative Descriptions of the Range and Adequacy of Functioning

- Can reflect on (i.e., observe and experience at the same time) a full range of own and others' feelings or experiences (including subtle variations in feelings). Can reflect both in the present and with respect to a longer-term view of self, values, and goals. Can reflect on multiple relationships between feelings and experiences, across the full range of age-expected experiences in the context of new challenges.
- Can reflect on feelings or experiences of self and others both in the present and with reference to a longer-term view of a sense of self, values, and goals for some age-expected experiences, but not others. Cannot be reflective in this way when feelings are strong.
- Can reflect on moment-to-moment experiences, but not with reference to a longer-term sense of self and experiences, values, and goals.
- Unable to reflect genuinely on feelings or experiences, even in the present. Self-awareness consists often of polarized feeling states or simple basic feelings without an appreciation of subtle variations in feelings. Self-awareness is lacking, and there may be a tendency toward fragmentation.

Related studies include: Almond, 1999; Arnold, et al., 2004; Bouchard & Lecours, 2004; Epstein, 1990; Gabbard, 2005; Glickauf-Hughes, Wells, & Chance, 1996; Grossman, 2002; Josephs, 2003; Levenson, 2004; Morin, 2005; Wilson, 2003.

Capacity to Construct or Use Internal Standards and Ideals: Sense of Morality

Illustrative Descriptions of the Range and Adequacy of Functioning

- Internal standards are flexible and integrated with a realistic sense of one's capacities and social contexts. They provide opportunities for meaningful striving and feelings of self-esteem. Feelings of guilt are used as a signal for reappraising one's behavior.
- Internal standards and ideals tend to be rigid. They are not sufficiently sensitive to one's own capacities and social contexts. Feelings of guilt are experienced more as self-criticism than as a signal for reappraising one's behavior.
- Internal standards, ideals, and sense of morality are based on harsh, punitive expectations. Feelings of guilt are denied and associated with acting out, depression, or both.
- Internal standards, ideals, and a sense of morality are, for the most part, absent.

Related studies include: Bouchard & Lecours, 2004; Bristol, 2004; Chasseguet-Smirgel, 1989; Eisnitz, 1991; Frank, 1999; Glenn, 1989; Grotstein, 2004; Josephs, 2000; Kilborne, 2004; Kissen, 1992; Lansky, 2004; Lax, 1990; Lax, 1994; Lichtenberg, 2004; Mendoza, 2004; Merkur, 2001; Milch & Orange, 2004; Novick & Novick, 2004; O'Shaughnessy, 1999; Reich, 1993; Tyson, 1991; Ury, 1997; Wurmser, 2004.

SUMMARY OF BASIC MENTAL FUNCTIONING

To summarize mental functioning, consider the descriptions of all of the categories of basic mental functions, e.g., regulation, relationships, quality of internal experience, affective expression, etc., and use those to summarize mental functioning as outlined in the following table. The descriptions under each broad level are meant to be illustrative of types of limitations.

M201.	**Optimal Age- and Phase-Appropriate Mental Capacities with Phase-Expected Degree of Flexibility and Intactness**
M202.	**Reasonable Age- and Phase-Appropriate Mental Capacities with Phase-Expected Degree of Flexibility and Intactness**
M203.	**Age- and Phase-Appropriate Mental Capacities with Phase-Specific Conflicts or Transient Developmental Challenges**
M204.	**Mild Constrictions and Inflexibility** **M204.1 – Encapsulated character formations, e.g.,** ■ Mild impairments in self-esteem regulation ■ Mild limitations in internalizations necessary for regulation of impulses, affect, mood, and thought ■ Mild externalization of internal events (e.g., conflicts, feelings, thoughts) ■ Mild alterations and limitations in pleasure orientation ■ Encapsulated limitation of experience of feelings, thoughts, in major life areas (i.e., love, work, play) **M204.2 – Encapsulated symptom formations, e.g.,** ■ Mild limitations and alterations in experience of affects and moods (e.g., obsessional isolation, depressive turning of feelings against the self, etc.) ■ Mild limitations and alterations in experience of areas of thought (hysterical repression, phobic displacements, etc.)
M205.	**Moderate Constrictions and Alterations in Mental Functioning** Moderate versions of major constrictions listed below.
M206.	**Major Constrictions and Alterations in Mental Functioning, e.g.,** ■ Limited tendencies toward fragmentation of self-object differentiation ■ Impairments in self-esteem regulation ■ Limitations in internalizations necessary for regulation of impulses, affect, mood, and thought ■ Major externalizations of internal events, e.g., conflicts, feelings, thoughts ■ Alterations and limitations in pleasure orientation ■ Limitation of experience of feelings and/or thoughts in major life areas (i.e., love, work, play)
M207.	**Defects in Integration and Organization and/or Differentiation of Self- and Object Representations**

M208.   **Major Defects in Basic Mental Functions**

For example,

- Major structural psychological defects and defects in mental functions
  - Perception and regulation of affect
  - Integration of affect and thought
  - Reality testing and organization of perception, thought, and capacity for human affective engagement
- Major defects in basic physical, organic integrity of mental apparatus (e.g., perception, integration, motor, memory, regulation, judgment, etc.)

REFERENCES

Bellak, L., & Hurvich, M. (1969). A systematic study of ego functions. *Journal of Nervous and Mental Disease, 48,* 569-585.

Bellak, L., Hurvich, & Crawford, P. (1970). Psychotic egos. *Psychoanalytic Review, 56,* 526-542.

Bellak, L., Hurvich, M., & Gediman, H. (1973). *Ego functions in schizophrenics, neurotics, and normals.* New York: Wiley.

Bellak, L., & Goldsmith, L. A. (Eds.) (1984). *The broad scope of ego function assessment.* New York: Wiley.

Blatt, S. J., & Auerbach, J. S. (2001). Mental representation, severe psychopathology, and the therapeutic process. *Journal of the American Psychoanalytic Association, 49,* 113-159.

Blatt, S. J., Auerbach, J. S., & Levy, K. N. (1997). Mental representations in personality development, psychopathology and the therapeutic process. *Review of General Psychology, 1,* 351-374.

Blatt, S. J., Chevron, E. S., Quinlan, D. M. Schaffer, C. E., & Wein, S. J. (1988). *The assessment of qualitative and structural dimensions of object representations.* Unpublished research manual, Yale University.

Blatt, S. J., Stayner, D., Auerbach, J. S., & Behrends, R. S. (1996). Change in object and self representation in long-term, intensive, inpatient treatment of seriously disturbed adolescents and young adults. *Psychiatry, 59,* 82-107.

Clarkin, J., Caligor, E., Stern, B.L., & Kernberg, O.F. (2004). *The structured interview of personality organization.* Unpublished manuscript, Weill Medical College of Cornell University.

DeWitt, K. N., Hartley, D. E., Rosenberg, S. E., Zilberg, N. J., & Wallerstein, R. S. (1991). Scales of psychological capacities: Development of an assessment approach. *Psychoanalysis and Contemporary Thought, 14,* 343-361.

Diamond, D., Blatt, S. J. Stayner, D.& Kaslow, N. (1991). *Self-other differentiation of object representation.* Unpublished research manual, Yale University.

Jones, E. E. (2000). *Therapeutic action: A guide to psychoanalytic therapy.* Northvale, NJ: Jason Aaronson.

Miller, T. J., McGlashan, T. H., Rosen, J. L., Cadenhead, K., Cannon, T., Ventura, J., et al. (2003). Prodromal assessment with the structured interview for prodromal syndromes and the scale of prodromal symptoms: Predictive validity, interrater reliability, and training to reliability. *Schizophrenia Bulletin, 29,* 703-715.

Stern, B.L., Clarkin, J., Caligor, E., & Kernberg, O.F. (2005). The structured interview of personality organization. In B. Strauss & J. Schumacher (Eds.), *Klinische interviews und ratingskalen [Clinical interviews and rating scales].* Goettingen, Germany: Hogrefe & Huber.

Waldron, S., Scharf, R., Crouse, J., Firestein, S. K., Burton, A., & Hurst, D. (2004). Saying the right thing at the right time: A view through the lens of the Analytic Process Scales (APS). *Psychoanalytic Quarterly, 73*, 1079-1125.

Waldron, S., Scharf, R.D., Hurst, D., Firestein, S.K., & Burton, A. (2004). What happens in a psychoanalysis? A view through the lens of the Analytic Process Scales (APS). *International Journal of Psychoanalysis, 85*, 443–466.

Wallerstein, R. S. (1988). Assessment of structural changes in psychoanalytic therapy and research. *Journal of American Psychoanalytical Association, 36*(S):241-262.

Weinryb, R. M., Rossel, R. J., & Asberg, M. (1991). The Karolinska Psychodynamic Profile: I. Validity and dimensionality. II. Interdisciplinary and cross-cultural reliability. *Acta Psychiatry Scandinavia, 83*, 64-72, 73-76.

Zilberg, N. J., Wallerstein, R., S., DeWitt, K. N., Hartley, D., & Rosenberg, S. E. (1991). A conceptual analysis and strategy for assessing structural change. *Psychoanalytical and Contemporary Thought, 14*, 317–342.

RELATED STUDIES

Almond, R. (1999). The patient's part in analytic process: The influence of the analyst's expectations. *Journal of the American Psychoanalytic Association, 47*, 519-541.

Arnold, E. G., Farber, B. A., & Geller, J. D. (2004). Termination, posttermination, and internalization of therapy and the therapist: Internal representation and psychotherapy outcome. In D. P. Charman (Ed.), *Core Processes in Brief Psychodynamic Psychotherapy: Advancing Effective Practice* (pp. 289-308). Mahwah, NJ: Erlbaum.

Bates, G. C. (2000). Affect regulation. *International Journal of Psychoanalysis, 81*, 317-379.

Bell, M. D. (2001). Object-relations and reality-testing deficits in schizophrenia. In P. W. Corrigan & D. L. Penn (Eds.), *Social Cognition and Schizophrenia* (pp. 285-311). Washington, DC: American Psychological Association.

Blatt, S. J., & Auerbach, J. S. (2001). Mental representation, severe psychopathology, and the therapeutic process. *Journal of the American Psychoanalytic Association, 49*, 113-159.

Blatt, S. J., Auerbach, J. S., & Levy, K. N. (1997). Mental representations in personality development, psychopathology and the therapeutic process. *Review of General Psychology, 1*, 351-374.

Blatt, S. J., Chevron, E. S., Quinlan, D. M. Schaffer, C. E., & Wein, S. J. (1988). *The assessment of qualitative and structural dimensions of object representations.* Unpublished research manual, Yale University.

Blatt, S. J., Stayner, D., Auerbach, J. S., & Behrends, R. S. (1996). Change in object and self representation in long-term, intensive, inpatient treatment of seriously disturbed adolescents and young adults. *Psychiatry, 59*, 82-107.

Blum, H. P., & Schneider, J. (2000). Dreams and affect: A hundred years later. *International Journal of Psychoanalysis, 81*, 789-792.

Boesky, D. (2000). Affect, language and communication. *International Journal of Psycho-analysis, 81*, 257–262.

Bouchard, M., & Lecours, S. (2004). Analyzing forms of superego functioning as mentalizations. *International Journal of Psychoanalysis, 85*, 879-896.

Bristol, R. C. (2004). History of a childhood neurosis and its relation to the adult superego. *Psychoanalytic Inquiry, 24*, 286-308.

Bucci, W. (1985). Dual coding: A cognitive model for psychoanalytic research. *Journal of the American Psychoanalytic Association, 33*, 571-608.

Bucci, W. (2000). Biological and integrative studies on affect. *International Journal of Psychoanalysis, 81*, 141-144.

Chasseguet-Smirgel, J. (1989). Thinking and the superego: Some interrelations. In E. M. Wein-shel, H. P. Blum, & F. R. Rodman (Eds.), *The psychoanalytic core: Essays in honor of Leo Rangell, MD* (pp. 207-223). Madison, CT: International Universities Press.

Clarkin, J., Caligor, E., Stern, B. L., & Kernberg, O. F. (2004). *The structured interview of personality organization.* Unpublished manuscript, Weill Medical College of Cornell University.

Coen, S. J. (2000). Affect, somatization and symbolization. *International Journal of Psychoanalysis, 80,* 159-161.

Cooper, A. M. (2005). The representational world and affect. *Psychoanalytic Inquiry, 25,* 196-206.

Corona, P. C., & Levinson, N. A. (2000). Affect and development. *International Journal of Psychoanalysis, 81,* 313-317.

Cramer, P. (1999). Ego functions and ego development: Defense mechanisms and intelligence as predictors of ego level. *Journal of Personality, 67,* 735-760.

De Folch, T. E., & Kavka, J. (2000). Affect and clinical technique. *International Journal of Psychoanalysis, 81,* 793-796.

DeWitt, K. N., Hartley, D. E., Rosenberg, S. E., Zilberg, N. J., & Wallerstein, R. S. (1991). Scales of psychological capacities: Development of an assessment approach. *Psychoanalysis and Contemporary Thought, 14,* 343-361.

Diamond, D., Blatt, S. J. Stayner, D., & Kaslow, N. (1991). *Self-other differentiation of object representation.* Unpublished research manual, Yale University.

Eisnitz, A. J. (1991). Some superego issues. In T. Shapiro (Ed.), *The Concept of Structure in Psychoanalysis* (pp. 137-163). Madison, CT: International Universities Press.

Epstein, L. (1990). Some reflections on the therapeutic use of the self. *Group, 14,* 151-156.

Frank, G. (1999). Freud's concept of the superego: Review and assessment. *Psychoanalytic Psychology 16,* 448-463.

Gabbard, G. O. (2005). Reflective function, mentalization, and borderline personality disorder. In B. D. Beitman (Ed.), *Self-awareness Deficits in Psychiatric Patients: Neurobiology, Assessment, and Treatment* (pp. 213-228). New York: Norton.

Glenn, J. (1989). Synthetic and conflictual aspects of the superego: A case study. In E. M. Weinshel, H. P. Blum, & F. R. Rodman (Eds.), *The psychoanalytic core: Essays in honor of Leo Rangell, MD* (pp. 225-241). Madison, CT: International Universities Press.

Glickauf-Hughes, C., Wells, M., & Chance, S. (1996). Techniques for strengthening clients' observing ego. *Psychotherapy: Theory, Research, Practice, Training, 33,* 431-440.

Green, A. (1999). On discriminating and not discriminating between affect and representation. *International Journal of Psychoanalysis, 80,* 277-310.

Greenspan, S. I. (1989). *The development of the ego: Implications for personality theory, psychopathology, and the psychotherapeutic process.* New York: International Universities Press.

Greenspan, S. I., & Shanker, S. G. (2004). *The first idea: How symbols, language, and intelligence evolved from our primate ancestors to modern humans.* Cambridge, MA: Da Capo.

Grossman, W. I. (2002). Hartmann and the integration of different ways of thinking. *Journal of Clinical Psychoanalysis, 11,* 271-293.

Grotstein, J. S. (2004). Notes on the superego. *Psychoanalytic Inquiry, 24,* 257-270.

Hartmann, H. (1964). Essays on ego psychology: Selected problems in psychoanalytic theory. New York: International Universities Press

Hernández, M. (1999). Affect, language and communication: Loose ends. *International Journal of Psychoanalysis, 80,* 341-346.

Jappe, G., & Lebe, D. M. (2000). Holocaust: Affect and memory. *International Journal of Psychoanalysis, 81,* 145-148.

Josephs, L. (2000). Self-criticism and the psychic surface. *Journal of the American Psychoanalytic Association, 48,* 255-280.

Josephs, L. (2003). The observing ego as voyeur. *International Journal of Psychoanalysis, 84,* 879-890.

Kantrowitz, J. L., Katz, A. L., Paolitto, F., Sashin, J., & Solomon, L. (1987a). Changes in the level and quality of object relationships in psychoanalysis: Follow-up of a longitudinal prospective study. *Journal of American Psychoanalytical Association, 35,* 23-46.

Kantrowitz, J. L., Katz, A. L., Paolitto, F., Sashin, J., & Solomon, L. (1987b). The role of reality testing in psychoanalysis: Followup of 22 cases. *Journal of American Psychoanalytical Association, 35,* 367-385.

Kantrowitz, J. L., Paolitto, F., Sashin, J., Solomon, L., & Katz, A. L. (1986). Affect availability, tolerance, complexity, and modulation in psychoanalysis: Followup of a longitudinal, prospective study. *Journal of American Psychoanalytical Association, 34,* 529-560.

Kilborne, B. (2004). Superego dilemmas. *Psychoanalytic Inquiry, 24,* 175-182.

Kissen, M. (1992). Gender and superego development. In M. Kissen (Ed.), *Gender and psychoanalytic treatment* (pp. 48-58). Philadelphia: Brunner/Mazel.

Krystal, H. (1974). The genetic development of affects and affect regulation. *Annual of Psychoanalysis, 2,* 98-126.

Krystal, H. (1975). Affect tolerance. *Annual of Psychoanalysis 3,* 179-219.

Lansky, M. R. (2004). Conscience and the project of a psychoanalytic science of human nature: Clarification of the usefulness of the superego concept. *Psychoanalytic Inquiry, 24,* 151-174.

Lax, R. F. (1990). The role of internalization in the development of certain aspects of female masochism: Ego psychological considerations. In R. Lax (Ed.), *Essential papers on character neurosis and treatment* (pp. 310–330). New York: New York University Press.

Lax, R. F. (1994). Thou shalt not kill: Some aspects of superego pathology. In A. K. Richards and A. D. Richards (Eds.), *The Spectrum of Psychoanalysis: Essays in Honor of Martin S. Bergmann* (pp. 243-255). Madison, CT: International Universities Press.

Levenson, L. N. (2004). Inhibition of self-observing activity in psychoanalytic treatment. *Psychoanalytic Study of the Child, 59,* 167-187.

Levy, I. (2001). Superego issues in supervision. In S. Gill (Ed.), *The supervisory alliance: Facilitating the psychotherapist's learning experience* (pp. 91-106). Northvale, NJ: Jason Aronson.

Lichtenberg, J. D. (2004). Commentary on "The superego—A vital or supplanted concept?" *Psychoanalytic Inquiry, 24,* 328-339.

Mariotti, P. (2000). Affect and psychosis. *International Journal of Psychoanalysis, 80,* 149-153.

McGaugh, J. L. (2003). *Memory and emotion: The making of lasting memories.* New York: Columbia University Press.

Meissner, W. W. (2000a). The self as structural. *Psychoanalysis and Contemporary Thought, 3,* 373-416.

Meissner, W. W. (2000b). The self-as-person in psychoanalysis. *Psychoanalysis and Contemporary Thought, 23,* 479–524.

Meissner, W. W. (2000c). The self-as-relational in psychoanalysis: I. Relational aspects of the self. *Psychoanalysis and Contemporary Thought, 23,* 177—204.

Meissner, W. W. (2000d). The structural principle in psychoanalysis: I. The meaning of structure. *Psychoanalysis and Contemporary Thought, 23,* 283-330.

Meissner, W. W. (2000e). The structural principle in psychoanalysis: II. Structure formation and structural change. *Psychoanalysis and Contemporary Thought, 23,* 331-371.

Meissner, W. W. (2005a). The dynamic unconscious: Psychic determinism, intrapsychic conflict, unconscious fantasy, dreams, and symptom formation. In E. S. Person, A. M. Cooper, & G. O. Gabbard (Eds.), *American Psychiatric Publishing Textbook of Psychoanalysis* (pp. 21-37). Arlington, VA: American Psychiatric Publishing.

Meissner, W. W. (2005b). [Review of the book *The internal world and attachment*]. *Bulletin of the Menninger Clinic, 69*, 98-113.

Mendoza, S. P. (2004). Sex, death and the superego: Experiences in psychoanalysis. [Review of the book *Sex, death and the superego: Experiences in psychoanalysis*]. *British Journal of Psychotherapy, 21*, 331-335.

Merkur, D. (2001). *Unconscious Wisdom: A Superego Function in Dreams, Conscience, and Inspiration*. Albany, NY: State University of New York Press.

Mikulincer, M., & Shaver, P. R. (2004). Security-based self-representations in adulthood: Contents and processes. In W. S. Rholes & J. A. Simpson (Eds.), *Adult attachment: Theory, Research, and Clinical Implications* (pp. 159-195). New York: Guilford.

Milch, W. E., & Orange, D. M. (2004). Conscience as the reappearance of the other in self-experience: On using the concepts superego and conscience in self psychology. *Psychoanalytic Inquiry, 24*, 206-231.

Miller, L. (1998). Ego autonomy and the healthy personality: Psychodynamics, cognitive style, and clinical applications. *Psychoanalytic Review, 85*, 423-448.

Moretti, M. M. (1999). Internal representations of others in self-regulation: A new look at a classic issue. *Social Cognition, 17*, 186-208.

Morin, A. (2005). Possible links between self-awareness and inner speech: Theoretical background, underlying mechanisms, and empirical evidence. *Journal of Consciousness Studies, 12*, 115-134.

Nagera, H. (2001). Reflections on psychoanalysis and neuroscience: Normality and pathology in development, brain stimulation, programming, and maturation. *Neuropsychoanalysis, 3*, 179-191.

Novick, J., & Novick, K. K. (2004). The superego and the two-system model. *Psychoanalytic Inquiry, 24*, 232-356.

O'Shaughnessy, E. (1999). Relating to the superego. *International Journal of Psychoanalysis, 80*, 861-871.

Reich, A. (1993). Early identifications as archaic elements in the superego. In G. H. Pollock (Ed.), *Pivotal papers on identification* (pp. 177-195). Madison, CT: International Universities Press.

Safyer, A. W., & Hauser, S. T. (1995). A developmental view of defenses: Empirical approaches. In H. R. Conte & R. Plutchik (Eds.), *Ego defenses: Theory and measurement* (pp. 120-138). Oxford, England: Wiley.

Sandell, R., Blomberg, J., Lazar, A., Carlsson, J., Broberg, J., & Schubert, J. (2000). Varieties of long-term outcome among patients in psychoanalysis and long-term psychotherapy: A review of findings in the Stockholm Outcome of Psychoanalysis and Psychotherapy Project (STOPP). *International Journal of Psychoanalysis, 81*, 921–942.

Schlessinger, N., & Robbins, F. P. (1975). The psychoanalytic process: Recurrent patterns of conflict and changes in ego functions. *Journal of American Psychoanalytical Association, 23*, 761-782.

Schore, A. N. (1994). *Affect regulation and the origin of the self: The neurobiology of emotional development*. Hillsdale, NJ: Earlbaum.

Stern, B. L., Clarkin, J., Caligor, E., & Kernberg, O. F. (2005). The structured interview of personality organization. In B. Strauss & J. Schumacher (Eds.), *Klinische interviews und ratingskalen [Clinical interviews and rating scales]*. Goettingen, Germany: Hogrefe & Huber.

Symons, D. K. (2004). Mental state discourse, theory of mind, and the internalization of self-other understanding. *Developmental Review, 24*, 159-188.

Szecsody, I., Varvin, S., Amadei, G., Stoker, J., Beenen, F., Klockars, L., et al. (1997, August). *The European Multi Site Collaborative Study of Psychoanalysis (Sweden, Finland, Norway,*

Holland, & Italy). Paper presented at the Symposium on Outcome Research, International Psychoanalytical Association Congress, Barcelona, Spain.

Tyson, P. (1991). Psychic structure formation: The complementary roles of affects, drives, object relations, and conflict. In T. Shapiro (Ed.), *The concept of structure in psychoanalysis* (pp. 73-98). Madison, CT: International Universities Press.

Ury, C. (1997). The shadow of object love: Reconstructing Freud's theory of preoedipal guilt. *Psychoanalytic Quarterly, 66,* 34-61.

Waldron, S., Scharf, R., Crouse, J., Firestein, S. K., Burton, A., & Hurst, D. (2004). Saying the right thing at the right time: A view through the lens of the Analytic Process Scales (APS). *Psychoanalytic Quarterly, 73,* 1079-1125.

Waldron, S., Scharf, R. D., Hurst, D., Firestein, S. K., & Burton, A. (2004). What happens in a psychoanalysis? A view through the lens of the Analytic Process Scales (APS). *International Journal of Psychoanalysis, 85,* 443–466.

Wallerstein, R. S. (1988). Assessment of structural changes in psychoanalytic therapy and research. *Journal of American Psychoanalytical Association,* 36(S):241-262.

Wallerstein, R. S. (2001). The generations of psychotherapy research: An overview. *Psychoanalytic Psychology, 18,* 243-267.

Wallerstein, R. S., Robbins, L. L., Sargent, H. D., & Luborsky, L. (1956). The psychotherapy research project of the Menninger Foundation. *Bulletin of the Menninger Clinic, 20,* 221-278.

Weinryb, R. M., Rossel, R. J., & Asberg, M. (1991). The Karolinska Psychodynamic Profile: I. Validity and dimensionality. II. Interdisciplinary and cross-cultural reliability. *Acta Psychiatry Scandinavia, 83,* 64-72, 73-76.

Wilson, S. N. (2003). Attack of the inward eye: Self-observing and aggression. *Psychoanalytic Review, 90,* 699–708.

Wurmser, L. (2004). Superego revisited: Relevant or irrelevant? *Psychoanalytic Inquiry, 24,* 183-205.

Zilberg, N. J., Wallerstein, R., S., DeWitt, K. N., Hartley, D., & Rosenberg, S. E. (1991). A conceptual analysis and strategy for assessing structural change. *Psychoanalytical and Contemporary Thought, 14,* 317–342.

Symptom Patterns:
The Subjective Experience
S Axis

WORK GROUP MEMBERS

Héctor Ferrari, MD
Buenos Aires, Argentina

Paul Fink, MD
Philadelphia, Pennsylvania

Abby Herzig, PsyD
New York, New York

Stanley I. Greenspan, MD
Bethesda, Maryland

Marvin Hurvich, PhD, ABPP
Brooklyn, New York

Judy Ann Kaplan, LCSW, BCD
New York, New York

Thomas K. Kenemore, PhD, LCSW
Chicago, Illinois

Edward J. Khantzian, MD
Cambridge, Massachusetts

Martha Kirkpatrick, MD
Los Angeles, California

Jodi Licht, PsyD
New York, New York

Malkah Notman, MD
Cambridge, Massachusetts

David G. Phillips, DSW
New York, New York

CONSULTANTS TO THE SYMPTOM PATTERNS WORK GROUP

Rachel Barbanel-Fried, PsyD
Edward Dewey, PsyD
Nadine Khoury, PsyD
Rachel Miller, PsyD
Sarah Sarkis, PsyD

Symptom Patterns:
The Subjective Experience
S Axis

This section builds on the symptom descriptions of DSM-IV-TR. In it, we attempt to elaborate on the patient's subjective experience of the symptom pattern. We depict individual subjectivity in terms of affective patterns, mental content, accompanying somatic states, and associated relationship patterns. In some instances, notably those in which there has been longstanding psychoanalytic scholarship in a particular area, we comment briefly on psychodynamic understandings of a given symptom pattern and include general implications for treatment. Although we have reservations about the current DSM's characterization and groupings of psychological problems in terms of overly discrete disorders, we feel it is valuable as a starting point for elucidating aspects of mental and emotional suffering.

The symptom-pattern section is placed third in our overall diagnostic profile because such patterns can be understood only in the context of the patient's overall personality structure and profile of mental functioning. In the experience of psychodynamic practitioners, symptom patterns are not simply disorders in their own right but are, rather, overt expressions of the ways in which individual patients characteristically cope with experience. In other words, a person may have symptoms such as anxiety, depression, and/or impulse-control problems as part of an overall emotional challenge. For example, problems with impulse control and mood regulation are common in patients with the larger developmental deficit of being unable to represent (symbolize) a wide range of affects and wishes (Greenspan, 1997).

Our approach includes consideration of the biological contributions to these patterns and may even facilitate meaningful exploration of biological correlates for a variety of mental health disorders. Despite evidence of biological contributions to many mental health problems, however, we do not assume that the presence of multiple symptom expressions inevitably constitutes "comorbidity" between different mental health disorders; we believe that more commonly, they are expressions of a basic complex disturbance of mental functioning. We also note that even in adults, there are developmentally relevant aspects of symptom patterns that interact with personality variables. A depression in an elderly woman may be experienced quite differently from a depression in a woman in her thirties, and it may consequently call for a different therapeutic approach (Thompson, Gallagher, & Czirr, 1988). Formulation and treatment plan should recognize such age-related differences.

Each person's symptom patterns, while sharing common features with others who have similar patterns, have a unique signature. The following clinical illustrations are intended to provide examples of types of internal experiences of some patients. They are not meant to comprise a definitive or exhaustive listing. The clinician is encouraged to capture the patient's unique subjective experience in a narrative form by considering the applicable descriptive patterns. In some instances, there are research findings that support the observations that follow; in others, in the absence of empirical work on the topic, we have drawn on the combined clinical experience of therapists with expertise in each area covered.

S301. Adjustment Disorders
S302. Anxiety Disorders S302.1 Psychic Trauma and Posttraumatic Stress Disorders S302.2 Phobias S302.3 Obsessive-Compulsive Disorders
S303. Dissociative Disorders
S304. Mood Disorders S304.1 Depressive Disorders S304.2 Bipolar Disorders
S305. Somatoform (Somatization) Disorders
S306. Eating Disorders
S307. Psychogenic Sleep Disorders
S308. Sexual and Gender Identity Disorders S308.1 Sexual Disorders S308.2 Paraphilias S308.3 Gender Identity Disorders
S309. Factitious Disorders
S310. Impulse-Control Disorders
S311. Addictive/Substance Abuse Disorders
S312. Psychotic Disorders
S313. Mental Disorders Based on a General Medical Condition

S301. Adjustment Disorders

The diagnosis of adjustment disorder covers a wide range of maladaptive responses to psychological stress, whether acute, chronic, or repeated. Such reactions are considered to be adjustment disorders if they occur within three months of the stress and do not last for more than six months. They may be responses to challenges such as illness or changes in one's family, or to developmental milestones such as puberty, leaving for college or military service, marriage, changes in employment, or the development of new interests. Adjustment disorders are described in relation to anxious mood, depressed mood, conduct disturbances, physical complaints, withdrawal, work or academic inhibition, or mixtures of these.

DSM-IV-TR Classification
Adjustment Disorders

- ■ Adjustment Disorder
  - • With Depressed Mood
  - • With Anxiety
  - • With Mixed Anxiety and Depressed Mood
  - • With Disturbance of Conduct
  - • With Mixed Disturbance of Emotions and Conduct
  - • Unspecified – Specify if: Acute/Chronic

The Internal Experience of Adjustment Disorders

Affective states accompanying an adjustment disorder vary from individual to individual. Often an overriding affective feature is a vague uneasiness deriving from a sense of change or flux. In other words, at a deeper subjective level than the presenting anxiety, depression, or behavior change, there may be a pervasive feeling of uncertainty and apprehensiveness. Clearly, pre-existing personality patterns and affective tendencies further color the subjective experience. It is often helpful to facilitate the patient's detailed descriptions of the affects associated with the uncertainty and apprehension.

Cognitive patterns may be characterized by either a focus on the current stress or a marked avoidance of the changes that the patient needs to assimilate. In other words, individuals with adjustment disorders may be preoccupied with what they are facing or may be defensively avoiding it.

Somatic states may accompany the predominant reaction to the stress (depression or anxiety or behavior change) and the general state of tension and apprehensiveness. The nature of the somatic expression depends upon the affective response.

Relationship patterns may be characterized by either an expansion of expressions of dependency or attempts to distance from potentially helpful relationships because of shame about an increased sense of neediness.

Clinical Illustration

A 35-year-old married woman with a 4-year-old child had just learned that her father required bypass surgery. Her parents were divorced when she was 12 years old, and she recalled having felt betrayed by her father when he left her mother. Nonetheless, she continued to be close to him and tried to endear herself to him by being "even nicer than most teenagers." With the news of her father's illness and planned surgery, she found herself experiencing waves of anxiety, including nightmares filled with gory details and daytime preoccupations with images of "his heart being cut open and blood gushing all over." During moments when the anxiety was most acute, this woman tried to slow down her breathing and calm herself, an effort at which she was partly successful. Outside these symptoms, she continued to function well as a mother, wife, and part-time freelance writer. On becoming more fully aware of all the different feelings she had towards her father, she was able to shift gradually back to feeling calm, organized, and methodical (her personal style before the news of her father's diagnosis). This patient was able to return to her more typical level of functioning after four weekly consultations.

S302. Anxiety Disorders

Under the rubric of anxiety disorders, DSM-IV-TR includes panic attacks; agoraphobia, social phobia, and other specific phobias; obsessive-compulsive disorder; posttraumatic stress disorder (PTSD); acute stress disorder; generalized anxiety disorder; anxiety disorders due to a general medical condition; substance-induced anxiety disorder; and anxiety disorder not otherwise specified (NOS).

Anxiety is fear in the absence of obvious danger. Psychodynamically oriented clinicians, who have found anxiety lurking behind virtually all psychopathological symptoms, have distinguished carefully between potential danger and present danger, between the evaluation of danger and the response to danger, and between an adaptive response to actual danger (which may or may not include fear/anxiety) and an anxiety response, in which the human fight/flight system is activated in the expectation of disaster. In light of the fact that some individuals suffer pervasive, chronic, and disabling anxieties, we regard generalized anxiety disorder as a personality disorder rather than a symptom syndrome (see Personality Patterns and Disorders, **P111**).

The psychoanalytic literature identifies different kinds of anxiety, any of which can be conscious or unconscious. *Separation anxiety* is the fear of losing a love object. *Castration anxiety*, a term used generally by some and specifically by others, is fear of damage to the body and sometimes specifically to the genitals. *Moral anxiety* is fear of the consequences of transgressing one's values. *Annihilation anxiety* includes apprehensions of being catastrophically overwhelmed, merged, invaded, and destroyed. *Fragmentation anxiety* is fear of self-disintegration. In certain contexts, and in bearable amounts, all these anxieties are normal, but when unremitting or disproportionate, they constitute psychopathology. *Persecutory anxiety* and irrational fears of harm to loved ones are more intrinsically problematic; they are understood psychoanalytically as the outcome of denial and projection of one's own hostile feelings.

With the exception of obsessive-compulsive disorder and possibly social anxiety (which we have often seen conflated with schizoid personality manifestations), women have twice the risk for anxiety disorders as men. A number of variables may account for this disparity, including hormonal factors, cultural pressures on women to meet the needs of others before their own, and fewer self-restrictions on women in reporting anxiety to physicians and therapists.

Developmentally, anxiety has been seen to evolve from diffuse somatic excitation, to pervasive psychic anxiety, to a more mature signal function. *Signal anxiety*, a concept similar to "learned expectations" in contemporary learning theory, is a state of arousal signaling that past experience has identified an object or situation as a danger. It involves both anticipation and an attenuated affect level. This developmental progression is to some extent fluid and reversible. Thus, under sufficient psychic threat, the progressive desomatization of anxiety tends to revert to somatic expression or "resomatization."

Anxiety thus involves cognitive content as well as emotional experience. A goal of psychodynamic psychotherapy is the integration of the affective and the cognitive components, along with the reduction of any somatizing of anxiety or acting out of anxiety-based self-harm. Although anxiety may be treated with a variety of symptom-focused approaches, a psychoanalytically informed exploration of the nature and possible origins of anxiety can increase a patient's sense of mastery and may prevent future outbreaks of anxiety, somatic suffering, and self-destructive defenses against anxiety.

DSM-IV-TR Classification
Anxiety Disorders

- Panic Disorder without Agoraphobia
- Panic Disorder with Agoraphobia
- Agoraphobia without History of Panic Disorder
- Specific Phobias
- Social Phobias
- Obsessive-Compulsive Disorders
- Posttraumatic Stress Disorders
- Acute Stress Disorders
- Generalized Anxiety Disorders
- Anxiety Disorders Due to . . . *[Indicate General Medical Condition]*
- Substance-Induced Anxiety Disorders
- Anxiety Disorders not otherwise specified

The Internal Experience of Anxiety Disorders

Affective states are often related to Freud's four basic danger situations (Freud, 1926): (1) loss of a significant other, resulting in feelings of abandonment that express themselves as anger, anxiety, depression, and/or guilt; (2) loss of love, experienced as rejection, and usually accompanied by rage, anxiety, depression, guilt, and feelings of being unworthy and even unlovable; (3) loss of bodily integrity, often with associated fears of mutilation or damage to the genital organs; and (4) loss of affirmation by one's own conscience, resulting in anxiety, guilt, shame, or depressed feelings. In addition, fear of loss of self-regulation (e.g., loss of control of one's feelings, thoughts, sensations, movements, actions, etc.) should be considered. The anxiety associated with the anticipation of these dangers may be controlled or uncontrolled. When the anxiety is out of control, it may trigger annihilation concerns.

Cognitive patterns may include distractedness, confusion, and difficulty thinking. Anxiety can also produce specific fears of all sorts: separation, abandonment or rejection; being devoured or engulfed; losing mental or bodily control; falling; having multiple selves; injury; and dying. Some patients have fears of overwhelming catastrophe and report a disorganizing sense of confusion over their body boundaries and sense of identity. People with anxiety may suffer intense worry over losing financial security or the presence of someone they depend upon. Fear of fear itself is common among those who have had panic attacks; they begin avoiding certain things for fear they will have another attack.

Somatic states may include tension, sweaty palms, the sense of butterflies in one's stomach or a tight band around one's head, bladder and bowel urgency, breathing difficulties, or a feeling of being disconnected from one's body. Anxiety can be associated with varying degrees of autonomic or physiological arousal.

Relationship patterns may include expressions of fears of rejection, such as clinging and seeking reassurance; expressions of guilt, such as blaming, guilt assignment, and blame avoidance; and expressions of conflicts about dependency, such as feelings of being smothered or suffocating, drowning or choking, and vacillation between pulling others closer and pushing them away.

Clinical Illustrations

Descriptions of Anxiety by Individuals with Neurotic and Borderline Psychologies

- "My mind is deluged with all sorts of frightening thoughts and images. My body is all nerves. I can't sit down for any period of time; I'm constantly up and down. I feel like I'm going to crack up. At my job I can't do a thing; I just feel I can't go on."

- "My sense of self was hollow, like I didn't have a self, like I was outside myself. Like a ghost—I'm watching, like I have absolutely no impact on what's going on. I felt like I was being literally ripped apart. There are all these characters who feel separate, not part of me, and they start fighting, I can't stop them or integrate them."

- "I can't stand the fear; I need comfort. Once fear steps in, I can't see anything or do anything. There are so many things I do out of fear. I'm afraid I'll fall apart, lose control, be taken over, be shot down with a machine gun . . . . The fear is always of something extreme happening. I won't get smacked; I'll get bombed. Some people fight or run away. When I'm cornered, I crumble."

- "When I get involved [in a relationship], I feel I have no rights, no prerogatives. The other person can make decisions; I can't. They can do what they want; I can't. I feel like I can't maintain my separate existence; I can't be a person when I'm involved in a relationship. It makes me feel panicky."

Examples of Anxiety in Psychotic Individuals

- "My brain and body are being eaten away by parasites. That is why I can't think or move my bowels."

- "I have faded into nothingness. I am no longer alive."

- "They have been blowing poison gas through the keyhole. It's destroying me and obliterating my thoughts."

Example of Anxiety in a Patient with Circumscribed (e.g., Neurotic) Difficulties

A 31-year-old corporate lawyer was referred by the president of his company when he reported feeling "stressed" at work. The patient began his first visit by saying that what he had been going through was "pretty scary." He described a recent experience at work as follows: "I want to the meeting, and shortly after being there I felt a wave go through my head. I began to feel dizzy, like I was going to pass out—and I started to breathe fast and feel nauseous." He emphasized that it was a terrible experience yet added that recent blood tests, blood pressure, and an EKG were normal. He reportedly began to feel calmer as the day progressed, especially after going home. Several better days followed, marred only by stomach cramps. He was quick to remind the psychiatrist that he still did not feel quite right. He described an ongoing discomfort in social situations, wherein he would feel lightheaded and dizzy while engaged in conversation. He speculated about having an "anxiety condition," mentioning in this connection a "phobia for public speaking." He wondered if his condition was mental or physical and seemed to be asking for reassurance.

Related studies include: Beidel & Turner, 1998; Bonime, 1981; Chessick, 2001; Compton, 1992, 1998; Deutsch, 1929; Fairbairn, 1952; Francis, Last, & Strauss, 1992; Gabbard, 2001; Gassner, 2004; Gillett, 1996; Honig, Grace, Lindy, Newman, & Titchener, 1993; Hurvich, 2000, 2003; Klein, 1933; Kulish, 1988; Lang, 1997; Little, 1966; Miliora & Ulman, 1996; Milrod, 1998; Rangell, 1968; Rhead, 1969; Ritvo, 1981; Schneier, Blanco, Antia, & Liebowitz, 2002; Schur, 1953; Tyson ,1973; Yorke & Weisberg, 1976.

S302.1 Psychic Trauma and Posttraumatic Stress Disorders

Because psychic trauma has been important diagnostically and clinically for psychodynamic clinicians from the beginning of psychoanalytic observation, we include more material in this section than under other mental health disorders. In his Introductory Lectures, Freud (1917) wrote that the effect of a trauma on a person "shatters the foundations of his life [as a result of which] he abandons all interest in the present and future and remains permanently absorbed in mental concentration on the past " (p. 276). The concept, like most others, has undergone modification and evolution (Furst, 1967, Krystal, 1988). In recent decades, mental health professionals have recognized the high prevalence of trauma-related psychopathology, based on evidence of the severe and disabling effects of trauma in concentration camp survivors (Krystal, 1968) veterans of the Vietnam War (Wilson and Raphael, 1993), victims of childhood sexual and aggressive abuse (Shengold, 1989), victims of torture (Varvin, 2003), and most recently, victims of terrorism (Danieli, Brom and Sills, 2005).

Posttraumatic stress disorder (PTSD) has become a widely employed diagnosis for residua of psychic trauma. It needs to be emphasized that PTSD constitutes a spectrum of complex and multifaceted conditions with different levels of adaptive interference, and different meanings to the individual. PTSD is only one set of outcomes of psychic trauma; less than 40% of traumatized individuals receive this diagnosis (Yehuda & McFarlane, 1999). PTSD has been classified as an anxiety disorder, a dissociative disorder, and a stress disorder (Brett, 1993). The relations between anxiety and dissociation are in need of further clarification. There are justifications (Brenner, 2001; McWilliams, 1994; Varvin, 2003) for classifying posttraumatic stress disorder among the personality disorders,(as we have done in the personality section of this manual, at least with respect to chronic dissociative sequallae of repeated trauma), as it often has both a tendency toward chronicity and a marked influence on personality development and functioning.

The Internal Experience of Psychic Trauma and Posttraumatic Stress

Sufferers of anxiety, psychic trauma and posttraumatic stress disorders, respectively, may share certain subjective experiences, including feelings of being overwhelmed, the sense of having suffered a catastrophe, loss of a sense of security, and fears of injury and death. Intense apprehensions over details associated with the trauma, sometimes reaching the point of true phobic avoidance, have been frequently noted in patients with PTSD. The dissociation of affect, creating a state of profound emotional numbness, is frequent in posttraumatic disorders and variable in the other anxiety disorders.

Psychodynamic formulations have long stressed the shock, helplessness, vulnerability, and terror specific to trauma. Traumatic experience may overwhelm mental capacities, disturb affective experience and expression, and interfere with the capacity for symbolization and fantasy, thus contributing to the breakdown of meaning. It may also interfere with thinking and with the mental processing of trauma-related memories and fantasies. Psychic trauma effects changes in the sense of self (Ulman & Brothers, 1988) and in the quality of interpersonal relationships. Clinical literature has highlighted obligatory repetition and persistent re-experiencing of traumatic events, through recurring nightmares flashbacks/ reminiscences, and driven re-enactments of traumatic themes (Brenner, 2001, 2004; Davies & Frawley, 1994; van der Kolk, McFarlane & Weisaeth, 1996). Psychodynamic clinical observations have also emphasized the importance of individual meaning of traumatic experience, and the fact that psychic trauma may constitute an organizer in the mental sphere. Traumatic memories have been found to change over time.

Critical distinctions have been made between catastrophic or shock trauma, and cumulative or strain trauma; among infantile, childhood and adult-onset psychic trauma, and between the nature of the traumatic event, the traumatizing process, and the subject's response to it. Response to trauma varies also with a person's mental and physical state, personality resources, and the effect of previous trauma history.

Horowitz (1976) identified eight common subjective experiences that follow severe psychic trauma: (1) grief or sadness, (2) guilt about one's angry or destructive impulses, (3) fear that one will become destructive, (4) guilt about surviving, (5) fear that one will identify with the victims, (6) shame about feeling helpless and empty, (7) fear that the trauma will be repeated, and (8) intense anger directed toward the source of the trauma. Key areas relevant for adult-onset psychic trauma are war combat, torture, rape, terrorism, life-threatening accidents, and the unexpected death of a significant other.

In adults, essential features of posttraumatic conditions include the development of characteristic symptoms following exposure to an external traumatic stressor. These include intense fear or horror; obligatory repetition and persistent re-experiencing of the traumatic event (e.g., flashbacks, nightmares); avoidance of associated stimuli; internal numbing (e.g., attempts at self-medication with drugs or alcohol); and symptoms of increased arousal (e.g., irritability and hypervigilance). Victims may alternate between suffering internal intrusions, in which memories and feelings associated with the trauma are re-experienced, and using numbing mechanisms, such as dissociation and substance abuse. In an unconscious effort to master the traumatic experience, some individuals re-experience aspects of the trauma or turn a passive experience into an active one; that is, some sufferers of trauma re-enact elements of the traumatic situation, with themselves as either victim or perpetrator. Personality factors influence response to psychic trauma (Horowitz, 1976).

Clinical implications vary with individual differences; still, several overall approaches to the treatment of trauma-based psychopathology have been suggested. One recent model, for example, recommends gradual progression from accepting (as a needed strategy for mental survival) the patient's initial stance of warding off dealing with the trauma residues, to increasing efforts to clarify the traumatic response, to fostering greater degrees of integration and mastery (Varvin, 2003). Psychodynamic writers have emphasized the inevitability of enactments with the therapist of aspects of a trauma history. While reworking of traumatic experience may enhance mastery, enactments often exert pressure on the therapist to compromise professionalism and abandon an empathic stance for that of rescuer, advocate, sexual healer, persecutor, or another trauma-related role. Working with seriously traumatized patients may threaten the therapist's emotional status quo and thus requires regular monitoring and processing of the therapist's own reactions (Perlman, 1999).

Affective states related to traumatization include both unmanageably overwhelming feeling reactions (including rage, terror, and shame about having been traumatized) and the dissociation of affects (manifested by numbness, blankness, and inability to connect disturbing feelings with the events that gave rise to them). Handling of affect in general may be profoundly affected by trauma. Trauma in early childhood interferes with normal maturational progress in differentiating affect experiences and verbalizing feelings. Such impediments in affect development often result in anhedonia, alexithymia, and intolerance of affective experience—all consistent indicators of serious traumatic psychopathology (Krystal, 1988). While childhood trauma may create an arrest in affect development, adult-onset trauma may induce regression in the experience and handling of affects.

Cognitive patterns that seem unique to posttraumatic stress disorders are flashbacks and recurrent nightmares. The thinking of traumatized individuals may include: (1) a sense of betrayal that goes beyond feelings of loss of security found in other anxiety conditions; (2) guilt about actions taken or not taken, or about having survived when others did not (survivor guilt); and (3) justification of overwhelming anxiety combined with defensive detachment. Other cognitive outcomes of trauma include the inability to think about traumatic events, including total, partial, or recurrent dissociation of memory of them; or, contrastingly, the helpless sense of being able to think of nothing else. It is common for traumatized individuals to develop theories of how they could have avoided the trauma (Terr, 1995) or, even in response to unforeseen natural disasters, to generate ideas about how others are to blame. Such beliefs may counteract the terrifying experience of helplessness by attributing power to self or others, but they may become sources of ongoing suffering, as they lead to relentless self-criticism or efforts to punish assumed perpetrators. Although both posttraumatic and obsessive-compulsive disorders are characterized by intrusive thoughts, the former are traceable to traumatic experience, while the latter are more often associated with intrapsychic conflicts.

Critical ego functions (Bellak, Hurvich & Gediman, 1973), including reality testing, sense of reality, judgment, affect regulation, defense, and organization-integration of memory may be negatively affected by trauma. There may be a loss of, or substantial interference with, the capacities for self-reflection and organized action, and intentionality may be paralyzed. The distinction between past and present may be obliterated or blurred, so that the past is experienced as though it is happening now. There tends to be a decreased ability to integrate experiences, and there may be dissociation of consciousness and a reversion to magical thinking. Damage to ego functions varies, depending on both the prior stability of specific functions and the patient's particular defenses (flexible or rigid, adaptive or maladaptive). Also relevant are the extent of psychological regression, degree of structural disruption, security of attachment (Finkelhor, 1986), level and quality of object relations, and capacity for self-soothing (Krystal, 1988).

Somatic states characteristic of posttraumatic stress disorders (also frequently found in other anxiety conditions) include irritability, sleep disturbances, and efforts at self-medication through substance abuse. Psychosomatic complaints are frequent (Krystal, 1988), and some traumatized individuals find themselves re-experiencing bodily reactions that happened at the time of the trauma. For example, a woman forced as a child to give oral sex to an adult may, as she recalls the experience, feel strong sensations of choking or nausea. The patient may regard somatic conditions caused by the trauma (e.g., war injuries or infertility due to scarring from violent rape) with a particularly intense rage and grief or, alternatively, such conditions may be minimized in ways that suggest unconscious denial of the gravity of the disability. Research by Nelson (2002) suggests that there has been an underestimation of the physical damage caused by violent sexual abuse, which may be the cause of both physical and mental problems suffered by victims.

Relationship patterns may include changes in relating to others, based on decreased trust and increased insecurity, and states of numbness, withdrawal, chronic rage, and guilt. Relationships can suffer greatly from dissociation, substance abuse, and other consequences of trauma. Psychic trauma often increases sadomasochistic modes of interacting, leading to derailment of dialogue and ruptures in connectedness. There may be avoidance of people or situations that remind the victim of the trauma. For example, a man who had survived the Bergen-Belsen concentration camp reported that after coming to America, he was still terrified of any person wearing a uniform. Some combat veterans live post-war lives of almost total isolation from others.

Clinical Illustrations

- The dissociation and loss of bodily integrity experienced in PTSD is captured in the following statement from an analytic session with an adult woman: "I was trying to return to my body. I am a survivor of childhood sex abuse, and my body to me had been a machine, and I didn't want to live within it. An out-of-the-body experience I couldn't control. Couldn't. Wouldn't. Who knows? I don't know. But I wanted to return, although I wasn't thoroughly convinced I wasn't there all along. I couldn't recall being any other way. And I wanted to see, to find out if perhaps I wasn't wholly in myself." This patient never took showers, a behavior that her analyst related to her fantasy that she had no body beneath her neck.

- A 25-year-old woman with a history of sexual molestation by her stepfather had a pattern of chronic vocational problems and difficulty with authority figures. When she was assigned a new supervisor who criticized her at public meetings and would not permit her to leave the room while being criticized, she began to experience, for the first time in her life, symptoms of claustrophobia, severe rage, and eventually, overwhelming and debilitating panic attacks.

S302.2 Phobias

While DSM IV-TR defines phobias on the basis of excessive fear coupled with avoidant behavior, psychodynamic therapists see these features as insufficient to define a clinical phobia. To be considered a phobia in the traditional sense, there must be evidence that the exaggerated fear (symptom) expresses the way the individual organizes internal experience. Developmental requirements to form a true phobia include the abilities to symbolize and to create psychic connections with the feared object.

The psychodynamic view is that they involve a special way of dealing with anxiety. Phobic symptoms involve less suffering and better overall adaptation than intense states of free-floating anxiety (panic attacks). In phobias, defensive measures restrict and focus what is feared, allowing afflicted individuals to remain free of anxiety so long as they avoid specific objects or situations. Clinically, phobias have been found to derive from attempts to moderate anxieties over competition and feared retaliation (oedipal issues) as well as efforts to deal with fears of loss of control (autonomy issues). At a more basic level, they may defend against fears of abandonment by caregivers, represent concerns over body integrity, and involve loss of ego functions. At a still more primitive level, phobias may entail efforts to restore a lost sense of connection with others and to re-establish a lost sense of identity (Ferber, 1959).

Considerations in evaluating patients with phobias include (1) whether the person has one or many phobias, (2) whether the phobic concern is specific or general, (3) content of the phobia, and (4) level of psychic functioning reflected in the phobia. Multiple phobias, as well as those that require severe restrictions in daily life (e.g., fears of stepping across thresholds, of blushing, of talking in public, of being looked at, and of contamination) suggest borderline personality organization (Kernberg, 1967).

Counterphobic patterns are those in which, instead of being avoided, a frightening object or situation is actively pursued, evidently in an unconscious effort to master the fear rather than to endure it more passively (e.g., the acrophobe who skydives). Counterphobic repetitions rarely eventuate in mastery of phobic apprehensions but may lead to compulsive repetition of the counterphobic activity. Although this phenomenon has been reliably observed clinically, it has received little empirical investigation and is not a problem for which treatment is ordinarily sought. These factors may explain its absence from the DSM in spite of the fact that counterphobic behavior may be quite self-destructive.

The implications of phobic symptoms for psychotherapy depend on the assessment of the total phobic picture. Freud (1919) was the first to note, in effect, that exposure therapy can be the best treatment for uncomplicated phobic symptoms. While symptom removal has always been a goal in psychodynamic psychotherapy, other goals are equally important. These include, for phobic patients, an increase in the sense of safety and trust, the resumption of blocked emotional growth, improvement in anxiety tolerance and affect regulation, exploration and reduction of fears of prudent risk-taking, and greater interpersonal involvement. In the Menninger Psychotherapy Research Project (Wallerstein, 1986), 18 of the 42 patients studied had phobic attitudes and symptoms; in five, they were dominant and severe. All demonstrated significant improvement in psychoanalysis or psychoanalytic therapy.

S302.3 Obsessive-Compulsive Disorders

Obsessive-compulsive disorders, characterized by persistent intrusive thoughts (obsessions) and inflexible rituals (compulsions) may be understood as efforts to reduce severe anxiety. When individuals with obsessive-compulsive disorders are prevented from carrying out their compulsions, they may become diffusely terrified. Behind such symptoms, psychoanalytic clinical experience points to a range of unconscious concerns, including potential loss of control (especially with respect to contamination, aggression, and shame). Compulsive activity often betrays remnants of the magical thinking of early childhood, when impulses and actions are incompletely differentiated. Thus, individuals with obsessive-compulsive symptoms may be understood as having convicted themselves unconsciously of thought crimes (hostile, selfish cognitions), which may haunt them in the form of obsessive images and ideas, and then having tried to expiate their guilt with rituals of cleansing or undoing.

Children between roughly 6 and 9 frequently develop minor rituals, accompanied by magical ideas, in which efforts to control frightening aggressive ideas seem evident ("If I don't step on a crack, I won't break my mother's back"). Ordinarily, such rituals are short-lived and not at all incapacitating. The rarity of such behaviors, and of diagnosed obsessive-compulsive disorders, in the preschool years suggests that the capacities to take initiative and to feel guilt are prerequisites to obsessive-compulsive symptom-formation.

In addition to working on the symptom directly, it is valuable to investigate recent losses, stresses, and other possible precipitants of anxiety, especially those that may have affected a patient's fantasies of control. Conveying the message that hostile and selfish thoughts are understandable and not inherently dangerous may also be of help. Although notably challenging clinically, some obsessions and compulsions remit when the afflicted person can express the feelings connected with difficult experiences—especially normal disappointment, anger, and grief at the limits of what is controllable.

S303. Dissociative Disorders

Dissociative disorders listed in DSM-IV-TR include a range of mental health problems: dissociative identity disorder (in this volume considered a personality disorder, as noted previously), psychogenic fugue, psychogenic amnesia, and depersonalization phenomena. To understand the subjective experience of dissociative disorders, it may be helpful to contrast them with the integrated sense of self of more stable individuals. Healthier people experience their bodies' movements as parts of themselves; they synthesize the information from their various senses (e.g., sight, sound, smell, touch) into an integrated perception of what they are doing and/or what is happening to them. In the absence of dissociation, thoughts and ideas are invested with different affects that help determine their meaning, and these affectively meaningful cognitions are all integrated into a sense of self. Even complex social interactions and their associated affective states are assimilated in an integrated way; feelings can be mixed or ambivalent, but they are experienced as connected. In dissociative disorders, such processes, which seem automatic to individuals without dissociative tendencies, cannot be taken for granted; any or all of them can be split off and experienced as alien.

DSM-IV-TR Classification Dissociative Disorders
■ Dissociative Amnesia ■ Dissociative Fugue ■ Dissociative Identity Disorder ■ Depersonalization Disorder ■ Dissociative Disorder not otherwise specified

The Internal Experience of Dissociation

Affective states: In the various dissociative disorders, there are different kinds of compromises of patients' integrated affective organization. In depersonalization disorder, for example, there is often a loss of a sense of one's own body; the affective states related to sensations or movements become experienced as alien, as not part of a sense of self or "me." The loss of a sense of "me" may be accompanied by sharp anxiety, even to the point of panic, or by its polar opposite, a strange indifference or calm. It is often helpful to encourage individuals with dissociative disorders to describe their affective experiences in detail. In the context of a trusting therapeutic relationship (which may take a long time to develop if the traumatic experiences that gave rise to dissociative tendencies involved mistreatment by intimate authorities), such descriptions—even if they are descriptions of numbness or nothingness—can be a first step in re-integrating the different affective states that comprise a sense of self. It is usually valuable then to relate such accounts to stressful experiences that may have preceded the current dissociative reaction.

In psychogenic fugue and psychogenic amnesia we observe another type of fragmentation. In these conditions, specific behaviors or memories, respectively, are dissociated from the sense of self. This pattern may also be accompanied by a range of affective reactions, from panic to relative indifference. Frequently patients' implicit (nonverbal) affective communications provide important clues as to the nature of their inner experience.

The *cognitive, somatic, and relationship patterns* of patients with dissociative disorders tend to reflect the particular affective states involved in the dissociation. For example, anxiety and panic may manifest themselves as an intense preoccupation over what is happening in the moment. Feelings of indifference may be expressed by seemingly idle chatter. Somatic states may accompany the different degrees of anxiety or depression that are either affectively available or dissociated. Bodily states may also stand in for dissociated affects; a somatic numbness or anesthesia, for example, may represent the emotional numbness induced by trauma. Relationships vary considerably, but are often characterized by shallow, needy, emotionally hungry, inconsistent, and seemingly ambivalent patterns.

Clinical Illustration

A 25-year old single woman who had recently left home to take a job in a distant city began experiencing "feelings that I was looking at myself from somewhere above myself, like I lost a sense of who I was. I became very nervous, and for a few moments, I wasn't sure what I was doing, where I was going, or where I was." These experiences increased in duration and frequency. As they continued and the patient became more anxious, she reported, "I couldn't cope or take care of myself," and she returned to her family and to a more supportive treatment program.

A related study includes: Sarlin, 1962.

S304. Mood Disorders

The authors of DSM-IV-TR divided mood disorders into depressive disorders and bipolar disorders. Depressive (or unipolar) disorders are further subdivided into major depressive disorder, dysthymic disorder, and depressive disorder not otherwise specified. The bipolar disorders include bipolar I, bipolar II, and cyclothymic disorder. Diagnosis of each disorder depends on specific criteria. Despite this clear delineation, most clinicians find that their mood-disordered patients experience a range of manic, depressive, and manic-depressive patterns except for certain "textbook cases."

**DSM-IV-TR Classification
Mood Disorders**

Depressive Disorders
- Major Depressive Disorder
  - Single Episode
  - Recurrent
- Dysthymic Disorder
- Depressive Disorder not otherwise specified

Bipolar Disorders
- Bipolar I Disorder
  - Single Manic Episode
  - Most Recent Episode Hypomanic
  - Most Recent Episode Manic
  - Most Recent Episode Mixed
  - Most Recent Episode Depressed
  - Most Recent Episode Unspecified
- Bipolar II Disorder
- Cyclothymic Disorder
- Bipolar Disorder not otherwise specified
- Mood Disorder due to . . . *[Indicate General Medical Condition]*
- Substance-Induced Mood Disorder
- Mood Disorder not otherwise specified

S304.1 Depressive Disorders

Depression is common. Although major depressive disorder may begin at any age, it usually begins in young adulthood. Symptoms develop over days to weeks. Some people have only a single episode, with a full return to premorbid functioning. More than 50 percent of those who initially suffer a single major depressive episode, however, eventually develop another.

Depression is not just a form of extreme sadness. It is a disorder that affects both brain and body, including cognition, behavior, the immune system and peripheral nervous system. Unlike a passing sad mood, depression is considered a disorder because it interferes with ordinary functioning in work, school, or relationships. Unlike normal grief, which comes in waves, it is constant and oppressive. Depression also differs from ordinary mourning in that the mourner experiences the world as empty or bad, whereas clinically depressed individuals locate their sense of emptiness or badness in the self.

The medical definition of depression is a sustained abnormality in a person's mood, or feelings of despair, hopelessness, and self-hatred. A depressive episode is defined as a period lasting at least two weeks in which a person feels depressed or becomes unable to experience any pleasure, accompanied by some of the following: changes in sleep patterns, changes in appetite, changes in sexual desire, loss of interest in things that were previously interesting, loss of pleasure in life (anhedonia), loss of energy, inability to concentrate, slowing of reflexes and bodily movements (psychomotor retardation), feelings of guilt, and thoughts of suicide. The quality, intensity, and disruptive nature of the symptoms appear to be most relevant clinically. Depression is an affect state that can vary in intensity from relatively mild to profound, from a subtle experience to a severely disabling clinical disorder. Depression can be a relatively appropriate, if somewhat excessive, response to an accurate appraisal of reality, or it can be based on severe reality distortions.

A careful assessment includes screening for medical problems and asking questions about what else may be going on in a person's life that might produce depression-like symptoms. Numerous medical conditions (including diabetes, hypo- or hyper-thyroidism, multiple sclerosis, Parkinson's disease, head trauma, hepatitis, AIDS, and other infectious diseases) can cause symptoms that resemble depression. Use of steroids or withdrawal from cocaine, alcohol, or amphetamines can also produce depressive reactions. Finally, normal bereavement can look very much like depression.

Major depression is manifested by a combination of symptoms that interfere with the ability to work, study, sleep, eat, and enjoy aspects of life. Overt behavior and symptoms include crying spells, loss of interest in previously enjoyable activities, indifference to social interaction, neglect of personal care and physical appearance, passive or withdrawn behavior, restlessness, and slowed movement, thought, and/or speech.

Dysthymia involves long-term, chronic symptoms that do not disable, but keep one from functioning well or feeling good. Many people with dysthymia also experience major depressive episodes at some time in their lives.

Bipolar disorder, also known as manic depression, is an illness characterized by mood swings from depression to mania. The diagnostic criteria for bipolar depression are the same as for major depression, but bipolar patients tend to have atypical features. Bipolar patients who cycle rapidly can be up and down in a matter of minutes, and mixed states of depression and mania can be present together.

Psychotic depression is a rare form of depression characterized by delusions (e.g., the belief that one is someone else, or the belief that one must kill oneself to purge the world of evil) or hallucinations (e.g., hearing voices that savagely criticize the self or command one to die).

Seasonal affective disorder (SAD), thought to be related to lack of sunlight, is major depression that appears in the fall or winter and remits in the spring.

Postpartum depression is a mood disorder that occurs within four weeks of childbirth. Many new mothers suffer from some degree of the "baby blues." Postpartum depression, by contrast, is major depression, thought by most investigators to be related to changes in hormonal flows associated with childbirth.

Components of an Evaluation for Suicidal Risk

- Presence of suicidal or homicidal ideation, intent, or plans
- Ready access to means for suicide and the lethality of those means
- Presence of psychotic symptoms, especially command hallucinations
- Presence of serious alcohol or substance abuse
- History and seriousness of previous self-harm attempts
- Family history of, or recent exposure to, suicide

The Internal Experience of Depressive Disorders

Affective states experienced by individuals with depression include two general emotional orientations that have been described respectively, as anaclitic and introjective patterns (Blatt, 2004).

Anaclitic depressive patterns, frequently associated with the disruption of the relationship with a primary caregiver, are characterized by feelings of helplessness, weakness, inadequacy, and depletion; fears of being abandoned, isolated, and unloved; struggles to maintain direct physical contact with a need-gratifying person; wishes to be soothed, helped, fed, and protected; difficulty tolerating delay and postponement; difficulty expressing anger and rage (for fear of destroying the other as a source of satisfaction); and valuing caregivers only for their capacity to provide needed gratification.

Introjective depressive patterns are characterized by harsh, punitive, unrelenting self-criticism; feelings of inferiority, worthlessness and guilt; a sense of having failed to live up to expectations and standards; fears of loss of approval, recognition, and love from important others; and fears of the loss of acceptance of assertive strivings. Self-esteem suffers badly under such onslaughts of self-criticism and fear.

Cognitive patterns may include rationalized conviction of guilt, fantasies of loss of approval, recognition and love; inability to make decisions; low self-regard; suicidal ideas; and impaired memory. Patients with anaclitic depressions may be preoccupied with ways to get care from others. The cognitive symptoms of depression are harsher in introjective versions of the experience. The intensity of thoughts in depression may be disturbing by itself. William Styron described his own experience of major depression as "a storm in the brain."

Somatic states may include: loss of sexual desire; physical irritability (especially in men and adolescents); restlessness; headache, back pain, muscle pain, palpitations, fainting, or constipation, with no known pathophysiology to account for such complaints. Substance use or abuse, common ways in which depressed people attempt to reduce dysphoria, may have physical effects. Changes in appetite may cause weight loss or gain. Fatigue, low energy, and lethargy (motor slowness) caused by depression are divorced from emotional pain in some patients and thus are experienced as sheerly physical complaints. Insomnia or hypersomnia may put additional stress on the body.

Relationship patterns may be characterized by insatiable neediness and/or demanding hostility. Feelings of being unlovable and unworthy may cause depressed individuals to cling to, withdraw from, or antagonize people with whom they have previously had good relationships.

Clinical Illustrations

An avid football fan in his late 50s presented with low energy, apathy, and feelings of being a failure. "I know I have a lot to be proud of. My children are doing well, yet I don't feel good." He went on, "I have felt so bad that I only went to one football game this season, even though I have season tickets. I've lost all my enthusiasm . . . I usually look forward to going with my son . . . we used to have a blast." The same patient could not stop dwelling on a change in his job at work. He said, "I feel like I have brought shame on myself and my family. I always felt so proud of my job, and now I feel I've lost all respect at work, like I'm not needed there anymore."

A 55-year-old physician participating in group therapy missed two group sessions without notice or explanation. When her therapist caught up with her by phone, she explained that she had become so depressed she could not get out of bed. She described the depression as a "black cloud" enveloping her. In a hastily scheduled individual session, she recounted that over the previous two weeks she had begun to experience restless, unpleasant awakenings in the middle of the night. She also described "going through the motions at work . . . getting things done," but only with considerable effort to push past her fatigue and difficulty concentrating. What was most striking was how her troubled mood had affected her self-esteem and feelings of adequacy as a mother. She was especially self-conscious about the fact that her three children attended less prestigious colleges than her friends' children did. She felt like a failure, characterizing her children as "not good kids," and citing as evidence her belief that her older daughter smoked too much pot. This lament contrasted with several previous statements in the group about how pleased she was that her children were decent and kind individuals.

S304.2 Bipolar Disorders

Bipolar disorders are characterized by the presence of an episode with manic features (manic, mixed, or hypomanic) in addition to a depressive episode and/or milder depressive symptoms. Manic episodes are identified by a distinct time period in which the individual experiences an elevated and/or irritable mood, along with inflated self-esteem, difficulties sleeping, pressured speech, flights of ideas, difficulties concentrating and focusing, psychomotor agitation, and engagement in activities that, while pleasurable, have serious negative consequences (e.g., spending inordinate amounts of money, engaging in promiscuous and ill-considered sexual relations).

Bipolar I disorder is diagnosed when the patient meets the full diagnostic criteria for both a full manic episode and major depressive disorder. Bipolar II disorder is identified by the presence and/or history of at least one major depressive episode and the existence and/or history of hypomanic episodes (less severe manic episodes). Cyclothymic disorder is diagnosed when mood fluctuations are notable but not of sufficient severity to be considered bipolar. Although cyclothymic disorder can appear as early as adolescence, the average age of onset for the bipolar disorders is the early twenties for both men and women. Their course typically involves the sudden onset of manic symptoms that escalate rapidly over a few days. Bipolar disorder has a strong genetic influence.

The Internal Experience of Manic States

Affective states: In the various dissociative disorders, may include feelings of intense pleasure or euphoria. They may also involve intense irritability, often accompanied by transient anxiety, agitation, and a hypersensitivity to, and expectation of, insult and rejection. Mania is characterized by excessive energy that may be experienced negatively, as a disruptive and distracting internal pressure, or positively, as a sense of infinite power, ability and creativity. In either case, the internal hyperarousal is often accompanied by impulsive behavior. Patients experiencing manic states often report increased desire—even desperate cravings—for others, frequently accompanied by intense, constant sexual desire and social disinhibition.

Individuals with mania may alternate between feeling frayed, fractured, and anxious, and feeling perfectly complete and elated. The quick fluctuations in their moods are accompanied by equally rapid fluctuations in the sense of self. One minute the individual feels sullen, useless, and agitated; the next minute, like a conquering hero. These changes in mood are sudden, unpredictable, and uncontrollable. There can be feelings of loss when the mania dissipates—a yearning for the emotional intensity, ecstasy, and productivity. Many people with manic tendencies seek out "upper" drugs, such as cocaine or methamphetamines, to intensify or bring back the euphoria of mania.

Cognitive patterns may include fantasies of invincibility and exceptional talent; a sense of capacity to succeed at any task regardless of preparation or training; wishes for fame or adoration; and difficulty thinking clearly, logically, and linearly. Individuals may fear that they cannot hold onto their thoughts, which seem flighty and ungraspable. At times, individuals in manic states can feel highly disoriented, as they are often unable to identify which of their racing thoughts are important or relevant. At other times, they may experience the welter of thoughts as freeing and joyful. They frequently express the contents of their mind without self-censorship and inhibition.

Somatic states may include restlessness and sleeplessness. Some patients in a manic state insist that sleep is a needless waste of time. They may feel physically invigorated and aroused, and describe a need to "Keep going! Don't stop!" Sexual desire is frequent and intense. Physical exhaustion, which may evoke suicidal depression, is a serious danger.

Relationship patterns are often unpredictable, chaotic, impulsive, and sexualized. Some people with manic tendencies inspire followers and protégés, whose mood may be elevated by sharing in the grand schemes of the manic person.

Clinical Illustration

A 32-year-old, outgoing, highly dramatic, energetic young man with a history of anxiety and depression began feeling more "empty" and "low" as intimate relationships and clear career paths were not "falling into place" as he had expected. He found that lots of coffee and "herbal energies" lifted his mood. His efforts to attain "high-energy states" increased, and he gradually became quite manic—interspersed with periods of feeling quite depressed. Over three years, these mood vacillations increased in intensity until he became very agitated and was unable to sleep. Within a short time, convinced that he had a "special ability" to predict the stock market, he approached colleagues to invest in him, to "trust" him. As his thoughts became more delusional, he was unable to function. His family helped him enter an inpatient treatment program. He was unable, however, to sustain a psychotherapeutic relationship. Any effort to examine the utility of his efforts to overcome his depressions by "feeling powerful and at one with the universe" was rejected. One to two times per year he became depressed and then manic and required further inpatient care.

Related studies include: Aarons, 1990; Badal, 1962; Blank, 1954; Blatt, 1974; Bonime, 1967; Dietz, 1995; Jamison, 1995; Pao, 1968; Rochlin, 1953.

S305. Somatoform (Somatization) Disorders

The authors of DSM-IV-TR describe somatoform disorders as "the presence of physical symptoms that suggest a general medical condition . . . and are not fully explained by a general medical condition, by the direct effects of a substance, or by another mental disorder." In our view, their classification puts together several conditions that are psychologically quite disparate, as least one of which we view as characterological (see Somatizing Personality Disorder, p. 47). Nevertheless, we have organized the discussion of affective, cognitive, somatic, and relational patterns according to the DSM rubric.

Classical psychoanalytic understanding of conversion disorders, the most dramatic of the somatoform conditions, construed them as symbolic representations of unconscious conflicts. A conflict about *seeing* something might be expressed in blindness; a forbidden sexual or aggressive impulse might take the form of a physical paralysis. In contemporary Western cultures, somatic symptoms that seem to be simple symbolic representations of conflict have become comparatively rare. In addition, some conditions that in the past would have been attributed to unconscious conflict are currently more likely to be considered posttraumatic. (These two levels of explanations are, of course, not mutually exclusive: trauma can create unconscious conflict.) Patients with conversion symptoms were classically noted for an accompanying blasé attitude toward their symptoms (*la belle indifférence*), a puzzling emotional minimization of the seriousness of conditions as disabling as blindness or paralysis. It is unclear whether this lack of affect is a variant of alexythymia, the inability to formulate affective experience in words (see the section on Somatizing Personality Disorder, p. 47) or a posttraumatic dissociation of affect that can be formulated, but has been felt as too painful to integrate with overall experience.

The frequency with which sufferers of some symptom complexes whose origins are still somewhat unclear—e.g., chronic fatigue syndrome, irritable bowel syndrome, fibromyalgia—are drawn to self-help groups, advocacy groups, or political involvement suggests that many people with these conditions see the medical community as not taking them seriously. Their perception may be accurate. Some patients who somatize seem to be trying to connect with their doctors through their constant symptoms; physicians are especially likely to draw this conclusion when the relief of one complaint seems quickly to lead to another. Other patients with puzzling and unremitting symptoms may be misunderstood as using their illness to ensure a relationship because the physician has not diagnosed their problem accurately. Either way, the patient's physical suffering may be minimized by medical personnel who feel helpless to heal them. Doctors who are oriented toward action and symptom relief can become frustrated and irritated at their inability to cure or even localize a problem. Thus, when patients with somatoform disorders come for psychotherapy, they are often poised to see the therapist as another authority that does not really listen, does not really care.

The issue of secondary gain is also important. Understanding of any somatoform disorder should include an analysis of what benefits the illness may provide (for example, some individuals may feel that the only legitimate way to get dependent needs met is via the sick role). Secondary gain motivations are almost always unconscious and should be addressed, if at all, with the utmost tact. Again, when doctors are at a loss to diagnose or help patients, it is not uncommon for those patients to feel accused of remaining ill for the sake of some secondary gain.

Some of the DSM-classified somatoform disorders involve a drive to action. The anorexic patient, for example, feels "I must take action to control my body." In gender identity disorders, the patient may feel "I must take action against the misunderstanding that I am a woman."

In hypochondriasis the patient is characteristically preoccupied with his or her body, sometimes to the exclusion of all else. This preoccupation can have a paranoid-like intensity and is associated with a deep reluctance to relinquish physical symptoms or divert attention to other aspects of life. Many explanations have been suggested for this resistance to change, including that the symptoms represent a way of taking care of conscious or unconscious feelings of guilt; that they constitute ways of dealing with early and hostile caregivers; and that they justify being cared for. The persistence of symptoms is often felt by the patient as evidence of a physician's ineffectiveness. Hostility to physicians and other health professionals may be conscious or unconscious to the patient, but it is usually felt by the professionals. Attachment to the symptoms is often accompanied by powerful fears of death.

Somatically expressed symptom clusters involve a range of disorders that have to do with the somatic self, the bodily self. They are not well differentiated. There is considerable confusion as to how to understand many of these symptom complexes. Some conditions now considered somatoform may eventually prove to have etiologies in which psychological factors play virtually no role. In working with physically compromised patients, it is hard to know which psychological attributes preceded their physical suffering and which constitute the psychological *effects* of having an illness that defies attempts at cure. Eating disorders and gender identity disorders were included in this section of the DSM on the grounds that they also involve feelings about the body, but they seem to us rather different conditions from those in which physical suffering is the primary complaint.

There are clear empirical findings about some somatoform disorders; about others, the research is equivocal or insufficient. Authors of the DSM note that there is depression in over half of the patients with somatization disorders and that generalized anxiety disorder and panic disorders coexist with a somewhat lower number. There is also an unclear relationship between the various disorders and any precipitating stressors. Clinical experience suggests that precipitants may include loss, illness in someone else, anxiety about a life event, an experience that threatens the sense of self-esteem or mastery, and cultural influences.

**DSM-IV-TR Classification
Somatoform Disorders**

- Somatization Disorder
- Undifferentiated Somatoform Disorder
- Conversion Disorder
- Pain Disorder
  - Associated with Psychological Factors
  - Associated with Both Psychological Factors and a General Medical Condition
- Hypochondriasis
- Body Dysmorphic Disorder
- Somatoform Disorder not otherwise specified

The Internal Experience of Somatoform Disorders

Affective states include a characteristic sense that "There is something wrong with my body." This complaint can be specific, e.g., pain or otherwise symptomatic, such as, "My body is too fat." The subjective state varies, from those who are preoccupied and hypervigilant and react with intense anxiety to what are probably normal variations in internal sensations, to those who have an apparent lack of anxiety or concern. The extent to which this unconcern represents a denial of internal experience or some break in the linkage between somatic sensation and self-awareness is a pertinent question for therapists trying to understand the patient's experience.

Cognitive patterns vary across the different conditions. In hypochondriasis, for example, there is a general cognitive absorption with one's body. Thoughts may include the terrifying belief that each pain or symptom is life-threatening, that *this time* it is serious, even if in the past it turned out not to be. Such preoccupations can dominate the person's thinking and be accompanied by depressed affect and a sense of doom. Perceived symptoms can be varied and shifting (e.g., headaches, abdominal pain, cardiac symptoms, and discomfort in the chest, back, pelvis, or elsewhere). Sometimes, perhaps most notably in women with histories of pelvic pain, patients come to therapy with a history of surgeries that have attempted to relieve their suffering, but to no avail.

Somatic states include the physiological accompaniments of anxiety, such as rapid heartbeat, blood pressure increase, and muscle tensions that give rise to pain. These responses of the autonomic nervous system are part of the "fight or flight" reaction. Sometimes somatic symptoms are delusional. "I'm suffocating. I can't breathe around here. All these big breathers around me are using up all the air."

Relationship patterns, including relationships with doctors, may vary from an intense, persistent, and aggressive search for reassurance (which fails to reassure), to psychological remoteness and inaccessibility.

Clinical Illustrations

- A 45-year-old woman was convinced that she was pregnant. She had been amenorrheic for several months and reported nausea, fatigue, and breast tenderness. Repeated examinations led to a diagnosis of menopausal amenorrhea. She refused to accept the diagnosis and returned repeatedly. She had a strong wish to "give her mother a baby" before her mother died.

- Another female patient had been amenorrheic for several months and reported a sensation of a pelvic mass. She felt her abdomen expanding and felt that she was pregnant. Her medical visit resulted in a diagnosis of a large fibroid.

- A businessman from a working-class background was on a trajectory of success in which he was increasingly being asked to make presentations to groups. He became terribly anxious each time, convinced that his lack of "what it takes" would become visible. He could barely speak, and began to have chest pain each time he had to make a presentation.

- A young woman in her first year of college was dating a student in another college with whom she had her first, and rather ambivalent, experience of sexual intercourse. On the day before they were to meet again, she was in the biology laboratory working with a microscope and suddenly felt that she could not see. Hours later in the infirmary she recalled a microorganism that had reminded her of her boyfriend's penis.

Related studies include: Adams-Silvan & Silvan, 1994; Aisenstein & Gibeault, 1991; Aisenstein, 1993; Brickman, 1992; Broden & Myers, 1981; Coen & Sarno, 1989; Crawford, 1996; Hull, Okie, Gibbons, & Carpenter, 1992; Krystal, 1997; Kuchenhoff, 1998; McDougall, 1980; Meares, 1997; Meyer, 1988; Miliora, 1998; Perlman, 1996; Rodin, 1991; Yarom, 1997.)

S306. Eating Disorders

According to DSM-IV-TR, eating disorders are characterized by "severe disturbances in eating behavior" and include two specific diagnoses, anorexia nervosa, and bulimia nervosa. The essential feature of eating disorders is that one's self-esteem is intricately tied to body shape and weight. Anorexia nervosa is characterized by a significant weight loss resulting from excessive food restriction, often coexisting with purging. Because of an intense fear of becoming obese, people with anorexia nervosa refuse to maintain a minimally normal body weight. They often have a significant disturbance in the perception of their body (e.g., feeling fat when emaciated). Weight loss is experienced as an accomplishment and a sign of great self-control and discipline. Bulimia nervosa is characterized by a cycle of binge eating followed by purging to try to rid the body of unwanted calories and prevent weight gain. A binge is defined as eating large amounts of food in a short period of time (usually less than 2 hours), accompanied by a transient reduction in dysphoria, often followed by a depressed mood, severe self-criticism, and a sense of a lack of control over what one is eating. Purging methods usually involve vomiting and laxative abuse. Other forms of purging include excessive exercise, fasting, and use of diuretics, diet pills, and enemas.

Anorexia and bulimia appear to be more prevalent in industrialized societies, where there is an abundance of food and where conceptions of attractiveness involve being thin. Women and girls make up 90% of the reported cases, but there is some evidence that eating disorders are increasing among males. They usually begin in late adolescence or early adulthood, and the course and outcome are variable. There is an increased incidence of anorexia and bulimia, along with mood disorders, among first-degree biological relatives of individuals with the disorder.

Eating disorders are readily recognized by the behaviors described above. They represent more than simply a problem with food, however. They are complex psychological disorders with aspects that are often not obvious or discernable to the outside observer.

DSM-IV-TR Classification
Eating Disorders

- Anorexia Nervosa
- Bulimia Nervosa
- Eating Disorder not otherwise specified

The Internal Experience of Eating Disorders

The onset of anorexia is often associated with a stressful life event, such as leaving home for college, while bulimia frequently begins during or after an episode of dieting. Although both anorexic and bulimic patterns range from minor to life-threatening, most mental health professionals consider anorexia the more serious disorder, and the more difficult to treat. Because of the shame that typically accompanies eating disorders, clinicians should be careful to ask about eating patterns when taking a history from patients with disorders of mood or personality; the information is often not volunteered. What follows are descriptions of the unseen, internal experience of individuals with eating disorders, including emotional conflicts and concerns that manifestly have little to do with food.

Affective states in individuals with eating disorders may include depressive symptoms, such as depressed mood, social withdrawal, low self-esteem, and diminished interest in sex. In addition to depressive problems, anxiety symptoms are common. Such symptoms include fear of social situations and obsessive-compulsive features both related and unrelated to food (e.g., collecting recipes, developing grooming rituals, hoarding food). The following emotional concerns are common in anorexia and bulimia:

- Feelings of being starved for care and affection and longings to be protected and cherished

- Feelings of failure, weakness, and extreme shame

- Feelings of being unworthy and ineffective. For example, "I would feel like I couldn't eat, and then if I did, I would feel guilty, like I did something I wasn't supposed to or took in something I didn't deserve"

- Fears of being abandoned by others or that others will withdraw their love

- Feelings of anger and aggression, which feel frightening, dangerous and intolerable and therefore are denied, muted, or hated. For example, "I'm a bubbly person who never gets angry. It doesn't feel good to get angry and nobody around me feels good when I get angry. They would get hurt and you can't hurt the people you care about."

- Fears that experiencing one's emotions leads to being out of control. For example, an anorexic woman stated that if she were to talk freely about her feelings, she would find herself "blowing in the wind."

Cognitive patterns may include the following:

- A preoccupation with being inadequate, incompetent, and unloved, and the development of strategies to deal with this
- A focus on being young, "little," un-grownup, and innocent; the desire to remain a child. For example, "I go home every weekend to my parents' house because I don't have to worry what I look like there. My parents have seen me naked in dirty diapers."

Somatic states may include a sense of "numbness" in relationship to the sensations ordinarily accompanying eating and elimination. There may be confusion about bodily sensations, including an inability to sense whether one is full after eating. The feeling of physical emptiness in the stomach may be associated with the sense of an empty, depleted self. "I have a void that I can't seem to fill . . . It's a lonely existence."

Relationship patterns may be characterized by issues of control and perfectionism, especially in the family of origin. Individuals with eating disorders may go to great lengths to keep their problem secret, thus making genuine emotional intimacy impossible. They may relate to others superficially and in ways that seem immature for their chronological age. They may handle their fears that they are unlovable by compliance, politeness and ingratiating behavior, accompanied by difficulties accepting positive affirmation. For example, "I would much rather please people. I realize that I become dormant and let people walk all over me; I just thought if I did what he needed, he'd spend time with me," or, "Pleasing people gives me a sense of purpose."

Clinical Illustration

A 22-year-old woman, a former athlete and self-described tomboy, was the youngest of five and the only girl in her family. After graduating from college, she became increasingly preoccupied with "being thin enough to be a high-fashion model." She began a series of diets and reportedly experienced anxiety and nausea every time she went near food. She also noted that "even when I force myself to eat so I won't get sick, I can't tell if I'm hungry or not. I can never tell if I've eaten enough." In her family and during her athletic training, she had always been on very strict regimens of exercise, nutrition, study, and daily routines. As her anxiety around eating increased and she became more and more preoccupied with the thought that she was getting too fat, often coupled with fantasies of "looking pregnant," she avoided dating because "I don't want to get pregnant." Eventually, her symptoms became severe enough that she entered treatment.

Related studies include: Barrows, 1999; Bemporad, Beresin, Ratey, O'Driscoll, Lindem, & Herzog, 1992a; Bemporad, O'Driscoll, Beresin, Ratey, Lindem, & Herzog, 1992b; Beresin, Gordon, & Herzog, 1989; Birsted-Green, 1989; Bromberg, 2001; Bruch, 1973, 1978; Fischer, 1989; Guinjoan, Ross, Perinot, Maritato, Jorda-Fahrer, & Fahrer, 2001; Herzog, Franko, & Brotman, 1989; Kernberg, 1995; Lawrence, 2001; Lombardi, 2002, Lowenkopf & Wallach, 1985; O'Neill, 2001; Rozen, 1993; Sands, 2003; Schwartz, 1986; Shahly, 1987; Thompson-Brenner & Westen, 2005a; Thompson-Brenner & Westen, 2005b; Williams, 1997.

S307. Psychogenic Sleep Disorders

DSM-IV-TR groups sleep disorders into (1) primary sleep disorders, (2) sleep disorders related to a general medical condition, (3) sleep disorders due to another mental disorder, and (4) substance-induced sleep disorders. Diagnoses include primary insomnia, primary hypersomnia, narcolepsy, breathing-related sleep disorder, circadian rhythm sleep disorder, and dyssomnia not otherwise specified. Young adults are more likely to have difficulty falling asleep, while midlife and older adults are more likely to have trouble staying asleep. Sleep disorders tend to run in families.

Sleep disorders considered "primary" include dyssomnias and parasomnias. Dyssomnias are problems in initiating or maintaining sleep (insomnia) or experiences of excessive sleepiness (hypersomnia). The defining feature of primary insomnia is trouble falling or staying asleep, sleep that is not restful, or a combination of these, lasting at least one month, and causing clinically significant difficulties in social, occupational, or other areas of functioning. Primary insomnia has been found to be associated with physical or mental stimulation at nighttime in conjunction with negative conditioning for sleep. Significant preoccupation with the problem may exacerbate it: The more one tries to sleep, the more upset and angry one becomes, and the less likely one is to sleep. Chronic insomnia may lead to deterioration of mood and motivation, lowered energy and attention, and increased exhaustion and sickness. Insomnia is more prevalent with age and in women.

Primary hypersomnia is defined by extreme sleepiness, extended sleep periods, or excessive napping, for at least one month, causing clinically significant difficulty or impairment in social, occupational, or other areas of functioning. Individuals with hypersomnia often carry out routine automatic behavior with little or no recall. The true prevalence is unknown. Primary hypersomnia typically begins between ages 15 and 30, with gradual progression and a chronic and stable course.

The essential features of narcolepsy are repeated episodes of irresistible attacks of refreshing sleep, episodes of cataplexy (sudden loss of muscle tone, usually following an outburst of intense emotion), and intrusion of REM sleep. The sleepiness typically decreases after an attack, only to reappear later.

Breathing-related sleep disorders (sleep apneas) are sleep disruptions caused by ventilation abnormalities during sleep, leading to excessive sleepiness or insomnia. Symptoms may include nocturnal chest discomfort, a sense of choking or suffocation, intense anxiety, dryness of the mouth, extreme difficulty awakening, and inappropriate behavior. Breathing-related sleep disorders have an insidious onset, a gradual progression, and a chronic course.

Circadian rhythm sleep disorder is an ongoing pattern of sleep difficulty resulting from a difference between a person's individual sleep-wake cycle and the demands of the outer world. Individuals with this disorder may experience wakefulness at regular points in each 24-hour period (e.g., at 11:00 p.m.) and excessive sleepiness at other points (e.g., at 11:00 a.m.). Without intervention the symptoms may last for years or decades.

Parasomnias are characterized by abnormal behavioral or physiological events occurring in association with sleep, specific sleep stages, or sleep-wake transitions. These disorders involve activation of the autonomic nervous system, motor system, and/or cognitive processes during sleep or sleep-wake transitions, and include the following diagnoses: nightmare disorder, sleep terror disorder, sleepwalking disorder, and parasomnia not otherwise specified. The essential feature of nightmare disorder is the repeated occurrence of frightening dreams from which the sleeper wakes, resulting in significant distress and/or social or occupational dysfunction. The dreams typically involve severe anxiety about imminent physical danger. Nightmares are common between the ages of 3 and 6 and tend to remit as children get older; in some individuals they continue to disturb sleep.

Sleep terror disorder (*pavor nocturnus*) is characterized by abrupt awakenings from sleep, usually beginning with a panicky scream or cry, and lasting about ten minutes. The individual experiences intense anxiety and symptoms of autonomic arousal such as sweating, rapid breathing, flushing of the skin, and pupil dilation. In children, the disorder usually begins between ages 4 and 12 and resolves spontaneously in adolescence. In adults it begins between ages 20 and 30, and tends to become chronic.

Sleepwalking disorder is characterized by repeated episodes of complex motor behavior initiated during sleep (rising from bed and walking about). Episodes include a variety of behaviors, including sitting up; walking into closets, down stairs, or out of buildings; using the bathroom; eating; talking; and even operating machinery, all while asleep. Internal and external stimuli, psychosocial stressors, and alcohol or sedative use increase the likelihood of sleepwalking. Episodes occur between ages 4 and 8 and tend to peak at age 12. Most commonly, the pattern of sleepwalking includes repeated episodes occurring over a period of several years.

Many sleep disorders are secondary consequences of mood disorders and anxiety disorders, including posttraumatic syndromes. The pathophysiological mechanisms responsible for these disorders also affect sleep-wake regulation. Their course generally follows that of the underlying mental disorder. Sleep disturbances resulting from intoxication or withdrawal of a substance are distinguished from other sleep disorders by a consideration of their onset and course. Onset of a substance-related sleep disturbance can occur up to four weeks after cessation of substance use.

DSM-IV-TR Classification
Sleep Disorders

Primary Sleep Disorders

Dyssomnias
- Primary Insomnia
- Primary Hypersomnia
- Narcolepsy
- Breathing-Related Sleep Disorder
- Circadian Rhythm Sleep Disorder
- Dyssomnia not otherwise specified

Parasomnias
- Nightmare Disorder
- Sleep Terror Disorder
- Sleepwalking Disorder
- Parasomnia not otherwise specified

Sleep Disorders Related to Another Mental Disorder
- Insomnia Related to . . . *[Indicate the Mental Disorder]*
- Hypersomnia Related to . . . *[Indicate the Mental Disorder]*

Other Sleep Disorders
- Sleep Disorder Due to . . . *[Indicate the General Medical Condition]*
- Insomnia Type
- Hypersomnia Type
- Parasomnia Type
- Mixed Type
- Substance-Induced Sleep Disorder

The Internal Experience of Sleep Disorders

Affective states include feelings of helplessness, frustration, and anger about not being able to sleep: "I just lie there tossing and turning!" Sleep deprivation can cause depressed, demoralized, anxious, and irritable feelings: "I'm just so tired all day, it makes me annoyed and short-tempered with everyone around me."

Cognitive patterns include confusion, distractedness, and an inability to concentrate. For example, "I can't concentrate, I can't think. I just feel horrible." Sleep-disordered individuals may feel overwhelmed by their inability to think clearly while sleep-deprived. Thoughts are disproportionately concerned with getting to sleep or staying asleep and may include a series of theories about why sleep is so evasive.

Somatic states include fatigue, agitation, and irritability, as well as hypo- and hypervigilance.

Relationship patterns may suffer from the patient's preoccupation with sleep and feelings of fatigue, anxiety, anger, and/or agitation.

Clinical Illustration

A 45-year-old woman about to receive a promotion to a high executive position began finding it difficult to fall asleep at night. She was preoccupied with fears of being humiliated "when they find out I can't do the job." She would frequently picture her military officer father and her older brothers laughing at her. She worried that she was upsetting her husband by being more successful than he and was guiltily apprehensive that she would soon have even less time with her two children. As she lay awake in bed, finding it harder and harder to fall asleep, she became "anxious over being so tired that tomorrow I won't even be able to think." Soon, while trying to get to sleep, she found her heart pounding, her muscles tensing, and her breathing shallow, and she was flooded with images of being humiliated, with "everyone looking at me like I'm a failure."

Related studies include: dePraingy, Digneton, & Colin, 1982; Dowling, 1982; Hoffman, 1975; Meyer, 1979; Nielsen, 1990.

S308. Sexual and Gender Identity Disorders

DSM-IV-TR categorizes sexual and gender identity disorders in the following ways: sexual dysfunctions, the paraphilias, and gender identity disorders. Sexual dysfunctions are further divided into sexual desire disorders, sexual arousal disorders, sexual pain disorders, sexual dysfunction due to a general medical condition, substance-induced sexual dysfunction, and sexual dysfunction not otherwise specified. Paraphilias, once called perversions, are recurrent, intense sexual urges, fantasies, or behaviors that involve unusual objects, activities, or situations and cause clinically significant distress or impairment in social, occupational, or other important areas of functioning. Gender identity disorders are described in terms of consistent discomfort with one's gender assignment and consequent cross-gender identification.

Sexual inclinations and experiences are sufficiently diverse among human beings that we urge caution in diagnosis. In this area we are particularly uncomfortable with the categorical depiction of "disorders" in the DSM. Especially in the area of the paraphilias, it becomes easy to pathologize behavior that may simply be idiosyncratic. In contrast to categorizing specific *acts* as inherently pathological, irrespective of context and meaning, we recommend a thoughtful assessment of subjective factors, meanings, and contexts of variant sexualities. Psychodynamic writers have usually considered drivenness, rigidity of sexual pattern, and inability to feel sexual satisfaction via any other route, rather than the presence or absence of a particular behavior, as diagnostic criteria for sexual disorders. In pedophilia and other inclinations that can damage others when enacted, we note that it is possible to have such tendencies and inhibit acting on them. Patients who struggle against such sexual temptations may need to talk in depth with a therapist about their internal world, but they should not receive the diagnosis of a sexual problem in the absence of driven, recurrent, and inflexible behavior.

DSM-IV-TR Classification Sexual and Gender Identity Disorders	
Sexual Dysfunctions *Sexual Desire Disorders* ■ Hypoactive Sexual Desire Disorder ■ Sexual Aversion Disorder *Sexual Arousal Disorders* ■ Female Sexual Arousal Disorder ■ Male Erectile Disorder *Orgasmic Disorders* ■ Female Orgasmic Disorder ■ Male Orgasmic Disorder ■ Premature Ejaculation *Sexual Pain Disorders* ■ Dyspareunia (Not Due to a General Medical Condition) ■ Vaginismus (Not Due to a General Medical Condition) *Sexual Dysfunction Due to a General Medical Condition* ■ Female Hypoactive Sexual Desire Disorder Due to . . . [Indicate the General Medical Condition] ■ Male Hypoactive Sexual Desire Disorder Due to . . . [Indicate the General Medical Condition] ■ Male Erectile Disorder Due to . . . [Indicate the General Medical Condition] ■ Female Dyspareunia Due to . . . [Indicate the General Medical Condition] ■ Male Dyspareunia Due to . . . [Indicate the General Medical Condition]	*Sexual Dysfunction, Medical Condition* (continued) ■ Other Female Sexual Dysfunction Due to . . . [Indicate the General Medical Condition] ■ Other Male Sexual Dysfunction due to . . . [Indicate the General Medical Condition] ■ Substance-Induced Sexual Dysfunction ■ Sexual Dysfunction not otherwise specified *Paraphilias* ■ Exhibitionism ■ Voyeurism ■ Fetishism ■ Frotteurism (Rubbing) ■ Pedophilia ■ Sexual Masochism ■ Sexual Sadism ■ Transvestic Fetishism ■ Paraphilia not otherwise specified *Gender Identity Disorders* ■ Gender Identity Disorder ■ In Children ■ In Adolescents or Adults ■ Gender Identity Disorder not otherwise specified ■ Sexual Disorder not otherwise specified

S308.1 Sexual Disorders

The Internal Experience of Sexual Disorders

Affective states vary in relation to the wide range of sexual dysfunctions. Individuality is perhaps even more marked in sexual life than in other realms. Often, however, one observes in individuals with sexual dysfunctions a tendency towards anxiety and depression. It is not unusual for them to feel unsure of themselves and to be preoccupied and worried about their general adequacy. Even when the cause of a sexual dysfunction is strictly physical, such reactions are common.

Cognitive patterns may involve preoccupation with inadequacy or compensatory fantasies of power, or both.

Somatic states in some individuals include a type of sensory hyper-responsivity, in which certain types of touch feel irritating rather than comforting or arousing. This response may lead to additional feelings of anxiety and the sense that "something is wrong with my body." Other individuals may experience sensory hypo-responsivity, in which they feel a lack of sensation.

Relationship patterns are often characterized by avoidance of mature emotional and sexual intimacy or by themes of domination and power.

Clinical Illustration

A 48-year-old, single man who had had intermittent difficulties with maintaining an erection during sexual intercourse became increasingly anxious that he would not be able to "perform" with his next girlfriend. He became preoccupied with images of his father's "huge penis," in comparison to his own, which he viewed as "modest." His anxiety level grew to the point that whenever he was in the company of attractive women towards whom he would ordinarily have sexual fantasies, he would feel, "my muscles tensing up, my stomach churning. I can hardly sit still," and had thoughts that "they know I can't perform." His challenges became increasingly intense and he was unable to sustain an erection "even with women I really like." He began avoiding social situations and limited himself more and more to work and his apartment. He finally came into treatment and began working on these issues.

S308.2 Paraphilias

Internal Experience of the Paraphilias

Some paraphilias are quite circumscribed. The subjective experiences described below may, therefore, be limited to specific situations. Other paraphilias, however, tend to constitute much of an individual's internal life, and therefore characterize his or her subjective experience a great deal of the time.

Affective states associated with the paraphilias are highly various. Some overall patterns include feelings of impulsivity, opportunism, and temporary elation followed by depressive reactions after the paraphilia is enacted. Conscious anxiety and guilt may be notably absent.

Cognitive patterns may involve a tendency to be consumed by the specific sexual desire and its accompanying feelings, along with a preoccupation with planning ways to achieve satisfaction. Much energy may be invested in rationalizing one's behavior, sometimes at the cost of distorting reality. Concern for others is often not present in a meaningful sense, although some individuals with paraphilias maintain that because what they do is "out of love," it cannot have any serious negative effects on the objects of their desire. Others agonize over efforts to avoid acting out their sexual pattern.

Somatic states may include high levels of arousal and vigilance when engaged in sexual pursuit or behavior, and numbness and emptiness when not.

Relationship patterns may be exploitative with the desired sexual object and avoidant and superficial with others. Many people with paraphilic tendencies go to great lengths to keep their sexual practices secret from those close to them.

Clinical Illustration

A 68-year-old successful businessman was preoccupied with exposing his genitals to preteen children in seemingly "accidental" ways (e.g., by wearing loose bathing suits). He experienced excitement while both contemplating and enacting these scenarios, which had an addictive quality. He felt superior when fooling his wife, colleagues, and the world at large, who saw him as a leader in the community. During long-term therapy, as he dealt with a history that included repeated humiliations by his mother and sexual activities with an older sibling, he began to reduce his paraphilic behavior and support his self-esteem in less destructive ways.

S308.3 Gender Identity Disorders

Ever since Hippocrates included transvestism in his list of mental diseases in the 5th century BCE, sexual behaviors and experiences have been subject to medical scrutiny and typology. This effort has been complicated and of limited success. A society's inclusion or exclusion of particular sexual variations has burdened our understanding of divergent sexualities and our efforts to help people who suffer, or cause others to suffer, because of their sexual psychology. Differentiating disease states from normal human variability is hampered by the popularity or demonization that a diagnosis acquires in a particular society at a particular time, by theories that generalize about a biologically determined goal of maturity applicable to every individual, and by phenomena of fluidity and adaptation that may create different sexual responses at different ages and in different situations.

The first DSM (American Psychiatric Association, 1952), representing the mainstream sensibility of its era and culture, mentioned only two sexual phenomena as disorders, paraphilias and homosexuality. Both were listed under sociopathic personality disturbance. DSM III, which included homosexuality as a disorder only if ego-dystonic (i.e., if the patient rejects his or her sexual orientation), reflected the outcome of the debate in the 1960s and 1970s about whether homosexuality is a mental disorder or a normal variant of human sexuality. In that edition, there was also evidence of an appreciation that sexual orientation (object of desire) and gender identity (sense of one's own gender) are separate phenomena. In the 1987 DSM-III-R, gender identity disorder was not listed under sexual disorders. In 2000, however, DSM-IV-TR placed sexual and gender identity disorders in separate sections of the same chapter. Because in lay usage the term gender has replaced sex, this seems unfortunate: "Sex" refers to a physiologic state, while "gender" connotes a psychological experience.

The DSM-IV-TR Study Guide emphasizes caution in making an early diagnosis of a gender identity disorder on the basis of gender role explorations in childhood and adolescence. We would add that many transgendered individuals do not report significant psychological suffering and do not cause suffering to others; therefore, there is debate among professionals regarding whether or not such individuals warrant a diagnosis. Clinician's should weigh all the aspects of an individual's mental functioning before ascribing psychopathology with respect to gender.

We do not adequately understand gender identity formation. Chromosomes, hormones, and anatomical genital organs are only part of a picture that includes many other factors. Assuming that some expressions of sexuality may be reasonably considered disorders, they seem to be much more common in males than females. Diagnosis and advice must be provided only with caution to patients whose problems involve sexuality or gender, but respect for the pain and confusion of such individuals is mandatory.

The Internal Experience of Gender Identity Disorders

In the clinical setting, patients with these disorders are frequently in a state of acute distress. Children may become socially withdrawn or desperately antagonistic; adolescents may be suicidal; and adults may perform genital self-mutilating acts. The belief that one has been born in the wrong body can be a constant and tormenting obsession.

Young children of both genders may wish to have the organs or capacities of the other. Sometimes such desires reduce over time, and sometimes they are relatively permanent. Mild disappointment in one's gender seems to be common and transient; more intense and lasting disappointment seems to compromise the core gender identity of boys more than girls. Many adult women who enjoy being female report having had strong wishes to be boys during childhood; they may have had "tomboy" personas that persisted into early adolescence. Comparable memories of childhood wishes to be female in adult men who identify as masculine are rare.

Cultural patterns of sexism may play a significant role in this disparity. It will be interesting to note whether, if girls' freedom and opportunities continue to expand, more aggressive behaviors in childhood will still be associated with maleness in their minds.

Gender identity disorders are to be differentiated from psychotic delusions of being the other gender or having the sexual organs of the other gender.

Affective states often include a depressed mood, and may reach despair of suicidal proportions. Negative and aggressive feelings toward gendered body parts are common (e.g., "I hate my breasts and want to cut them off!"). Individuals who cross-dress on occasion report that they feel different internally when in a female versus male persona. One male transvestite, for example, commented on how soft, warm, and receptive he felt when in drag, whereas when dressed as a man, he felt more angular, aggressive, and impatient.

Cognitive patterns of individuals with gender identity disorders generally do not show loss of reality testing. People who suffer on the basis of the disparity between their psychological and morphological gender may be deeply and constantly preoccupied with that discordance.

Somatic states may include intense focus on and discomfort with selected body parts that are viewed as "not me." The suffering that may accompany their psychological dilemma makes individuals with gender identity disorders highly susceptible to substance abuse and addiction.

Relationship patterns vary over a wide range from those who are isolated to those with deep and enduring ties. The interwoven and disjunctive relationships among sexual orientation, gender identity, and gender role in the individual patient demonstrate the complexity of human sexuality.

Clinical Illustrations

A 46-year-old electrical engineer gave a history of life-long episodes of depression and alcoholism. His wife of sixteen years had left him two years earlier. Balding, stocky, and heavily muscled, he had been a bomber pilot in a recent war and enjoyed watching the destruction below after dropping his bombs. Now, he felt, was the time to assume his real persona, a female who could receive the care that he felt was precluded by his male presentation. He explained that he had no interest in a male sexual partner, but believed that only as his true female self could he realize an intimate relationship with a female partner. He began living as a woman not only on weekends, as he had for some time, but after work as well. He had electrolysis and took hormones to develop breasts but did not pursue sex re-assignment surgery. His depression lifted, and he stopped drinking. He began long-neglected proper medical and dental treatments. He gave up his career and began working as a secretary. He had a few brief romances with women. From age 50 until his death at 68 he lived a stable and satisfying life as a woman.

This man did not show evidence of schizophrenia or the other conventionally diagnosed psychotic disorders. He was intent on changing his body to attain congruence with an inner experience of great intensity. While the same drive is seen in women requesting sex change, relationships seem to play a greater role in their decisions.

A 30-year-old woman had lived as a man since the age of 17, when she had been discovered in a sexual relationship with another girl. Her devoutly religious father beat her, and when she refused to repent and to promise to agree to an arranged marriage, he disowned her and banished her from the home. She assumed a male identity, found work as a carpenter's assistant, and eventually became a skilled cabinet-maker in a furniture factory. After several years of alcoholism she, now he, joined AA. Sober now for four years and in a committed relationship with a woman, he wanted a double mastectomy to relieve him of having to flatten his breasts with a binder. He took male hormones, which gave him some facial hair. He was not interested in an attempt to construct a penis, but expressed his concern to provide his lover with an appropriately male-looking partner for the small town to which they had recently moved.

S309. Factitious Disorders

Sometimes called Münchausen's syndrome, factitious disorders are mental health conditions in which a patient intentionally produces or feigns physical or psychological symptoms. Little is known about the etiology, family patterns, or predisposing factors except that individuals with this diagnosis typically have a prior history of early (and possibly traumatizing) medical treatment. Psychoanalytic experience suggests that not infrequently factitious phenomena may be understood as a variant of posttraumatic stress disorder, in which patients reenact painful illnesses or surgeries in an effort to feel that *this* time, they are in control of what in childhood was inflicted on them. They may also have defined their sense of self in terms of their physical suffering. Individuals with factitious disorders are famously difficult to treat medically and are highly refractory to psychotherapy.

In recent years, there has been attention to a variant of this psychology, often called "Munchausen by Proxy Syndrome," in which individuals (usually parents but sometimes a nurse or other caretaker) repeatedly cause illness or physical harm to their child or a person in their care (Schreier & Libow, 1993). Perpetrators of these acts deny their role in the damage—sometimes even in the face of videotaped evidence of their destructive activity—and present themselves to medical personnel in states of great distress over the health crisis of the person they have harmed.

DSM-IV-TR Classification
Factitious Disorders

- Factitious Disorder
  - With Predominantly Psychological Signs and Symptoms
  - With Predominantly Physical Signs and Symptoms
  - With Combined Psychological and Physical Signs and Symptoms
  - Factitious Disorder not otherwise specified

Internal Experience of Factitious Disorders

Individuals with factitious disorders may exhibit a wide range of *affective states*, from anxiety over an alleged physical symptom to hostile expectations that medical professionals do not believe them. The overriding affective tone, however, is one of superficiality rather than emotional depth. A manipulative, opportunistic quality is often present. Despite the patient's seemingly sincere insistence on the seriousness of a physical or psychological ailment, it may be difficult for the clinician to feel empathy or concern.

Cognitive patterns involve the physical or psychological complaint of the moment coupled with ruminations about how to get medical professionals to take the complaint seriously. Patients with factitious disorders may be chronically preoccupied cognitively with persuading themselves as well as others of the reality of their suffering. They may be more or less obsessed with their connection to physicians and others on whom they feel medically dependent.

Somatic states may include chronic tension when desired care is not forthcoming. Some patients with factitious disorders, in their quest for attention from doctors or hospital personnel, inflict serious injury upon themselves. Others have succeeded in persuading previous physicians to do unnecessary surgeries. In such instances, the body may be permanently compromised. In a condition known as "Munchausens by Proxy Syndrome" (a disorder on which there had not been enough research for it to be included in the last edition of the DSM), patients deliberately damage the body of someone else, usually their children, evidently out of an unconscious wish to enact a personal drama and to reinforce the strength of a relationship with a medical professional who figures into their fantasy life.

Relationship patterns tend to be needy and dependent, with a great deal of negativism and dissatisfaction underlying an initial overt compliance. In their effort to get their complaints taken seriously, patients may exaggerate the symptom description, thereby eliciting irritation from others. It is common for others to experience the individual with this disorder as unreliable, manipulative, self-dramatizing, and difficult.

Clinical Illustration

A 42-year-old woman with a history of multiple surgeries for congenital abnormalities expressed the firm conviction that "I need surgery for my gall bladder because I have pain in my stomach all the time." Multiple complete medical evaluations, including full gastrointestinal workups, were negative. During a course of intensive psychotherapy, she was able to experience feelings of anger, fear, and helplessness associated with her childhood surgeries. She complained poignantly about her parents "handling me like a fragile piece of glass." She gradually was able to explore her potential for more assertiveness. Eventually, she confessed, "I ate spicy foods that gave me pain because I felt like my stomach pain was a friend."

S310. Impulse-Control Disorders

In DSM-IV-TR, the impulse-control disorders not classified elsewhere in the manual include the following diagnoses: intermittent explosive disorder, kleptomania, pyromania, pathological gambling, trichotillomania, and impulse-control disorders not otherwise specified. The essential feature of impulse-control disorders is the failure to resist the temptation to perform an act that is harmful to oneself or others. In addition, for most of these disorders, the individual feels an increasing sense of tension or arousal before committing the act; experiences pleasure, gratification, or relief at the time of committing the act; and may feel regret, self-reproach, or guilt following the act.

Intermittent explosive disorder is characterized by a failure to resist aggressive impulses, resulting in serious physical assaults or destruction of property. Individuals with explosive tendencies may feel deep contrition about their episodes of rage and violence, or they may rationalize them as warranted by the situation they were in.

Kleptomania is characterized by the recurrent failure to resist impulses to steal objects not needed for any personal or monetary value. Many individuals with kleptomania experience the impulse to steal as ego-dystonic and morally problematic. They fear being apprehended and may feel depressed or guilty about the thievery.

Pyromania is characterized by a pattern of fire-setting for pleasure or relief of tension, often with advance planning and preparation. Fire-setting incidents are episodic and may wax and wane in frequency.

Pathological gambling includes recurrent, persistent, and maladaptive gambling behavior, which disrupts personal, family, or vocational pursuits. Individuals who gamble in highly self-destructive ways report experiencing a "rush" when gambling and may show cognitive distortions such as denial, superstition, overconfidence, and a sense of grandiose power and control. Pathological gambling typically begins in early adolescence in males and later in females. For most, the course is insidious, with the urge to gamble increasing during periods of stress. States of dysphoria, depression, and boredom often precede and precipitate episodes of gambling, but they can also come as an aftermath of a gambling run. Frequent consequences of binge gambling (most often associated with losing) are anxiety (often rising to panic), agitation, shame, guilt, and feelings of doom. Not infrequently, the repetitious gambling cycles are linked to painful childhood experiences.

Trichotillomania involves recurrent, compulsive hair-pulling at a frequency that causes noticeable hair loss. The pulling gives a sense of gratification and/or relief of tension. Individuals with this disorder may also examine the hair root, twirl the strand, pull it between the teeth, or eat it (trichophagia). The most common sites are the scalp, eyebrows, and eyelashes. Despite the overt evidence of their disorder, those afflicted with trichotillomania typically pull out their hair only in private and deny that they do so. They may go to great lengths to conceal their behavior and its effects. This secrecy may reflect a deep shame or an unawareness (based on dissociation) when the act is occurring, or both. The age of onset for trichotillomania is usually before young adulthood, with peaks at 5 to 8 years old and around age 13. Some individuals have continuous symptoms for decades, while in others the disorder may remit for weeks, months, or years at a time.

Impulse-control disorders are chronic and episodic, and rates of spontaneous remission are unknown. Patients tend to be refractory to treatment and have a reputation among mental health professionals for poor insight and cooperation. Because the impulsive behavior is psychologically rewarding and even "addictive" (because of its self-stimulating or self-soothing effects), it is unlikely that patients with such behaviors will be motivated for treatment until they run into severe negative consequences of their acts. Epidemiological studies suggest that afflicted individuals (and their relatives) are at high risk for alcohol and other substance abuse disorders, obsessive-compulsive disorder, anxiety disorders, mood disorders, and other diagnoses. Except for trichotillomania and klepto-mania, these diagnoses are more common in men. There is limited information available on the course of most of the impulse disorders.

DSM-IV-TR Classification
Impulse-Control Disorders Not Elsewhere Classified

- Intermittent Explosive Disorder
- Kleptomania
- Pyromania
- Pathological Gambling
- Trichotillomania
- Impulse-Control Disorder not otherwise specified

The Internal Experience of Impulse-Control Disorders

Affective states observed in impulse-control disorders often include vacillations between feelings of emptiness or apathy, longing for the excitement or soothing that the behavior provides, and shame, fear, and depression. A young woman with trichotillomania, for example, may feel intensely stressed internally until she pulls out some hair, after which she may feel a diffuse relief. Often absent is a mature sense of regret that motivates change. Instead, affective states are more typical of those experienced by a young child and are not well integrated with thoughts.

Cognitive patterns are more notable for absence of thought than presence of problematic thoughts. The behaviors may have an automatic quality, reflecting dissociation from thinking processes that involve long-term considerations. Early personal memories may be curiously vague or lacking. There may be obsessive concern with getting opportunities to enact the impulsive behavior.

Somatic states that accompany these disorders may include hypo- and hyper-arousal as well as gastrointestinal symptoms and palpitations.

Relationship patterns often suffer from the disorders themselves and the psy-chology that tends to accompany them. People living with someone who sets fires or steals or explodes in violence or gambles away the family nest egg are rarely tolerant and forgiving; most of these disorders take a severe toll on rela-tionships. Individuals with impulse disorders tend to be reluctant patients; they

are frequently seen by court order or when confronted with the legal consequences of their actions. Genuine therapeutic relationships are, as a result, difficult to make in the absence of strong internal motivation to change, and require
patience with patients' reluctance to try to understand and control obviously
problematic behaviors.

Clinical Illustrations

Trichotillomania

A 22-year-old woman in therapy described some of her experiences quite vividly. "I was feeling weird, almost like when you have an itch that you need to
scratch. It just wouldn't go away, and it got worse and worse until I just had to
do it, I pulled at my eyelashes, pulled out a few. And then I felt a sense of peace,
the itch was gone. I felt really good, actually." She went on to elaborate, "I just
can't help it; it's like there is something inside me that makes me do it and then
I do it. When I'm done, it's like I can't even remember that I felt that way, until I
have to do it again."

Thus, she felt a complete disconnection between the action and the realization that she had done it. She also experienced intense feelings of shame and
embarrassment: "I was watching TV. I guess I was pulling out my hair. I didn't
really notice until this morning, when I saw that it was thinner over here." She
went on to say, "I don't know why I do it. I can't help it. But then I see the mirror the next day and it's so bad I have to spray some stuff onto my scalp so it
doesn't look so thin in certain spots. I'm sure people notice anyway. It's so
embarrassing; I look terrible."

Pathological Gambling

An articulate psychologist, who had been traumatized by his father's violent
suicide when he was 13 years old, described how his gambling cycles repeated the
feelings of loss, loneliness, and gloomy mood he experienced as a teen in the
aftermath of that loss. There seemed to be an element of a search for mastery
("I'm suffering again, but this time I'm in charge of what happens to me") in his
gambling behavior. He said, "I feel better for a while, anticipating going to the
casino, figuring the odds at the tables, placing my bets—but then I lose. I feel
horrible, guilty that I've lost control again . . . like I'll never recover from my
[mounting] debt . . . I panic." Spontaneously, he added, "It's like I retraumatize
myself . . . I feel like I felt as a teenager, all alone in my room, everything so dark
and gloomy, so hopeless."

Related studies include: Castelnuovo-Tedesco, 1974; Chadwick, 1925; Chused, 1990; Greenberg, 1966; Novick & Novick, 1987, Ornstein, Gropper, & Bogner, 1983; Rotenberg, 1997; Sperling, 1968; Swift & Cody, 1998; Zavitzianos,
1971, 1982.

S311. Addictive/Substance Use Disorders

Substance use disorders are among the most prevalent mental disorders in our society. Except for nicotine dependence, addiction to alcohol continues to be the most common substance-related disorder, followed by marijuana dependence. Abuse of cocaine, heroin, prescription pain relievers, and, increasingly, metham-phetamines is also common.

Acute and chronic distress is at the heart of addictive behavior. There is significant variation among individuals in the degree to which the distress is experienced consciously. At one extreme, painful affects are intense and intolerable; at the other, distressed affect is experienced as only vaguely dysphoric, confusing, and inarticulable. The range of psychopathology involved may also be highly variable. Underlying personality disturbance may be as severe as pervasive borderline-level personality disorders, or may be limited to vulnerabilities in specific sectors of personality organization. Psychotic and neurotic processes and the associated negative affects may also be involved; many individuals with diagnosed or undiagnosed mental pain attempt self-medication with substances. In all cases, self-care functions are notable for their absence or deterioration; painful affects interact with diminished cognitive and emotional capacities to anticipate dangers. Continued use precipitates physiologic and addictive mechanisms.

In the main, addictive vulnerabilities are the result of developmental deficits in ego and self-organization related to neglectful, abusive, and chaotic family environments that often include substance abuse by others. Capacities for regulating emotions, self-esteem, relationships, and self-care are deeply affected by these deficits. Substances are employed to ameliorate, control, change, or mute affective experiences that are too intense or confusing.

In taking a history from any patient, it is important to ask about substance use. If the therapist inquires in an open manner, free of moralizing or critical overtones, the patient is more likely to be honest about the kind and amount of substances regularly ingested. Denial of dependency on substances is ubiquitous among addicted individuals.

The DSM-IV-TR sections on substance-induced disorders are not included in this section. They include toxic and withdrawal reactions for all the substance-related disorders listed in the following table. The substance-induced disorders principally involve pharmacologic toxicity and physiologic reactions, whereas the substance-related disorders reviewed in this section address the psychodynamics of substance use and dependence.

DSM-IV-TR Classification Substance-Related Disorders	

■ Alcohol-Related Disorders
  • Alcohol Use Disorders
  • Alcohol-Induced Disorders
■ Amphetamine (or Amphetamine-Like)-Related Disorders
  • Amphetamine Use Disorders
  • Amphetamine-Induced Disorders
■ Caffeine-Related Disorders
  • Caffeine-Induced Disorders
■ Cannabis-Related Disorders
  • Cannabis Use Disorders
  • Cannabis-Induced Disorders
■ Cocaine-Related Disorders
  • Cocaine Use Disorders
  • Cocaine-Induced Disorders
■ Hallucinogen-Related Disorders
  • Hallucinogen Use Disorders
  • Hallucinogen-Induced Disorders
■ Inhalant-Related Disorders
  • Inhalant Use Disorders
  • Inhalant-Induced Disorders
	■ Nicotine-Related Disorders
	  • Nicotine Use Disorders
	  • Nicotine-Induced Disorders
	■ Opioid-Related Disorders
	  • Opioid Use Disorders
	  • Opioid-Induced Disorders
	■ Phencyclidine (or Phencyclidine-Like)-Related Disorders
	  • Phencyclidine Use Disorders
	  • Phencyclidine-Induced Disorders
	■ Sedative-, Hypnotic-, or Anxiolytic-Related Disorders
	  • Sedative, Hypnotic, or Anxiolytic Use Disorders
	  • Sedative-, Hypnotic-, or Anxiolytic-Induced Disorders
	■ Polysubstance-Related Disorder
	  • Polysubstance Dependence
	■ Other (or Unknown) Substance-Related Disorders
	  • Other (or Unknown) Substance Use Disorders
	  • Other (or Unknown) Substance-Induced Disorders

The Internal Experience of Addictive/Substance Use Disorders

In terms of *affective states*, drugs, including alcohol, change or make more bearable the distressing feelings experienced by people who become dependent upon addictive substances. Depending on the affects that are most painful for the individual, a particular class of drugs may be preferred. Opiates help a person to feel "calm, mellow or normal." Stimulants counter low energy, feelings of weakness, and feelings of being unloved; they may also be employed by high-energy individuals to augment a preferred hypomanic adaptation. Sedatives (e.g., alcohol, benzodiazepines, barbiturates) in high doses drown out negative, unwelcome feelings; in low doses, they can overcome feelings of isolation and allow feelings of closeness and warmth (e.g., "I can feel like one of the guys ... I can join the human race").

Following are some of the main ways that addiction-prone individuals experience their emotional life.

- Feelings of boredom and depression, of unworthiness alternating with demandingness are common.

- Intense feelings of rage or anger can fester or erupt. Such feelings may be associated with agitation or a sense of falling apart. Individuals dependent on opiates, for example, say the drug acts to calm or contain their feelings or to make them feel normal.

- Continued, chronic use causes physical need and desire for drugs. Patients report feeling awful without their drug of choice; they may feel panic if they cannot obtain the drug to which they have become addicted.

- As physical dependence develops, many of the feelings relieved by drugs are made more intense and intolerable when the drugs are abruptly withdrawn.

Cognitive patterns are notable for centering on rationalizations that support addiction. The dangers of addiction are denied, via comments such as, "I never thought about it." The fact of addiction is often disavowed via protests such as, "I can stop at any time." When confronted with the realities of their condition, substance-abusing individuals tend to respond with comments prefaced by denial, such as, "No, I'm not afraid when I shoot drugs."

Relationship patterns may include intense feelings of neediness alternating with protests that one has no such needs. Life may feel unmanageable and unregulated to both the substance-dependent person and those close to him or her. Relationships may be described as shaky or untrustworthy or disappointing. Partners who put pressure on the substance abuser to get help are typically put off and devalued.

Clinical Illustration

The following patient suffered with intense emotions, chronic depression, and difficult interpersonal relations. His impulsive and risky behaviors revealed poor self-care in that he invariably failed to anticipate the dangers of his actions. The case also illustrates the short-term adaptive effects of addictive drugs, demonstrating how they can relieve emotional suffering and counter certain restricting personality characteristics.

The patient first came to therapy at age twenty-nine, having just started treatment in a methadone maintenance program. Starting in early adolescence, he heavily used and abused sedatives and stimulants (amphetamines). In his words, "I was less afraid . . . I felt I could take on anyone when I was speeding." His longstanding shaky self-esteem and tenuous capacity to relate to others lent a self-effacing and reticent quality to his interpersonal dealings, including the way he related in psychotherapy. He described how dating was difficult because he feared rejection, and he worried about how awkward he would appear if he showed his needs. His combination of charm and vulnerability made him highly appealing.

At the same time, a more brutal, violent, sadistic side was evident in the intensity of his boast that nobody could or would "screw me over." When describing his day-to-day encounters, he could adopt a chilling veneer of self-sufficiency and disdain for other peoples' needs and feelings. He was not reluctant to convey to the therapist how much he enjoyed stalking younger or weaker kids "to beat on them and hurt them." In contrast to his generally gentle and solicitous veneer, his penchant for aggression was also suggested by a keen attraction to risky versions of athletics, martial arts, and high-performance motorcycles and automobiles. He was quick to dismiss with bravado the seriousness of injuries sustained in such activities. If asked about a visible wound or any associated pain, he would say, "Nah, doc, it doesn't bother me," even while he was wincing or moving about in a guarded manner.

In his adolescence he used both depressants and amphetamines to overcome his shyness. He reported that speed "made me feel strong and sure of myself." It made him feel powerful and helped him to overcome feelings of vulnerability and "weakness" in social situations and contact sports. Barbiturates "made me feel less shy and uptight." He emphasized that they would loosen him up so that he could more easily relate to his peers. As he continued to use amphetamines, he realized that they also helped to counter his low self-esteem and inertia, indications of a longstanding depression. Progressive reliance on stimulants empowered him ("I felt twice as powerful") and frequently led to brutal, punishing fights. As time went on, he realized that amphetamines caused him profound dysphoria and fear and heightened his sadism, which took the form of beating someone up or being cruel to his pet cats. He shyly described how ashamed he felt about losing his temper and throwing a cat against the wall.

As he approached his mid-twenties, his uncontrolled violence and rage was interfering with his friendships, work, and life in general. At that point, he discovered heroin and quickly became dependent on it. In contrast to the amphetamines and sedatives, narcotics immediately impressed him as calming and containing. When asked what heroin did for him, he said "I felt calm and more normal than I had ever felt in my life." He acknowledged a marked diminution in his rage and aggressiveness and reported feeling more organized, in control, and able to work.

Related studies include: Dodes, 1990, 1996; Khantzian, 1978, 1985, 1997; Krystal, 1988; Krystal & Raskin, 1970; McDougall, 1984; Milkman & Frosch, 1973; Wilson, Passik, Faude, Abrams, & Gordon, 1989; Wurmser, 1974.

S312. Psychotic Disorders

DSM-IV-TR lists the following under the heading of psychotic disorders: schizophrenia; schizophreniform disorder; schizoaffective disorder; delusional disorder; brief psychotic disorder; shared psychotic disorder; psychotic disorder due to a general medical condition (previously called an organic psychosis); substance-induced psychotic disorder; and psychotic disorder not otherwise specified. While individuals with these disorders all have psychotic symptoms, there are many features that distinguish these illnesses from one another.

Schizophrenia includes the constellation of both positive symptoms (e.g., delusions, hallucinations, disorganized thinking and speech, disorganized or catatonic behavior) and negative symptoms (e.g., flattened affect, apathy, withdrawal, and anhedonia). To meet the DSM criteria for the disorder, these symptoms should have persisted for at least one month and have impaired a person's functioning at work (or school), in interpersonal relations, or with self-care. There are five defined subtypes: paranoid, disorganized (previously hebephrenic), catatonic, undifferentiated, and residual. Among other possible features of schizophrenia are inappropriate affect, depression, anxiety, phobias, difficulties sleeping, poor insight, somatic concerns, violent behavior, and a high rate of suicide attempts.

Onset of schizophrenia usually occurs between the late teens and mid-thirties and may be abrupt or insidious. Most people with the disorder experience a prodromal phase, when those to whom they are close describe them as "slipping away." The outcome of schizophrenia varies. Some patients with the disorder get progressively worse, some experience a partial or full remission, and others remain stable yet chronically ill. Although research indicates a genetic contribution to the etiology of schizophrenia, there is also much evidence for the significance of personal experiences and environment (Read & Ross, 2003; Read, Mosher, & Bentall, 2004; Karon, 2003). Interaction of biological and experiential factors has engaged many researchers.

Schizophreniform disorder is an illness identical to schizophrenia except for its short course and lower degree of impairment in social and occupational functioning. If symptoms persist beyond six months, the diagnosis is changed to schizophrenia. Some studies suggest that one-third of the patients diagnosed this way recover within six months, retaining the diagnosis of schizophreniform disorder, while the remaining two-thirds progress to a final diagnosis of schizophrenia or schizoaffective disorder. These patterns must be regarded with caution because it is difficult to control for the effects of optimal treatment approaches. Most studies are not able to ascertain whether each case is approached in a truly optimal manner (e.g., psychosocial and family support; psychotherapeutic work; medication; reduction of likely precipitants, and so on).

Developing countries have higher prevalence rates of schizophreniform disorder than developed countries.

Schizoaffective disorder is defined by the concomitant occurrence of both a mood disorder episode (major depressive, manic, or mixed) and symptoms of schizophrenia. Additionally, the individual experiences either hallucinations or delusions without mood symptoms for at least two weeks. The DSM specifies two types, determined by the nature of the mood symptoms: bipolar type (manic or mixed episode) and depressive type (major depressive episode). Onset can occur anywhere between adolescence and late in life, but schizoaffective disorder most commonly begins in early adulthood. Although the condition appears to be less common than schizophrenia, prevalence rates for schizoaffective disorder are unknown. As with schizophrenia, there are strong indications of a genetic component to the etiology of the illness.

Delusional disorder is diagnosed when an individual has nonbizarre delusions (delusions with plausible themes and situations; e.g., of being followed) for at least one month. Symptoms of schizophrenia are not present unless related directly to the delusion(s), and mood episodes, if present, are brief. Levels of functioning and behavior vary, but generally are less impaired and disorganized compared with levels of functioning in those diagnosed with schizophrenia.

A particular variant of delusional disorder reported in the psychoanalytic literature, but never specifically noted in DSM, is that of hysterical psychosis, occurring usually (but not only) in individuals of hysterical character, and emerging within the context of specific severe stress and traumata, or within the transference reactions in intensive psychoanalytic therapy (and then called transference psychosis) (Wallerstein, 1967). This consists of severe distortions of reality testing including rigidly held delusions and even hallucinations, but without signs pathognomic of schizophrenia, such as thought disorder. When this occurs in a treatment context, it may be confined there or it may spill over into the patient's ongoing life outside. It is an eminently psychotherapeutically treatable psychotic disorder.

DSM-IV-TR includes seven subtypes of delusional disorder: erotomanic, grandiose, jealous, persecutory, somatic, mixed, and unspecified. The persecutory type is the most common. Depending on the subtype, other symptoms commonly observed in those with delusional disorders are ideas of reference, irritable or dysmorphic mood, violent behavior, litigious behavior, and somatic complaints. Delusional disorders tend to be found in individuals with personality disorders in the low borderline range. Age of onset is variable, ranging from adolescence to late in life. The course of the illness is also variable, ranging from full remissions to continual relapses. Delusional disorder is relatively uncommon. Prior to DSM III, delusional disorders were usually designated as paranoid schizophrenia.

Brief psychotic disorder is identified by the presence of symptoms of schizophrenia (e.g., delusions, hallucinations, disorganized thinking, speech, or behavior) for at least one day but less than one month, followed by a return to premorbid levels of functioning. Although brief, this disorder can be severe and presents a high risk for suicide. Personality disorders at the borderline level of organization may predispose the individual to the development of this condition. Average age of onset is the late 20s to early 30s. During World War II, psychotic collapses under combat stress, which were often reversed with intensive hypnoanalytic or narcoanalytic treatments, were designated as "three-day schizophrenia."

A shared psychotic disorder (*folie à deux*) occurs when an individual begins to take on the delusion of someone with whom he or she is involved, who already has a psychotic disorder. Typically, the psychotic person (the "primary case") is more dominant in the relationship and insinuates the disorder into the more passive and previously non-psychotic individual. The delusional beliefs of the submissive person often disappear when the relationship is terminated. Very little is known about the prevalence of this disorder; some argue that many cases go unrecognized. The course is variable, often depending upon the length of the relationship in which it occurs.

DSM-IV-TR Classification
Schizophrenia and Other Psychotic Disorders

- Schizophrenia
  - Paranoid Type
  - Disorganized Type
  - Catatonic Type
  - Undifferentiated Type
  - Residual Type
- Schizophreniform Disorder
- Schizoaffective Disorder
- Delusional Disorder
- Brief Psychotic Disorder
- Shared Psychotic Disorder
- Psychotic Disorder Due to . . . *[Indicate the General Medical Decision]*
- With Delusions
- With Hallucinations
- Substance-Induced Psychotic Disorder
- Psychotic Disorder not otherwise specified

The Internal Experience of Psychosis

While the previous depictions of the various psychotic disorders identify qualities that are observable in those afflicted, they do not capture the internal world of someone suffering from any of these illnesses. Below is a list of subjective experiences expressed by those grappling with schizophrenia and other psychotic disorders.

Affective states may include:

- Feelings of being empty, numb, adrift, and detached from emotions and from other people, often accompanied by difficulty expressing or identifying any feelings
- Intense feelings of anxiety, nervousness, and wishes to withdraw into sleep or isolation
- Intense anger in response to perceived threats from others
- Urgent neediness and fears of being left alone, often accompanied by anxiety and intense urges to cling to anyone available

Other possible affective patterns include feelings of extreme isolation, suspicion, and withdrawal. Individuals suffering a psychotic breakdown may retreat to an inner world in preference to remaining attached to the outer world.

Cognitive patterns may include being distracted, unable to focus, or overwhelmed by pressing thoughts that do not make sense to other people. Sometimes these reactions are accompanied by difficulties remembering recent events. Feelings of being disoriented or out of synch with other people may be pervasive. The experience of hearing, seeing, feeling, or smelling things that are not present in reality can be deeply disturbing. Such hallucinations are usually experienced as intrusive, uncomfortable, degrading or threatening, but on occasion they may be experienced as calming or interpreted as evidence of specialness. A sense of being transparent, vulnerable, and easily invaded, of being an open book, may precipitate severe anxiety or, in extreme cases, terror that other people can read or control one's mind. Delusions of omnipotence (feelings of great power and importance that have gone unnoticed by other people, or feelings of special powers of prophecy, mind-reading, and mind-control) and ideas of reference (feeling that everything that happens pertains to oneself) may be both comforting and terrifying, as such power is expected to evoke attacks by envious others. In addition, there can be shame, deep sadness, and jealousy, often momentary but intolerably intense. A psychotic person may have deep convictions of being unlikable or toxic and may, on that basis, be suicidal. Intense self-disgust may lead to the beliefs that one will inevitably be rejected or abandoned. Individuals with psychotic disorders often believe that other people feel as they do, or that they know what other people are feeling. In the absence of such certainty, they may feel ungrounded, unsure of their own corporeal reality; e.g., "Do I really exist? Am I really here?"

Somatic states include a range of sensations, often related to particular delusional beliefs (e.g., "my guts are rotting," "my head is exploding," "I am not human and have no body"). Sleeping, eating, gastrointestinal, and cardiovascular symptoms are common.

Relationship patterns vary from needy and clinging (especially with a trusted person such as a family member, therapist, or friend) to avoidant and suspicious. People who are close to the psychotic person may feel frightened, helpless, or exasperated, as their efforts to calm the patient fail, and their attempts to persuade the patient of their own version of reality are rejected.

Clinical Illustration

A 21-year-old woman who was outgoing, fearful, anxious, and slightly fragmented in her thought patterns engaged in her first sexual relationship with a man she did not know well. Over the next week, she experienced agitation and hyperarousal, and began believing that he was now controlling her thoughts. A few days later, she began believing that two of her professors were following her and that other students were talking about her. She began hearing voices. She was hospitalized and experienced recurrent episodes of hallucinations and delusions.

Related studies include: Abramson, 2001; Auerbach & Blatt, 1996; Mariotti, 2000; Beneditti, 1999; Cohen, 1995; Feinsilver, 1980; Fowler, Hilsenroth, & Piers, 2001; Karon, 1989; Robbins, 2002; Salonen, 2000, 2002; Searles 1965, 1979, 1986; Stolorow & Stolorow, 1989.

S313. Mental Disorders Based on a General Medical Condition

Mental disorders based on a general medical condition cover a wide range of conditions from degenerative dementia of the Alzheimer's type to disorders produced by various substance-abuse patterns. The category also covers a wide range of reactions, from gradual changes in memory, mood, thinking, and behavior, to acute states of delirium. DSM-IV-TR describes in detail each of these different types, along with their associated symptoms. There follows a brief description of the subjective states that may accompany these disorders and some vignettes that may encourage clinicians to try to capture the distinctive qualities of their patients' experiences with organic compromise.

DSM-IV-TR Classification
Delirium, Dementia, Amnestic, and Other Cognitive Disorders

Delirium
- Delirium Due to . . . *[Indicate the General Medical Condition]*
- Substance Intoxication Delirium
- Substance Withdrawal Delirium
- Delirium Due to Multiple Etiologies
- Delirium not otherwise specified

Dementia
- Dementia of the Alzheimer's Type, With Early Onset
  - Without Behavioral Disturbance
  - With Behavioral Disturbance
- Dementia of the Alzheimer's Type, With Late Onset
  - Without Behavioral Disturbance
  - With Behavioral Disturbance
- Vascular Dementia
  - Uncomplicated
  - With Delirium
  - With Delusions
  - With Depressed Mood
- Dementia Due to HIV Disease
- Dementia Due to Head Trauma

Dementia (continued)
- Dementia Due to Parkinson's
- Dementia Due to Huntington's
- Dementia Due to Pick's Disease
- Dementia Due to Creutzfeldt-Jakob Disease
- Dementia due to . . . *[Indicate the General Medical Condition not listed above]*
- Substance-Induced Persisting Dementia
- Dementia Due to Multiple Etiologies
- Dementia not otherwise specified
- Amnestic Disorders
- Amnestic Disorder Due to . . . *[Indicate General Medical Condition]*
- Substance-Induced Persisting Amnestic Disorder
- Amnestic Disorder not otherwise specified

Other Cognitive Disorders
- Cognitive Disorder not otherwise specified

The Internal Experience of Mental Disorders Based on a General Medical Condition

With the most common types of gradual-onset organicity associated with memory loss, *affect states* may include a combination of anxiety, fear, and depression. Depression or sadness often emerges with intimate awareness of lost capacities. Extreme feelings of helplessness and resignation can not only intensify depressive mood states, but may lead to secondary memory loss. Along with memory loss, there are often compromises in the individual's capacity to sequence actions and ideas, to follow directions, or to carry out novel problem-solving activities. These problems may further lead to feelings of helplessness, inadequacy, loss, and depression.

Not infrequently, individuals also experience significant fear and anxiety because of their difficulties in carrying out what in the past had been effortless daily activities. The anxieties range from fear of being alone and unprotected, to fear of injury, and fear of losing control and hurting others. Outright panic and agitation can occur in especially challenging situations without adequate and familiar support. Acute states of delirium are often accompanied by catastrophic affective reactions involving intense fear, panic, and agitation. Affective states are often so intense and overwhelming that only the provision of supportive soothing structure, along with appropriate medical management, can alter them.

Cognitive patterns associated with organic problems tend to parallel the affective states. Depressive states, for example, are often accompanied by preoccupation with helplessness, further loss, and, in some individuals, intermittent anger and suspiciousness (sometimes secondary to compromised reality testing). An inability to accept or comprehend, and a need to deny lessening mental capacities, may also characterize thoughts (e.g., individuals may insist on the reality of their immediate perceptions, ignoring the evidence that they have gotten something wrong). As memory loss progresses, individuals may live more and more in the affective states and mental content of the moment, sometimes showing immediate insight and cleverness without a sense of continuity to the recent past. During states of delirium, there are often rapidly shifting mental contents expressed in a fragmented manner.

Somatic states may mirror the affective patterns. They include chest pain, palpitations, headaches, gastrointestinal symptoms, and sleeping and eating difficulties, as well as agitation and apathy.

Relationship patterns also tend to be governed by mood states. They range from needy and dependent to unrealistically independent and abusive. Supportive relationships that provide continuity, soothing guidance, and appropriate levels of challenge are often needed and appreciated (even if not acknowledged verbally).

Clinical Illustration

A 77-year-old man living in a retirement village began having frequent lapses of memory. He became more and more anxious. He began developing compulsive rituals to make sure he did basic things like turning off the stove and locking the door. Increasingly, however, he began worrying, "I must have a physical illness," even though he had had a recent complete evaluation by his internist, in which he was told that he was in good health and that his memory lapses appeared to be gradual and associated with aging rather than with any acute or new medical disorder. Over time, however, he became more convinced that there was something seriously wrong with his body. He frequently called his children to discuss various physical ailments, and he began making weekly visits to a gradually enlarging group of physicians. As his anxiety grew, he became increasingly preoccupied with thoughts of "skin cancers," "bone thinning," and other physical dangers.

Related studies include: Cohen & Jay, 1996; Hirsch, 2001; Kasl-Godley & Gatz, 2000; Kilchenstein, 1999; Orr-Andrawes, 1987; Palombo, 1993; Richartz & Frank, 2004; Wasson & Grunes, 1998; Willick, 1990.

REFERENCES

Bellak, L., Hurvich, M., & Gediman, H. (1973). *Ego functions in schizophrenics, neurotics, and normals*. New York: Wiley

Blatt, S. J. (2004). *Experiences of depression: Theoretical, research and clinical perspectives*. Washington, DC: American Psychological Association Press.

Bowlby, J. (1960). Separation anxiety. *International Journal of Psycho-Analysis, 41*, 89-113

Brenner, I. (2001). *Dissociation of trauma: Theory, phenomenology and technique*. Madison, CT: International Universities Press.

Brenner, I. (2004). *Psychic trauma: Dynamics, symptoms, and treatment*. Oxford: Rowman & Littlefield.

Brett, E. A. (1993). Classification of PTSD in DSM IV: Anxiety disorder, dissociative disorder, or stress disorder. In Davidson, R. T. & Foa, E. B. (Eds.), *Posttraumatic stress disorder: DSM-IV and beyond* (pp. 191–204). Washington DC: American Psychiatric Press.

Compton, A. (1992). The psychoanalytic view of phobias—Part IV: General theory of phobias and anxiety. *Psychoanalytic Quarterly, 61*, 426-446.

Danieli, Y., Brom, D., & Sills, J. (Eds.) (2005). *The trauma of terrorism*. New York: Haworth Maltreatment & Trauma Press.

Davies, J. M., & Frawley, M. G. (1994). *Treating the adult survivor of childhood sexual abuse: A psychoanalytic perspective*. New York: Basic Books.

Ferber, A. (1959) (Reporter). Phobias and their vicissitudes. *Journal of the American Psychoanalytic Association, 7*, 182-192.

Finkelhor, D. (Ed.) (1986). *A sourcebook on child sexual abuse*. Thousand Oaks, CA: Sage.

Freud, S. (1917). Fixation to traumas: The unconscious. Introductory Lectures on Psychoanalysis, Lecture XVIII. *Standard Edition, 16*, 273-285.

Freud, S. (1919). Lines of advance in psychoanalytic therapy. *Standard Edition, 17*, 159-168.

Freud, S. (1926). Inhibitions, symptoms and anxiety. *Standard Edition, 29*, 75-175, 1959.

Greenspan, S. I. (1997). *Developmentally based psychotherapy*. Madison, CT: International Universities Press.

Furst, S. (Ed.) (1967). *Psychic trauma*. New York: Basic Books.

Horowitz, M. J. (1976). *Stress response syndromes*. New York: Jason Aronson Press.

Karon, B. P. (2003). The tragedy of schizophrenia without psychotherapy. *Journal of the American Academy of Psychoanalysis and Dynamic Psychiatry, 31*, 89-118.

Kernberg, O. F. (1967). Borderline personality organization. *Journal of the American Psychoanalytic Association, 15*, 641-685.

Krystal, H. (Ed.) (1968). *Massive psychic trauma*. New York: International Universities Press.

Krystal, H. (1978). Trauma and affects. *Psychoanalytic Study of the Child, 33*, 81-116.

Krystal, H. (1988). *Integration and self-healing: Affect, trauma and alexithymia*. Hillsdale NJ: The Analytic Press.

McWilliams, N. (1994). *Psychoanalytic diagnosis: Understanding personality structure in the clinical process*. New York: Guilford Press.

Nelson, S. (2002). Physical symptoms in sexually abused women: Somatization or undetected injury? *Child Abuse Review, 11,* 51-64.

Perlman, S. D. (1999). *The therapist's emotional survival: Dealing with the pain of exploring trauma.* Northvale, NJ: Jason Aronson.

Read, J., Mosher, L. R., & Bentall, R. P. (Eds.) (2004). *Models of madness: Psychological, social, and biological approaches to schizophrenia.* East Sussex/New York: Brunner-Routledge.

Read, J., & Ross, C. A. (2003). Psychological trauma and psychosis: Another reason why people diagnosed schizophrenic must be offered psychological therapies. *Journal of the American Academy of Psychoanalysis and Dynamic Psychiatry, 31,* 247-268.

Schreier, H. A., & Libow, J. A. (1993). *Hurting for love: Munchausen by proxy syndrome.* New York: Guilford Publications

Shengold, L. (1989). *Soul murder: The effects of childhood abuse and deprivation.* New York: Ballantine.

Terr, L. (1995). *Unchained memories: True stories of traumatic memories, lost and found.* New York: Basic Books.

Thompson, L., Gallagher, D., & Czirr, R. (1988). Personality disorder and outcome in the treatment of late-life depression. *Journal of Geriatric Psychiatry, 21,* 133-146.

Ulman, R. B., & Brothers, J. (1988). *The shattered self: A psychoanalytic study of trauma.* Hillsdale, NJ: The Analytic Press.

van der Kolk, B. A., McFarlane, A. C., & Weisaeth, L. (Eds.) (1996). *Traumatic stress: The effects of overwhelming experience on mind, body, and society.* New York: Guilford Press.

Varvin, S. (2003). *Mental survival strategies after extreme traumatisation.* Copenhagen: Multivers..

Wallerstein, R. S. (1967). Reconstruction and mastery in the transference psychosis. *Journal of the American Psychoanalytic Association, 15,* 551–583.

Wallerstein, R. S. (1986). *Forty-two lives in treatment: A study of psychoanalysis and psychotherapy.* New York: Guilford.

Wilson, J. P., & Raphael, B. (Eds.) (1993). *International handbook of traumatic stress syndromes.* New York: Plenum.

Yehuda, R., & McFarlane, A. C. (1999). Conflict between current knowledge about posttraumatic stress disorder and its original conceptual basis. In M. Horowitz (Ed.), *Essential papers on posttraumatic stress disorder* (pp. 41-60). New York: New York University Press.

RELATED STUDIES

Aarons, Z. A. (1990). Depressive affect and it ideational content: A case study of dissatisfaction. *The International Journal of Psychoanalysis, 71,* 285-296.

Abramson, R. (2001). A cost-effective psychoanalytic treatment of a severely disturbed woman. *Journal of the American Academy of Psychoanalysis, 29,* 245-264.

Adams-Silvan, A., & Silvan, M. (1994). Paradise lost: A case of hysteria illustrating a specific dynamic of seduction trauma. *International Journal of Psycho-Analysis, 75,* 499-510.

Aisenstein, M. (1993). Psychosomatic solution or somatic outcome: The man from Burma. Psychotherapy of a case of haemorrhagic rectocolitis. *International Journal of Psycho-Analysis, 74,* 371-381.

Aisenstein, M., & Gibeault, A. (1991). The work of hypochondria: A contribution to the study of the specificity of hypochondria, in particular in relation to hysterical conversion and organic disease. *International Journal of Psycho-Analysis, 72,* 669-681.

Auerbach, J. S., & Blatt, S. J. (1996). Self-representation in severe psychopathology: the role of reflexive self-awareness. *Psychoanalytic Psychology, 13,* 297-341.

Badal, D. W. (1962). The repetitive cycle in depression. *International Journal of Psychoanalysis, 43,* 133–141.

Barrows, K. (1999). Ghosts in the swamp: Some aspects of splitting and their relationship to parental losses. *International Journal of Psycho-Analysis, 80,* 549-561.

Beidel, D.C., & Turner, S.M. (1998). *Shy Children, phobic adults: the nature and treatment of social phobia.* Washington, D.C.: American Psychological Association Books.

Bemporad, J. R., Beresin, E., Ratey, J. J., O'Driscoll, G., Lindem, K., & Herzog, D. B. (1992). A psychoanalytic study of eating disorders: I. A developmental profile of 67 cases. *Journal of the American Academy of Psychoanalysis, 20,* 509-531.

Bemporad, J. R., O'Driscoll, G., Beresin, E., Ratey, J. J., Lindem, K., & Herzog, D. B. (1992). A psychoanalytic study of eating disorders: II. Intergroup and intragroup comparisons. *Journal of the American Academy of Psychoanalysis, 20,* 533-541.

Beneditti, G. (1999). Interpretation and schizophrenia. *Journal of the American Academy of Psychoanalysis, 27,* 551-562.

Beresin, E. V., Gordon, C., & Herzog, D. B. (1989). The process of recovering from anorexia nervosa. *Journal of the American Academy of Psychoanalysis, 17,* 103-130.

Birsted-Breen, D. (1989). Working with an anorexic patient. *International Journal of Psycho-Analysis, 70,* 29-40.

Blank, H. R. (1954). Depression, hypomania, and depersonalization. *Psychoanalytic Quarterly, 23,* 20-37.

Blatt, S. (1974). Levels of object representation in anaclitic and introjective depression. *Psychoanalytic Study of the Child, 29,* 107-157.

Bonime, W. (1967). A case of depression in a homosexual young man. *Contemporary Psychoanalysis, 3,* 1-14.

Bonime, W. (1981). Anxiety: Feared loss of functional effectiveness. *The Journal of Contemporary Psychoanalysis, 17,* 69-90.

Brickman, B. (1992). The desomatizing selfobject transference: A case report. In W. J. Coburn (Series Ed.) & A. Goldberg (Vol. Ed.), *Progress in self psychology: Vol. 8. New therapeutic visions* (pp. 93-108). Hillsdale, NJ: Analytic Press.

Broden, A. R., & Myers, W. A. (1981). Hypochondriacal symptoms as derivatives of unconscious fantasies of being beaten or tortured. *Journal of the American Psychoanalytic Association, 29,* 535-557.

Bromberg, P. M. (2001). Treating patients with symptoms and symptoms with patience; Reflections on shame, dissociation, and eating disorders. *Psychoanalytic Dialogues, 11,* 891-912.

Bruch, H. (1973). *Eating disorders: Obesity, anorexia nervosa, and the person within.* New York: Basic Books.

Bruch, H. (1978). *The golden cage: The enigma of anorexia nervosa.* Cambridge: Harvard University Press.

Castelnuovo-Tedesco, P. (1974). Stealing, revenge and the Monte Cristo complex. *International Journal of Psycho-Analysis, 55,* 169-181.

Chadwick, M. (1925). A case of kleptomania in a girl of ten years. *International Journal of Psycho-Analysis, 6,* 300-312.

Chessick, R. D. (2001).OCD, OCPD: Acronyms do not make a disease. *Psychoanalytic Inquiry, 21,* 183-207.

Chused, J. F. (1990). Neutrality in the analysis of action-prone adolescents. *Journal of the American Psychoanalytic Association, 38,* 679-704.

Coen, S. J., & Sarno, J. E. (1989). Psychosomatic avoidance of conflict in back pain. *Journal of the American Academy of Psychoanalysis, 17,* 359-376.

Cohen, M. (1995). Schizophrenia, perception, and empathy. *Journal of American Academy of Psychoanalysis, 23,* 603-617.

Cohen, D., & Jay, S. M. (1996). Autistic barriers in the psychoanalysis of borderline adults. *International Journal of Psychoanalysis, 77*, 913-933.

Compton, A. (1992). The psychoanalytic view of phobias. *The Psychoanalytic Quarterly, 61*(2), 206-229

Compton, A. (1998). An investigation of anxious thought in patients with DSM-IV agoraphobia/panic disorder: Rationale and design. *Journal of the American Psychoanalytic Association, 46*, 691-721.

Crawford, J. (1996). The severed self: Gender as trauma. In W. J. Coburn (Series Ed.) & A. Goldberg (Vol. Ed.), *Progress in self psychology: Vol. 12. Basic ideas reconsidered* (pp. 269-283). Hillsdale, NJ: Analytic Press.

De Praingy, M., Digneton, J., Colin, F. (1982). Hypersomnias. Myth and reality. Global approach. *Ann Med Psychol (Paris), Sep-Oct;0*(8):829-41

Deutsch, H. (1929). The genesis of agoraphobia. *International Journal of Psychoanalysis, 10*:51-56

Dietz, I. J. (1995). The self-psychological approach to the bipolar spectrum disorders. *The Journal American Academy of Psychoanalysis, 23*, 475-492.

Dodes, L. M. (1990). Addiction, helplessness, and narcissistic rage. *Psychoanalytic Quarterly, 59*, 398-419.

Dodes, L. M. (1996). Compulsion and addiction. *Journal of the Psychoanalytic Association, 44*, 815-836.

Dowling, S. (1982). Mental organization in the phenomena of sleep. *The Psychoanalytic Study of the Child, 37*, 285-302.

Fairbairn, W. R. D. (1952) *Psychoanalytic study of personality*. London: Rutledge

Feinsilver, D. B. (1980). Transitional relatedness and containment in the treatment of a chronic schizophrenic patient. *International Review of Psycho-Analysis, 7*, 309-318.

Fischer, N. (1989). Anorexia nervosa and unresolved rapprochement conflicts. A case study. *International Journal of Psychoanalysis, 70*, 41-54.

Fowler, J. C., Hilsenroth, M. J., & Piers, C. (2001). An empirical study of seriously disturbed suicidal patients. *Journal of the American Psychoanalytic Association, 49*, 161-186.

Francis, G., Last, C. G., & Strauss, C. C. (1992). Avoidant personality disorder and social phobia in children and adolescents. *Journal of the American Academy of Child and Adolescent Psychiatry, 31*,1086.1089.

Gabbard, G. O. (2001). Psychoanalytically informed approaches to the treatment of obsessive-compulsive disorder. *Psychoanalytic Inquiry, 21*, 208-22.

Gassner, S. M. (2004). The role of traumatic experience in panic disorder and agoraphobia. *Psychoanalytic Psychology, 21*, 222-243.

Gillett, E. (1996). Learning theory and intrapsychic conflict. *International Journal of Psycho-Analysis, 77*, 689-707.

Greenberg, H. (1966). Pyromania in a woman. *Psychoanalytic Quarterly, 35*, 256-262.

Guinjoan, S. M., Ross, D. R., Perinot, L., Maritato, V., Jorda-Fahrer, M., & Fahrer, R.D. (2001). The use of transitional objects in self-directed aggression by patients with borderline personality disorder, anorexia nervosa, or bulimia nervosa. *Journal of the American Academy of Psychoanalysis, 29*, 457-467.

Herzog, D. B., Franko, D. L., & Brotman, A. W. (1989). Integrating treatments for bulimia nervosa. *Journal of the American Academy of Psychoanalysis, 17*, 141-150.

Hirsch, R. D. (2001) [Socio- and psychotherapy in patients with Alzheimer disease.] *Zeitschrift fur Gerontologie und Geriatrie, 34*, 92-100.

Hoffman, S.O. (1975). Psychoanalytic interpretation of sleep-disturbances. Model of a structural-theoretical classification. Translated from the German. *Psychotherapie medizinische Psychologie (Stuttg), March, 25*(2): 51–58.

Honig, R. G., Grace, M. C., Lindy, J. D., Newman, C. J., & Titchener, J. S. (1993). Portraits of survival: A twenty-year follow up study of the children of Buffalo Creek. *Psychoanalytic Study of the Child, 48,* 327-355.

Hull, J. W., Okie, J., Gibbons, B., & Carpenter, D. (1992). Acting up and physical illness: Temporal patterns and emerging structure. *Journal of the American Psychoanalytic Association, 40,* 1161-1183.

Hurvich, M. (2000). Fear of being overwhelmed and psychoanalytic theories of anxiety. *Psychoanalytic Review, 87,* 615-649.

Hurvich, M. (2003). The place of annihilation anxieties in psychoanalytic theory. *Journal of the American Psychoanalytic Association, 51,* 579-616.

Jamison, K. R. (1995). *An unquiet mind: A memoir of moods and madness.* New York: Vintage Books.

Karon, B. (1989). On the formation of delusions. *Psychoanalytic Psychology, 6,* 169-185.

Kasl-Godley, J., & Gatz, M. (2000). Psychosocial interventions for individuals with dementia: An integration of theory, therapy, and a clinical understanding of dementia. *Clinical Psychology Review, 20,* 755-82.

Kernberg, O. (1995). Technical approach to eating disorders with borderline personality organization. J. A. Winer (Ed.), *Annual of psychoanalysis* (Vol. 23, pp. 33-48). Hillsdale, NJ: Analytic Press.

Khantzian, E. J. (1978). The ego, the self and opiate addiction: Theoretical and treatment considerations. *International Review of Psychoanalysis, 5,* 189-198.

Khantzian, E. J. (1985). The self-medication hypothesis of addictive disorders: Focus on heroin and cocaine dependence. *American Journal of Psychiatry, 142,* 1259-1264.

Khantzian, E. J. (1997). The self-medication hypothesis of substance use disorders: A reconsideration and recent applications. *Harvard Review of Psychiatry, 4,* 231-244.

Kilchenstein, M. W. (1999). The psychoanalytic psychotherapy of a mentally retarded man. *International Journal of Psychoanalysis, 80,* 739-753.

Klein, M. (1933). The early development of conscience in the child. In S. Lorand (Ed). *Psychoanalysis Today.* New York: Covici-Friede.

Krystal, H.(1988). *Integration and self-healing: Affect, trauma, alexithymia.* Hillsdale, NJ: Analytic Press.

Krystal, H. (1997). Desomatization and the consequences of infantile psychic trauma. *Psychoanalytic Inquiry, 17,* 126-150.

Krystal, H., & Raskin, H. A. (1970). *Drug dependence: Aspects of ego functions.* Detroit, MI: Wayne State University Press.

Kuchenhoff, J. (1998). The body and ego boundaries: A case study on psychoanalytic therapy with psychosomatic patients. *Psychoanalytic Inquiry, 18,* 368-382.

Kulish, N. (1988). Precocious ego development and obsessive compulsive neurosis. *Journal of the American Academy of Psychoanalysis, 16,* 167-87.

Lang, H. (1997).Obsessive-compulsive disorders in neurosis and psychosis. *Journal of the American Academy of Psychoanalysis, 25,* 143-150.

Lawrence, M. (2001). Loving them to death: The anorexic and her objects. *International Journal of Psycho-Analysis, 82,* 43-55.

Little, R. (1966). Umbilical cord symbolism of the spider's dropline. *Psychoanalytic Quarterly, 35,* 587.

Lombardi, R. (2002). Primitive mental states and the body: A personal view of Armando B. Ferrari's concrete original object. *International Journal of Psycho-Analysis, 83,* 363-381.

Lowenkopf, E. L., & Wallach, J. D. (1985). Bulimia: Theoretical conceptualizations and therapies. *Journal of the American Academy of Psychoanalysis, 13,* 489-503.

Mariotti, P. (2000). Affect and psychosis. *International Journal of Psycho-Analysis, 81,* 149-152.

McDougall, J. (1980). A child is being eaten: I. Psychosomatic states, anxiety neurosis and hysteria: A theoretical approach. II. The abysmal mother and the cork child: A clinical illustration. *Contemporary Psychoanalysis, 16,* 417-459.

McDougall, J. (1984). The "dis-affected" patient: Reflections on affect pathology. *Psychoanalytic Quarterly, 53,* 386-409.

Meares, R. (1997). Stimulus entrapment: On a common basis of somatization. *Psychoanalytic Inquiry, 17,* 223-234.

Meyer, J. K. (1988). A case of hysteria, with a note on biology. *Journal of the American Psychoanalytic Association, 36,* 319-346.

Meyer, R. (1979). [Psychodynamics of psychogenic somnolence (secondary narcolepsy): Case report.] *Zeitschrift fur Psychosomatische Medizin und Psychoanalyse, 25,* 64-83.

Miliora, M. T. (1998). Trauma, dissociation, and somatization: a self-psychological perspective. *Journal of the American Academy of Psychoanalysis, 26,* 273-293.

Miliora, M. T., & Ulman, R. B. (1996) Panic disorder: A bioself-psychological perspective. *Journal of the American Academy of Psychoanalysis, 24,* 217-256.

Milkman, H., & Frosch, W. A. (1973). On the preferential abuse of heroin and amphetamine. *Journal of Nervous and Mental Disease, 156,* 242-248.

Milrod, B. (1998). Unconscious pregnancy fantasies as an underlying dynamism in panic disorder. *Journal of the American Psychoanalytic Association, 46,* 673-690

Nielsen, G. (1990). Brief integrative dynamic psychotherapy for insomnia: Systematic evaluation of two cases. *Psychotherapy and Psychosomatics, 54,* 187-92.

Novick, K. K., & Novick, J. (1987). The essence of masochism. *Psychoanalytic Study of the Child, 42,* 353-384.

O'Neill, S. (2001). The psychotherapy of a male anorectic. *International Journal of Psycho-Analysis, 82,* 563-581.

Ornstein, A., Gropper, C., & Bogner, J. (1983). Shoplifting: An expression of revenge and restitution. In *Annual of psychoanalysis* (Vol. 11, pp. 311-331). Chicago: Chicago Institute for Psychoanalysis.

Orr-Andrawes, A. (1987). The case of Anna O.: A neuropsychiatric perspective. *Journal of the American Psychoanalytic Association, 35,* 387-419.

Palombo, J. (1993). Neurocognitive deficits, developmental distortions, and incoherent narratives. *Psychoanalytic Inquiry, 13,* 85-103.

Pao, P. N. (1968). On manic-depressive psychosis: A study of the transition of states. *Journal of the American Psychoanalytic Association, 16,* 809-832.

Perlman, S. D. (1996). Psychoanalytic treatment of chronic pain: The body speaks on multiple levels. *Journal of the American Academy of Psychoanalysis, 24,* 257-271.

Rangell, L. (1968). A further attempt to resolve the "problem of anxiety." *Journal of the American Psychoanalytic Association, 16,* 371-404.

Rhead C., (1969), The role of pregenital fixation in agoraphobia. *International Journal of Psycho-Analysis, 17,* 848-861

Richartz, E. R., & Frank, C. (2004). [A psychodynamic approach in counseling vulnerable persons for Chorea Huntington: A case report.] *Psychiatrische Praxis, 31,* 255-8.

Ritvo, S. (1981). Anxiety, symptom formation, and ego autonomy. *Psychoanalytic Study of the Child, 36,* 339-364

Robbins, M. (2002). The language of schizophrenia and the world of delusion. *International Journal of Psycho-Analysis, 83,* 383-405.

Rochlin, G. (1953). The disorder of depression and elation: A clinical study of the changes from one state to another. *Journal of the American Psychoanalytic Association, 1,* 438-457.

Rodin, G. M. (1991). Somatization: A perspective from self psychology. *Journal of the American Academy of Psychoanalysis, 19,* 367-384.

Rotenberg, C. T. (1997). Vengeance and transformation in Daniel Deronda. *Journal of the American Academy of Psychoanalysis, 25,* 473-492.

Rozen, D. L. (1993). Projective identification and bulimia. *Psychoanalytic Psychology, 10,* 261-273.

Salonen, S. (2000). Recovery of affect and structural conflict. *Scandinavian Psychoanalytic Review, 23,* 50–64.

Salonen, S. (2002). Understanding Psychotic Disorder. *Scandinavian Psychoanalytic Review, 25,* 143-146.

Sands, S. H. (2003). The subjugation of the body in eating disorders: A particularly female solution. *Psychoanalytic Psychology, 20,* 103-116.

Sarlin, C. N. (1962). Depersonalization and derealization. *Journal of the American Psychoanalytic Association, 10*: 784-804.

Schneier F, Blanco C, Antia S, Liebowitz M. (2000). The social anxiety spectrum. *Psychiatric Clinics of North America, 25*(4):757-74.

Schur, M. (1953) The ego in anxiety. In R. M. Loewenstein (Ed.), *Drives, affects, and behavior* (pp. 67-100). New York: International Universities Press.

Schwartz, H. J. (1986). Bulimia: psychoanalytic perspectives. *Journal of the American Psychoanalytic Association, 34,* 439-462.

Searles, H. F. (1965). *Collected papers on schizophrenia and related subjects.* New York: International Universities Press

Searles, H. F. (1979). *Countertransference and related subjects.* New York: International Universities Press.

Searles, H. F. (1986) *My Work with Borderline Patients.* Northvale, NJ: Jason Aronson Publishers.

Shahly, V. (1987). Eating her words—food as a metaphor as transitional symptom in the recovery of a bulimic patient. *Psychoanalytic Study of the Child, 42,* 403-421.

Sperling, M. (1968). Trichotillomania, trichophagy, and cyclic vomiting: A contribution to the psychopathology of female sexuality. *International Journal of Psycho-Analysis, 49,* 682-690.

Stolorow, D. S., & Stolorow, R. D. (1989). My brother's keeper: Intensive treatment of a case of delusional merger. *International Journal of Psychoanalysis, 70,* 315-326.

Swift, W. J., & Cody, G. (1998). Gilda: fear and loathing of the exquisite object of relentless desire. *Gender and Psychoanalysis, 3,* 301-330.

Thompson-Brenner, H., & Westen, D. (2005a). Personality subtypes in eating disorders: Validation of a classification in a naturalistic sample. *British Journal of Psychiatry, 186,* 516-24.

Thompson-Brenner, H., & Westen, D. (2005b). A naturalistic study of psychotherapy for bulimia nervosa: Part 1. Comorbidity and therapeutic outcome. *Journal of Nervous and Mental Disease, 193,* 573-84.

Thompson-Brenner, H., & Westen, D. (2005c). A naturalistic study of psychotherapy for bulimia nervosa, part 2: therapeutic interventions in the community. *Journal of Nervous and Mental Disease, 93*(9):585-95.

Tyson, R. L. (1978), Notes on the analysis of a prelatency boy with a dog phobia. *Psychoanalytic Study of the Child, 33*:427-460.

Wasson, W., & Grunes, J. (1998). Attachment behavior in dementia: Parent orientation and parent fixation (POPFiD) theory. In G. Pollock & S. I. Greenspan (Eds.), *The course of Life: Vol. VII. Completing the journey* (pp. 197-230). Madison, CT: International Universities Press.

Williams, G. (1997). Reflections on some dynamics of eating disorders: "No entry" defences and foreign bodies. *International Journal of Psycho-Analysis, 78,* 927-941.

Willick, M. S. (1990). Psychoanalytic concepts of the etiology of severe mental illness. *Journal of the American Psychoanalytic Association, 38,* 1049-1081.

Wilson, A., Passik, S. D., Faude, J., Abrams, J., & Gordon, E. (1989). A hierarchical model of opiate addiction: Failures of self-regulation as a central aspect of substance abuse. *Journal of Nervous and Mental Diseases, 177,* 390-399.

Wurmser, L. (1974). Psychoanalytic considerations of the etiology of compulsive drug use. *Journal of the American Psychoanalytic Association, 22,* 820-843.

Yarom, N. (1997). A matrix of hysteria. *International Journal of Psycho-Analysis, 78,* 1119-1134.

Yorke, C., & Wiseberg, S. (1976). A developmental view of anxiety: Some clinical and theoretical considerations. *Psychoanalytic Study of the Child, 31,* 107-135.

Zavitzianos, G. (1971). Fetishism and exhibitionism in the female and their relationship to psychopathy and kleptomania. *International Journal of Psycho-Analysis, 52,* 297-305.

Zavitzianos, G. (1982). The perversion of fetishism in women. *Psychoanalytic Quarterly, 51,* 405-425.

Case Illustrations of the PDM Profile with Adult Mental Health Disorders

The three case descriptions that follow illustrate how to apply the PDM profile to clinical material. Clinicians differ in how they construct a clinical narrative, as will be evident in the different styles exemplified below. The PDM provides a systematic framework by which to organize such a description without diminishing the personal writing style and individuality of the therapist. We hope that it will help practitioners to capture unique qualities and essential attributes of each patient and thereby increase the depth and accuracy of clinical communications between colleagues. Readers may note that while all the patients are arguably diagnosable, according to DSM-IV-TR, with dysthymic disorders, their personality structures, maturational achievements, individual assets and deficits, and ways of relating suggest significant differences that have important implications for effective psychotherapy.

CASE ILLUSTRATION I

A 40-year-old multi-talented lawyer is successful up to a point, the point at which his firm would expect to consider him seriously as a senior partner, a status he has never officially let on is not one of his ambitions. He presents for evaluation out of a sense that although his life is one anyone could envy, he is not really happy and sees no possibility of being happy. He is very good at making do insofar as his own needs are concerned, feeling he has enough money to live his comfortable but not extravagant life style, and he does not want to do what he would have to do to make significantly more money.

His ability to be easily satisfied in this way infuriates his wife, who also has a career at which she works hard and cannot understand why he would "settle for so little," why he would "waste his talents" by stopping short of getting to the top. He is a partner in the firm, promoted early some years ago because he "obviously" would become a "rainmaker," but he has never lived up to this promise; being promising is a main characteristic. He is not an especially good fit in his firm as he is utterly (and in his partners' views, excessively) ethical, unwilling to cut corners to make a deal for himself or to help a client to do so. Thus he has become a "lawyer's lawyer," a prized consultant rather than an advocate.

Friendly, warm, and open in relationships, he inspires trust and never lets others down. Cautious in manner and unobtrusive, he does not put himself forward, but waits to be discovered as the expert. Others soon find out that he knows the right answer, but they have to ask him for it. Swift and certain when called upon to solve the problem of another, he is close to being obsessionally paralyzed when the problem is his own and he senses that he may have to make a decision. Then, if he can, he procrastinates until it is too late. He commonly does not balance his checkbook or pay taxes on time. Bills pile up. While he is advanced in his career, he recognizes that he has never fully decided what he would like to be, but he dreams of a life as an undersea explorer, at which he is an accomplished amateur, much valued on expeditions. While he has all the credentials he would need for that field, he has never allowed himself to make a serious move in that direction, certain (as in all important matters concerning himself) that if he were to make that decision, it likely would prove to be humiliatingly wrong—quite in contrast with his swift and certain decisions on behalf of clients and colleagues.

He has always been in the right place when someone was looking for a person with his skills or attributes. Thus he has managed to keep the fiction alive that he always was chosen and did not himself choose, as by his law firm and his wife, who picked him out and married him. Now with several children, of whom he is a good and fond parent, he merely endures his marriage, though his wife is very much in love with him, if frequently exasperated. He dreams instead of the "one that got away," a woman who excited him but whom he could not choose to marry. He behaved with her in the same hot and cold fashion he displays on his job, and she soon caught on that he would always be like that and dropped him. While he knows he never could have chosen her, he holds her as the ideal, the only one for whom he has truly felt love.

While he has been a chronic nail-biter for years, he does not complain of anxiety and denies feeling anxious other than when external circumstances would justify anxiety, and even then, he keeps his cool. Neither does he become angered when it would be justified, preferring to back off and mollify. He submits to his wife's tirades about his work habits, biting his tongue, fearing to make her angrier. He has never had much interest in sex, but accommodates his wife when she makes up to him. She recognizes that he is a "good man"; unlike the husbands of friends, he does not smoke, drink, gamble or seek other women. She says, "if only he would be more ambitious."

DIAGNOSTIC PROFILE

Personality Patterns

Though professionally successful, this man is passive and inhibited, living a kind of muted life, accommodating to happenstance and shrinking from taking the initiative. In terms of personality, he seems to be a depressive character with masochistic features, at the neurotic level of severity. It is hard to tell yet whether introjective or anaclitic trends predominate. **PDM Code: P107.1, with features of P106.2 and P112.1**

Profile of Mental Functioning

Capacity for Regulation, Attention, and Learning

The patient's capacity for attention and learning is unimpaired, as evidenced by his insightfulness at work. It is in the area of regulation that he inhibits himself and undermines his own interests. He suppresses resentments when berated by his wife for his lack of ambition, lest he further fuel her anger.

Capacity for Relationships

He is able to relate readily to his wife, his children, and the interviewer, though mostly in a passive, diffident manner. When advising colleagues on professional issues, however, he is friendly and open, inspiring trust by his competence and reliability. He does not allow his interactions to reach deeper and more problematic realms, such as engaging more meaningfully with his wife. Thus, although warm, he is not deeply intimate.

Quality of Internal Experience

Here the evidence is ambiguous. When dealing with the problems of others, he can be direct and decisive; when dealing with his own, he is passive and indecisive, preferring to withdraw and accept, seemingly without anger, his wife's censure and exasperation. How he feels this internally is hard to say, though he acknowledges that he stifles any response out of fear of heightening her angry distress. There is no evidence of any conscious, passive-aggressive satisfaction in frustrating her. His confidence and self-regard outside a limited work role seem minimal at best.

Affective Experience, Expression, and Communication

Here he is passive, constricted, and anhedonic, though not clinically depressed. He feels that he can't really be happy; he can only endure. He has never expressed much ambition or made efforts to fulfill the promise suggested by his having achieved partner status early. He shows little interest in developing a gratifying sexual life; instead, he accommodates to his wife's initiatives.

Defensive Patterns and Capacities

The patient's defensive style is avoidant. Except when addressing others' needs professionally, he withdraws from active engagement and coasts, becoming obsessional to the point of paralysis when engagement is demanded. He rationalizes and intellectualizes in the service of avoidance.

Capacity to Form Internal Representations

Here the evidence is minimal. He gives few clues about the inner price he may feel he pays for his cautious, unobtrusive manner. He seems content to be discovered rather than to offer himself. It is of interest that he also harbors adventurous fantasies, such as being an undersea explorer or reconnecting romantically with his "true love," the one that got away.

Capacity for Differentiation and Integration

The patient here seems split. Though his capacity to differentiate fantasy from reality is well established, he appears to lack the ability to differentiate and integrate the full range of adult emotions and wishes. He does not seem overtly troubled by the dichotomy between his functioning at work and at home, and he covers over this disparity by making do, getting along, and withdrawing when anything is demanded of him domestically.

Self-Observing Capacities

Though this man's intelligence and thoughtfulness indicate considerable psychological-mindedness, it seems mostly latent. His chronic nail-biting suggests anxiety, but he seems oddly devoid of felt anxiety—or even curiosity—about his character discrepancies or the gulf between his capacities and his achievements. He denies anger about his inhibited life and his curtailed accomplishments, which he must, at some level, know are self-generated. Despite his passivity, I feel that with an appropriate therapy, his capacity for self-observation could emerge and thrive.

Capacity for Internal Standards and Ideals

This is clearly a "good man," as his wife, even when angry, readily acknowledges. In fact, he irritates colleagues by being "excessively ethical," suggesting a mild degree of moral masochism. My preliminary impression is that he is guided by rigid internal standards that foster inhibition.

Summary of Profile of Mental Functioning

This patient appears to have moderate constrictions in the range and flexibility of age-expected functioning. Overall he is inhibited and anhedonic, managing and enduring life but not really enjoying it. His aim seems to be to get along, and he seems to extract some contentment from doing so. **PDM Code: M205**

Symptom Patterns

The patient complains of no specific symptoms, though it is easily inferred that he is a depressive personality. But symptomatically, he is neither significantly depressed nor significantly anxious, and his withdrawals are not overtly phobic. At times he could be considered to be mildly depressed. **PDM Code: S304.1 (tentative)**

CASE ILLUSTRATION II

A 35-year-old man comes for consultation, complaining of feeling "depressed, empty, hollow inside . . . bad about myself . . . I can't fall asleep. I wake up early in the morning, and at times I feel so bad, I think life is not worth living." He begins to talk about himself almost at once, with little hesitancy. He speaks clearly and appears surprisingly undepressed. He is stylishly dressed, well groomed, pleasant, and relaxed, with a warm smile and comfortable eye contact. There is a great deal of apparent personal engagement, yet, at the same time, paradoxically, an impersonal quality.

He reveals that a longstanding relationship with a woman had ended for reasons hard to specify, except that they were fighting and she complains that he wasn't committed enough. Subsequently, he had begun to feel "empty, hollow, at times like life isn't worth living," and had experienced problems with sleeping. He is an advertising executive and is still functioning quite well at his work. He indicates that much of the success of the whole company, in fact, was due to his natural flair for choosing successful promotional themes. He seems to be the only one who could consistently orchestrate winning campaigns.

After this opening statement, he sits with a blank look and after about 20 seconds of silence asks, "What shall I talk about next? What would you like to know?" The clinician asks how it is that, although he presents himself so readily and easily, he is unclear on where to go from here. He reveals then that he is "very good at superficial conversation, but I find it hard to really talk about myself." The interviewer sympathetically encourages him to make an attempt. After another silence, he wonders if the interviewer had ever felt depressed like him and whether or not psychiatry could "be of any help." The interviewer empathizes that he is aware that one might be reluctant to talk about difficult personal issues when one is not sure how helpful it would be. He quickly responds, "Oh, I know I'm supposed to talk about myself. I guess I should tell you about my relationship with my girlfriend." He then goes on to describe the relationship in superficial terms of things they had done together (e.g., dinner, movies). There is little talk of intimacy or the nature of the emotional involvement. He does observe that he has great difficulty expressing or even experiencing any anger at her. In the last few months, she has repeatedly failed to appreciate what he was accomplishing in his work and at times seems to be indifferent to him. The interviewer finds it hard to formulate a lifelike picture of the young lady.

Following this, the man comments spontaneously, "Did you see in the newspaper today that there is concern about radiation from energy plants? This is a much graver danger than people realize. I've had headaches and stomach pains, and I am worried that they may be caused by radiation." When the interviewer inquires about these pains and their relationship to radiation, he for the first time shows real engagement and involvement, going on to describe a series of "minor physical irregularities which may be due to cancer."

He then talks about saving money and tells the interviewer how much he has made and how much he is saving because, "I am afraid of not being able to work and having to support myself; I'd better save my money now." His associations oscillate between "protecting myself for my future" and accounts of physical ailments that he suspects are related to radiation in the atmosphere. He says, "I guess I'm going off into an irrelevant area. I should get back to talking about myself." He then glances toward a plant in the room and says, "You know, occasionally I've seen people being recorded without their knowing it," and follows by asking the interviewer, "What do you think of me so far?" The interviewer suggests that he seems to feel uneasy about what he is talking about, that he is also concerned about whether he is being taped and about what the interviewer is thinking of him. He seems somewhat relieved at this point and remarks, "I guess I'm being silly. I am very nervous, though."

He then says, "I guess I should tell you more about myself. I know psychiatrists are not supposed to direct the patient, but I guess I should start with my childhood history." He then recounts in some detail, though without much emotion, a childhood history in which he is the only son of middle-class parents, his father a bookkeeper, his mother a housewife and part-time nurse. He describes having a "normal childhood, with lots of friends, doing well in school, and being a class officer in high school." He does reasonably well in college and "had no emotional problems" until recently. While he observes in passing that he "always had good relationships with people," he does not describe any relationship with much depth or share with the interviewer the nature of any of his childhood or early adult relationships. The interviewer comments that it is hard to get much of a sense of the emotional qualities involved in his growing up. He acknowledges, "I'm not a very emotional person, but I do care for people." At this point he appears to become anxious and looks off in the other direction.

He also indicates that as a child, and now as an adult, he is sensitive to certain kinds of sounds and touch, avoiding, for example, loud or high-pitched music, as well as wool clothing. In addition, he reports that he is always better at reading and talking than at math and physics. He does not have a very good sense of direction, saying, "I usually get lost in a new city."

He goes on to recall having been depressed periodically but "never like this before." In the preceding 10 years, he has had many relationships with women, and frequently after one ended, and before the next one began, he goes through a period of "loneliness and sadness." But, he repeats, "Never like this." Near the end of the interview, there are references to people "getting older." He mentions that his father had died three years earlier, as a relatively young man, of a heart attack. He says little about his mother, except that she is now living in Florida and seems to be enjoying herself. Other family members include an aunt, who had chronic depressive episodes, and a second cousin, who has been hospitalized with "psychosis." Other than that, "nobody had had any emotional problems in my family."

DIAGNOSTIC PROFILE

Personality Patterns

The patient complains of symptoms of depression. Yet, he describes and interacts with the interviewer in a way that suggested a pattern of engaging the world characterized by emptiness and lack of awareness or experience of deeply felt feelings, coupled with superficial social skills and a creative flair to come up with new ad ideas at work. At times during the interview, his thoughts focus on physical ailments, half-believed theories that use magical, rather than realistic thinking (from which he was able to regroup quickly), and an overall sense of emotional isolation. His depressive qualities seem much more anaclitic than introjective, despite the fact that his need for others is not available to his awareness.

The personality pattern that captures this man's ongoing way of experiencing the world is Narcissistic Personality Disorder of the more depressed and depleted variety, characterized by a sense of inner emptiness and meaninglessness and mild tendencies toward hypochondriasis and paranoid thinking. His functioning is generally in the borderline range. **PDM Code: P104.2**

Profile of Mental Functioning

Capacity for Regulation, Attention, and Learning

The patient's capacity for attention is reasonably developed. During the interview, he focuses, shows good recall for details, sequences his information, and provides a history of having done well at school and in work. There is a history of mild sensitivities to sounds and certain types of touch, and relatively stronger auditory-verbal than visual-spatial processing capacities.

Capacity for Relationships

The patient reports and demonstrates constrictions in the depth and range of his relationships. For example, he relates to the interviewer with whom he is beginning a new relationship, without demonstrating a range of feelings or a growing depth. As he describes his relationship with his girlfriend and other prior girlfriends, a similar quality comes through—a lack of intimate depth and, instead, a superficial social pattern. At the same time, however, he reports, and conveys in the way he related to the interviewer and described his work history, the ability to stay with relationships and persist. Therefore, he evidences a capacity for relationships, but with marked constrictions in their depth.

Quality of Internal Experience

The patient's internal experience is mostly characterized by an empty and hollow feeling. His self-esteem appears to hinge on the events of the moment. One of the few times he seemed to feel positive about himself during the interview was in reporting that he is one of the few people at work who could be truly original with his ad ideas. For the most part, his internal experience came through as one of confusion and emptiness. He evidenced difficulty in forming a consistent pattern of self-regard and seemed to lack the psychological capacity for this level of internal organization.

Affective Experience, Expression and Communication

His affective experiences are characterized by moderate to severe constrictions at two levels. At the most basic level, he doesn't appear to experience the full range of feelings one would expect at his age, including in his current situation, deep sadness, longing, or regret. Nor does he appear to experience great joy, intimacy, pleasure, anger, and other nuanced affects. These feelings are not evidenced in his facial expressions or other affective gestures. As the interviewer attempted empathic gestures in response to his communications, he didn't appear to respond to the interviewer at this basic level of emotional communication, either.

He evidences the same constrictions at the level of experiencing emotions symbolically (as would be expected). When basic affective experiences are not mobilized at presymbolic levels, the individual does not have the fundamental affective experiences to represent and subsequently verbalize. His severe constrictions in his affective range and depth appear to be at the heart of his malaise.

Defensive Patterns and Capacities

The patient's defenses appear to work superficially well when he isn't challenged. There were a few points during the interview, however, where illogical thought patterns and somatic preoccupations briefly emerged (for example, when he was concerned about being taped and when he verbalized his theory about how his somatic complaints arose). In both these instances, however, he was able to regroup quickly.

Capacity to Form Internal Representations

The patient evidences moderate to marked constrictions in his capacity to represent the full range of expected internal experience. Deeper feelings, including those of intimacy, loss, and anger, were, at the time of his initial meeting, not accessible to being represented. He could eloquently describe surface aspects of his work and relationships. These accounts were mostly descriptions of events, actions, or interactions, rather than "represented" wishes or feeling states (i.e., "She left me and I don't have anything to do now," rather than "She left me and I feel devastated and lonely and, for the first time, I really miss her").

Capacity for Differentiation and Integration

The patient evidences transient vulnerabilities in his capacities for integration and differentiation, as well as moderate to marked constrictions in the range of internal experience that he can integrate and differentiate. There were a few instances in the interview of illogical thinking, suggesting a not-fully-differentiated sense of self and other. While he could be highly logical and reality-based at the level of superficial social adaptation, in attempting to explore his inner world, he showed more constrictions in the range of experience he could integrate. He also had difficulty sustaining highly differentiated thought patterns in these emotional areas (e.g., his illogical theories and his preoccupation with somatic complaints).

Self-Observing Capacities

He could observe his patterns of behavior and report, for example, some of his strengths (e.g., creative thinking) and some of his difficulties (e.g., being aware of his feelings). However, he has little or no self-observing capacity with regard to his deeper wishes and feelings. His limitations in self-observation are, in part, based on his inability to experience deeper levels of emotional life.

Capacity for Internal Standards and Ideals

The patient is able to adapt his behavior to the implicit rules of the consulting room and is adept at both reading and responding to guidelines at work and in his larger community. Yet, except for a wish to be a better advertising executive, he shows little capacity for guiding himself towards meaningful internal standards in the core themes of emotional life. For example, in the interview there was no mention of future relationships, plans or non-plans for marriage and family, or concern for others (other than how they affect his day-to-day world). He appears to live predominantly in moment-to-moment experiences, focusing on his immediate sense of security, physical well-being, and immediate satisfaction.

Summary of Profile of Mental Functioning

The patient shows moderate constrictions and alterations in mental functioning characterized by significant constrictions in the range of emotional experiences he mobilizes and organizes, coupled with tendencies toward fragmented or illogical thinking and somatic preoccupation. **PDM Code: M205**

Symptom Patterns

The patient presented with a range of symptoms that most closely approximates the category of depressive disorder. His internal experience includes feelings of emptiness and hollowness, sleep problems, vague intimations of "feeling bad" and thinking "life is not worth living." There was little follow-up on these complaints; instead, he offered descriptions of interactive patterns characteristic of an individual with little experience of, or capacity to experience and communicate, deeper levels of feelings. **PDM Code: S304.1**

CASE ILLUSTRATION III

Ms. R. is a 41-year-old African American mother of three living with her husband in a middle-class suburb. She has a college education and has sometimes worked part-time in clerical positions. Currently, she is not working outside the home. There are three previous contacts with mental health professionals. She is self-referred, is the main informant, and impressed the interviewer as a reliable source of information. She is on no medications.

Chief Complaint

Ms. R has what she describes as "very whimsical" mood swings. She is depressed for two or three days, during which she becomes irritable and self-reproaching. She finds herself unsatisfied with everything she does, feels keenly that her children deserve a "better mother; one who can keep her spirits up no matter what." In her depressed state, she also feels that she abandons her role as disciplinarian and finds herself happy "just not to be bothered" by her children. In these depressive episodes, her sleeping becomes disturbed and she wakes up early despite feeling continuing exhaustion. Her appetite declines and she feels no energy for life tasks. She withdraws from family members because she feels that her bad mood must be contagious. She refuses her husband's overtures for sexual contact. These episodes tend to last for several days. Then for the next few days she feels quite good. This up-and-down sequence has been particularly noticeable to her in the past four months. She has previously had depressive episodes, but in her earlier low periods she could always identify a precipitant; at this time, she cannot. She is reportedly seeking therapy in hopes of understanding and controlling her emotional lability.

History of Current Difficulties

The first time Ms. R experienced symptoms severe enough to impel her to seek therapy was around age 25, when she became both anxious and depressed about the prospect of getting married. She saw a clinical psychologist once a week for several months and felt considerable relief from her premarital symptoms. Her next bout of depression came after the birth of her first child, when she was 28. She saw a social worker once a week for about a year to deal with this postpartum experience and felt she got considerably better, but then after the birth of her second child two years later, she again became depressed and worked with the same therapist for another one and a half years. When her third child was born, she did not have a depressive reaction. A year and a half ago, as her mother was dying, she entered group therapy and again reports a good experience.

Personal History

Ms. R was born in a small Midwestern city, the second of two daughters born to a working-class family. Her father was a bus driver and part-time landscaper who died 10 years ago after a two-year struggle with cancer. She described him as "bright, super-controlled, tyrannical, and very frightening to a child." He would go into sudden rages followed by abject guilt, and Ms. R remembers his occasionally shutting himself in the bathroom and crying when things became overwhelming for him. In the face of death, he was "very much a fighter," and she admires him for the dignity with which he died.

Her mother, a housewife who worked part-time cleaning houses when the family was under financial strain, is remembered as perpetually and artificially cheerful, never depressed, always needing to deny unpleasant realities and romanticize whatever happened. She accepted uncomplainingly her husband's frequent derogatory comments (he would call her a stupid housewife, a spendthrift who didn't contribute anything to the family). Ms. R was close to her mother and remembers confiding "everything" to her, even explicit sexual material that she now thinks it odd for a daughter to have shared with a parent. She recalls how her mother would tell her father these secrets despite her own pleas to keep them to herself. She added, "Maybe I really wanted him to know."

From both parents Ms. R felt a strong pressure to "keep up appearances." Things were often difficult financially, but her mother would keep empty cans on the top of her refrigerator so that her neighbor would admire her ample food supply. She would nag her daughter not to wear her glasses in public, lest she be found unattractive, and she took great pains to avoid others finding out that she sometimes worked as a cleaning woman. Ms. R's father criticized other black men for being lazy and unreliable and made a point of working hard to a fault. She remembers that it was taboo in her family to "have problems." She was raised in a mainstream Protestant church that she sees as having supported the values of self-reliance and not feeling sorry for oneself.

Discipline in the home was inconsistent. The children were not expected to have any responsibilities in the family, but they were sometimes made to feel guilty that they did not contribute anything. Ms. R feels she was clearly the favorite child, yet her ambivalence toward her parents, especially her father, was so great that she still bears grudges that she feels are disproportionate.

Ms. R's sister Samantha is five and a half years older. As children they perpetually bickered and fought, but their relationship now is friendly. Samantha has become a successful attorney in California, where she lives with her husband and children. Ms. R described her as "a real world beater . . . her outlet is achieving." Samantha went to college at age 16 on a scholarship for exceptional minority students, and Ms. R seems to envy her for having escaped the family early. Samantha has had extensive psychotherapy and considers it to have been deeply valuable. It was at her urging that her sister first sought help.

There is evidence of depressive illness in the family history. Ms. R's father married her mother when he was 31 and she was 19. Within the first year of their marriage, both his mother and her father committed suicide. Ms. R feels that both of her parents' descriptions of their opposite-sex parent suggest some inappropriate boundaries. After her father's mother killed herself, he went into a severe depression.

Ms. R's first memory, from about age 4, is of her father hitting her on the rear end, in exasperation. This is her only memory of corporal punishment. Also at age 4, she hugged a puppy so hard that it died. She can remember her mother teasing, "We have a murderer in the house." Other early recollections include watching her parents get dressed to go out. Holidays are remembered as times of great unpleasantness; any unexpected event, such as a child spilling her milk, would cause a major family upset. She also remembers her father's overprotectiveness and excessive worries that she would be hurt physically. A traumatic memory from about age 9 involves her father's threat that if she and her sister did not stop fighting by a certain date, she would be sent to an orphanage. Her mother would tease both her and her sister, saying that they were really adopted and thus could be "sent back."

In school, Ms. R was bright and popular. She was consistently and deliberately precocious and rebellious and began smoking marijuana and experimenting sexually at about 14. She started menstruating at 14 and was so embarrassed to be so "late" that she lied to her classmates, claiming to have gotten her period at 11. First intercourse was at 15 with an older boy toward whom she felt very little. "We just went about the mechanics."

Although Ms. R's marriage is described as a good one, she and her husband have not developed a satisfying sexual relationship. Previously, she says, they approached sex "as a chore." She attributes this change to her therapy experiences, which reduced her defensiveness toward men. Her only complaint about her husband, a high school teacher, is that he tends to withdraw when he is upset. The couple have three children, ages 14, 12, and 7, whom she says they enjoy very much. Their son, the 12-year-old, had some school problems in the past for which he got effective help from a school counselor.

Further Observations and Mental Status

Ms. R is an attractive, personable, well-dressed woman who relates in a friendly and even eager way. For example, despite her depressive affect, she smiles frequently and states that she is relieved to be talking to a therapist, emphasizing how much her previous therapies had helped her. Her affect is appropriate, mood slightly labile, and her tone often self-deprecating. For example, she states about herself, "I guess I'm screwed up enough that I ought to be in therapy for life!" At another point, she states about her 14-year-old daughter, "I hope she has enough sense to stay out of bed with the first guy who comes along—unlike her mother!"

She has been quite introspective about her problems and seems frustrated that she cannot figure out why her current moods are unstable. At one point she comments, "I've figured a lot of things out, so I should be able to control these moods." At another point she remarks, "It's not really all about depression; I run hot and cold about sex the same way. I can never predict when I'm going to be in the mood." She contrasts this erratic pattern to that of men, about whom she generalizes, "They're always ready." She also comments that after so much therapy she is still not able to "keep control of my feelings."

Her speech is coherent, colorful, sometimes humorous, and very intelligent. For example, she refers to herself as a "frustrated librarian—not the 'Marian the librarian' type, but the type who wishes she could have a job surrounded by good books." When she is asked how it feels to be talking with an interviewer of another race, she responds, "I don't care if you're black, white, or green, honey; if you can help me smooth out this roller coaster ride, I'll be grateful." When pressed about whether there were any areas she would assume the interviewer might not be familiar with, she comments, "I'll be glad to translate for you if I start 'talkin' black.'" She seemed notably nondefensive in this area, and there was a quality in her reassurances that racial differences would not be a problem of her reversing roles and reassuring the interviewer.

At times, however, Ms. R. seems tangential. For example, when she expresses some worry about her 12-year-old son, who had difficulty adapting to middle school, she associates that with her father and his wish to have had a better education, and then she goes on to talk about how she wishes she had gone to a better college. Soon she is giving details about her college sorority and how strongly she feels against hazing. When reined in from tangents such as this, she reports that her thoughts occasionally race by "too fast for me to grasp" and explains that she is trying not to leave anything out. She seems to feel criticized when called back to the thread of the conversation.

Her emotional range is characterized by expressing affects of warmth, excitement, surprise, sadness, and disappointment, but there is a slightly intellectual quality to her expression of these feelings. It is as if she were giving a report on herself rather than directly expressing herself. Her descriptions seem notably lacking in anxiety, anger, envy and the negative affects other than sadness. For example, when the interviewer suggests that she might feel skeptical or apprehensive about whether therapy could help her, given that she had had previous treatment that did not protect her from this bout of difficulty, she is very quick to state how helpful the other therapies were and how much confidence she has in mental health professionals. When it came to difficult thoughts, such as her worry about her sex life or her son, she would joke and change the subject. It was hard to tell whether she was in touch with her feelings and containing them because of not yet feeling comfortable with the interviewer, or whether she was out of touch. She has a slight quality of self-dramatization that seems to represent an attempt to convey that she did not want to be thought of as taking herself too seriously. For example, she commented, "I thought I was the first woman ever to be having a baby, I was so excited. And then, I crashed so badly I felt like the village idiot!"

Eye contact was good. Capacity to reflect on her experience seems substantial, though intellectualized. There is no evidence of delusions, hallucinations, or ideas of reference. Her motivation for treatment seems to be high.

DIAGNOSTIC PROFILE

Personality Patterns

Ms. R has a mild personality disorder with prominent depressive features and some hysterical and hypomanic tendencies, characterized by lots of energy being put into saying the "right things" in an intellectualized way and, at the same time, feeling periodically depressed and depleted. She conveys an ongoing mood of pessimism and an empty sadness just behind the "appropriate front," while denying and/or rationalizing underlying feelings of anger, competition, and disappointment. Her personality structure seems to be mainly in the neurotic range, marked by a striking tendency to use introjective mechanisms. **PDM Code: P107.1**

Profile of Mental Functioning

Capacity for Regulation, Attention, and Learning

Ms. R functions well psychologically, as evidenced by her ability to understand complex questions, provide organized and logical responses, maintain her focus, and modulate her behavior in keeping with the expectations of the interview. In addition, her memory, both recent and historical, is excellent.

Capacity for Relationships

Ms. R shows a capacity for intimacy and trust, but with a notably constricted range of feelings.

Quality of Internal Experience

This client struggles to put a "good face" on. She seems to have a fundamentally negative picture of herself, which underlies her expectations of criticism, sensitivity to being criticized, and tendency to make fun of herself in a pre-emptive way.

Affective Experience, Expression and Communication

Ms. R has a constricted range of affects at both preverbal and verbal levels. Exuberant joy, anger, competition, and disappointment are avoided, and a type of dutiful, vulnerable attempt at assertive mastery is pursued. There is a capacity for some empathy and compassion, and lots of commitment.

Defensive Patterns and Capacities

Intellectualization, rationalization, self-deprecating humor, idealization and some denial around a number of basic wishes and feelings seem to be her main strategies for handling conflict and felt deficit, with periodic breakthroughs of depressive affect.

Capacity to Form Internal Representations

Ms. R can represent wishes and feelings, but with significant constrictions in their range and depth. For example, there is little to no expression of pleasure, joy, or anger. Thus, she seems able (or perhaps safe enough?) to give verbal representation to only a limited range of wishes and affects.

Capacity for Differentiation and Integration

Ms. R is able to integrate and differentiate internal experience into stable configurations of self and non-self and to maintain reality testing and impulse control. She is, however, unable to maintain a stable mood (related to constrictions in the range of wishes and feelings that can be differentiated and integrated).

Self-Observing Capacities

This woman can observe and reflect on only a limited range of wishes and affects. Because the fundamental ability is present, however, she should be able to broaden her self-observing capacity during the course of treatment.

Capacity for Internal Standards and Ideals

Ms. R is able to follow high standards of behavior, but with a harsh and rigid set of internal prohibitions, evidenced by an acute sensitivity to criticism and a strong need to put on a positive front and say the "appropriate" things. This tendency sustains a negative self-image that may be exacerbated by sensitivity to issues of race and culturally negative images of African Americans.

Summary of Profile of Mental Functioning

Ms. R. has mild to moderate constrictions in the range of wishes and feelings experienced and expressed, with stable basic mental functions (e.g., relationships, reality testing, and impulse control). **PDM Codes: M204-M205.**

Symptom Patterns

Ms. R suffers from episodic bouts of clinical depression of the introjective type. Her internal experience centers on concern and self-criticism about not being in control of "my moods." She handles her depressive episode with efforts to turn negative thoughts and feelings into positive ones, thus never fully owning, evaluating, and grieving negative experiences with a depth that would allow recovery from her depressive tendencies. **PDM Code: S304.1**

Part II
Classification of Child and Adolescent Mental Health Disorders

Child and Adolescent Mental Health Disorders

INTRODUCTION

In this section, we consider (1) children and adolescents and (2) infants and very young children. In the child and adolescent subsection, we begin by taking a microscopic look at the child's specific mental functions, such as the way he or she experiences relationships and emotions and copes with anxiety (MCA Axis). Next, we look through a low-power lens at the child's broad patterns of engaging the world (personality tendencies—PCA Axis). Finally, we characterize the child's symptoms in the context of those understandings (SCA Axis). Symptoms are construed as one dimension of the child's way of dealing with his or her world. While symptom patterns may have biological and experiential origins, and often have admixtures of both, we believe they are only understandable in the broader context of the child's mental functioning and developing personality. We thus include here the same dimensions as in Part I, but in a different order.

Because children develop and change rapidly and are best described by their unique capacities and contexts, we begin the description of a child's functioning with a detailed narrative that discusses processing capacities, relationships, emotional patterns, behavior tendencies, and similar observations. Once the child's mental functioning profile is derived, emerging personality tendencies may be assessed. Our review of personality patterns in young people takes a developmental perspective and assumes that many children show a mixture of patterns and that these may change at different developmental stages. Then we consider symptom patterns, highlighting the child's subjective experience, characterized in terms of affects, mental content, somatic states, and relationship proclivities. In addition to the DSM-IV-TR descriptions of symptom patterns in children, this section has been informed by the clinical experience of seasoned child therapists and by members of the Group for the Advancement of Psychiatry.

In an effort to emphasize the developmental context of psychopathology in infants, children, and adolescents, we describe some symptom patterns that are not included in the DSM system as well as some that appear in the adult section of DSM-IV-TR. Therefore, rather than listing the DSM categories and subcategories at the beginning of each major section, we indicate the corresponding DSM category, where appropriate, in a chart and then in the text. As in the adult section, we view symptom patterns as one part of the child's mental life rather than as discrete disorders and hence do not automatically regard the coexistence of different patterns as comorbidity (see Part III—Conceptual and Research Foundations, for discussions of problems with this assumption). Because reliability between clinicians in real practice settings using existing diagnostic systems is poor, the current state of our knowledge favors a broad framework for understanding children, with reliance on the judgment of experienced practitioners.

In order to characterize a child along the three dimensions explicated here, the clinician must conduct a comprehensive evaluation that includes a detailed developmental history, review of concerns and symptoms, evaluation of biomedical factors, and exploration of family, school, and community patterns. Direct observations, interviews (including interactive play), and observations of parent-child interactions are necessary features of such an evaluation. While conducting it, the clinician can form impressions about the child's

- Information-processing (sight, sound, touch, movement, etc.)
- Self-regulation
- Engagement in relationships
- Expression and comprehension of age-appropriate affects
- Use of words, pictures, or play to represent wishes, affects, conflicts, and experiences
- Organization of internal life (e.g., reality testing)
- Internalized limits
- Emerging values.

These impressions should be informed by an understanding of age-expected capacities and should not emphasize psychopathology to the exclusion of the child's assets and strengths. We note that children sometimes use symptoms adaptively, in the service of protecting against interferences with their functioning. In addition, some children show impressive resilience or an ability to compensate for adverse environments that may protect them from serious psychopathology even when they are periodically symptomatic.

This section is based on a developmental biopsychosocial model that considers multiple factors interacting at each stage of maturation to create relatively healthy or compromised patterns of functioning. The biopsychosocial context—including cultural, social, and family influences within which children and adolescents organize their world—is critical to their adaptation to life's challenges. Poverty, hunger, illness, injury, neglect, abuse, and catastrophic events may interact with high divorce rates, family dysfunction, and an insufficiency of ongoing nurturing relationships to put youngsters under chronic and severe stress. Cultural and social expectations that challenge a child beyond the coping capacities realistic for his or her age must also be taken into consideration when one seeks to understand a child's symptoms, feelings, thoughts, and actions.

The organization of childhood disorders in the PDM does not parallel that of the adult disorders. Although the two sections share some labels (mostly because of tradition rather than as a result of scientific investigation), childhood disorders should be considered distinct patterns in their own right. Children develop and change rapidly, and the qualities that characterize their mental functioning, personalities, symptom patterns, and internal experiences are, as previously noted, highly dependent on their developmental context. In addition, while many adult disorders had their origins in childhood, a number of developmental transformations in mediating developmental-biopsychosocial processes occur between childhood and adulthood. A specific childhood disorder should therefore not be assumed to be a precursor of the adult disorder with the same name. The goal of the PDM is to provide a framework that facilitates description of the idiosyncratic pattern of problems and assets of each child and adult whose mental health is evaluated.

Profile of Mental Functioning for Children and Adolescents MCA Axis

WORK GROUP MEMBERS

Joseph Palombo, MA, Co-Chair
Chicago, Illinois

Bernard Friedberg, MD, Co-Chair
Voorhees, New Jersey

Amy Eldridge, PhD
Chicago, Illinois

Theodore Fallon, Jr., MD, MPH
Philadelphia, Pennsylvania

Paul Fink, MD
Philadelphia, Pennsylvania

Ruth Fischer, MD
Philadelphia, Pennsylvania

Stanley I. Greenspan, MD
Bethesda, Maryland

Leon Hoffman, MD
New York, New York

Thomas K. Kenemore, PhD
Chicago, Illinois

Paulina Kernberg, MD (deceased)
Westchester, New York

Stuart G. Shanker, DPhil
Toronto, Ontario, Canada

Serena Wieder, PhD
Silver Spring, Maryland

Profile of Mental Functioning for Children and Adolescents
MCA Axis

The following describes categories of basic mental functions for children and adolescents. The goal is to use these categories to help capture the richness and individuality of the patient. For each category, there are some vignettes describing different levels of healthy-to-impaired functioning. These descriptions are not intended to be used for ratings; they serve to amplify what might be considered in each category.

The descriptions cover a variety of areas of mental functioning. While no profile can hope to capture the full panoply of mental life, the following categories highlight a number of crucial areas. The first category on *regulation, attention, and learning* concerns fundamental processes that enable human beings to attend to and learn from their experiences. The second category focuses on the capacity for *interpersonal relationships (object relationships)—including depth, range, and consistency*. The third category, the *quality of internal experience*, attempts to capture the level of confidence and self-regard with which an individual relates to others and the larger world. The fourth delineates the basic nature of the individual's *affective experience, expression and communication (affect tolerance)*, and his or her ability express the full range of pre-representational and representational patterns of affects. The fifth category, *defensive patterns and capacities*, highlights the way the individual attempts to cope with and alter wishes, affects, and other experiences, and the degree to which he or she distorts experience in the process. The sixth category, the *capacity to form internal representations*, focuses on the individual's capacity to symbolize meaningful experience affectively (i.e., to organize experience in a mental, rather than somatic or behavioral, form). This capacity to represent or mentalize enables the individual to use ideas to experience, describe, and express internal life. The seventh category, the *capacity for differentiation and integration (ego strength, self-cohesion, stability of reality-testing)*, focuses on the individual's ability to build logical bridges between internal representations (i.e., to separate logical fantasy from reality and construct connections between internal representations of wishes, affects, self and object relationships, fantasy and reality, and the past, present, and future). The next category, *self-observing capacities (psychological mindedness, emotional insight)*, concerns the individual's ability to observe his or her own internal life. This category is an extension of the capacity for differentiation and integration but is a significant enough advance to warrant its own description. The last category focuses on the *capacity to construct or use internal standards and ideals (e.g., superego integration, mature ego ideal)*. An outgrowth of other mental functions and an integration of a number of them, the capacity to formulate internal values and ideals reflects a consideration of one's self in the context of current and future experiences.

Mental functions include very basic capacities that do not depend on verbal exchanges, such as engaging in relationships and using gestures to express and respond to affects (i.e., the affects are not represented, symbolized, mentalized), as well as more mature and elaborated capacities that we usually communicate verbally, such as self-observation.

By necessity, some of these categories overlap. Each category, however, highlights an important feature of mental functioning that cannot quite be described by the others. Critical human features cannot be accounted for without reference to these categories or some similar constructs. We emphasize again, however, that the following profile of mental functioning is simply an attempt to systematize the richness of human emotional experience. Any such attempt will always be an approximation of infinitely complex processes.

The following categories can be applied to describing infants, children, and adolescents, as well as adults. Infants and very young children, however, are often just developing the capacities described in these categories. Older children and adolescents normally develop many of these basic capacities further. Therefore, in characterizing a particular child or adolescent, the clinician should always consider the age-expectations for each capacity. The descriptors presented below provide some general guidance for older children and adolescents.

In describing a child's profile of mental functioning, especially the aspects dealing with perception, memory, language, sequencing, and organizing actions, it is easy to assume that these are largely based on constitutional and maturational variations. Yet we have often observed that variations in these capacities are secondary to early infant/caregiver interactions and that different affective organizations may significantly influence these capacities in any given child (e.g., anxiety may disrupt the capacity for attention or sequencing). The profile of mental functioning does not include a discussion of the causes of different profiles. The clinician, however, should consider all relevant possibilities when attempting to explore the basis for a child's unique profile.

Capacity For Regulation, Attention, and Learning[1]

Consider constitutional and maturational contributions, including:

- Auditory processing and language
- Visual-spatial processing
- Motor planning and sequencing
- Sensory modulation

and related capacities for

- Executive functioning
- Memory (working, declarative, and non-declarative)
- Attention
- Intelligence
- Processing of affective and social cues

Illustrative Descriptions of the Range and Adequacy of Functioning

The child or adolescent:

- Can be focused, organized, and able to learn most of the time, even under stress.
- Can be focused, organized, calm, and able to learn except: when over-stimulated or under-stimulated (e.g., in a noisy, active, or very dull setting); when challenged to use a vulnerable skill (e.g., when a person with weak fine motor skills is asked to write rapidly), or when ill, anxious, or under stress.
- Can attend, be calm, and learn for short periods (e.g., 30 to 60 seconds) and to a limited degree (i.e., problems with language, motor, or visual-spatial processing) only when very interested, motivated, or captivated.
- Has fleeting attention (a few seconds here or there) and/or is very active or agitated or mostly self-absorbed and/or lethargic or passive. Learning capacity is severely limited due to multiple "processing" difficulties.

Related studies include: Aronen, Vuontela, Steenari, Salmi, & Carlson, 2005; Beebe, Jaffe, Feldstein, Mays, & Alson, 1985; Beebe & Lachmann, 1988; Bucci, 1985, 1997; Fonagy, Gergely, Jurist, & Target, 2002; Fonagy & Target, 2002; Greenspan & Shanker, 2004; ICDL-DMIC Diagnostic Classification Task Force, 2005; Mattson & Riley, 1999; McGaugh, 2003; Schore, 1994; Vicari, Caravale, Carlesimo, Casadei, & Allemand, 2004.

[1] For further clarification of the meanings of the terms used in this set of functions, please refer to the "Selected Definitions Related to Attention, Regulation, and Learning" at the end of this section.

Capacity for Relationships and Intimacy
(Including Depth, Range, and Consistency)

Note: The following descriptors apply to children aged 3 and older. For infants, as well as for older children, a chart describing age expectations in more detail is available in the Infancy and Early Childhood section.

Illustrative Descriptions of the Range and Adequacy of Functioning

The child or adolescent has:

- A deep, emotionally rich capacity for intimacy, caring, and empathy, even when feelings are strong or under stress in a variety of expectable contexts.
- A capacity for intimacy, caring, and empathy, but those capacities are disrupted by strong emotions and wishes, such as anger or fear, or by stress, such as separation (e.g., the child withdraws or acts out).
- A superficial and need-oriented capacity for intimacy and caring; relationships lack intimacy and empathy.
- An indifference to others or a more or less complete withdrawal from others.

Related studies include: Burgner & Edgcumbe, 1972; Edgcumbe & Burgner, 1972, 1975; Fonagy, 2001; Freud, S., 1905; Freud, A., 1937, 1962, 1965; Greenberg & Mitchell, 1983

Quality of Internal Experience
(Level of Confidence and Self-Regard)

Illustrative Descriptions of the Range and Adequacy of Functioning

The child or adolescent has

- A sense of well-being, vitality, and realistic self-esteem that is present even when under stress.
- A sense of well-being, vitality, and realistic self-esteem that is disrupted by strong emotions or stress, but can eventually be recovered.
- Feelings of depletion, emptiness, and incompleteness, along with self-involvement that tend to occur unless experiences are nearly "perfect." Self-esteem is vulnerable.
- Feelings of depletion, emptiness, incompleteness and self-involvement that dominate self-experience.

Related studies include: Buie, 1981; Ferenczi, 1933; Kohut, 1959, 1982; Olden, 1953; Stern, 1984; Trevarthen & Aitken, 1994; Tyson, 1988.

Affective Experience, Expression, and Communication

Note: The following descriptions combine the individual's capacity to experience, comprehend and express affects. Some individuals will be relatively stronger or weaker in either affect comprehension or affect expression. Similarly, individuals will differ in the way they express or comprehend affects through nonverbal cues (e.g., gestures, facial expressions, and voice tone) as well as with words. These unique patterns should be captured in the narrative.

Illustrative Descriptions of the Range and Adequacy of Functioning

The child or adolescent:

- Uses a wide range of subtle emotions and wishes in a purposeful manner most of the time, even under stress. Reads and responds to most emotional signals flexibly and accurately even under stress (e.g., comprehends safety vs. danger, approval vs. disapproval, acceptance vs. rejection, respect vs. humiliation, partial anger, etc.).

- Is often purposeful and organized, but not does not show a full range of emotional expressions (e.g., seeks out others for closeness and warmth with appropriate glances, body postures, and the like). Often accurately reads and responds to a range of emotional signals, except in circumstances involving selected emotions and wishes, or very strong emotions and wishes, or stress. For example, becomes chaotic, fragmented or aimless when very angry.

- Gives expression to some need-oriented, purposeful islands of behavior and emotional expressions. However, there are no cohesive larger integrated emotional patterns. In selected relationships can read basic intentions of others (such as acceptance or rejection) but is unable to read subtle cues (e.g., respect or pride or partial anger).

- Is mostly aimless or fragmented, with unpurposeful emotional expressions (e.g., no purposeful smiles or reaching out with body posture for warmth or closeness). Distorts the intents of others (e.g., misreads cues and therefore feels suspicious, mistreated, unloved, angry, etc.).

Related studies include: Amini, Lewis, Lannon, Louie, Baumbacher, McGuinness, et al., 1996; Davidson, 2003a, 2003b; Demos, 1981; Emde, 1989a, 1989b, 1999, 2000; Pally, 1998; Mayer, Salovey, & Caruso, 2000; Schore, 1994; Stern, 1984, 1988; Tomkins, 1962, 1963; Tronick, 1989, 2002.

Defensive Patterns and Capacities

Illustrative Descriptions of the Range and Adequacy of Functioning

The child or adolescent:

- Demonstrates an optimal capacity to experience a broad range of thoughts, affects and relationships and handles stresses with minimal use of defenses that suppress or alter feelings and ideas. Tends to use defenses and coping strategies that support flexibility and healthy emotional functioning, including sublimations, altruism, humor, etc.

- Makes use of defenses to keep potentially threatening ideas, feelings, memories, wishes, or fears out of awareness, without significant distortion of experiences. May use defenses such as intellectualization and rationalization, and, to a limited degree, repression, reaction formation, and displacement.

- Makes extensive use of defenses that distort experience and/or limit the experience of relationships to deal with internal and external stressors and to keep feelings and thoughts out of awareness. Uses defenses such as disavowal, denial, projection, somatization, dissociation, and acting out.

- Demonstrates a generalized failure of defensive regulation leading to a pronounced break with reality through the use of delusional projection and psychotic distortion.

Related studies include: Bronnec, Corruble, Falissard, Reynaud, Guelfi, & Hardy, 2005; Burns, 1991; Cramer, 2000; Conte, Plutchik, & Draguns, 2004; Davidson, MacGregor, Johnson, Woody, & Chaplin, 2004; Fraiberg, 1982; Freud, 1937, 1965; Gottschalk, Fronczek, & Bechtel, 2004; Holmes, 1996; Jones, 1993; Kline, 2004; Nesse, 2005; Schafer, 1968; Shill, 2004.

Capacity to Form Internal Representations

Illustrative Descriptions of the Range and Adequacy of Functioning

The child or adolescent:

- Constructs and uses internal representations to experience and express the full range of emotions and wishes and a sense of self and others. Able to use internal representations to regulate impulses and behavior.

- Often uses internal representations to experience and express a range of emotions and wishes and a sense of self and others except when experiencing selected conflicts or difficult emotions and wishes. Able to use internal representations to inhibit impulses.

- Uses representations or ideas in a concrete way to convey desire for action or to get basic needs met. Does not express feelings as such (e.g., "I want to hit but can't because someone is watching" rather than "I feel mad"). Often puts wishes and feelings into action (i.e., impulsive behavior) or into somatic states ("my stomach hurts").

- Is unable to use internal representations to experience a sense of self and others or to elaborate wishes and feelings (e.g., acts out or demands excessive physical closeness when needy).

Related studies include: Beebe, 1986; Beebe, Lachmann & Jaffe, 1997; Coates, 1998; Dahl, 1995; Diamond & Blatt, 1994; Fonagy, 2005; Fonagy & Target, 1998; Fraiberg, 1969; Linnell, 1990; Sandler & Rosenblatt, 1962; Slade, 1999; Stern, 1989.

Capacity for Differentiation and Integration

Illustrative Descriptions of the Range and Adequacy of Functioning

The child or adolescent:

- Is able to connect (i.e., create bridges between) internal experiences of self and non-self; self and others; fantasy and reality; past, present and future; and a range of wishes, emotions, and feelings states (i.e., can separate and comprehend differences in these patterns of internal experiences).

- Has the capacity to differentiate and integrate experience (i.e., create connections between experiences), but is constricted. Strong emotions and wishes, or selected emotions and wishes, or stresses can lead to the temporary fragmentation or polarization (all-or-nothing extremes) of internal experience.

- Has the capacity for differentiation and integration (i.e., to connect experiences), but is limited to just a few emotional realms (e.g., very superficial relationships). Challenges outside these limited areas often lead to the fragmentation or polarization (all-or-nothing extremes) of internal experience.

- Internal experience is fragmented most of the time. For example, is unable to make emotionally meaningful differentiations of experiences of self and non-self, past and present, or different wishes and feelings.

Related studies include Fonagy & Target, 1996; Greenspan & Shanker, 2005; Greenspan & Wieder, 1997; Target & Fonagy, 1996.

Self-Observing Capacity (Psychological-Mindedness)

Illustrative Descriptions of the Range and Adequacy of Functioning

The child or adolescent:

- Can reflect on (i.e., observe and experience at the same time) a full range of own and others' feelings or experiences, including subtle variations in feelings. At the same time, can compare them to a longer-term view of a sense of self, values, and goals. Can reflect on multiple relationships between feelings and experiences and be reflective in this way across the full range of age-expected experiences in the context of new challenges.

- Can reflect on feelings or experiences of self and others in the present and, at the same time, compare them to a longer-term view of a sense of self, values, and goals for some age-expected experiences, but not others. Cannot be reflective in this way when feelings are strong or when under significant stress.

- Can reflect on moment-to-moment experiences, but not in relationship to a longer-term sense of self and experiences, values, and goals.

- Is unable to reflect on feelings or experiences, even in the present. Self-awareness may be limited to polarized feeling states, or simple basic feelings without an appreciation of emotional subtlety. Or self-awareness may be lacking, and there may be a tendency toward fragmentation.

Related Studies include: Kantrowitz, 1999; Spacal, 1990.

Capacity to Construct or Use Internal Standards and Ideals: Sense of Morality

Illustrative Descriptions of the Range and Adequacy of Functioning

The child or adolescent:

- Has internal standards that are flexible and integrated with a realistic sense of his or her capacities and social contexts. They provide opportunities for meaningful striving and feelings of self-esteem. Feelings of guilt are used as a signal for reappraising one's behavior.

- Has internal standards and ideals that tend to be rigid. Is not sufficiently sensitive to his or her own capacities and social contexts. Feelings of guilt are experienced more as self-criticism than as a signal for reappraising one's behavior.

- Has internal standards, ideals, and sense of morality that are based on harsh, punitive expectations. Feelings of guilt are denied and are manifested by somatization, acting out, and/or depression.

- Internal standards, ideals, and a sense of morality are, for the most part, absent.

Related studies include Anderson, Bechara, Damasio, Tranel, & Damasio, 1999; Frank, 1999; Hartmann & Lowenstein, 1962; Joseph, 2000; O'Shaughnessy, 1999; Poland, 2000; Ury, 1997.

SUMMARY OF BASIC MENTAL FUNCTIONING

To summarize mental functioning, consider the descriptions of all the categories of basic mental functions; e.g., regulation, relationships, quality of internal experience, affective expression, etc., and use those to summarize mental functioning as outlined in the following table. The descriptions under each broad level are meant to be illustrative of types of limitations. Consider age-expectations in summarizing.

MCA201.	**Optimal Age- and Phase-Appropriate Mental Capacities with Phase-Expected Degree of Flexibility and Intactness**
MCA202.	**Reasonable Age- and Phase-Appropriate Mental Capacities with Phase-Expected Degree of Flexibility and Intactness**
MCA203.	**Age- and Phase-Appropriate Capacities with Phase-Specific Conflicts or Transient Developmental Challenges**
MCA204.	**Mild Constrictions and Inflexibility** **MCA204.1 – Encapsulated character formations, e.g.,** ■ Mild impairments in self-esteem regulation

- Mild limitations in internalizations necessary for regulation of impulses, affect, mood, and thought
- Mild externalization of internal events (e.g., conflicts, feelings, thoughts)
- Mild alterations and limitations in pleasure orientation
- Encapsulated limitation of experience of feelings and thoughts in major life areas (love, work, play)

MCA204.2 Encapsulated symptom formations, e.g.,

- Mild limitations and alterations in experience of affects and moods (e.g., obsessional isolation, depressive turning of feelings against the self, etc.)
- Mild limitations and alterations in experience of areas of thought (e.g., hysterical repression, phobic displacements, etc.)

MCA205. Moderate Constrictions and Alterations in Mental Functioning
Moderate versions of major constrictions listed below.

MCA206. Major Constrictions and Alterations in Mental Functioning, e.g.,
- Limited tendencies toward fragmentation of self-object differentiation
- Impairments in self-esteem regulation
- Limitations in internalizations necessary for regulation of impulses, affect, mood, and thought
- Major externalizations of internal events (conflicts, feelings, thoughts)
- Alterations and limitations in pleasure orientation
- Limitation of experience of feelings and/or thoughts in major life areas (love, work, play)

MCA207. Defects in Integration and Organization and/or Differentiation of Self- and Object Representations

MCA208. Major Defects in Basic Mental Functions
For example,
- Major structural psychological defects and defects in mental functions
  - Perception and regulation of affect
  - Integration of affect and thought
  - Reality testing and organization of perception and thought and capacity for human affective engagement
- Major defects in basic physical, organic integrity of mental apparatus (e.g., perception, integration, motor, memory, regulation, judgment, etc.)

RELATED STUDIES

Amini, F., Lewis, T., Lannon, R., Louie, A., Baumbacher, G., McGuinness, T., et al. (1996). Affect, attachment, memory: Contributions toward psychobiologic integration. *Psychiatry, 59,* 213-239.

Anderson, S. W., Bechara, A., Damasio, H., Tranel, D., & Damasio, A. R. (1999). Impairment of social and moral behavior related to early damage in human prefrontal cortex. *Nature Neuroscience, 2,* 1032-1037.

Aronen, E. T., Vuontela, V., Steenari, M. R., Salmi, J., & Carlson, S. (2005). Working memory, psychiatric symptoms, and academic performance at school. *Neurobiology of Learning & Memory, 83,* 33-42.

Beebe, B. (1986). Mother-infant mutual influence and precursors of self- and object represen- tation. In J. Masling (Ed.), *Empirical Studies of Psychoanalytic Theories* (Vol. 2, pp. 27-48). Hills- dale, New Jersey: Analytic Press

Beebe, B., Jaffe, J., Feldstein, S., Mays, K., & Alson, D. (1985). Interpersonal timing: The appli- cation of an adult dialogue model to mother-infant vocal and kinesic interactions. In T. Field & N. Fox (Eds.), *Social perception in infants* (pp. 217-247). Norwood, NJ: Ablex.

Beebe, B. and F. M. Lachman (1988). 'The contribution of mother-infant mutual influence to the origins of self- and object representations'. *Psychoanalytic Psychology, 5:* 305-337.

Beebe, B., Lachmann, F. M., & Jaffe, J. (1997). Mother-infant structures and presymbolic self and object representations. *Psychoanalytic Dialogues, 7,* 133-182.

Bronnec, M., Corruble, E., Falissard, B., Reynaud, M., Guelfi, J. D., & Hardy, P. (2005). Reports on defense styles in depression. *Psychopathology, 38,* 9-15.

Bucci, W. (1985). Dual coding: A cognitive model for psychoanalytic research. *Journal of the American Psychoanalytic Association, 33,* 571-607.

Bucci, W. (1997). *Psychoanalysis and cognitive science: A multiple code theory.* New York: Guilford Press.

Buie, D. H. (1981). Empathy: Its nature and limitations. *Journal of the American Psychoanalytic Association, 29,* 281-307.

Burgner, M. & Edgcumbe, R. (1972), Some problems in the conceptualization of early object relationships. Part II: The concept of object constancy. *The Psychoanalytic Study of the Child, 27,* 315-333.

Burns, D. P. (1991). Focusing on ego strengths. *Archives of Psychiatric Nursing, 54,* 202-208.

Coates, S. (1998). Having a mind of one's own and holding the other in mind: A discussion of "Changing aims and priorities of psychoanalytic intervention" by Peter Fonagy and Mary Target. *Psychoanalytic Dialogues, 8,* 115–148.

Conte, H. R., Plutchik, R., & Draguns, J. G. (2004). The measurement of ego defenses in clini- cal research. In U. Hentschel, G. Smith, J. G. Draguns, & W. Ehlers (Eds.), *Defense mecha- nisms: Theoretical, research and clinical perspectives* (Vol. 136, pp. 393-214). Oxford: Elsevier Science.

Cramer, P. (2000). Defense mechanisms in psychology today: Further processes for adapta- tion. *American Psychologist, 55,* 637-646.

Dahl, E. K. (1995). Daughters and mothers: Aspects of the representational world during ado- lescence. *Psychoanalytic Study of the Child, 50,* 187-204.

Davidson, K. W., MacGregor, M. W., Johnson, E. A., Woody, E. Z., & Chaplin, W. F. (2004). The relation between defense use and adaptive behavior. *Journal of Research in Personality, 38,* 105-129.

Davidson, R. J. (2003a). Affective neuroscience: A case for interdisciplinary research. In F. Kes- sel, P. L. Rosenfield, & N. B. Anderson (Eds.), *Expanding boundaries and social science: Case studies in interdisciplinary innovation* (pp. 99-121). London: Oxford University.

Davidson, R. J. (2003b). Affective neuroscience and psychophysiology: Toward a synthesis. *Psychophysiology, 40*, 655-665.

Demos, E. V. (1981). Affect in early infancy: Physiology or psychology? *Psychoanalytic Inquiry, 1*, 533-574.

Diamond, D., & Blatt, S. J. (1994). Internal working models and the representational world in attachment and psychoanalytic theories. In M. B. Sperling and W. H. Berman, *Attachment in adults: Clinical and developmental perspectives* (pp. 2-97). New York: Guilford Press.

Edgcumbe, R., & Burgner, M. (1972). Some problems in the conceptualization of early object relations. Part I: The need satisfying relationships. *The Psychoanalytic Study of the Child, 27*, 283-314.

Edgcumbe, R., & Burgner, M. (1975). The phallic-narcissistic phase: A differentiation between preoedipal and oedipal aspects of phallic development. *The Psychoanalytic Study of the Child, 30*, 161-180.

Emde, R. N. (1989a). Toward a psychoanalytic theory of affect: I. The organizational model and its propositions. In S. I. Greenspan & G. H. Pollock (Eds.), *The course of life: Psychoanalytic contributions towards understanding personality development* (pp. 165-191). Madison, CT: International Universities.

Emde, R. N. (1989b). Toward a psychoanalytic theory of affect: II. Emerging models of emotional development in infancy. In S. I. Greenspan & G. H. Pollock (Eds.), *The course of life: Psychoanalytic contributions towards understanding personality development* (pp. 193-227). Madison, CT: International Universities.

Emde, R. N. (1999). Moving ahead: Integrating influences of affective processes for development and for psychoanalysis. *International Journal of Psychoanalysis, 80*, 317-339.

Emde, R. N. (2000). Commentary on emotions: Ongoing Discussion: Affect dialogue. *Neuro-Psychoanalysis, 2*, 69-74.

Ferenczi, S. (1933). Confusion of tongues between adults and the child: The language of tenderness and passion. In M. Balint (Ed.), *Final contribution to the problems and methods of psychoanalysis* (pp. 156-167). New York: Brunner/Mazel, 1955.

Fonagy, P. (2001). *Attachment theory and psychoanalysis*. New York: Other Press.

Fonagy, P. (2005). An overview of Joseph Sandler's Key contributions to theoretical and clinical psychoanalysis. *Psychoanalytic Inquiry, 25*, 120-147.

Fonagy, P., Gergely, G., Jurist, E. L., & Target, M.. (2002). *Affect regulation, mentalization, and the development of the self*. New York: Other Press.

Fonagy, P., & Target, M. (1996). Playing with reality: I. Theory of mind and the normal development of psychic reality. *International Journal of Psychoanalysis, 77*, 217-233.

Fonagy, P., & Target, M. (1998). Mentalization and the changing aims of child psychoanalysis. *Psychoanalytic Dialogues, 8*, 87-114.

Fonagy, P., & Target, M. (2002). Early intervention and the development of self-regulation. *Psychoanalytic Inquiry, 22*, 307-335.

Fraiberg, S. H. (1969). Libidinal object constancy and mental representation. *The Psychoanalytic Study of the Child, 24*, 9-47.

Fraiberg, S. (1982). Pathological defenses in infancy. *Psychoanalytic Quarterly, 51*, 612-635.

Frank, G. (1999). Freud's concept of the superego: Review and assessment. *Psychoanalytic Psychology, 16*, 448–464.

Freud, A. (1936). *The ego and the mechanisms of defense*. New York: International Universities Press.

Freud, A. (1962). Assessment of childhood disturbances. *The Psychoanalytic Study of the Child, 17*, 149-158.

Freud, A. (1965). Normality and pathology in childhood: Assessments of development. *The Writings of Anna Freud* (Vol. VI). New York: International Universities.

Freud, S. (1905). Three essays on the theory of sexuality. *Standard Edition, 7*, 136-243.

Gottschalk, L. A., Fronczek, J, & Bechtel, R. J. (2004). Defense mechanisms and hope as protective factors in physical and mental disorders. In U. Hentschel, G. Smith, J. G. Draguns, & W. Ehlers (Eds.), *Defense mechanisms: Theoretical, research and clinical perspectives* (Vol. 136, pp. 453-476). Oxford: Elsevier Science.

Greenberg, J. R., & Mitchell, S. A. (1983). *Object relations in psychoanalytic theory.* Cambridge, MA: Harvard University.

Greenspan, S. I., & Shanker, S. G. (2004). *The first idea: How symbols, language, and intelligence evolved from our primate ancestors to modern humans.* Cambridge, MA: Da Capo Press.

Greenspan, S. I., & Shanker, S. G. (2005). Developmental Research. In E. S. Person, A. M. Cooper, & G. O. Gabbard, *American psychiatric publishing textbook of psychoanalysis* (pp. 335-360). Washington, DC: American Psychiatric Publishing.

Greenspan, S. I., & Wieder, S. (1997). Developmental patterns and outcomes in infant and children with disorders in relating and communicating: A chart review of 200 cases of children with autistic spectrum diagnosis. *Journal of Developmental and Learning Disorders, 1,* 87-141.

Hartmann, H., & Lowenstein, R. (1962). Notes on the super-ego. *The Psychoanalytic Study of the Child, 17,* 42–81.

Holmes, D. E. (1996). Emerging indicators of ego growth and associated resistances. *Journal of the American Psychoanalytic Association, 44,* 1101-1119.

ICDL-DMIC Diagnostic Classification Task Force. (2005). *Interdisciplinary Council on Developmental and Learning Disorders Diagnostic manual for infancy and early childhood mental health disorders, developmental disorders, regulatory-sensory processing disorders, language disorders, and learning challenges: ICDL-DMIC.* Bethesda, MD: ICDL.

Jones, B. P. (1993). Repression: the evolution of a psychoanalytic concept from the 1890's to the 1990's. *Journal of the American Psychoanalytic Association, 41,* 63-93.

Joseph, L. (2000). Self-criticism and the psychic surface. *Journal of the American Psychoanalytic Association, 48,* 255-280.

Kantrowitz, J. L. (1999). Pathways to self-knowledge: Private reflections and mutual supervision and other shared communications. *International Journal of Psychoanalysis, 80,* 111-132.

Kline, P. (2004). A critical perspective on defense mechanisms. In U. Hentschel, G. Smith, J. G. Draguns, & W. Ehlers (Eds.), *Defense mechanisms: Theoretical, research and clinical perspectives* (Vol. 136, pp. 43-54). Oxford: Elsevier Science.

Kohut, H. (1959). Introspection, empathy and psychoanalysis: An examination of the relationship between mode of observation and theory. *Journal of the American Psychoanalytic Association, 7,* 459-483.

Kohut, H. (1982). Introspection, empathy, and the semi-circle of mental health. *International Journal of Psychoanalysis, 63,* 395-407.

Linnell, Z. M. (1990). What is mental representation? A study of its elements and how they lead to language. *Journal of the American Psychoanalytic Association, 38,* 131-194.

Mattson, S. N., & Riley, E. P. (1999). Implicit and explicit memory functioning in children with heavy prenatal alcohol exposure. *Journal of the International Neuropsychological Society, 5,* 462-471.

Mayer, J. D., Salovey, P., & Caruso, D. (2000). Models of emotional intelligence. In R. J. Sternberg (Ed.), *Handbook of intelligence* (pp. 396-420). New York: Cambridge University.

McGaugh, J. L. (2003). *Memory and emotion: The making of lasting memories.* New York: Columbia University.

Nesse, R. M. (2005). Natural selection and the regulation of defenses: A signal detection analysis of the smoke detector principle. *Evolution and Human Behavior, 26,* 88-105.

Olden, C. (1953). On adult empathy with children. *The Psychoanalytic Study of the Child, 8,* 111-126.

O'Shaughnessy, E. (1999). Relating to the superego. *International Journal of Psychoanalysis, 80,* 861-870.

Pally, R. (1998). Emotional processing: The mind-body connection. *International Journal of Psychoanalysis, 79,* 349-362.

Poland, W. S. (2000). The analyst's witnessing and otherness. *Journal of the American Psychoanalytic Association, 48,* 16-35.

Sandler, J., & Rosenblatt, B. (1962). The concept of the representational world. *The Psychoanalytic Study of the Child, 17,* 128-145.

Schafer, R. (1968). The mechanisms of defence. *International Journal of Psychoanalysis, 49,* 49-62.

Schore, A. N. (1994). *Affect regulation and the origin of the self: The neurobiology of emotional development.* Hillsdale, NJ: Erlbaum.

Shill, M. A. (2004). Signal anxiety, defense, and the pleasure principle. *Psychoanalytic Psychology, 21,* 116–133.

Slade, A. (1999). Representation, symbolization and affect regulation in the concomitant treatment of a mother and child: Attachment theory and child psychotherapy. *Psychoanalytic Inquiry, 19,* 797-830.

Spacal, S. (1990). Free association as a method of self-observation in relation to other methodological principles of psychoanalysis. *Psychoanalytic Quarterly, 59,* 420-436.

Stern, D. N. (1984). Affect attunement. In J. D. Call, E. Galenson, & R. L. Tyson (Eds.), *Frontiers of Infant Psychiatry* (Vol. 1, pp. 3-14). New York: Basic Books.

Stern, D. N. (1988). Affect in the context of the infant's lived experience: Some considerations. *International Journal of Psychoanalysis, 69,* 233-238.

Stern, D. N. (1989). The representation of relational patterns: developmental considerations. In A. J. Sameroff & R. N. Emde (Eds.), *Relationship disturbances in early childhood* (pp. 52-69). New York: Basic Books.

Target, M., & Fonagy, P. (1996). Playing with reality: II. The development of psychic reality from a theoretical perspective. *International Journal of Psychoanalysis, 77,* 459-479.

Tomkins, S. S. (1962). *Affect, imagery, consciousness: Vol. I. The positive affects.* New York: Springer.

Tomkins, S. S. (1963). *Affect, imagery, consciousness: Vol. II. The negative affects.* New York: Springer.

Trevarthen, C., & Aitken, K. J. (1994). Brain development, infant communication, and empathy disorders: Intrinsic factors in child mental health. *Development and Psychopathology, 6,* 597-633.

Tronick, E. Z. (1989). Emotions and emotional communication in infants. *American Psychologist, 44,* 112-119.

Tronick, E. Z. (2002). A model of infant mood states and Sandarian affective waves. *Psychoanalytic Dialogues, 12,* 73-99.

Tyson, P. (1988). Psychic structure formation: The complementary roles of affects, drives, object relations, and conflict. *Journal of the American Psychoanalytic Association 36(Suppl.),* 73-98.

Ury, C. (1997). The shadow of object love: Reconstructing Freud's theory of preoedipal guilt. *Psychoanalytic Quarterly, 66,* 34-62.

Vicari, S., Caravale, B., Carlesimo, G. A., Casadei, A. M., & Allemand, F. (2004). Spatial working memory deficits in children at ages 3-4 who were low birth weight, preterm infants. *Neuropsychology, 18,* 673-678.

SELECTED DEFINITIONS RELATED TO ATTENTION, REGULATION, AND LEARNING

Attention

According to William James (1890), "Everyone knows what attention is. It is the taking possession by the mind, in clear and vivid form, of one out of what seems several simultaneously possible objects or trains of thought." Attention is a psychological process that allows people to be selectively aware of a part or aspect of the sensory environment and respond selectively to a class of stimuli. A disturbance in attention may be manifested by easy distractibility, difficulty in finishing tasks, or difficulty in concentrating on work. Certain behaviors can be performed with little, if any, attention, whereas others are highly sensitive to the allocation of attention.

Related studies include: Baron-Cohen, 1993; Barkley, 1996a; Lyon & Krasnegor, 1996; Sergeant, 1996.

Auditory Processing

Bryan and Bryan (1986) define auditory perception as:

"... a system specialized for dealing with temporal (serially organized) stimulus patterns. To the extent that the verbal symbolic system is linked to the auditory sensory modality, it must be characterized as a sequential processing system ... [The] verbal system is also sequentially organized as a symbolic system by virtue of its syntactical nature; the grammar of a language involves a temporal ordering of its elements. All language has a form which requires us to string out ideas even though their objects rest one with the other ... There is flexibility in the sequential order.. the information conveyed depends on what came before and what is yet to come in the sequence." (p. 97)

Auditory information processing is involved in speech comprehension. It consists of the following steps: analysis of the sound images of words or expressions, matching that sound image with a memory of the words or expressions, and deriving meaning from the words or expressions. Deficits in this capacity may result in a central auditory processing disorder, a condition in which comprehension of speech discourse is impaired.

Related studies include: Bryan & Bryan, 1986; Pascoe, Stackhouse, & Wells, 2005.

Cognitive Deficits (see also Learning Disabilities)

Broadly speaking, cognitive deficits are brain-based dysfunctions that manifest themselves as processing deficits or impairments in one or more of the following domains: sensorimotor function, intelligence, attention, memory, executive function, affect processing, nonverbal communication, language processing, and social interactions. These may be caused by brain lesions or, as in the case of some learning disorders, may be of unknown etiology. Cognitive deficits often give rise to learning disorders, including those in attention, perception, thinking, learning, memory, and executive functioning. Neuropsychological assessment, used to diagnose these disorders, is designed to achieve quantifiable and reproducible results that can be compared to the test scores of normal people whose age and demographic background are similar to those of the patient tested. Standardized techniques for assessing cognitive, behavioral, and emotional functioning include psychological and neuropsychological tests, scales that rate behavior, and controlled interviews. Clinical neuropsychological assessment is indicated to identify cognitive deficits, to differentiate depression from dementia, to determine the course of an illness, to assess neurotoxic effects (e.g., a memory deficit caused by substance abuse), to evaluate the effects of treatment (e.g., surgery for epilepsy or psychopharmacology), and to evaluate learning disorders.

Executive Functions

Executive functions are cognitive abilities necessary for complex goal-directed behavior and adaptation to a range of environmental changes and demands. Functions include the ability to plan and anticipate outcomes (cognitive flexibility), the ability to direct attentional resources to meet the demands of non-routine events, and self-monitoring and self-awareness, which are necessary for appropriateness of behavior and behavioral flexibility.

Related studies include: Barkley, 1996b; Baron-Cohen & Swettenham, 1997; Borkowski & Burke, 1996; Denckla, 1994, 1996; Eslinger, 1996; Gioia, Isquith, Guy, & Kenworthy, 2000; Goldberg, 2001; Lyon & Krasnegor, 1996; Palombo, 2001; Torgesen, 1994; Welsh, Pennington, & Grossier, 1991.

Intelligence

Intelligence is regarded as an index of a person's capacity to process information. It is generally measured through IQ tests. The most common of those tests was the WISC-III for children. A new edition, the WISC-IV, is currently in use. In the WISC-III the full scale score (FSIQ) that is generated by the results of this test is given as a ratio of the child's performance on the test and his or her chronological age. It is represented by the Bell curve ranging from zero to 200 with a mean or average of 100. Higher scores indicate greater than average processing ability, while lower scores indicate less than average processing ability. The FSIQ is made up of two subscores, each derived from several subtests: the Verbal IQ (VIQ) and the Performance IQ (PIQ). The VIQ measures overall verbal abilities, while the PIQ measures overall nonverbal abilities. In general, the VIQ and the PIQ ought to be within one standard deviation of one another, that is of at most 15 points from each other. Disparities greater than the standard deviation would flag the child as having a problem. Thus, the child with a VIQ of 90 and a PIQ of 110 would be suspected of having difficulties in the area of verbal language, while the child with a VIQ of 110 and a PIQ of 90 would be suspected of having problems in the area of visual-spatial processing—a situation not uncommon in children with a nonverbal learning disability. Disparities with the subscores of the VIQ and PIQ would indicate cognitive problems that require further investigation.

Gardner (1987) regards these IQ measures as too narrow and unreflective of the full range of a person's competencies. He proposes eight different intelligences that account for a broader range of human potential in children and adults. These include:

- Linguistic intelligence ("word smart")
- Logical-mathematical intelligence ("number/reasoning smart")
- Spatial intelligence ("picture smart")
- Bodily-kinesthetic intelligence ("body smart")
- Musical intelligence ("music smart")
- Interpersonal intelligence ("people smart")
- Intrapersonal intelligence ("self smart")
- Naturalist intelligence ("nature smart")

See Gardner (1987) for related concepts.

Language

Verbal language has these basic levels: phonemes, morphemes, syntax, semantics, pragmatics, discourse, and prosody. *Phonemes* are the smallest units of sounds in a language that are perceived as linguistically similar. Phonemes, when appropriately combined, form words. *Morphemes* are the smallest combination of speech sounds that have meaning. *Syntax* refers to the set of rules that specify how words should be combined to produce meaningful phrases and sentences. *Semantics* refers to the capacity to relate a word's meaning to objects or events in the world. *Pragmatics* refers to the implicit rules for using language effectively. *Discourse* refers to sentences that are combined into a text. *Prosody* includes intonation, rhythm, pauses, and variations in speech rate or amplitude.

Nonverbal communication, which can contain significant information, should be distinguished from verbal language. Nonverbal communication occurs through an array of four or more channels: the auditory, visual, tactile, and kinesic. It uses a variety of codes such as gestures, body language, facial signals, gaze, prosody, touch, proximics (spatial proximity), and chronimics (sense of time). Nonverbal signs are not organized into systems in the same way as verbal signs. Nonverbal signs have no general syntax or grammar that guides the sequence in which expressions must be ordered for meaningful communication. Although facial expressions of the basic emotions are similar across cultures (Ekman, 1999a, 1999b), the pragmatics of nonverbal communication are highly influenced by social and cultural factors.

Language disorders may range from the inability to decode written materials to disorders of thinking.

Related works include: Bashir & Scavuzzo, 1992; Beeman & Chiarello, 1998; Borod, Bloom, & Hayward, 1998; Britton & Pellegrini, 1990; Bruner, 1975, 1983; Bucci, 1985; Cantwell & Baker, 1977; Edelson, 1975; Forrester, 1996; Greenspan & Shanker, 2004; Gualtieri, Koriath, Van Bourgondien, & Saleeby, 1983; Lewis, 1977; Makari & Shapiro, 1993; Nelson, 1990; Olinick, 1984; Pinker, 1994; Ruhlen, 1994; Tager-Flusberg, 1996; Vygotsky, 1986; Wilson & Weinstein, 1992.

Learning Disabilities (see also Cognitive Deficits)

Learning disabilities are diagnosed when achievement on standardized tests in reading, mathematics, or written expression is substantially below what is expected for age, schooling, and level of intelligence. To be diagnosable as such, a learning problem must significantly interfere with academic achievement or everyday activities. Demoralization, low self-esteem, and social skills deficits are associated with learning disorders. Approximately 5% of students in public schools in the United States have a diagnosable learning disorder. These disorders have their onset during infancy or early childhood and are related to the biological maturation of the central nervous system. Learning disorders are distinguished from "normal variations in cultural attainment," and from academic difficulties arising from lack of opportunity, poor teaching, cultural factors, and vision and hearing problems. Disorders include: reading disorder, mathematics disorder, disorder of written expression, and learning disorder not otherwise specified (e.g., a spelling skills deficit).

Related studies include: Bryan & Bryan, 1986; Bryan, Burstein, & Ergul, 2004; Cohen, 1985; Cosden, Elksnin & Elksnin, 2004; Elliott, Noble, & Keleman, 1999; Hammill, Johnson & Myklebust, 1967; Leigh, McNutt, & Larsen, 1987; Osman, 2000; Palombo, 2001; Reiff, Gerber, & Ginsberg, 1997; Rothstein, Glenn, & Barrett, 1999; Torgesen, 1986.

Learning Disorders (see Cognitive Deficits, Learning Disabilities)
Memory

The following components are one way to comprise memory: working memory, declarative memory, and non-declarative memory.

- *Working memory* is a short-term memory buffer that retains auditory inputs and/or visual images. It is guided by a "central executive," the mechanism that directs attention toward one stimulus or another and determines which items are stored in working memory.

- *Declarative memory* consists of episodic memory and semantic memory. For the most part, declarative memory is conscious memory. Episodic memory is tied to specific moments in one's life. It refers to the memory of things personally experienced, as opposed to the knowledge of facts one has learned. Semantic memory is memory for facts; it is our dictionary memory.

- *Non-declarative memory* is the storage area for nonconscious memories. It consists of procedural memory, priming, associative, and non-associative learning.

  - *Procedural memory* is the storage area of non-conscious memories such as motor skills and associations. Memories are inflexibly stored in a manner related to the context in which they were first acquired.

  - *Priming* assists retrieval when a partial stimulus serves to elicit the entire memory of an event.

  - *Associative learning* is conditioned or operant learning.

  - *Non-associative learning* manifests itself primarily in reflexes.

Related studies include: Amini, Lewis, Lannon, Louie, Baumbacher, McGuinness, et al., 1996; Howe & Courage, 1997; Lewis, 1995; Loewald, 1977; Lyon & Krasnegor, 1996; Nelson, 1992, 1993; Pally, 1997; Schacter, 1996; Siegel, 2001; Stern, 1988; Torgesen, 1996.

Motor Planning

Motor planning is thought to develop from tactile and proprioceptive input to the body/brain, and from the laying down of "maps" which let the individual "know" internally the possibility for movement or manipulation of objects/tools. Effective planning utilizes feed forward (anticipation of the event) and feedback. *Postural praxis* is the ability to replicate body positions. *Bilateral motor coordination* reflects the child's ability to plan, coordinate, and integrate bilateral motor movements. *Sequencing praxis* is the ability to plan and execute sequential movements with the hands and fingers.

Motor planning can be assessed by the Praxis on Verbal Command test, a timed test requiring the child to assume various positions, and the Constructional Praxis test, a block construction test measuring the capacity to duplicate an already formed construction and the capacity to construct from the "picture in your head."

Related studies include: DeGangi & Balzer-Martin, 1999; Fraiberg, 1977; Lewis, 1995; Wieder, 1994.

Sequencing

Sequencing is the ability to place motor patterns, visually perceived images, events, objects, ideas, and other stimuli in logical and/or consecutive order.

Sensory Integration

Sensory integration is the ability to receive, interpret, sort, and integrate sensory information from touch, gravity and movement (vestibular) receptors, muscle and joint (proprioceptive) receptors, and visual, auditory, taste, and smell receptors so as to respond appropriately to the environment. The capacity to modulate or regulate the levels of inputs is required to avoid over- or under-stimulation. (See Ayres [1972] for related information.)

Speech

Speech involves the mechanical production of verbal language. Examples of speech disorders are articulation problems and dysfluencies such a stammering or stuttering.

Related studies include: Baker & Cantwell, 1987; Cantwell & Baker, 1977; Freedman, Cannady, & Robinson, 1971; Luria, 1959; Nelson, 1977.

Visual-Spatial Processing

Visual-spatial processing refers to a set of functions mediated by the right hemisphere that include facial recognition, recognition of facial emotional expression, right-left orientation, mental rotation of shapes, and comprehension of nonverbal communication cues. Visual perception involves visual sequential memory, figure-ground discrimination, visual memory, visual closure, and visual form constancy. Spatial processing involves comprehension of the spatial dimensions of one's body and physical environment.

Related studies include: Beebe & Gerstman, 1980; Edelman, 1995; Forrest, 1981; Getman, 1981; Harnadek & Rourke, 1994.

REFERENCES

Ayres, A. J. (1972). *Sensory integration and learning disorders.* Los Angeles: Western Psychological Services.

Bryan, T. H., & Bryan, J. H. (1986). *Understanding learning disabilities* (3rd Ed.). Palo Alto, CA: Mayfield.

Ekman, P. (1999a) Basic emotions. In T. Dalgleish and T. Power (Eds.) *The handbook of cognition and emotion* (pp. 45-60). Sussex, UK: John Wiley & Sons.

Ekman, P. (1999b) Facial expressions. In T. Dalgleish and T. Power (Eds.) *The handbook of cognition and emotion* (pp. 301-320). Sussex, UK: John Wiley & Sons.

Gardner, H. (1987). The theory of multiple intelligences. *Annals of Dyslexia, 37,* 19-35.

James, W. (1890). *The Principles of Psychology.* New York: Dover (reprinted 1950).

RELATED STUDIES

Amini, F., Lewis, T., Lannon, R., Louie, A., Baumbacher, G., McGuinness, T., et al. (1996). Affect, attachment, memory: Contributions toward psychobiologic integration. *Psychiatry, 59,* 213-239.

Baker, L., & Cantwell, D. P. (1987). A prospective psychiatric follow-up of children with speech/language disorders. *Journal of the American Academy of Child and Adolescent Psychiatry, 26,* 546-553.

Barkley, R. A. (1996a). Critical issues in research on attention. In G. R. Lyon & N. A. Krasnegor (Eds.), *Attention, memory, and executive function* (pp. 45-56). Baltimore: Brookes.

Barkley, R. A. (1996b). Linkages between attention and executive function. In G. R. Lyon & N. A. Krasnegor (Eds.), *Attention, memory, and executive function* (pp. 307-325). Baltimore: Brookes Publishing.

Baron-Cohen, S. (1993). From attention-goal psychology to belief-desire psychology: The development of a theory of mind, and its dysfunction. In S. Baron-Cohen, H. Tager-Flusberg, & D. J. Cohen (Eds.), *Understanding other minds: Perspectives from autism* (pp. 59-82). Oxford: Oxford University Press.

Baron-Cohen, S., & Swettenham, J. (1997). Theory of mind in autism: Its relationship to executive function and central coherence. In D. J. Cohen & F. R. Volkmar (Eds.). *Handbook of autism and pervasive developmental disorders* (pp. 880-893). New York: Wiley.

Bashir, A. S., & Scavuzzo, A. (1992). Children with language disorders: Natural history and academic success. *Journal of Learning Disabilities, 25,* 53-65.

Beebe, B., & Gerstman, L. (1980). The "packaging" of maternal stimulation in relation to infant facial-visual engagement. A case study at four months. *Merrill-Palmer Quarterly, 26,* 321-339.

Beeman, M., & Chiarello, C. (Eds.). (1998). Right hemisphere language comprehension: Perspectives from cognitive neuroscience. Mahwah, NJ: Erlbaum.

Borkowski, J. G., & Burke, J. E. (1996). Theories, models, and measurements of executive functioning: An information processing perspective. In G. R. Lyon & N. A. Krasnegor (Eds.), *Attention, memory, and executive function* (pp. 235-261). Baltimore: Brookes Publishing.

Borod, J. C., Bloom, R. L., & Hayward, C. S. (1998). Verbal aspects of emotional communication. In M. Beeman & C. Chiarello (Eds.), *Right hemisphere language comprehension: Perspectives from cognitive neuroscience* (pp. 285-307). Mahwah, NJ: Lawrence Erlbaum Publishing.

Britton, B. K., & Pellegrini, A. D. (Eds.). (1990). *Narrative thought and narrative language.* Mahwah, NJ: Lawrence Erlbaum Publishing.

Bruner, J. S. (1975). From communication to language: A psychological perspective. *Cognition, 3*, 255-287.

Bruner, J. S. (1983). *Child's talk: Learning to use language.* New York: Norton.

Bryan, T., Burstein, K., & Ergul, C. (2004). The social-emotional side of learning disabilities: A science-based presentation of the state of the art. *Learning Disabilities Quarterly, 27*, 43-51.

Bryan, T. H., & Bryan, J. H. (1986). *Understanding learning disabilities* (3rd Ed.). Palo Alto, CA: Mayfield.

Bucci, W. (1985). Dual coding: A cognitive model for psychoanalytic research. *Journal of the American Psychoanalytic Association, 33*, 571-607.

Cantwell, D. P., & Baker, L. (1977). Psychiatric disorders in children with speech and language retardation: A critical review. *Archives of General Psychiatry, 34*, 583-591.

Cohen, J. (1985). Learning disabilities and adolescence: Developmental considerations. *Adolescent Psychiatry, 12*, 177-196.

Cosden, M., Elliott, K., Noble, S., & Keleman, E. (1999). Self-understanding and self-esteem in children with learning disabilities. *Learning Disabilities Quarterly, 22*, 279-290.

DeGangi, G. A., & Balzer-Martin, L. A. (1999). The sensorimotor history questionnaire for preschoolers. *The Journal of Developmental and Learning Disabilities, 3*, 59-82.

Denckla, M. B. (1994). Measurement of executive function. In G. R. Lyon (Ed.), *Frames of reference for the assessment of learning disabilities: New views on measurement issues* (pp. 117-142). Baltimore: Brookes Publishing.

Denckla, M. B. (1996). A theory and model of executive function: A neuropsychological perspective. In G. R. Lyon & N. A. Krasnegor (Eds.), *Attention, memory, and executive function* (pp. 263-278). Baltimore: Brookes Publishing.

Edelman, G. M. (1995). The wordless metaphor: Visual art and the brain. K. Kertess (Ed.), *Whitney Museum Catalogue* (pp. 33-47). New York: Harry N. Abrams Publishing.

Edelson, M. (1975). *Language and interpretation in psychoanalysis.* New Haven: Yale University Press.

Elksnin, L. K., & Elksnin, N. (2004). The social-emotional side of learning disabilities. *Learning Disabilities Quarterly, 27*, 1-6.

Eslinger, P. J. (1996). Conceptualizing, describing, and measuring components of executive function: A summary. In G. R. Lyon & N. A. Krasnegor (Eds.), *Attention, memory, and executive function* (pp. 367-395). Baltimore: Brookes Publishing.

Forrest, E. B. (1981). Visual imagery as an information processing strategy. *Journal of Learning Disabilities, 14*, 584-586.

Forrester, M. A. (1996). Psychology of language: A critical introduction. London: Sage Publishing.

Fraiberg, S. H. (1977). Congenital sensory and motor deficits and ego formation. In Chicago Institute for Psychoanalysis (Ed.), *The annual of psychoanalysis* (Vol. V, pp. 169-194). New York, International Universities Press.

Freedman, D. A., Cannady, C., & Robinson, J. S. (1971). Speech and psychic structure: A reconsideration of their relation. *Journal of the American Psychoanalytic Association, 19*, 765-779.

Getman, G. N. (1981). Vision: Its role and integrations in learning processes. *Journal of Learning Disabilities, 14*, 577-580.

Gioia, G. A., Isquith, P. K., Guy, S. C., & Kenworthy, L. (2000). Behavior rating inventory of executive function. *Child Neuropsychology, 6*, 235-238.

Goldberg, E. (2001). *The executive brain: Frontal lobes and the civilized mind.* New York: Oxford University Press.

Greenspan, S. I., & Shanker, S. G. (2004). The first idea: How symbols, language, and intelligence evolved from our primate ancestors to modern humans. Cambridge, MA: Da Capo Press.

Gualtieri, C. T., Koriath, U., Van Bourgondien, M., & Saleeby, N. (1983). Language disorders in children referred for psychiatric services. *Journal of the American Academy of Child Psychiatry, 22,* 165-171.

Hammill, D. D., Leigh, J. E., McNutt, G., & Larsen, S. C. (1987). A new definition of learning disabilities. *Journal of Learning Disabilities, 20,* 109-113.

Harnadek, C. S., & Rourke, B. P. (1994). Principal identifying features of the syndrome of nonverbal learning disabilities in children. *Journal of Learning Disabilities, 27,* 144-154.

Howe, M. L., & Courage, M. L. (1997). The emergence and early development of autobiographical memory. *Psychological Review, 104,* 499-523.

Johnson, D. J., & Myklebust, H. R. (1967). *Learning disabilities: Educational principles and practices.* New York: Grune & Stratton.

Lewis, M. (1977). Language, cognitive development, and personality: A synthesis. *Journal of the American Academy of Child Psychiatry, 16,* 646-661.

Lewis, M. (1995). Memory and psychoanalysis: A new look at infantile amnesia and transference. *Journal of the American Academy of Child and Adolescent Psychiatry, 34,* 405-417.

Loewald, H. W. (1977). Perspectives on memory. In M. M. Gill & P. S. Holzman (Eds.), *Psychology versus metapsychology* (No. 9, pp. 298-325). New York: International Universities Press.

Luria, A. R. (1959). The directive function of speech in development and dissolution: Part 1. Development of directive function of speech in early childhood. *Word, 15,* 341-352.

Lyon, G. R., & Krasnegor N. A. (Eds.) (1996). *Attention, memory, and executive function.* Baltimore: Brookes Publishing.

Makari, G., & Shapiro, T. (1993). On psychoanalytic listening: Language and unconscious communication. *Journal of the American Psychoanalytic Association, 41,* 991-1020.

Nelson, K. (1990). Language development in context. *Annals of the New York Academy of Sciences, 583,* 93-108.

Nelson, K. (1992). Emergence of autobiographical memory at age 4. *Human Development, 35,* 172-177.

Nelson, K. (1993). The psychological and social origins of autobiographical memory. *Psychological Science, 4,* 7-14.

Nelson, K. E. (1977). Aspects of language acquisition and use from age 2 to age 20. *Journal of the American Academy of Child Psychiatry, 16,* 584-607.

Olinick, S. L. (1984). Psychoanalysis and Language. *Journal of the American Psychoanalytic Association, 32,* 617–653.

Osman, B. B. (2000). Learning disabilities and the risk of psychiatric disorders in children and adolescents. In L. L. Greenhill (Ed.), *Learning disabilities: Implications for psychiatric treatment* (pp. 33-57). Washington, DC: American Psychiatric Press.

Pally, R. (1997). Memory: Brain systems that link past, present and future. *International Journal of Psychoanalysis, 78,* 1223-1234.

Palombo, J. (2001). *Learning disorders and disorders of the self in children and adolescents.* New York: Norton Publishing.

Pascoe, M., Stackhouse, J., & Wells, B. (2005). Phonological therapy within a psycholinguistic framework: Promoting change in a child with persisting speech difficulties. *International Journal of Language & Communication Disorders, 40,* 189-220.

Pinker, S. (1994). The language instinct: How the mind creates language. New York: William Morrow Publishing.

Reiff, H. B., Gerber, P. J., & Ginsberg, R. (1997). *Exceeding expectations: Successful adults with learning disabilities.* Austin, TX: PRO-ED.

Rothstein, A. A., Glenn, J., & Barrett, D. (1999). *Learning disabilities and psychic conflict: A psychoanalytic casebook.* Madison, CT: International Universities Press.

Ruhlen, M. (1994). *The origin of language: Tracing the evolution of the mother tongue.* New York: Wiley Publishing.

Schacter, D. L. (1996). *Searching for memory: The brain, the mind, and the past.* New York: Basic Books.

Sergeant, J. (1996). A Theory of Attention: An information processing perspective. In G. R. Lyon & N. A.. Krasnegor (Eds.), *Attention, memory, and executive function* (pp. 57-69). Baltimore: Brookes Publishing.

Siegel, D. J. (2001). Memory: An overview, with emphasis on developmental, interpersonal, and neurobiological aspects. *Journal of the American Academy of Child and Adolescent Psychiatry, 40*, 997-1011.

Stern, D. N. (1988). The dialectic between the "interpersonal" and the "intrapsychic": With particular emphasis on the role of memory and representation, case presentation. *Psychoanalytic Inquiry, 8*, 505-512.

Tager-Flusberg, H. (1996). Language acquisition and theory of mind: Contributions from the study of autism. In L. B. Adamson & M. A. Romski (Eds.), *Communication and Language Acquisition: Discoveries from Atypical Development* (pp. 135-160). Baltimore: Brookes Publishing.

Torgesen, J. K. (1986). Learning disabilities theory: Its current state and future prospects. *Journal of Learning Disabilities, 19*, 399-407.

Torgesen, J. K. (1994). Issues in the assessment of executive function: An information-processing perspective. In G. R. Lyon (Ed.), *Frames of reference for the assessment of learning disabilities: New views on measurement issues* (pp. 143-162). Baltimore: Brookes Publishing.

Torgesen, J. K. (1996). A model of memory from an information processing perspective: The special case of phonological memory. In G. R. Lyon & N. A. Krasnegor (Eds.), *Attention, memory, and executive function* (pp. 157-184). Baltimore: Brookes.

Vygotsky, L. (1986). *Thought and language.* A. Korzulin (Ed.). Cambridge, MA: MIT Press.

Welsh, M. C., Pennington, B. F., & Grossier, D. B. (1991). A normative-developmental study of executive function: A window on prefrontal function in children. *Developmental Neuropsychology, 7*, 131-149.

Wieder, S. (1994). The separation-individuation process from a developmental-structuralist perspective: Its application to infants with constitutional differences. *Psychoanalytic Inquiry, 14*, 111-127.

Wilson, A., & Weinstein, L. (1992). Language and the psychoanalytic process: Psychoanalysis and Vygotskian psychology. II. *Journal of the American Psychoanalytic Association, 40*, 725-759.

Child and Adolescent Personality Patterns and Disorders
PCA Axis

WORK GROUP MEMBERS

Joseph Palombo, MA, Co-Chair
Chicago, Illinois

Bernard Friedberg, MD, Co-Chair
Voorhees, New Jersey

Amy Eldridge, PhD
Chicago, Illinois

Theodore Fallon, Jr., MD, MPH
Philadelphia, Pennsylvania

Ruth Fischer, MD
Philadelphia, Pennsylvania

Stanley I. Greenspan, M.D
Bethesda, Maryland

Leon Hoffman, MD
New York, New York

Thomas K. Kenemore, PhD LCSW
Chicago, IL

Paulina Kernberg, MD (deceased)
Westchester, New York

Stuart G. Shanker, DPhil
Toronto, Ontario

Serena Wieder, PhD
Silver Spring, Maryland

Child and Adolescent Personality Patterns and Disorders
PCA Axis

EMERGING PERSONALITY STYLES IN CHILDREN AND ADOLESCENTS

Personality patterns form during childhood and continue to further develop throughout the course of life. Depending on a number of factors, including biological dispositions, age and developmental stage of the child, the nature of the family and broader cultural influences, life events, and other factors, they may continually change or remain relatively stable.

To characterize children's mental health and mental health disorders, it is important to describe both emerging and relatively formed personality patterns. These patterns exist on a continuum from relatively healthy to compromised. Severity of personality problems in children may be evaluated via the profile of mental functioning in the previous section and a number of other factors, including:

- The age-expected depth, range, and flexibility of relationships with caregivers, other adults, and peers
- The age-expected experience, comprehension, and expression of emotions
- The age-expected quality and stability of self-esteem and a sense of well-being
- The age-expected range and structure of internal fantasies, thoughts, and related affects
- The flexibility and age-appropriateness of coping and/or defensive strategies to deal with conflicts, strong affects, or stressful experiences
- The depth and stability of age-expected levels of reality testing
- The age-expected capacities for regulating impulses, internalizing prohibitions, and forming values
- The age-expected capacities for self-observation and observing and understanding the emotional life of others

At the healthy end of the personality continuum, all above capacities are working together in a healthy, flexible, age-expected manner, and the child employs one or a number of personality traits or patterns to support healthy functioning. For example, the child may become a bit more compulsive when challenged by a difficult school assignment in order to master it. At the same time, he may be able to relax and be silly with his friends.

At the other end of the continuum are children who evidence personality patterns characterized by rigid or limited capacities for relationships, emotional range, imagination, and so forth. Such patterns are often viewed as personality disorders. A teenager who is chronically involved in antisocial behavior, has little awareness or concern about the feelings of others, relating to them largely as things rather than people, may show considerable compromises in all the capacities above and might be legitimately considered to have a psychopathic (antisocial) personality.

For children, the assessment of personality disorder is more difficult than with adults because we must take into account the child's age and developmental stage, the enormous flexibility children have to change, the sensitivity of children to changing family and environmental patterns, and the need for more research on the relationship between early personality patterns and later ones. Ultimately the decision about whether a child's personality patterns are sufficiently rigid and maladaptive to constitute a personality disorder depends on the clinician's consideration of all the factors outlined above. If there is not compelling evidence that a pattern is significantly compromising the above capacities, the clinician may characterize a relatively stable personality pattern as the child's unique personal signature of strengths and vulnerabilities.

Child and adolescent personalities emerge as a result of ongoing mutual interactions among a number of factors.

- Each baby is born with certain biological dispositions, such as activity level and ability to be soothed. The baby's unique neuropsychological state develops over time in response to interactions with the environment.

- Within the activities of daily life, unique caregiver-infant patterns develop that ideally allow the child to master, modulate, and regulate his affective responses. As development proceeds, the field of important relationships widens. Later in childhood, adolescence and adulthood, there may be a tendency to repeat earlier patterns of interaction.

- There is a gradual development of a conscious and unconscious intrapsychic picture in the child, a pattern of inner experience and behavior that continues to affect and be affected by the interactions with and responses of the people in the child's interpersonally expanding environment. The child's self esteem develops as a result of the conscious and unconscious meanings the individual attaches to these experiences.

■ During development, a variety of adaptive and defensive operations (conscious and unconscious) emerge as ways of mastering both unusual or traumatic experiences and the normal frustrations of growing up. For example, children with high levels of aggression and irritability are often in chronic conflict with parents, teachers, and peers. They may respond to these conflicts with even more aggression. In contrast, children with behavioral inhibition who invest others with too much power often elicit over protective responses, which, in turn, increase their inhibition and their consequent feelings of inferiority.

Below are four common, general patterns of engaging the world, arranged from healthiest to most disturbed.

"Normal" Emerging Personality Patterns

Some children and adolescents engage the world with patterns reflecting a cohesive emerging personality organization in which their biological endowments, including their temperamental vulnerabilities are managed adaptively within developmentally appropriate relationships with families, peers, and others. They have an organized sense of self comprised of healthy internalizations, mature coping skills, and empathic, conscientious ways of dealing with feelings about self and others. Barring unforeseen, unmanageable adversities, such children and adolescents likely grow into the rich array of healthy characters.

Related studies include: Anthony & Cohler, 1987; Becker, 1974; Blos, 1979; Chess & Thomas, 1977, 1986; Chused, 1999; Dahl, 1995; Dowling, 1989; Emde, 1988; Erikson, 1959; Fajardo, 1988; Fischer, 1991; Fischer & Balsam, 2004; Fischer & Fischer, 1991; Freud, 1963, 1965, 1981; Frenkel, 1993; Greenspan, 1988, 1989a, 1989b, 2003; Greenspan & Pollock, 1991a, b, c, d; Grigsby & Stevens, 2000; Horowitz, Gorfinkle, Lewis, & Phillips, 2002; Hughes, 1988; Kendler, 1993; Kendler & Eaves, 1986; Leckman & Mayes, 1998; Lichtenberg, 1983, 1989; Mahler, 1968; Mahler, Pine, & Bergman, 1975; Mayer, 1991; Meers, 1966, 1973; Nagera, 1963; Offer, Ostrow, & Howard, 1981; Palombo, 1987, 1988, 1990; Parens, Ollock, Stern, & Kramer, 1976; Pine, 1985; Pruett, 1992; Rutter, 1966; Sander, 1985, 1987; Sandler, 1972; Sarnoff, 1976; Shapiro, 1976; Siegel, 1999; Spitz, 1965; Stern, 1985, 2004; Tyson & Tyson, 1990; Weil, 1970; and Winnicott, 1953, 1965, 1992.

Mildly Dysfunctional Emerging Personality Patterns

Some children and adolescents engage the world with patterns that suggest a less cohesive emerging personality organization in which their biological endowments, including their temperamental vulnerabilities are managed less adaptively. Early in life, their primary caregivers may have trouble helping them manage these constitutional dispositions. Thus, relationships with families, peers, and others are more fraught with problems. Such children do not navigate the various developmental levels, enumerated below, as successfully as those with less problematic endowments and/or more responsive caregivers. However, their sense of self and their sense of reality are pretty solid. As development proceeds their adaptive mechanisms may fixate in moderately rigid defensive patterns, and their reactions to adversities may be somewhat dysfunctional.

Related studies include: Cytryn, 1998; Freud, 1962, 1965, 1970; Gabbard, 2005; Kernberg, Weiner, & Bardenstein, 2000.

Moderately Dysfunctional Emerging Personality Patterns

Other children engage the world in ways that suggest vulnerabilities in reality testing and sense of self. Such problems may be manifested by recurrent losses of confidence and maladaptive ways of dealing with feelings about self and others. Their defensive operations may distort reality (e.g., one's own feelings may be perceived in others, rather than in oneself; the intentions of others may be misperceived, etc.).

Related studies include: Fraiberg, 1975; Greenspan, 1981; Kernberg, Weiner, & Bardenstein, 2000.

Severely Dysfunctional Emerging Personality Patterns

Finally, some children show significant deficits in their capacity for reality testing and forming a sense of self, manifested by persistent loss of confidence and consistently maladaptive ways of dealing with feelings about self and others. Their defensive operations interfere with basic capacities to relate to others and to separate one's own feelings and wishes from those of others.

Related studies include: Coker & Widiger, 2005; Kernberg, Weiner, & Bardenstein, 2000; Winnicott, 1960.

DEVELOPMENTAL ASPECTS OF EMERGING PERSONALITY PATTERNS

Within the broad developmental parameters outlined above (from a "normal" emerging personality pattern to a severely dysfunctional one), there are a variety of distinct emerging personality organizations. Each personality organization, of course, may be expressed from the "normal" range to the most dysfunctional range.

Normal Range of Patterns

1. At first a baby is totally dependent on its caregivers, not only for sustenance but also for affect regulation and soothing. The unique match between

the primary caregiver and the baby marks the beginning of the development of a unique personality style. Although perceptual and cognitive functioning can be demonstrated from the earliest days of life, it is during the first year and a half to two years that there is a clear-cut emergence of the child as a person in his or her own right. Motor development and language development are important markers in that they permit the child control of the body in space and a means of communicating likes and dislikes. During this period one normally sees a range of synchronous and reciprocating ways of relating to others, including the capacities to attend and be calm, to engage with progressive intimacy, to exchange emotional and social gestures, and to use these to engage in shared problem-solving.

2. Between 1½ and 3 years of age, the child becomes able to navigate and communicate more effectively and experiences a greater need for independent action, resulting in potential willful battles with caregivers. The word "no" becomes an important part of the child's vocabulary. The child gains significant control over body functions, including toileting. Strivings toward independence alternate with sudden, helpless demands to be cared for. Messiness alternates with neatness, provocativeness with submissiveness, and power and glory with fearfulness. During this time, the toddler learns to represent (symbolically), comprehend, and verbalize feelings; to express wishes and ideas in pretend play; and to construct representations and their associated wishes and feelings into logical patterns. Autonomy, agency, and interdependence are preeminent issues for the toddler.

3. From 3 or 4 until 5 or 6 years of age, the child's world expands and he is able to participate more socially with peers and other adults in a variety of settings. Within the family as well as in the larger community, the child becomes increasingly aware of difference and tends to generalize about gender and role. Curiosity is at a high level as the child begins to puzzle out the nature of life—of where babies come from, how coupling occurs among adults, and what is the nature of death. Typically during this time the child is a true investigator. A pregnancy or an adoption triggers excitement, concerns, and questions. Concerns about these investigations into central human issues may lead to even greater curiosity and expression of interests, as well as anxiety and conflict with resulting sleep disruptions, fears of animals, and worries about monsters, ghosts, and other common phantasms. Fantasies of glory alternate with fearfulness.

4. The elementary school years, when the intensity of the above concerns abates or becomes "latent," are considered the period of latency. Energy is directed toward the development of social, cognitive, motor, and academic skills. During this time, children develop independent friendships and judge their own and other people's actions via the lens of their developing sense of morality. Dangerous and unacceptable feelings and impulses are normally contained with

obsessional defenses. Fairness, tact, and empathy for others are important achievements of this period. In times of stress, these qualities may alternate with unfairness, excessive rivalry, and egocentrism. As children move beyond all-or-nothing thinking, they better understand and tolerate differences and "shades of gray." Behavior is under better control. Because of their obsessional defenses and their emerging moral sensibilities, latency-age children tend to be pliable and educable. Differences between boys and girls may be emphasized and exaggerated, both internally and externally. Boys tend to engage in group interactions with specific rules. Girls tend to cultivate exclusive relationships and may experience an abundance of jealousies and rivalries for best-friend status. Children with significant cross-gender and minority sexual orientations may find this period notably stressful.

5. Puberty ushers in a period of expansion and potential inner turmoil. Most adolescents manage to navigate this period successfully, without undue storminess, so that by the end of adolescence and early adulthood a more or less stable, dignified, and respectful personality is established. During adolescence, the young person has to accomplish three major tasks:

- Coming to terms with hormonal and other changes in the body;
- Beginning the slow process of transferring attachment from the family of origin to other love objects; and
- Constructing a more nuanced and competent capacity to compare and evaluate experiences realistically in the context of an emerging, ever more complex sense of self.

In moving away from the family as the major objects of affection, and in abandoning identifications with parents, adolescents may show a variety of patterns: identifications with (and imitation of) a range of peers and adults; sexual experimentation and/or a hyper-moralistic stance; obsessive involvement in idealistic or intellectual pursuits and/or egocentric hedonism. The adolescent may deny vulnerability and mortality with counterphobic, impulsive actions or may withdraw avoidantly from action in the world.

Temporary identifications, ranging from healthy to unhealthy, assist the adolescent in forming an identity and relationships separate from the family of origin. The need to be more reliant on peers exposes the adolescent to whatever risks characterize his or her peer group (promiscuity or asceticism, drug abuse or moralistic abstinence, the pursuit of physical "perfection" or the rejection of concern for the body).

Body issues may also arise, ranging from mild to more extreme as adolescents integrate the physical changes associated with puberty. As one example, some girls may hide themselves in baggy clothes or wear overly revealing outfits. Some boys may become overfocused on evidence of masculinity or withdraw into a more cerebral stance. Ways of coping with physical changes will vary enormously, however. Old identifications are modified and intermixed with new identifications as the post-adolescent personality emerges. Understandably, different cultural and family patterns are crucial to an appropriate clinical formulation.

At the end of this section, we present a table of concordance with PDM and DSM-IV-TR personality disorders.

Dysfunctional Personality Patterns

PCA101. Fearful of Closeness/Intimacy (Schizoid) Personality Disorders
PCA102. Suspicious/Distrustful Personality Disorders
PCA103. Sociopathic (Antisocial) Personality Disorders
PCA104. Narcissistic Personality Disorders
PCA105. Impulsive/Explosive Personality Disorders
PCA106. Self-Defeating Personality Disorders
PCA107. Depressive Personality Disorders
PCA108. Somatizing Personality Disorders
PCA109. Dependent Personality Disorders
PCA110. Avoidant/Constricted Personality Disorders PCA110.1 Counterphobic Personality Disorder
PCA111. Anxious Personality Disorders
PCA112. Obsessive-Compulsive Personality Disorders
PCA113. Histrionic Personality Disorders
PCA114. Dysregulated Personality Disorders
PCA115. Mixed/Other

PCA101. Fearful of Closeness/Intimacy (Schizoid) Personality Disorders

Although they may also crave relationships, schizoid children and adolescents have a pervasive pattern of detachment from social relationships and have a very restricted range of expression of emotions in interpersonal settings. They seem to avoid social interactions very actively and are seen by others as loners. In contrast to avoidant and constricted children, who may be likeable and popular, they have few or no friends. Either because of a severe inhibition or lack of social skills, schizoid children cannot spontaneously interact appropriately with others. When asked about their withdrawals, they may assert that others do a variety of ills to them. Clinical experience suggests that they may have learned to fear the negative consequences of their need for love.

Related studies include: Battalia, Bernardeschi, Franchini, Bellodi, & Smeraldi, 1995; Caplan & Guthrie, 1992; McGlashan, 1986; Nagy & Szatmari, 1986; Olin, Raine, Cannon, Parnas, Schulsinger, & Mednick, 1997; Wolff, 1991; Wolff & Barlow, 1979; Wolff, Townshend, McGuire, & Weeks, 1991.

PCA102. Suspicious/Distrustful Personality Disorders

A pervasive pattern of distrustfulness and suspiciousness is relatively rare in childhood. In adolescence it is less rare, but is often part of another emerging personality pattern, such as an antisocial pattern or multi-dimensionally impaired (borderline) clinical picture. These children and adolescents have mild to moderate to pervasive distrust and suspiciousness of others, whose motives they interpret as malevolent. Shame and humiliation are important predeterminants to this emerging personality pattern. In interactions with peers and adults, such children expect shame and humiliation to occur. They therefore project, avoid, and attack in a preemptive fashion, in words and/or in actions.

Related studies include: Carstairs, 1992; Juni, 1979; Kernberg, 1987.

PCA103. Sociopathic* (Antisocial) Personality Disorders

Children and adolescents with significant sociopathic tendencies show some degree of disregard for, and violation of, the rights of others, and are notable for deceitfulness and lack of remorse. Their disregard may be expressed intermittently in explosions when rules and limits are imposed, or in more flagrant, pervasive antisocial actions. They may be mistrustful and suspicious and thus need to assert their power over others directly or manipulatively in order to get what they want. Most sociopathic children have not developed sufficiently intimate and stable relationships with primary caregivers and consequently have not developed even minimal degrees of empathy or concern for others. Some have made a strong identification with a psychopathic parent. On the more adaptive end of the spectrum such children and adolescents may achieve success at the expense of meaningful mutually enhancing relationships. At the most maladaptive end, criminality is a danger.

---

*Although the adult section of the PDM uses the term "psychopathic" to describe the psychologies of antisocial individuals, the tendency in the scholarly literature on children has been to use "sociopathic," probably because of a reluctance to label young people with the more definite, more stigmatizing term.

Related studies include: Blair, Budhani, Colledge, & Scott, 2005; Houghton, West, & Tan, 2005; Lahey, Loeber, Burke, & Applegate, 2005; Loeber & Schmaling, 1985; Moffitt 1993; Moffitt, Caspi, Dickson, Silva, & Stanton, 1996; Pajer, 1998; Rygaard, 1998.

PCA104. Narcissistic Personality Disorders

There is a full range of patterns of narcissistic issues in children and adolescents. At the healthier end of the narcissistic spectrum, children are highly focused on realistic pride in accomplishment. Toward the more dysfunctional end, narcissistically motivated children and adolescents may show pervasive patterns of grandiose fantasy and/or behavior. They may exhibit arrogance, entitlement, need for admiration, and lack of empathy for others. Or, they may seem depressed, irritated, and full of complaints, behind which are frustrated grandiose aspirations. Although some narcissistic children and adolescents seem "spoiled" and entitled, most are clearly defending against feelings of low self-esteem and are trying to avoid shame and humiliation.

Related studies include: Bene, 1979; Bleiberg, 1984; Egan & Kernberg, 1984; Kernberg, 1989, 1999; Rinsley, 1980; Robbins, 1982; Weise & Tuber, 2004; Willock, 1987.

PCA105. Impulsive/Explosive Personality Disorders

Children with this pattern tend to experience a need to take action and have difficulty using thoughts or fantasies to cope with elaborate feelings. Fears, anxieties, as well as humiliations are often dealt with through aggressive acts. (See **IEC104. Disruptive Behavior and Oppositional Disorder** in The Classification of Mental Health and Developmental Disorders in Infancy and Early Childhood, p. 319, for further description.) Babies and toddlers with "hard to socialize sensory craving" patterns, as well as children growing up in environments providing poor, disruptive, or inconsistent emotional responsiveness are vulnerable to a variety of impulsive and explosive behavior patterns. In childhood and adolescence, inadequate and impaired relationships with primary caregivers are typical. Such children need special assistance via appropriate limits, empathetic responsiveness, and help with affect-regulation and behavioral containment. A therapist can help them associate self-esteem with self-control.

Related studies include: Greene, 1998.

PCA106. Self-Defeating Personality Disorders

Children and adolescents with overly self-defeating tendencies repeatedly create situations in which they clearly undermine their success. The tendency may be part of a larger problem of feeling inferior and being overly sensitive, pessimistic, perfectionistic, and dysphoric but not actually clinically depressed. It may express an underlying concern that one's capabilities will have hurtful consequences, such as attack, punishment, abandonment, or other harm to self or to others. Academic success may be regularly followed by failure; winning in competitive events may be followed by losing. While masochistic children may be very competitive, victory always seems to be taken away at the last minute. They may sabotage their relationships with peers and others. Guilt over success is often clearly inferable and pride in accomplishments is either lacking or defended against. Many self-defeating children verbalize the beliefs that they will not be abandoned if they demonstrate their suffering, and that people pay attention only when they are suffering.

Related studies include: Pezzarossa, Della Rosa, & Rubino, 2002; Rubino, Pezzarossa, Della Rosa, & Siracusano, 2004.

PCA107. Depressive Personality Disorders

Children and adolescents with depressive personalities suffer intermittent or chronic dysphoric affect. Their unhappiness may be expressed mainly in terms of emptiness and loneliness or in terms of guilt. They have an irrationally negative estimation of themselves, are highly reactive to loss and rejection, and hold themselves to scrupulous standards from which they consistently feel they fall short. Because many depressive children have never had a significant depressive episode, they are unlikely to have been diagnosed with a mood disorder. Rather than blaming others, they attribute their suffering to their own badness. Taking on this responsibility allows them a sense of control, leaving them with the feeling that they have the power to change that which feels unchangeable. They work hard to be "nice" and "good." In treatment it is vital to elicit the buried, defended-against, negative feelings of these children and adolescents. They typically try to be good patients, idealize the therapist, and assume that the therapist's noncritical acceptance indicates that he has not noticed how bad they really are. In treatment, it is important that they come to appreciate that this belief in their badness is a misplaced effort to protect themselves from other dangers, such as the fact that one's life is not always under one's control.

Related studies include: Huprich & Frisch, 2004; Klein, et al., 1999.

PCA108. Somatizing Personality Disorders

Some children and adolescents with this pattern have an excessive preoccupation with body concerns. Expectable developmental challenges, such as new feelings, peer relationships, and body changes, as well as strong feelings, conflicts, or anxieties, tend to be associated with (or dealt with) through an overfocus on one or another bodily concern. This personality pattern may be related to a constitutional disposition to illness, a reaction to early medical interventions, attachment problems, and/or an identification with a somatizing caregiver. They tend to be alexithymic (inability to feel and express affects), and they see themselves as vulnerable. In its extreme form, this pattern may disrupt participation in age-expected peer, school, and family activities and cause excessive medical care.

Related studies include: Abbass, 2005; Abbey, 2005; Brown, Schrag, & Trimble, 2005; Chapman, 2005; Eifert & Zvolensky, 2005; Keenan & Wakschlag, 2004; Proner, 2005.

PCA109. Dependent Personality Disorders

Children and adolescents with excessively dependent personalities experience a compelling need to be taken care of. They fear separation, either recurrently or pervasively, and typically engage in submissive and clinging behavior. They are often anxious in new situations and shrink from taking risks or new steps. Fears of being hurt are common, which, along with a general sense of inadequacy, results in a desire for others to protect them. They may appear infantile and may regress frequently to a more passive state. Difficulty with independent action and assertion often reflects a problem in mastering aggressive impulses and wishes, based on either a constitutional impairment or conflicts over rage and destructiveness. They may become homesick when away from the primary caregivers. Alternatively, they may compensate by developing dependent relationships with other adults. As adolescents, they may become overly dependent followers of the leaders of their peer groups.

Related studies include: Bornstein, 1996, 2005a, 2005b.

PCA110. Avoidant/Constricted Personality Disorders

Children with avoidant or constricted personalities may have been born with a temperament described as "slow to warm up." Alternatively, they may be children who have been overwhelmed with stimulation from the environment and who avoid or constrict to avoid further inundation. They are often highly sensitive, easily overstimulated, and markedly shy. In many instances, during early childhood, parents may inadvertently support their withdrawal by overprotecting them from or overexposing them to conflictual, frustrating, and over-challenging situations. In their interactions with other children, they avoid conflict and respond to others' potential aggression by inhibiting their own aggression and submitting. They may become anxious or frightened enough to withdraw from their environment or tend towards phobic patterns. When forced to interact, however, they often do participate in activities. Unlike dependent children, they usually are not homesick when away from their families. A selectively mute child, a child with school avoidance, or a child who avoids play dates may develop such a personality structure. In adolescence, such children may be painfully shy, often avoid peers, especially in relation to peers of the gender to which they are attracted. The pattern of social inhibition and shyness, feelings of inadequacy, and hypersensitivity to negative evaluation may be occasional or pervasive. Avoidant children may interact and express themselves quite well in a safe, comfortable, well-known milieu, such as their own home or that of relatives.

At the adaptive end of the continuum, children with this pattern may be very sensitive, sweet, empathetic, thoughtful, and creative, with a few close friends and a capacity to pursue interests in depth. At the maladaptive end of the continuum, children may limit themselves emotionally and intellectually to a degree where they avoid or retreat from many age-expected peer and school activities.

Related studies include: Alden, Laposa, Taylor, & Ryder, 2002; Francis & D'Elia 1994; Francis, Last, & Strauss, 1992; Horowitz, 2004; McLean & McLean, 2004; Rettew, Zanarini, Yen, Grilo, Skodol, Shea, et al., 2003; Taylor, Laposa, & Alden, 2004; Tillfors, Furmark, Ekselius, & Fredrikson, 2004.

PCA110.1 Counterphobic Personality Disorders

Some children and adolescents seem to have a high threshold for stimulation (probably a temperamental variation of "sensory craving" or a reaction to emotional deprivation) and/or a need to deny any fear. Clinicians describe them as "kids who can't swim but jump into the deep end of the pool." Particularly during adolescence, they take unusual risks—driving recklessly, taking drugs indiscriminately, and engaging in high-risk sexual behavior. Counterphobia is a common reaction in younger children also, when they are faced with an intolerable sense of powerlessness or fear of passivity. On the more adaptive end of the counterphobic spectrum, children and adolescents with this psychology become involved in risky activities, but in a controlled way. At the most maladaptive end of the spectrum they flirt with potentially suicidal behavior.

Related studies include: de Young, 1984; Holmes, 1982; Robertiello, 1988.

PCA111. Anxious Personality Disorders

Children and adolescents with overly anxious personalities show recurrent to pervasive anxiety. They are generally fearful about new situations, resist taking risks, and feel in constant danger from unknown forces. Other people may be perceived as either sources of danger or protection from danger. Anxiety may be secondary to a fear of impulsiveness or expressive explosiveness. These children tend to be cautious and avoid situations associated with anxiety. While children with this pattern have some of the characteristics described for the dependent personality, children with anxious personality disorder may employ a variety of ways of engaging the world, from avoidance to periodic impulsivity and negativism.

Related studies include: Bernstein, Borchardt, & Perwien, 1996; Goodwin, Brook, & Cohen, 2005; Hofer, 1995; Last, 1989; Strauss, 1990; Warren, Emde, & Sroufe, 2000.

PCA112. Obsessive-Compulsive Personality Disorders

Children and adolescents with obsessive and compulsive personalities are preoccupied with orderliness, perfectionism, and mental and interpersonal control, at the expense of flexibility, openness, and efficiency. They may be countering unconscious or pre-conscious aggression. On the more disturbed end of the spectrum, they may be defending against overwhelming anxiety, wishes to regress, loss of reality testing, or loss of impulse control. On the healthy end of the obsessive-compulsive spectrum are obedient children who follow rules and are very conscientious about such duties as school work and house chores. At the most maladaptive end are children whose need for control has a stubborn quality that oppresses their family and their environment. Obsessive children handle anxiety with isolation of affect, compartmentalization, and intellectualization. During adolescence they may avoid impulsivity by an over-focus on intellectual and idealistic pursuits. Compulsive children handle anxiety with repetitive perfectionistic behavior that may have the meaning of "undoing" their fantasied badness.

Related studies include: Chused, 1999; Clark and Bolton, 1985; Flament, Koby, Rapoport, Berg, Zahn, Cox, et al., 1990; Francis & Gragg, 1996; March & Leonard, 1996.

PCA113. Histrionic Personality Disorders

In contrast to obsessive children and adolescents who may be mortified by impulsive exhibitionistic actions, histrionic children and adolescents demonstrate a pattern of self-dramatizing, attention-seeking, provocative behavior, which is often both sexual and aggressive. During the pre-school years, the play activities of these children may have already demonstrated a marked theatricality. During the school years, the exhibitionism of children at the healthier end of the histrionic spectrum may be expressed in socially rewarded activities such as school plays and other performances. Children in the more maladaptive range may respond to frustrations with theatrics that provoke anger and frustration in those around them. Underlying the display of histrionic children is frequently a concern with the power of others, especially those of the opposite gender. During adolescence, heterosexual histrionic girls may act seductively, yet be frightened and surprised at reciprocation by boys. Some adolescent boys with histrionic psychologies may be considered effeminate because of their version of self-dramatization; others adopt hyper-masculine personas seemingly intended to counteract such attributions.

Related studies include: Bleiberg, 2004; Sigmund, Barnett, & Mundt, 1998; Widiger & Bornstein, 2001; Gibson, 2004.

PCA114. Dysregulated Personality Disorders

What we prefer to call dysregulated personality disorder is consistent with descriptions of children with "borderline" personality disorders. It includes vulnerable reality testing, judgment, and impulse control (i.e., aggressive behavior with sensory craving). The clinical picture is characterized by a mixture of pathology on several dimensions—externalizing, internalizing, and cognitive. "These children are highly impulsive but may also be suicidally depressed and/or have micropsychotic symptoms" (Paris, 2003, pg. 34). They may have some paranoid tendencies, along with instability in interpersonal relationships, self-image, and affects (especially anger). In childhood it is difficult to distinguish where this symptom cluster ends and a personality disorder begins.

Related studies include: Bemporad, Smith, Hanson, & Cicchetti, 1982; Bleiberg, 2000; Blum, 1974; Greenman, Gunderson, Cane, & Saltzman, 1986; Kernberg, 1983, 1988; Lubbe, 2000; Mahler, 1971; Mahler & Kaplan, 1977; Masterson, 1980; Palombo, 1982, 1983, 1985, 1987; Paul, Cohen, Klin & Volkmar, 1999; Petti & Vela 1990; Pine, 1974; Rinsley, 1980; Robson, 1983; Zanarini, Gunderson, Marino, Schwartz, & Frankenberg, 1989.

PCA115. Mixed/Other

This category is included to describe children and adolescents presenting with a mixture of the above emerging personality features and/or other patterns not described, such as sadism, dissociation, hypomania, counter-dependency, and passive-aggressive patterns, to name a few.

Concordance of PDM PCA Axis and DSM IV-R Axis II Personality Disorders in Children and Adolescents

PDM Code	PDM Disorder	DSM IV Description
PCA101	Fearful of Closeness/Intimacy (Schizoid) Personality Disorder	Schizoid Personality Disorder
PCA102	Suspicious/Distrustful Personality Disorder	Paranoid Personality Disorder
PCA103	Sociopathic (Antisocial) Personality Disorder	Antisocial Personality Disorder
PCA104	Narcissistic Personality Disorder	Narcissistic Personality Disorder
PCA105	Impulsive/Explosive Personality Disorder	Disruptive Behavior Disorder, NOS or Impulse Control Disorder NOS
PCA106	Self-Defeating Personality Disorder	
PCA107	Depressive Personality Disorder	
PCA108	Somatizing Personality Disorder	
PCA109	Dependent Personality Disorder	Dependent Personality Disorder
PCA110	Avoidant/Constricted Personality Disorder ■ PCA110.1 Counterphobic Personality Disorder	Avoidant Personality Disorder
PCA111	Anxious Personality Disorder	
PCA112	Obsessive-Compulsive Personality Disorder	Obsessive-Compulsive Personality Disorder
PCA113	Histrionic Personality Disorder	Histrionic Personality Disorder
PCA114	Dysregulated Personality Disorder	Borderline Personality Disorder
PCA115	Mixed/Other	Personality Disorder NOS

REFERENCES

Paris, J. (2003). *Personality disorders over time: Precursors, course, and outcome.* American Psychiatric Publishing.

RELATED STUDIES

Abbass, A. (2005). Somatization: Diagnosing it sooner through emotion-focused interviewing. *Journal of Family Practice, 54,* 231-239, 243.

Abbey, S. E. (2005). Somatization and somatoform disorders. In J. L. Levenson (Ed.), *Textbook of psychosomatic medicine* (pp. 271-296). Arlington, VA: American Psychiatric Publishing.

Alden, L. E., Laposa, J. M., Taylor, C. T., & Ryder, A. G. (2002). Avoidant personality disorder: Current status and future directions. *Journal of Personality Disorders, 16,* 1-29.

Anthony, E. J., & Cohler, B. J. (Eds.). (1987). *The invulnerable child.* New York: Guilford.

Battalia, M., Bernardeschi, L., Franchini, L., Bellodi, L., & Smeraldi, E. (1995). A family study of schizotypal disorder. *Schizophrenia Bulletin, 21,* 33-45.

Becker, T. (1974). On latency. *Psychoanalytic Study of the Child, 29,* 3-11.

Bemporad, J. R., Smith, H. F., Hanson, G., & Cicchetti, D. (1982). Borderline syndromes in childhood: Criteria for diagnosis. *American Journal of Psychiatry, 139,* 596-602.

Bene, A. (1979). The question of narcissistic personality disorders: Self pathology in children. *Bulletin of the Hampstead Clinic, 2,* 209-218.

Bernstein, G. A., Borchardt, C. M., & Perwien, A. R. (1996). Anxiety disorders in children and adolescents: a review of the past 10 years. *Journal of the American Academy of Child & Adolescent Psychiatry, 35,* 1110–1119.

Blair, R. J., Budhani, S., Colledge, E., & Scott, S. (2005). Deafness to fear in boys with psychopathic tendencies. *Journal of Child Psychology and Psychiatry, 46,* 327-336.

Bleiberg, E. (1984). Narcissistic disorders in children. *Bulletin of the Menninger Clinic, 48,* 501-517.

Bleiberg, E. (2000). Borderline personality disorder in children and adolescents. In T. Lubbe (Ed.), *The borderline psychotic child: A selective integration* (pp. 39-68). London: Routledge.

Bleiberg, E. (2004). Treatment of dramatic personality disorders in children and adolescents. In J. J. Magnavita (Ed.), *Handbook of personality disorders: Theory and practice* (pp. 467-497). New York: Wiley.

Blos, P. (1979).*The adolescent passage: Developmental issues.* New York: International Universities Press.

Blum, H. P. (1974). The borderline childhood of the Wolf Man. *Journal of the American Psychoanalytic Association, 22,* 721-742.

Bornstein, F. 1999. Oxford textbook of psychopathology. T. Millon and P. H. Blaney. London, Oxford University Press: 535-554.

Bornstein, R. F. (1996). Beyond orality: Toward an object relations/interactionist reconceptualization of the etiology and dynamics of dependency. *Psychoanalytic Psychology, 13,* 177-203.

Bornstein, R. F. (2005a). Diagnosis. In *Dependent patient: A practitioner's guide* (pp. 91-109). Washington, DC: American Psychological Association.

Bornstein, R. F. (2005b). An integrated treatment model. In *Dependent patient: A practitioner's guide* (pp. 151–171). Washington, DC: American Psychological Association.

Brown, R. J., Schrag, A., & Trimble, M. R. (2005). Dissociation, childhood interpersonal trauma, and family functioning in patients with somatization disorder. *American Journal of Psychiatry, 162,* 899-905.

Bucci, W. (1997). *Psychoanalysis and cognitive science: A multiple code theory*. New York: Guilford.

Caplan, R., & Guthrie, D. (1992). Communication deficits in childhood schizotypal personality disorder. *Journal of the American Academy of Child and Adolescent Psychiatry, 31*, 961-967.

Carstairs, K. (1992). Paranoid-schizoid or symbiotic? *International Journal of Psychoanalysis, 73*, 71-85.

Chapman, M. V. (2005). Neighborhood quality and somatic complaints among American youth. *Journal of Adolescent Health, 36*, 244-252.

Chess, S., & Thomas, A. (1977). Temperamental individuality: from childhood to adolescence. *Journal of the American Academy of Child Psychiatry, 16*, 218-226.

Chess, S., & Thomas, A. (1986). *Temperament in clinical practice*. New York: Guilford Press.

Chused, J. (1999). Obsessional manifestations in children. *Psychoanalytic Study of the Child. 54*, 219-232.

Clark, D., & Bolton, D. (1985). Obsessive-compulsive adolescents and their parents: A psychometric study. *Journal of Child Psychology and Psychiatry, 26*, 267-276.

Coker, L. A. and T. A. Widiger (2005). Personality disorders. In J. E. Maddux & B. A. Winstead (Eds.), *Psychopathology: Foundations for a contemporary understanding* (pp. 201-228). Mahwah, NJ: Lawrence Erlbaum Publishing.

Cytryn, L. (1998). Classification of childhood disorders: The need for developmental-dimensional approaches. A personal-historical perspective. *The Journal of Developmental and Learning Disabilities, 2*, 139-153.

Dahl, E. K. (1995). Daughters and mothers: Aspects of the representation world during adolescence. *Psychoanalytic Study of the Child, 50*, 187-204.

de Young, M. (1984). Counterphobic behavior in multiply molested children. *Child Welfare 63*, 333-339.

Dowling, S. (1989). The significance of infant observations for psychoanalysis in later states of life: A discussion. In S. Dowling & A. Rothstein (Eds.), *The significance of infant observational research for clinical work with children, adolescents and adults* (pp. 213-226). Madison, CT: International Universities Press.

Egan, J., & Kernberg, P. F. (1984). Pathological narcissism in childhood. *Journal of the American Psychoanalytic Association, 32*, 39-62.

Eifert, G. H., & Zvolensky, M. J. (2005). Somatoform disorders. In J. E. Maddux & B. A. Winstead (Eds.), *Psychopathology: Foundations for a contemporary understanding* (pp. 281-300). Mahwah, NJ: Lawrence Erlbaum Publishing.

Emde, R. N. (1988). Development terminable and interminable. *International Journal of Psycho-Analysis, 69*, 23–42.

Erikson, E. H. (1959). *Identity and the life cycle: Selected papers*. Psychological Issues Monograph (1, Serial No. 1). New York: International Universities Press.

Fajardo, B. (1988). Constitution in infancy: Implications for early development and psychoanalysis. In A. Goldberg (Ed.), *Progress in self psychology: Learning from Kohut* (Vol. 4, pp. 91-100). Hillsdale, NJ: Analytic Press.

Fischer, R. (1991). Pubescence: A psychoanalytic study of one girl's experience of puberty. *Psychological Inquiry, 11*, 457-479.

Fischer, R. S., & Balsam, R. H. (Eds.). (2004). Mothers and daughters [whole issue]. *Psychological Inquiry, 24*(5).

Fischer, N., & Fischer, R. (1991). Adolescence, sex, and neurogenesis: A clinical perspective. In S. Akhtar & H. Parens (Eds.), *Beyond the symbiotic orbit: Advances in separation-individuation theory. Essays in honor of Selma Kramer, M.D.* (Chap. 10). Hillsdale: Analytic Press.

Flament, M. F., Koby, E., Rapoport, J. L., Berg, C. J., Zahn, T., Cox, C., et al. (1990). Childhood obsessive-compulsive disorder: A prospective follow-up study. *Journal of Child Psychology and Psychiatry, 31*, 363-380.

Fonagy, P., Gergely, G., Jurist, E. L., & Target, M. (2002). *Affect regulation, mentalization, and the development of the self.* New York: Other Press.

Fraiberg, S. H. (1975). Ghosts in the nursery: A psychoanalytic approach to the problem of impaired infant-mother relationships. *Journal of the American Academy of Child Psychiatry, 14,* 387-421.

Francis, G., & F. D'Elia (1994). Avoidant disorder. In M. C. Roberts (Series Ed.) & T. H. Ollendick, N. J. King, & W. Yules (Vol. Eds.), *Issues in clinical child psychology: International handbook of phobic and anxiety disorders in children and adolescents* (pp. 131-143). New York: Plenum.

Francis, G., & Gragg, R. A. (1996). *Childhood obsessive compulsive disorder.* In Developmental Clinical Psychology and Psychiatry Series (Vol. 35). Thousand Oaks, CA: Sage Publishing.

Francis, G., Last, C., & Strauss, C. (1992). Avoidant disorder and social phobia in children and adolescents. *Journal of the American Academy of Child and Adolescent Psychiatry, 31,* 1086-1089.

Frenkel, R. S. (1993). Problems in female development. Comments on the analysis of an early latency-age girl. *The Psychoanalytic Study of the Child,* 171-192

Freud, A. (1962). Assessment of childhood disturbances. *The Psychoanalytic Study of the Child, 17,* 149-158.

Freud, A. (1963). The concept of developmental lines. *Psychoanalytic Study of the Child, 18,* 245-265.

Freud, A. (1965). *Normality and pathology in childhood: Assessments of development.* New York: International Universities Press.

Freud, A. (1970). The symptomatology of childhood: A preliminary attempt at classification. *The Psychoanalytic Study of the Child, 25,* 19-44.

Freud, A. (1981). The concept of developmental lines: Their diagnostic significance. *Psychoanalytic Study of the Child, 36,* 129-136.

Gabbard, G. O. (2005). Mind, brain, and personality disorders. *American Journal of Psychiatry, 162,* 648-655.

Gibson, P. R. (2004). Histrionic personality. In P. G. Caplan & L. Cosgrove (Eds.), *Bias in psychiatric diagnosis* (pp. 201-206). Northvale, NJ: Jason Aronson.

Goodwin, R. D., Brook, J. S., & Cohen, P. (2005). Panic attacks and the risk of personality disorder. *Psychological Medicine,35,* 227-235.

Greene, R. W. (1998). *The explosive child: A new approach for understanding and parenting easily frustrated, "chronically inflexible" children.* New York: Harper Collins.

Greenman, D. A., Gunderson, J. G., Cane, M., & Saltzman, P. R. (1986). An examination of the borderline diagnosis in children. *American Journal of Psychiatry, 143,* 998-1003.

Greenspan, S. I. (1981). Psychopathology and adaptation in infancy and early childhood: Principles of clinical diagnoses and preventive intervention. *Clinical Infant Reports* (No. 1). Madison, CT: International Universities Press.

Greenspan, S. I. (1988). The development of the ego: Insights from clinical work with infants and young children. *Journal of the American Psychoanalytic Association, 36(suppl.),* 3-55.

Greenspan, S. I. (1989a). The development of the ego: Biological and environmental specificity in the psychopathological developmental process and the selection and construction of ego defenses. *Journal of the American Psychoanalytic Association, 37,* 605-638.

Greenspan, S. I. (1989b). *The development of the ego: Implications for personality theory, psychopathology, and the psychotherapeutic process.* Madison, CT: International Universities Press.

Greenspan, S. I. (2003). *The clinical interview with the child* (3rd Ed.). Arlington, VA: American Psychiatric Publishing.

Greenspan, S. I. & Pollock, G. H. (Eds.). (1991a). *The course of life: Vol. I Infancy.* Madison, CT: International Universities Press.

Greenspan, S. I. & Pollock, G. H. (Eds.). (1991b). *The course of life: Vol. II Early childhood*. Madison, CT: International Universities Press.

Greenspan, S. I. & Pollock, G. H. (Eds.). (1991c). *The course of life: Vol. III Middle and late childhood*. Madison, CT: International Universities Press.

Greenspan, S. I. & Pollock, G. H. (Eds.). (1991d). *The course of life: Vol. IV. Adolescence*. Madison, CT: International Universities Press.

Grigsby, J., & Stevens, D. (2000). *Neurodynamics of personality*. New York: Guilford Press.

Hofer, M. A. (1995). An evolutionary perspective on anxiety. In S. P. Rose & R. A. Glick (Eds.), *Anxiety as symptom and signal* (pp. 17-38). Hillsdale, NJ: Analytic Press.

Holmes, J. (1982). Phobia and counterphobia: Family aspects of agoraphobia. *Journal of Family Therapy, 4*, 133–152.

Horowitz, L. M. (2004). The dependent and avoidant personality disorders. In *Interpersonal foundations of psychopathology* (pp. 103-129). Washington, DC: American Psychological Association.

Horowitz, K., Gorfinkle, K., Lewis, O., & Phillips, K. (2002). Body dysmorphic disorder in an adolescent girl. *American Academy of Child and Adolescent Psychiatry, 14*, 1503-1509.

Houghton, S., West, J., & Tan, C. (2005). The nature and prevalence of psychopathic tendencies among mainstream school children and adolescents: Traditional and latent-trait approaches. In R. F. Waugh (Ed.), *Frontiers in educational psychology* (pp. 259-280). Hauppague. NY: Nova Science Publishers.

Hughes, A. (1988). The use of manic defence in the psycho-analysis of a 10-year-old girl. *International Review of Psychoanalysis, 15*, 13-24

Huprich, S. K., & Frisch, M. B. (2004). The Depressive Personality Disorder Inventory and its relationship to quality of life, hopefulness, and optimism. *Journal of Personality Assessment, 83*, 22-28.

Juni, S. (1979). Theoretical foundations of projection as a defence mechanism. *International Review of Psychoanalysis, 6*, 115-121.

Keenan, K., & Wakschlag, L. S. (2004). Are oppositional defiant and conduct disorder symptoms normative behaviors in preschoolers? A comparison of referred and nonreferred children. *American Journal of Psychiatry, 161*, 356-358.

Kendler, K. S. (1993). Twin studies of psychiatric illness: Current status and future directions. *Archives of General Psychiatry, 50*, 905-915.

Kendler, K. S., & Eaves, L. J. (1986). Models for the joint effect of genotype and environment on liability to psychiatric illness. *American Journal of Psychiatry, 143*, 279-289.

Kernberg, O. F. (1987). Projection and projective identification: Developmental and clinical aspects. *Journal of the American Psychoanalytic Association, 35*, 795-819.

Kernberg, O. F. (1999). A severe sexual inhibition in the course of the psychoanalytic treatment of a patient with a narcissistic personality disorder. *International Journal of Psycho-Analysis, 80*, 899-908.

Kernberg, P. F. (1983). Borderline conditions: Childhood and adolescent aspects. In K. S. Robson (Ed.), *The borderline child: Etiology, diagnosis, and treatment* (pp. 101-119). New York: McGraw Hill.

Kernberg, P. F. (1988). Children with borderline personality organization. In C. J. Kestenbaum & D. T. Williams (Eds.), *Handbook of clinical assessment of children and adolescents* (pp. 604-625). New York: New York University Press.

Kernberg, P. F. (1989). Narcissistic personality disorder in childhood. *Psychiatric Clinics of North America, 112*, 671-693.

Kernberg, P. F., Weiner, A.S., & Bardenstein, K. K. (2000). *Personality disorders in children and adolescents*. New York: Basic Books.

Klein, D. N., Schatzberg, A. F., McCullough, J. P., Dowling, F., Goodman, D., Howland, R. H., et al. (1999). Age of onset in chronic major depression: Relation to demographic and clinical variables, family history, and treatment response. *Journal of Affective Disorders, 55,* 149-157.

Lahey, B. B., Loeber, R., Burke, J. D., & Applegate, B. (2005). Predicting future antisocial personality disorder in males from a clinical assessment in childhood. *Journal of Consulting and Clinical Psychology, 73,* 389-399.

Last, C. G. (1989). Anxiety disorders of childhood or adolescence. In C. G. Last & M. Hersen (Eds.), *Handbook for child psychiatric diagnosis.* New York: Wiley.

Leckman, J. F., & Mayes, L. C. (1998). Understanding developmental psychopathology: How useful are evolutionary accounts? *Journal of the American Academy of Child and Adolescent Psychiatry, 37,* 1011-1021.

Lichtenberg, J. D. (1983). *Psychoanalysis and infant research.* Hillsdale, NJ: Analytic Press.

Lichtenberg, J. D. (1989). *Psychoanalysis and motivation.* Hillsdale, NJ: Analytic Press.

Loeber, R., & Schmaling, K. B. (1985). The utility of differentiating between mixed and pure forms of antisocial child behavior. *Journal of Abnormal Child Psychology, 73,* 315-335.

Lubbe, T. (2000). The borderline concept in childhood: Common origins and developments in clinical theory and practice in the USA and the UK. In T. Lubbe (Ed.), *The borderline psychotic child: A selective integration* (pp. 3-38). London: Routledge.

Mahler, M. S. (1968). *On human symbiosis and the vicissitudes of individuation.* New York: International Universities Press.

Mahler, M. S. (1971). A study of the separation-individuation process and its possible application to borderline phenomena in the psychoanalytic situation. *The Psychoanalytic Study of the Child, 26,* 403-424.

Mahler, M. S., & Kaplan, L. (1977). Developmental aspects in the assessment of narcissistic and so-called borderline personalities. In P. Hartocollis (Ed.), *Borderline personality disorders: The concept, the syndrome, the patient* (pp. 71-89). New York: International Universities Press.

Mahler, M. S., Pine, F., & Bergman, A.(1975) *The psychological birth of the human infant: Symbiosis and individuation.* New York: Basic Books.

March, J. S., & Leonard, H. L. (1996). Obsessive-compulsive disorder in children and adolescents: A review of the past 10 years. *Journal of the American Academy of Child and Adolescent Psychiatry, 34,* 1265-1273.

Masterson, J. F. (1980). *From borderline adolescent to functioning adult.* New York: Brunner/ Mazel, Inc.

Mayer, E. L. (1991). Towers and enclosed spaces: A preliminary report on gender differences in children's reactions to block structures. *Psychological Inquiry. 11,* 480-510.

McGlashan, T. H. (1986). Schizotypal personality disorder. Chestnut Lodge follow-up study: VI. Long term follow-up perspectives. *Archives of General Psychiatry, 43,* 329-334.

McLean, P. D., & McLean, C. P. (2004). Family therapy of avoidant personality disorder. In M. M. MacFarlane (Ed.), *Family treatment of personality disorders: Advances in clinical practice* (pp. 273-303). Binghamton, NW: Haworth Clinical Practice Press.

Meers, D. R. (1966). A diagnostic profile of psychopathology in a latency child. *Psychoanalytic Study of the Child, 21,* 483-526.

Meers, D. R. (1973).Psychoanalytic research and intellectual functioning of ghetto-reared black children. *Psychoanalytic Study of the Child,* 28:395-417.

Moffitt, T. E. (1993). Adolescence-limited and life course-persistent antisocial behavior: A developmental view. *Psychological Review, 100,* 674-701.

Moffitt, T., Caspi, A., Dickson, N., Silva, P., & Stanton, W. (1996). Childhood-onset versus adolescent-onset antisocial conduct problems in males: Natural history from ages 3 to 18 years. *Development and Psychopathology, 8,* 399-425.

Nagera, H. (1963). The developmental profile: notes on some practical considerations regarding its use. *Psychoanalytic Study of the Child, 18*, 511-540.

Nagy, J., & Szatmari, P. (1986). A chart review of schizotypal personality disorders in children. *Journal of Autism and Developmental Disorders, 16*, 351-367.

Offer, D., Ostrow, E., & Howard, K. I. (1981). *The adolescent: A psychological self-portrait.* New York: Basic Books.

Olin, S., Raine, A., Cannon, T. D., Parnas, J., Schulsinger, F., & Mednick, S. A. (1997). Childhood behavior precursors of schizotypal personality disorder. *Schizophrenia Bulletin, 23*. 93-103.

Pajer, K. A. (1998). What happens to "bad" girls? A review of the adult outcome of antisocial adolescent girls. *American Journal of Psychiatry, 155*, 862-870.

Palombo, J. (1982). Critical review of the concept of the borderline child. *Clinical Social Work Journal, 10*, 246-264.

Palombo, J. (1983). Borderline conditions: A perspective from self psychology. *Clinical Social Work Journal, 11*, 323-338.

Palombo, J. (1985). The treatment of borderline neurocognitively impaired children: A perspective from self psychology. *Clinical Social Work Journal, 13*, 117-128.

Palombo, J. (1987). Self-object transferences in the treatment of borderline neurocognitively impaired children. In J. S. Grotstein, M. F. Solomon, & J. A. Lang (Eds.), *The borderline patient: Emerging concepts in diagnosis, psychodynamics, and treatment* (Vol. 2, pp. 317-345). Hillsdale, NJ: Analytic Press.

Palombo, J. (1988). Adolescent development: A view from self psychology. *Child and Adolescent Social Work Journal, 5*, 171-186.

Palombo, J. (1990). The cohesive self, the nuclear self, and development in late adolescence. *Adolescent Psychiatry, 17*, 338-359.

Parens, H., Pollock, L., Stern, J., & Kramer, S. (1976). On the girl's entry into the Oedipus complex. *Journal of the American Psychoanalytic Association, 24S*, 79-107.

Paul, R., Cohen, D. J., Klin, A., & Volkmar, E. (1999). Multiplex developmental disorders: The role of communication in the construction of a self. *Child and Adolescent Psychiatric Clinics of North America, 8*, 189–202.

Petti, T. A., & Vela, R. M. (1990). Borderline disorders in childhood: An overview. *Journal of the American Academy of Child and Adolescent Psychiatry, 29*, 327-337.

Pezzarossa, B., Della Rosa, A., & Rubino, I. A. (2002). Self-defeating personality and memories of parents' child-rearing behaviour. *Psychological Reports 91*, 436-438.

Pine, F. (1974). On the concept "borderline" in children: A clinical essay. *Psychoanalytic Study of the Child, 29*, 341-368.

Pine, F. (1987). *Developmental theory and clinical practice.* New Haven, CT: Yale University Press.

Proner, B. D. (2005). Bodily states of anxiety: the movement from somatic states to thought. *Journal of Analytical Psychology, 50*, 311-331.

Pruett, K. D., & Litzenberger, B. (1992). Latency development in children of primary nurturing fathers: Eight-year follow-up. *Psychoanalytic Study of the Child, 47*, 85-101.

Rettew, D. C., Zanarini, M. C., Yen, S., Grilo, C. M., Skodol, A. E., Shea, M. T., et al. (2003). Childhood antecedents of avoidant personality disorder: A retrospective study. *Journal of the American Academy of Child and Adolescent Psychiatry, 42*, 1122-1130.

Rinsley, D. B. (1980). Diagnosis and treatment of borderline and narcissistic children and adolescents. *Bulletin of the Menninger Clinic, 44*, 147-170.

Robbins, M. (1982). Narcissistic personality as a symbiotic character disorder. *International Journal of Psycho-Analysis, 63*, 457-473.

Robertiello, R. C. (1988). A rare diagnosis: The counterphobic personality. *Journal of Contemporary Psychotherapy, 18*, 329-332.

Robson, K. S. (Ed.) (1983). *The borderline child: Etiology, diagnosis, and treatment.* New York: McGraw-Hill.

Rubino, I. A., Pezzarossa, B., Della Rosa, A., & Siracusano, A. (2004). Self defeating personality and memories of parents' child rearing behaviour: A replication. *Psychological Reports, 94,* 733-735.

Rutter, M. (1966). *Children of sick parents: An environmental and psychiatric study* (Institute of Psychiatry Maudsley Monograph No. 16). London: Oxford University Press.

Rygaard, N. P. (1998). Psychopathic children: Indicators of organic dysfunction. In T. Millon, E. Simonsen, M. Burket-Smith, & R. D. Davis (Eds.), *Psychopathy: Antisocial, criminal, and violent behavior.* New York: Guilford.

Sander, L. W. (1985). Toward a logic of organization in psychobiological development. In H. Klar & L. Siever (Eds.), *Biologic response styles: Clinical implications* (pp. 20-36). Washington, DC: American Psychiatric Association.

Sander, L. W. (1987). A 25-year follow-up: Some reflections on personality development over the long term. *Infant Mental Health Journal, 8* [Special Issue: Papers from the Third Congress of the World Association for Infant Psychiatry and Allied Disciplines], 210-220.

Sandler, J. (1972). The role of affects in psychoanalytic theory. *Ciba Foundation Symposium, 8,* 31-46.

Sarnoff, C. (1976). *Latency.* New York: Jason Aronson.

Schore, A. N. (1994). *Affect regulation and the origin of the self: The neurobiology of emotional development.* Hillsdale, NJ: Lawrence Erlbaum Publishing.

Shapiro, T. (1976). Latency revisited: The age 7 plus or minus 1. *Psychoanalytic Study of the Child, 31,* 79-105.

Siegel, D. J. (1999). *The developing mind: Toward a neurobiology of interpersonal experience.* New York: Guilford.

Sigmund, D., Barnett, E., & Mundt, C. (1998). The hysterical personality disorder: A phenomenological approach. *Psychopathology, 31,* 318-330.

Spitz, R. A. (1965). *The first year of life: A psychoanalytic study of normal and deviant development of object relations.* New York: International Universities Press.

Stern, D. N. (1985). *The interpersonal world of the infant: A view from psychoanalysis and developmental psychology.* New York: Basic Books.

Stern, D. N. (2004). *The present moment in psychotherapy and everyday life.* New York: Norton.

Strauss, C. C. (1990). Overanxious disorder in childhood. In M. Hersen & C. G. Last (Eds.), *Handbook of child and adult psychopathology: A longitudinal perspective.* New York: Pergamon.

Taylor, C. T., Laposa, J. M., & Alden, E. (2004). Is avoidant personality disorder more than just social avoidance? *Journal of Personality Disorders, 18,* 571-594.

Tillfors, M., Furmark, T., Ekselius, L., & Fredrikson, M. (2004). Social phobia and avoidant personality disorder: One spectrum disorder? *Nordic Journal of Psychiatry, 58,* 147-152.

Tyson, P. (1988). Psychic structure formation: The complementary roles of affects, drives, object Relations, and conflict. *Journal of the American Psychoanalytic Association, 36(S),* 73-98

Tyson, P., & Tyson, R. L. (1990). *Psychoanalytic theories of development: An integration.* New Haven, CT: Yale University.

Warren, S. L., Emde, R. N., & Sroufe, L.A. (2000). Internal representations: Predicting anxiety from children's play narratives. *Journal of the American Academy of Child and Adolescent Psychiatry, 39,* 100-107.

Weil, A. P. (1970). The basic core. *Psychoanalytic Study of the Child, 25,* 442-460.

Weise, K. L., & Tuber, S. (2004). The self and object representations of narcissistically disturbed children: An empirical investigation. *Psychoanalytic Psychology, 21,* 244-258.

Widiger, T. A., & Bornstein, R. F. (2001). Histrionics, dependent, and narcissistic personality disorders. In P. B. Sutker & H. E. Adams (Eds.), *Comprehensive handbook of psychopathology* (3rd ed., pp. 509-531). New York: Plenum.

Willock, B. (1987). The devalued (unloved, repugnant) self: A second facet of narcissistic vulnerability in the aggressive, conduct-disordered child. *Psychoanalytic Psychology, 3,* 219-240.

Winnicott, D.(1953). Transitional objects and transitional phenomena: A study of the first not-me possession. *International Journal of Psychoanalysis, 34,* 89-97.

Winnicott, D. W. (1960). Ego distortion in terms of true and false self. In D. W. Winnicott (Ed.), *The maturational processes and the facilitating environment* (pp. 140-152). New York: International Universities Press.

Winnicott, D. W. (1965). *The maturational processes and the facilitating environment: Studies in the theory of emotional development.* New York: International Universities Press.

Winnicott, D. (1992). Primary maternal preoccupation. In D. Winnicott, *Paediatrics to psychoanalysis: Collected papers* (pp. 300-305). New York: Brunner-Routledge.

Wolff, S. (1991). "Schizoid" personality in childhood and adult life: III. The childhood picture. *British Journal of Psychiatry. 159,* 629-635.

Wolff, S., & Barlow, A. (1979). Schizoid personality in childhood: A comparative study of schizoid, autistic and normal children. *Journal of Child Psychology and Psychiatry. 20,* 29-46.

Wolff, S., Townshend, R., McGuire, R. J., & Weeks, D. J. (1991). "Schizoid" personality in childhood and adult life: II. Adult adjustment and the continuity with schizotypal personality disorder. *British Journal of Psychiatry, 159.* 620-629.

Zanarini, M. C., Gunderson, J. G., Marino, M. F., Schwartz, E. O., & Frankenberg, E. R. (1989). Childhood experiences of borderline patients. *Comprehensive Psychiatry, 30,* 18-25.

Child and Adolescent Symptom Patterns: The Subjective Experience SCA Axis

WORK GROUP MEMBERS

Joseph Palombo, MA, Co-Chair
Chicago, Illinois

Bernard Friedberg, MD, Co-Chair
Voorhees, New Jersey

Alex Burland, MD (deceased)
Philadelphia, Pennsylvania

Amy Eldridge, PhD
Chicago, Illinois

Theodore Fallon, Jr., MD, MPH
Philadelphia, Pennsylvania

Ruth Fischer, MD
Philadelphia, Pennsylvania

Stanley I. Greenspan, MD
Bethesda, Maryland

Leon Hoffman, MD
New York, New York

Thomas K. Kenemore, PhD
Chicago, Illinois

Paulina Kernberg, MD (deceased)
Westchester, New York

Stuart G. Shanker, DPhil
Toronto, Ontario

Serena Wieder, PhD
Silver Spring, Maryland

Child and Adolescent Symptom Patterns: The Subjective Experience SCA Axis

Symptom patterns in children, as in adults, are best viewed in a developmental, dynamic context. Clinicians who work with children are reminded daily of the multiple factors that contribute to different symptom patterns as well as the unique developmental pathways that lead to various symptoms. Consider the example of a child evidencing anxiety. Family factors, events at school, biologically based tendencies to be overresponsive to sensations such as touch or sound, and a developmental history characterized by frightening experiences and insufficient opportunities to learn to cope with conflict may all contribute to varying degrees.

Similarly, each child's subjective experience of his or her symptoms is unique. For one child, anxiety may be experienced predominantly as a "gurgling tummy," or expressed as "my muscles hurt," and in another child as "I'm scared of being kidnapped." In addition, children develop rapidly and therefore experience changes in their behaviors, feelings, thoughts, fantasies, and symptom patterns. The meaning or subjective level of a symptom pattern may be quite different for a child at different developmental stages.

This section describes the most common symptom patterns observed in children. Some of these are also described in the DSM-IV-TR system, but without comment on the child's subjective experience. Some are described only in the adult sections of DSM-IV-TR, and yet we believe that their childhood manifestations deserve separate consideration because of the developmental processes that inform and influence the child's experience and expression of symptoms. At the end of this section, we include a chart showing the concordance between the PDM and the DSM-IV-TR, respectively, in the area of symptom patterns. Because of the divergent preferences of the different work groups and because of some differences between children and adults, the disorders in this section appear in a different order from that of the comparable conditions in the adult section.

Healthy Response
Developmental crises Situational crises
Anxiety Disorders
SCA301. Anxiety Disorders SCA302. Phobias SCA303. Obsessive-Compulsive Disorders SCA304. Somatization (Somatoform) Disorders
Affect/Mood Disorders
SCA305. Prolonged Mourning/Grief Reaction SCA306. Depressive Disorders SCA307. Bipolar Disorders SCA308. Suicidality
Disruptive Behavior Disorders
SCA309. Conduct Disorders SCA310. Oppositional-Defiant Disorders SCA311. Substance Abuse Related Disorders
Reactive Disorders
SCA312. Psychic Trauma and Posttraumatic Stress Disorder SCA313. Adjustment Disorders (other than developmental)
Disorders of Mental Functions

SCA314. Motor Skills Disorders
SCA315. Tic Disorders
SCA316. Psychotic Disorders
SCA317. Neuropsychological Disorders
    SCA317.1 Visual-Spatial Processing Disorders
    SCA317.2 Language and Auditory Processing Disorders
    SCA317.3 Memory Impairments
    SCA317.4 Attention Deficit/Hyperactivity Disorders (AD/HD)
    SCA317.5 Executive Function Disorders
    SCA317.6 Severe Cognitive Deficits
SCA318. Learning Disorders
    SCA318.1 Reading Disorders
    SCA318.2 Mathematics Disorders
    SCA318.3 Disorders of Written Expression
    SCA318.4 Nonverbal Learning Disabilities
    SCA318.5 Social-Emotional Learning Disabilities

Psychophysiologic Disorders
SCA319. Bulimia **SCA320. Anorexia**
Developmental Disorders

SCA321. Regulatory Disorders
SCA322. Feeding Problems of Childhood
SCA323. Elimination Disorders
    SCA323.1 Encopresis
    SCA323.2 Enuresis
SCA324. Sleep Disorders
SCA325. Attachment Disorders
SCA326. Pervasive Developmental Disorders
    SCA326.1 Autism
    SCA326.2 Asperger Syndrome
    SCA326.3 Pervasive Developmental Disorder (PDD) not
        otherwise specified

Other Disorders
SCA327. Gender Identity Disorders

HEALTHY RESPONSE

Developmental Crises

In a healthy response to a developmental challenge, the child's maturation is interrupted temporarily by an arrest or regression to a prior phase with no obvious external precipitant. Such reactions follow a stable period of adjustment and are time-limited. Developmental crises occur as a normal part of maturation and vary in how visible they are to others. In an effort to resolve earlier unresolved crises before moving on, children typically regress to the psychological issues associated with earlier phases. This process is particularly notable in adolescence (Blos, 1967; Noshpitz, 1991; Offer, 1991).

Affective states may include the child's feeling shame, and/or blaming self or others for painful feelings. Anger, sadness, and shame may be expressed in outbursts. The child's mood may be subdued or highly charged, inappropriate or euphoric. He or she may express acute distress by crying, rage, or destructive behavior The child may understand what has occurred but be upset nevertheless, or may refuse to acknowledge the meaning of the developmental event yet come to terms with it over time. Responses are highly variable depending on the age of the child, the child's resilience, the nature of the developmental problem, the support that is available from caregivers, and other factors.

Thoughts and fantasies may include the child's puzzlement at the destabilization of a previously unproblematic sense of self. The child may deny or disavow the existence of a problem, or project and displace his feelings onto others.

In terms of *somatic states,* the child's sleep patterns may be disturbed. He may complain of not feeling well. Appetite may increase or be suppressed.

The child's capacity for *relationships* is intact and age-appropriate in a healthy response to a developmental challenge. But the child may become more clingy and demanding while struggling with the imbalance created by the crisis. There may be bouts of resentment and anger at caregivers who are felt to be unhelpful. Siblings may become targets of displaced anger and hostility. The child may be responsive to restorative interventions from caregivers.

Case Illustration

A 13-year-old boy who began developing secondary sexual characteristics was embarrassed and refused to go to school for a few days for fear that his erection would be noticed by the girls in his class. The father's empathic, patient, and supportive attitude allowed him to feel more comfortable with his physical changes. Within a brief period of time he was able to go back to school and gradually resumed his activities. Interestingly, he then learned from his friends the tactic of using his backpack or book to cover his genital area.

Related studies include: Anthony 1987.

Situational Crises

In a situational crisis, the child's development is interrupted by a relatively minor precipitant. The child's reaction follows a stable period of adjustment and is time-limited. Examples of precipitants of a normal situational crisis include a mother's pregnancy, the arrival of a sibling, first day of day care, loss of a transitional object, illness, medical procedure, separation at the beginning of school, caregiver's withdrawal following the death of a relative, or other changes and stresses that fall short of constituting a significant trauma.

Affective states, thoughts and fantasies, somatic states, and relationship patterns are similar to those found in children with developmental crises.

Case Illustrations

- A 5-year-old girl was brought for an evaluation because of a variety of fears and some separation issues at nursery school. After a few meetings with the therapist, her symptoms ameliorated. It became clear that the little girl was responding to her younger brother's having been moved out of her room to another bedroom.

■ A 17-year-old girl was about to go to college. Although she had had some previous therapy for anxious and depressive reactions when a sibling was born during her pre-school years, she functioned well, had friends, and did well in school. She became very worried about leaving home and reported that the impending separation reminded her of her homesickness during camp. She was homesick during her first month of college but soon adjusted well.

SCA301. Anxiety Disorders

Manifestations of anxiety in children may include feelings of overwhelming fear, panic states accompanied by somatic symptoms, school refusal, and acute anxiety states. (Please see The Classification of Mental Health and Developmental Disorders in Infancy and Early Childhood, p. 319, for further discussion of anxiety disorders, including developmental anxiety disorders and separation anxiety.) While there are expectable transient anxieties associated with development and new experiences (going to school, being in a peer group, separating from parents, etc.), an anxiety disorder is characterized by continuing anxiety that may interfere with full mastering of age-expected experiences.

Anxiety is the affective signal of danger. The content of what is dangerous may be conscious or unconscious, real or unreal. In children it is often associated with basic safety issues; e.g., fear of illness, injury, loss of or damage to a caregiver, or even the imagined consequences of a successful accomplishment. Although anxiety appears very early in development, the individual's ability to regulate responses and metabolize the anxiety increases and changes with psychological development. As children grow, they are increasingly able to manage greater amounts of anxiety. The course of an anxiety disorder is highly variable depending on the child and the family. In some instances it is transient and episodic, while in others it is so intense that it interferes with the child's functioning. Family patterns, peer relationships, the school environment, and the child's internal stability can play significant roles in its course.

The signs of anxiety vary with the child's age and stage of development. *Affective states* include both pervasive fear and a heightened state of alertness. The subjective experience of anxiety is a sense of danger. In its extreme form, there is dread of impending doom. In its less extreme form, children describe a vague worry, and nervousness. When the experience is more chronic, adolescents will sometimes use the words "stress" and "tension." These states may be handled with defense mechanisms ranging from denial to sublimation. When defensive function is not sufficient to contain the anxiety, there may be a repetitive, even compulsive replaying of anxiety-producing situations or events until the anxiety is neutralized and the child feels a sense of mastery over the imagined threat.

A mild-to-moderate anxiety may stimulate cognitive activity while moderate-to-severe anxiety can disrupt cognitive processes and thinking in general. Anxiety can also interfere with sleep, eating, learning, and peer relations. Performance anxiety, for example, may include mild apprehension about giving a book report or stage fright so extreme as to be paralyzing.

Thoughts and fantasies may be inferred from the repetitive play of children with anxiety disorders. On the other hand, the narrative around the disorder can be completely disrupted due to the cognitively disruptive effects of anxiety. Sometimes with severe anxiety, children will repetitively and compulsively play out the perceived threat while simultaneously dissociating any awareness of the meaning of the play.

Somatic states may include decreased or increased motor activity and changes in posture. Physiological responses may include increased heart rate, increased or decreased respiration, dilated pupils, increased muscle tension, and increases in galvanic skin responses. Chronic states of anxiety contribute to a variety of physical maladies, including most notably eczema and neurodermatitis. Unmanaged anxiety may also be manifested as disorders of skin, muscle, or joints, and may affect gastrointestinal functioning and evacuation. There can also be physiological responses such as palpitations and sweating.

Gross motor activity may increase in an effort to discharge anxiety, but this discharge usually provides only temporary relief and does not contribute significantly to mastery. Nightmares, eating and sleeping disorders, and regressive behaviors are common in highly anxious children.

Relationships may be interrupted, burdened, or compromised by anxiety disorders. Social and learning activities may suffer. When a child or adolescent has little or no capacity to cope with fears realistically, the result can be a complete breakdown in psychological functioning. In a vicious cycle of anxiety and failed efforts to master it, this breakdown leaves the anxiety unchecked, leading to an escalation of the breakdown and further escalation of anxiety. Relationships in this situation become disrupted by the child's inability to attend to anything but the anxiety and the efforts to reduce it.

Clinical Illustrations

- A 13-year-old girl was brought for assessment because she had recently developed severe panic attacks. A psychopharmacologist prescribed an antidepressant and an anxiolytic and recommended attention to the dynamics of the girl's anxiety. This young adolescent was a straight-A student, popular among her peers, and active in sports. While two clear precipitants could be found to the specific anxiety attacks, it appeared that their onset related to her concern about weight gain and attractiveness to boys. Although she clearly did not have a weight problem, she made several unsuccessful attempts at dieting. Her mother was concerned about her worries, but her father teased her for being "fat." She felt enraged at her father and alienated from her mother, who did not protect her from the teasing. It was at the point when she began to feel isolated from her parents that she experienced her first anxiety attack. At first, the parents did not take the attacks seriously, even though the girl was extremely distressed. In time the attacks recurred and escalated in intensity. At that point, her parents became overly concerned, and the daughter felt vindicated in having convinced them of her distress. In therapy, she focused increasingly on the issues of independence and autonomy. When the attacks diminished in intensity and became more manageable, the girl was able to move on developmentally.

■ A 6-year-old boy who was otherwise doing well in school would become disruptive to other children's play at recess. When he was observed on the playground, he would initially stand on the outside. After a time, he would jump into the middle of the play, disrupt it, and sometimes taunt others. Further observation established that he played well with his peers in one-on-one situations, including sharing and turn taking. His play with action figures during therapy (who enacted numerous fears) elaborated how he would become anxious in group interactions, felt awkward when attempting to negotiate with more than one peer, and would respond to these situations by either withdrawing or becoming disruptive.

Related studies include: Bernstein, Borchardt, & Perwien, 1996; Goodwin, Brook, & Cohen, 2005; Hofer, 1995a, 1995b; Little, 1990; Strauss, 1990; Warren, Emde, & Sroufe, 2000.

SCA302. Phobias

Phobias are also discussed in the adult section of this manual (see p. 104).

A phobia may develop when a child's anxiety is displaced onto an object or situation that is not ordinarily considered dangerous. The process by which the object becomes associated with danger is generally not readily accessible. That is, the individual with the phobia is usually not able to explain how he or she became afraid of this benign object, which we assume may unconsciously symbolize anxieties about separation, change, harm, or death. We assume that this process is held in unconscious memory by psychological defenses.

In phobias, anxiety from an original threat is displaced onto an object that is less threatening, either because it is inherently less dangerous or because of its decreased proximity. The displacement of the anxiety, however, makes it less likely that the phobic individual will direct activity toward decreasing the original threat. In this way, phobias work against dealing successfully with primal anxieties.

If this displacement sufficiently reduces the anxiety, then the established phobia remains stable. If, however, anxiety is not reduced to a tolerable level, it may become associated with other objects, in a process that spreads the phobia from one object to many (e.g., from snakes to all reptiles). The course of the disorder is extremely variable, lasting from days to years. A resolution to this disorder comes when the displacement is no longer necessary to address the source of the anxiety.

Affective states associated with phobias include fear when thinking about or when confronted with the phobic object or situation. As long as the child can avoid that stimulus, he or she experiences minimal anxiety. As the feared object or situation comes closer, the child characteristically experiences anxiety that escalates to panic. No amount of reassurance diminishes it. Some children, in the absence of phobic stimuli, are hypervigilant with respect to their environment, but they may experience this affective state as being "just the way I feel."

Thoughts and fantasies may be dominated by the phobic object and strategies to avoid it, or the phobic child may avoid thinking about the topic entirely. Overall, the child's ideational life is characterized by constrictions in certain age-expected emotional themes, such as competition and aggression, and an intensification of others, such as dependency ("Is my mother waiting for me at home?").

A phobic child may develop *somatic* symptoms associated with experiences of, or anticipation of, exposure to the object. These vary from child to child and may include a tightening in the chest, a hollow feeling in the tummy, rapid heartbeat, stomachaches, lack of appetite, frequent urges to urinate or defecate, and nausea and vomiting. Their intensity depends upon the intensity of the child's fear. The symptoms dissipate if the phobic object is removed or the situation is avoided.

Relationships tend to be approached with caution by phobic children and adolescents. New situations and people may be assimilated only gradually. Nonetheless, the capacity for intimacy tends to be undamaged in phobic children, who may be quite dependent on their caregivers when young and on close friends when older.

Clinical Illustration

After a fight with a girlfriend who had rejected her, an 11-year-old girl became phobic about going back to school. She was consciously afraid of getting into a physical fight there and also feared that something would happen to her mother while she was gone. These anxieties resulted in her avoiding school for a long time. Work with her repetitive dreams of killing vulnerable animals and being chased by angry females helped her to recognize that she had been feeling deeply guilty over the death of her 5-year-old brother from cancer when she was three. She recalled having felt very angry with her preoccupied mother and having had fleeting death wishes towards her brother, mother, and father. She learned that her fears of getting into fights and of something bad happening to her mother were her unconscious ways of keeping from feeling threatened or being reminded about her earlier murderous desires. She was also struggling to keep homoerotic desires, based on longing for her distracted mother, out of her mind. Behind these were heterosexual interests that felt even more threatening because of the incestuous meanings they had for her. It took her about six months to understand and work though these conflicts around aggression and sexuality, after which she re-entered school.

Related studies include: Beidel & Turner, 1998; Francis, Last, & Strauss, 1992; Schneider, Blanco, Antia, & Liebowitz, 2002.

SCA303. Obsessive-Compulsive Disorders

Obsessive-compulsive disorders require the hallmark symptoms of either excessive rumination (obsessions), compulsively repeated behaviors (rituals), or both. There seems to be a constitutional predisposition in most children who develop these disorders. In many individuals, the course waxes and wanes over a lifetime. The symptoms are accompanied by an anxiety in the child that is conveyed to, and sometimes magnified by, the parents. Together, the parents and the child are not able to quell the anxiety, which becomes acutely worse if the symptoms (ritual behaviors) are not allowed to be expressed. These symptoms can occur in children as young as 4, but more commonly they first appear between ages 6 and 9. Early adolescence and young adulthood are other common periods of new or recurrent onset, probably because these tend to be times of developmental stress.

As with the other anxiety disorders, the associated *affective states* involve pervasive anxiety. In obsessive-compulsive disorders, its source is usually not clear. Both parent and child tend to focus on the anxiety itself, rather than wishing to explore its origins. The characteristic patterns of symptom onset, together with case material, suggest that the sources of many obsessions and compulsions lie in developmental challenges facing the growing child and the parents. Anger and magical fears of loss of control may lie beneath the anxiety.

The child's *thoughts and fantasies* include a preoccupation with the obsessional ideation or ritual in the service of defending against the underlying anxiety.

The child may also develop *somatic* symptoms similar to those described for both anxiety and phobias. Obsessional thinking may make the child's preoccupation with sensations such as stomachache and headache much greater than it is in other anxiety disorders.

The excessive preoccupation with the obsessional idea or compulsive ritual, along with the underlying anxiety, may interfere with *relationships* and with functioning in daily life. Even when obsessional anxiety is not interfering in routine activities, it may be present as a more generalized affective state. Obsessive-compulsive children are noted for their attempts to control situations and relationships as they try to keep their anxieties at manageable levels. Relationships may thus be characterized by a tendency toward rigidity, control, and dependency (often unacknowledged). Nonetheless, and in spite of difficulties expressing vulnerable feelings, the child may be capable of a great deal of warmth and intimacy.

Clinical Illustration

A 17-year-old boy was exercising four hours per day, obsessively weighing and measuring everything he ate, and spending the rest of his day planning his eating and exercising. Although he had done well academically in previous years, he was ignoring his schoolwork and doing poorly. Over a period of four months he lost 50 pounds. Throughout his childhood he had been mildly obese; he was labeled a "brainiac" and was shunned by his peers. His compulsively regulated eating and exercising began when he had an e-mail liaison with a girl in another city. He began psychoanalysis and after four months attempted suicide by purposely losing control of the family car at a high rate of speed. This attempt revealed the extent of his rage toward his parents, who he felt had prepared him poorly for the world; he was angry at his mother for holding on to him and at his father for seemingly abandoning him. With this insight, his preoccupation with his eating and exercise diminished and he began to make friends, to engage more fully in exploring his feelings, and to form more healthy patterns of adaptation. While this case illustrates difficulties with regulating eating, it demonstrates obsessive and compulsive patterns that can manifest themselves in a variety of symptoms.

Related studies include: Chused, 1999; Clark & Bolton, 1985; Flament, et al., 1990; Francis & Gragg, 1996; March & Leonard, 1996; Rapoport, 1991.

SCA304. Somatization (Somatoform) Disorders

Children with somatization disorders complain about a variety of physical symptoms for which no medical condition can be found. They may suffer stomachaches, headaches, nausea, urgency to urinate or defecate, and other similar maladies. The symptoms appear to be related to situations that evoke anxiety in the child, although the child does not associate the symptoms with the situation. Somatization tends to occur in families with difficulties integrating physical sensations, feelings, and thoughts. The symptoms, which are not produced intentionally, may begin spontaneously or following a minor illness. The child is typically convinced that the ailment is purely physical. A pattern ensues in which the child progressively uses the symptoms in the service of avoidance. This pattern may become generalized to the point where the child appears debilitated by the symptoms.

The child's *affective state* is often characterized by anxiety and "neediness." The child appears distressed and in pain. The distress may be compounded if the child feels that caregivers question the reality of the illness. On feeling disbelieved, the child is likely to protest loudly, to feel injured, and to become enraged.

The child's *thoughts* often focus on the particular somatic symptoms, and there is often a narrowing of interests in age-expected domains. Some children with this pattern also experience numerous fears characteristic of younger children. The child's conviction of the gravity of the illness leads to concerns about dire physical consequences. Depending on the child's age and cognitive development, these concerns may be vague and ill-defined or specific and elaborate.

The child may feel that he or she is seriously ill and in danger of dying. In terms of *somatic states*, it is important not to ignore the possibility of undiagnosed medical illness. Whether or not such a condition can be found, taking seriously the child's pain and anxiety may prevent an escalation of complaint designed to demonstrate just how bad the suffering is.

Depending on the dynamics that trigger the somatic symptoms, the child's *relationships* may be reasonably intact or may demonstrate severe regressive features. In the latter case, the child may become excessively fearful of separating from caregivers or may become withdrawn and isolated. Relationships may be characterized by a great deal of dependency and by avoidance of new relationships, especially those that require exploration and curiosity.

Clinical Illustrations

- A 12-year-old girl came in completely paralyzed, unable to walk or move. There were no neurological findings to explain her paralysis. After six months in treatment, she began to move about the consultation room, and two years later she was back in school functioning normally. Her parents were immigrants. Psychoanalysis revealed that she was extremely conflicted about whether to identify with her new culture, implying a move away from parents, or to stay in the "old culture" with her parents and avoid anxieties about new challenges.

- A 9-year-old girl complained of abdominal pain and recurrent vomiting, though she would vomit mostly saliva. This seemed to occur mostly when her parents would argue. Because of her vomiting, they worried about her and kept her out of school. Extensive medical evaluation revealed no physiological reasons for the vomiting. It was later revealed that prior to the onset of the vomiting, the parents had been arguing frequently and threatening to divorce. Since the vomiting, however, the parents had come together to care for their child.

- A 14-year-old boy came in for trouble with swallowing. His ability or inability to swallow was situational. He would have trouble getting his breakfast down, for example, and could not take medicine, but in the therapist's office he had no trouble downing a hamburger. His parents had been in the midst of a contentious divorce for seven years. The boy had a highly conflicted relationship with his mother, who was raised in a military family and imposed strict discipline. He was an oppositional, rebellious child, who would provoke huge fights with her. During the course of the treatment, the therapist found that much of his swallowing problem was related to the tension and anxiety he experienced in relationship with his mother. His symptom was expressing the fact that he was having a hard time swallowing what she was "feeding" him. It remitted once he gave sufficient expression to the feelings associated with her harsh discipline. The therapist's influence on his mother to moderate her style may have also helped to reduce his swallowing problem.

Related studies include: Bonnard, 1963; Evans, 1975; Milrod, 2002.

SCA305. Prolonged Mourning/Grief Reaction

Grief is the normal reaction to the loss of a significant other. In childhood, prolonged mourning may accompany the loss of a parent or other caregiver through death, divorce, or extended separation. In its acute phase, the child may show severe distress, although some children do not display overt symptoms but instead show regression in cognitive function and in the nature of the attachment to the surviving caregiver. If the surviving caregiver is in mourning, the child may experience the loss of both caregivers, with the consequence of being in even greater distress. In young children, the emotional availability of the surviving caregiver, as well as the strength of the family support system, determines the child's response. In optimal circumstances the child grieves in an uncomplicated way and continus to function well. The effects of the loss may be more in evidence as the child matures and misses the specific functions the absent caregiver would have provided. Latency-age children often do not manifest overt symptoms of grief or mourning. This is not because they are incapable of grieving, as was thought in the past, but rather because their immature egos are too overwhelmed by the loss for them to be able to express their feelings. In the presence of an adult who can supportively share in their distress, they are able to give expression to their grief. The loss of a parent in adolescence will usually interfere with the adolescent's normal developmental process.

Affective states depend on the age and resilience of the child and on the strength of the relationship prior to the loss. At a young age, children evince severe distress at a loss or long separation. Bowlby's stages may be in evidence as the child goes through a phase of protest (and anger), then despair, and finally accommodation. Some latency-age children respond hypomanically, giving the impression that the trauma has not affected them. Only much later, in young adulthood, are they able to recall the extent of their distress and the meaning of the loss. Some adolescents openly grieve for a brief period of time. For the most part, their preoccupation with the developmental tasks they confront does not allow them to deal fully with the meaning of the loss. Generally a dysphoric mood accompanies the loss and persists for many months.

In terms of *thoughts and fantasies* accompanying childhood mourning, it is not uncommon for children to personalize the meaning of the loss. They may feel that they are the cause of the event or that they could have prevented its happening. Many children retain the fantasy of a special attachment to an idealized absent caregiver, whatever the nature of the prior relationship.

Children and adolescents in a state of grief may evidence various types of *somatic states* depending on the affects they experience. For example, some children or adolescents suffer a diminished appetite, low energy, and decreased interest in age-expected activities. In relationship to the same underlying feelings, other children, in an attempt to avoid feeling mournful, feel agitated and restless and may behave aggressively.

Generally, losses during childhood and adolescence play a critical role in shaping future *relationships*. The specific dynamics depend on the nature of the attachment the child had to the lost caregiver. In most cases, the child or adolescent has been deprived of the security and love that the lost caregiver would have provided and consequently may be left yearning for those benefits. These yearnings may turn into expectations that others provide the missing functions. When that does not occur, disillusionment may threaten the relationship.

Clinical Illustration

A 10-year-old child who lost his mother to cancer was brought to a therapist by relatives because he was not sleeping. For this child, going to sleep had come to represent his mother on her deathbed. He feared that he would end up on the deathbed himself, worrying that what had killed her would spread to him as he slept. His insomnia was also tied to his being angry about her death, with the associated fantasy that she had died because she had not taken good enough care of herself. When first seen, he was not feeling well and was exhausted from lack of sleep. He said that when he went to bed, his body felt wired and he could not get comfortable. Over several weeks in therapy, he began to wonder why his mother's dying should affect his sleep. He had some telling dreams of talking to his mother and being angry with her, but in general, he was befuddled about why he could not sleep. When he came in, he was tearful about losing his mother but had difficulty representing his emotions in words. Over time, he was slowly able to experience and give expression to feelings of sadness. First, he was able to do it in games he played with the therapist when he lost. Then he could do it with peers at school. He is still working on experiencing and verbalizing a deeper sense of loss.

Related studies include: Bowlby, 1961, 1969; Brown & Goodman, 2005; Doka, 1995; Fleming & Altschul, 1963; Frankiel, 1994; Freud, 1917; Furman, 1974, 1994; Hofer, 1984; McClowry, Davies, May, Kulenkamp, & Martinson, 1995; Palombo 1981; Parens, 2002a, 2002b; Pollock, 1961; Wallerstein, Lewis, Blakeslee, 2000.

SCA306. Depressive Disorders

Depression in children is characterized by either sadness or, especially in young children, irritability. It affects boys and girls equally. In adolescence, females are twice as likely as males to suffer depression. Changes in appetite or weight, sleep, and psychomotor activity frequently accompany the mood state. Usually, the depressed child is tired, loses interest in activities, feels guilty and worthless, and has difficulty concentrating. Suicidal thoughts, plans, or even attempts are not rare. Somatic complaints often accompany depression and sometimes mask it. Behavioral symptoms are observable in younger children, whereas adolescents may feel a deeper level of mood disturbance. The depressed adolescent is at risk for substance abuse, early sexual involvement, eating disorders, and suicide. Childhood depression entails a risk of recurring depression over the life cycle. Untreated childhood depression can severely derail social and emotional development and lead to a poor adult adjustment.

Affective states in depressed children include not feeling as loved and protected as children typically do, even when they are in loving, supportive circumstances. Their intense emotions may be beyond their capacity to understand or regulate. Some children experience more feelings of helplessness (e.g., "I can't do this alone") and others are more self-critical (e.g., "I am bad"), corresponding to the anaclitic and introjective patterns described by Blatt and discussed in the sections on depressive disorders in the adult disorders. Many children experience both patterns. In addition, some children suffer from intense feelings of vulnerability and emotional fragility, often together with helplessness. They are readily upset by circumstances and easily overcome by their intense dysphoria. Once upset, they have a very difficult time calming their feelings, which may linger as a persistent sadness. Other children experience intense, chronic irritability. They are easily provoked to angry outbursts that are not easily overcome. Once the anger is resolved, sadness and remorse may follow. Such children may feel assaulted by many features of their world. Consequently, they may feel unsupported, misunderstood, and victimized. Some depressed children defend against their negative self-estimation with an attitude of arrogant entitlement, while others feel an inordinate amount of guilt, self-blame, and insecurity, leading to repetitive pleas for reassurance. Because of their unmanageable mood states, self-regulation is an issue for children with depression. Episodes of dysregulation are common.

Their *thoughts and fantasies* tend to parallel their affective states. The child's ideas may constitute efforts to explain and justify depressive feelings. "Nobody likes me" and "I can't do anything right" are typical cognitions. The child may be preoccupied with fears that harm will befall a caregiver. Fantasies and drawings are somber, filled with blood and violence. The play of the depressed child reflects preoccupations with injury or death.

Children with depression often complain of *somatic symptoms*. They may be tired and lethargic and yet may have trouble sleeping. Appetite may be affected; depressed children often eat too much or too little. They may complain of vague or even specific discomforts and ailments for which no physical cause can be found. They are more likely than nondepressed children to contract physical illnesses.

Depression negatively affects childhood *relationships*. When depressed children experience intense episodes of dysphoria in the context of relationships, they may blame those who are with them for these episodes. They frequently feel both provoked and failed by significant others, including their parents. At the same time, they have an intense need for assistance with managing their mood. This pattern of upset and need may strain primary relationships.

Clinical Illustration

A very sad-looking 8-year-old boy was brought to treatment because of his withdrawal in school and frequent references to "being bad" and not being able "to do anything." Although he appeared ready to cry, he would often protest that everything was fine. When he went to his therapist's office for the first time, he had no trouble separating from his mother. While playing catch with the therapist, he told her that his mother had said she had brought him to see her to talk about his stomachaches and headaches, which occurred during school time and whenever he was reading. He was nervous about book reports and homework. He preferred the earlier grades in school because there was less writing and reading, and he liked it better when "you could play." Homework was no fun. Later, as he talked about his family, his intense sense of guilt and responsibility were evident in his describing how bad he felt when he became angry at his brother. As soon as he would get angry, he stated, he would feel sorry for him and would have to make up with him. In addition to suffering stomachaches and headaches, he had a very nervous feeling about school and reading. He had a difficult time acknowledging how sad he felt.

Related studies include: Allen-Meares, 1987; Birman, et al., 1996; Bostic, Rubin, Prince, & Schlozman, 2005; Diller, 2005; González-Tejera, et al., 2005; Harrington, 2001; Michael, Huelsman, & Crowley, 2005; Najman, et al., 2005; Ollendick, Shortt, & Sanders, 2005; Spitz, 1946; Wilcox & Anthony, 2004; Zetzel, 1965.

SCA307. Bipolar Disorders

The most striking features of bipolar disorder in children and adolescents are mood instability and intensity that seem impervious to attempts to soothe or correct them. Bipolar children are unpredictable in their reactions and shift states rapidly. They are at high risk for harm to self or others. This disorder severely compromises relationships, family life, self-image, school performance, and extra-curricular activities. Individuals who are diagnosed with the disorder in adolescence or later are often described as highly sensitive, irritable, inconsolable, active babies who did not require normal amounts of sleep. As children, they are prone to intense fears, phobias, and anxieties, and may engage in oppositional and disruptive behavior. They may have been given a number of diagnoses before the bipolar diagnosis is established. In adolescence, there is substantial risk for eating disorders, self-mutilation, substance abuse, and suicide. In childhood, it is less common to see the distinct mood patterns that characterize bipolar adults. Adolescents generally exhibit more distinct mood patterns and cycles. Children with bipolar disorder are often first seen as having behavior problems (e.g., silliness, euphoria, and impulsivity) and as being unmanageable and unreachable.

Bipolar disorders occur relatively infrequently and affect boys and girls equally. A significant proportion of children and adolescents diagnosed with depression are later re-diagnosed as having a bipolar spectrum disorder. Careful diagnosis is required before medication is considered.

In the realm of *affect*, children and adolescents with bipolar disorder suffer greatly. Their mood shifts are painful and beyond their control. These children are inconsolable and unreachable and do not understand why they feel or behave as they do. Their mood states are so varied and intense that their thinking and perception may be distorted. Thus, they are prone to grandiosity alternating with severely negative self-appraisals. They often appear quite self-referential and lacking in sensitivity to others. Many children with this disorder are overreactive to sensory stimuli such as touch and sound. Some crave movement, while others, especially when overstimulated, experience a sensory craving. Children with bipolar disorder are quickly moved to extreme mood states—often, but not always, in response to circumstances. For example, boredom can evoke a manic response. Most frequently, children with this disorder are prone to unpredictable and prolonged episodes of rage, sometimes with physical violence. Bipolar children also may undergo frequent and prolonged episodes of despair. These children are driven by impulses, may be hypersexual, and often exhibit poor judgment.

The *thoughts and fantasies* of the bipolar child tend to follow the mood of the moment and often are used to explain or justify the mood. For example, when agitated and angry, the child may believe "He tried to get me, so I got him first." When feeling despair, the child may say (to self or others), "I get blamed all the time. It's unfair. Everyone would be better off without me."

In terms of *somatic states*, children with bipolar disorder are often hyperactive; they appear uncomfortable in their own skin. They may develop nervous habits and are injury-prone. The disorder frequently disrupts sleep and eating patterns. Because self-regulation is a serious problem for children with bipolar disorder, their varied states may seem contradictory. For example, they may show a disregard for pain in one state and hypersensitivity in another.

Bipolar disorder is highly disruptive to children's *relationships*. Bipolar children often misconstrue and personalize other's motives and behaviors. Their unstable mood patterns dramatically affect the child's experience of being with others. Moments of closeness with a parent may lead to silliness that quickly gets out of hand, such that someone becomes angry. The unpredictability of the bipolar disorder child's behavior often markedly disturbs sibling and peer relationships.

Clinical Illustrations

- A 9-year-old boy who vacillated between being very agitated and being very angry would physically attack his sisters for "getting in my face and playing with my stuff." He felt justified and acted excited, "like I was a warrior defending my castle." (He also played a lot of video games.) When the parents would come home, they would criticize him for upsetting his sisters.

Then he would feel remorseful, threaten to jump out the window, and get very sad. In the "down" times, he would get angry at himself and talk about how bad he was. This pattern continued over many months. When he began brandishing a kitchen knife, his parents brought him in, fearing he would harm himself or family members. During the sessions, he would talk agitatedly about being mad, protest that people could not do this or that to him anymore, then move into states of self-recrimination in which he would exclaim that he should die like his recently deceased uncle.

- A 10-year-old child entered a school for children with emotional problems. He had a long history of disruptiveness and had been variously diagnosed with attention deficit/hyperactivity disorder, conduct disorder, oppositional defiant disorder, and impulsive disorder. Various medications were prescribed with limited success. He was expelled from several school programs because of his behavior, which lasted from ages 6 to 9. This child acted very "goofy" in class, climbing on desks, provoking the teacher and the other children, and acting like a kangaroo. He could not seem to stop his behavior, but he made it clear to a therapist that he wished he could. He described both chronic irritability and occasional paranoid ideation such as the belief that the other children were provoking and teasing him. The mother, who herself was somewhat hypomanic, ashamedly revealed that her father had been diagnosed with manic-depressive disorder twenty years earlier.

Related studies include: Dilsaver, Benazzi, Rihmer, Akiskal, & Akiskal, 2005; Faedda, Baldessarini, Glovinsky, & Austin, 2004; Galatzer-Levy 1987.

SCA308. Suicidality

Suicidal ideation occurs in a number of mental states. Understanding its meaning and implications in children requires an understanding of the individual child's concept of death. Young children, for example, do not see death as irreversible. They may also understand it as a opportunity to meet a deceased loved one. Older children or adolescents may see death in terms of the sadness, pain, and mourning of those left behind, and thus an option if they wish to hurt someone who cares about them. A child or adolescent may see death as a way of escaping pain or conflict. In adolescents, prodromal symptoms are depression, sleeplessness, hopelessness, and either the belief that no one cares or the belief that those who do care feel guilty and sorry for not having cared more. Some adolescents have clearly articulated plans, which they may share with peers, who are sworn to secrecy.

The child or adolescent may use his or her concept of death to discharge or defend against feelings. Evaluating the seriousness of the suicidal risk is made easier by understanding the underlying mental state. For example, a child suffering from the loss of a parent through death may contemplate joining the parent. An adolescent conflicted about the developmental challenge of greater independence may become distressed and withdrawn and regard suicide as a means to escape the conflict. An adolescent who feels unbearable shame may think about escaping it by dying.

Suicide may also express more aggressive dynamics. For example, the unbearably shamed adolescent may contemplate, consciously or unconsciously, killing the person who has shamed him. If this fantasy is unacceptable, the action may be redirected toward the self. Suicidal behaviors may occur out of awareness. For example, many car "accidents" that "happen" to adolescents express unconscious intentions to tempt death or end one's life. On the other hand, suicide is less likely to be seen as an acceptable option by someone who fully understands that death is final and permanent.

Although adolescent girls make ten times as many suicide attempts as adolescent boys do, boys die from suicide twice as often as girls do. This ratio is higher if one considers some car accidents as suicidal. Boys generally use more lethal means (e.g., firearms, rope) than girls, who prefer ingesting drugs. Often the less-than-lethal amounts that a girl ingests imply a suicide "gesture" rather than a determination to die, but there is always the danger that she will misjudge the lethality of whatever drug she takes. Some deaths from acetaminophen, for example, seem to have been intended as non-lethal acts.

Strong negative *affective states,* including anger, rage, sadness, and shame, should alert clinicians to the possibility of conscious or unconscious thoughts of suicide. Understanding the child's reaction to these states, including his or her ways of defending against or discharging the feelings, is a next step. Obtaining the child's thoughts about death and inquiring about how he or she would suicide may provide vital information about the child's understanding of death and therefore about potential lethality. Affective patterns may include underlying feelings of helplessness and/or hopelessness.

The *thoughts and fantasies* of the potentially suicidal child are closely tied to these painful feelings. The child may ruminate about a sense of worthlessness and an inability to improve school performance, relationships with peers, and relationships with family members. The child may see no possibility of feeling better or of restoring or attaining a sense of pride. Fantasies about what suicide would achieve (e.g., reunion with a lost loved one, remorse in those left behind) may be frequent and consuming. In some children, fantasies of some "special" meaning in the anticipated suicidal acts are prominent, as are fantasies that may be induced by drug use. Some adolescents do not indicate the extent of their despair, appearing normal to those who know them.

The *somatic states* often follow the mood of the child. Examples include physiologic responses associated with rage, such as muscle tightening and rapid heartbeat; tremulousness associated with fear; and sleeping or eating difficulties associated with despair.

Relationships with parents and/or peers of a suicidal child are typically unsatisfying. The child feels inadequately supported and thus bereft of feelings of being cared for, respected, and valued. Suicidal children who feel particularly angry may provoke hostile reactions from others.

Clinical Illustrations

- An 18-year-old, recently inducted male recruit shot himself with his military-issue rifle after being rejected from an elite special operations unit. His parents, who had been very proud of him, described him as a high achiever who had received straight "A's" in high school. His teachers described him as very conscientious. His suicide note described terrible shame and anger at not making the cut for the elite assignment.

- A young woman of eighteen came to treatment with a diagnosis of social anxiety disorder. She was being treated with Paxil, with limited results. She stopped the medication and refused any other antidepressants. The therapist was concerned that she might commit suicide. She was a loner who refused permission to the therapist to speak with her parents but allowed him to talk with an older married sister. A high school graduate, she had taken a year off before going to college and was living with a roommate and holding a job. When not at work, she would spend time in her room smoking marijuana. In the past, whenever she had been away from home, she had been unhappy and homesick.

  During the therapy, it became clear how angry she was with her mother, whom she described as overbearing and intrusive. She would rarely call home or visit. Despite the strength of her feelings that her family was suffocating her, shame was her most intense affect. She saw herself as hopelessly ugly. A recent rebuff by a young man had exacerbated her depression. As the holiday season approached, the patient discussed her ambivalence about going home for Thanksgiving, the first time she would see her parents in several months. She finally told the therapist that she had decided to visit her parents for Christmas. A few days later, the sister called and said the girl had "fallen" in front of a train and died.

Related studies include: Brent, et al., 1994; King & Apter, 1996; Kochman, et al., 2005; Pfeffer, 1982.

SCA309. Conduct Disorders

"Conduct disorder" is the umbrella term for a complicated group of provocative behavioral and emotional problems in youngsters. The hallmarks of conduct disorders are indifference toward others, impulsivity, and affective instability. Children and adolescents with conduct disorder have great difficulty following rules and behaving in a socially acceptable way. Many factors may contribute to the development of a conduct disorder, including brain damage, child abuse, genetic vulnerability, school failure, inadequate relationships, and traumatic life experiences. Many children with conduct disorders have coexisting symptomatology such as mood disorders, anxiety, posttraumatic syndromes, substance abuse, problems with attention and hyperactivity, learning problems, and thought disorders.

Conduct disorder is the most frequently diagnosed childhood disorder in outpatient and inpatient mental facilities. It is estimated that six percent of all children have some form of conduct disorder, which is far more common in boys than in girls. Girls are more likely to develop adolescent-onset conduct disorder, whereas for boys, onset is usually in childhood and involves more aggressiveness.

Other children, adults, and agency personnel often view children with conduct disorders as "bad" or delinquent rather than as mentally ill, largely because of the nature of their behavior. Among the symptoms manifested by a conduct-disordered child are:

- Aggression toward people and animals (the child bullies, threatens, or intimidates others; initiates physical fights; has used a weapon that could cause serious harm [e.g., a bat, brick, broken bottle, knife, or gun]; is cruel to people or animals; steals from victims while confronting them [i.e., commits assault]; or forces someone into sexual activity);
- Destruction of property (the child defaces buildings, damages automobiles, or sets fires intended to destroy others' property);
- Deceitfulness, lying, or stealing (the child breaks into someone else's building, house, or car; lies to obtain goods or favors or to avoid obligations; steals items without confronting a victim);
- Serious violations of rules (the child stays out at night despite parental objections; runs away from home; or is truant from school).

Research shows that youngsters with conduct disorder are likely to have ongoing problems if they and their families do not receive early and comprehensive treatment. Many youngsters with conduct disorder are unable to adapt to the demands of adulthood and continue to be antisocial, to have problems with relationships, to lose jobs, and to break laws.

These children and adolescents are remarkably unaware of their own *affective states* and are also remarkably unresponsive to the feelings of others. Because of this quality of being emotionally out of touch, some clinicians describe conduct-disordered children as experiencing excitement or pleasure in hurting others, as lacking remorse, and as being greedy and opportunistic. Some children experience these feelings, but many do not. In children and adolescents with this diagnosis, affect in general is labile and not well regulated; they are usually not able to tolerate even small amounts of frustration or delay of gratification. They can be observed expressing anger when they do not get their own way, and they tend to express satisfaction when they succeed. At times, they express feelings of fear, and they may also admit to deeper feelings of pain and resentment at not being cared for and at being mistreated by others. They commonly express a defeated attitude of having given up on people.

Thoughts and fantasies often involve the conviction of being frequently wronged. Conduct-disordered children may have a clearly defensive sense of invulnerability, and they tend to regard others with indifference. Their goals usually include material gain and power. Thoughts about any other aspects of interpersonal relationships are remarkably absent.

Somatic states most prominently seen in these individuals include arousal and hypervigilance.

Relationship patterns may be characterized by impulsivity and indifference toward others. Because others tend to be seen as objects to manipulate in the service of power, excitement, or material benefits, it is not surprising that relationships tend to be poor and short-lived.

Clinical Illustrations

- An 11-year-old boy would climb under or on top of his classroom desk, ostentatiously drooling, especially after being asked to quiet down by his teacher. At bedtime he would whisper in his 8-year-old brother's ear, "I'll kill you while you're asleep." Frequently, he would pack the family's water spigots with fecal matter. After the failure of outpatient daily psychotherapy, medication, family therapy, and various individual educational plans, he was institutionalized.

- A 16-year-old boy had failed eighth grade, had been stealing cars since age 12 and was acting very intimidating toward his peers. Eventually, he was arrested and sent to a detention center, where he was described as angry and entitled, with little regard for others. He also behaved in intimidating ways toward the staff—a significant problem, as he was 6'6" tall, weighing almost 300 pounds. An especially intuitive detention officer began talking sympathetically with him, often about his history of being treated unfairly, while at the same time setting limits on his excessive intimidation by giving him "time outs" in the county jail. After a year in this setting, he began to comply with its rules; within two years he became one of the best students in the detention center.

Related studies include: Blair, Budhani, Colledge, & Scott, 2005; Frick, O'Brien, Wootton, & McBurnett, 1994; Harrington, 2001; Kernberg & Chazen, 1991; Moffitt, 1993; Moffitt, Caspi, Dickson, Silva, & Stanton, 1996; Pajer, 1998; Parens, 1979, 1987, 1989a, 1989b, 1991, 1997.

SCA310. Oppositional-Defiant Disorders

While all children can be negative in the service of self-definition, openly provocative, uncooperative, and hostile behavior becomes a serious concern when it is a continuing pattern markedly more frequent and consistent than the behavior of other children of the same age and developmental level, and when it interferes with adaptive patterns in the major areas in the child's life. Symptoms such as temper tantrums, excessive arguing with adults, active defiance of requests and rules, deliberate attempts to annoy or upset people, blaming others, being touchy and easily annoyed by others, and expressing anger and resentment are frequent features of this problem. Although the causes of such behavior patterns are not fully known, the early history of oppositional and defiant children is often characterized by difficulty in fully meeting early emotional goals, including emotional regulation. Two-way affective signaling involving the full range of emotions, constructive assertiveness, and frustration and loss are particularly challenging. In addition, many parents report that their child with this diagnosis was more sensitive than others to a range of experiences, such as different sounds and types of touch, and seemed to need to try to control the environment, resulting in many battles over control.

A child with oppositional and defiant symptoms should have a comprehensive evaluation, as other disorders (e.g., difficulties with attention and hyperactivity, learning disabilities, mood disorders, and anxiety disorders) may be present. It may be difficult to improve oppositionality without working with the challenges that may contribute to the behavior. Some children with the diagnosis of oppositional-defiant disorder go on to develop a conduct disorder.

In terms of prevalence and sex ratio, the symptoms are usually seen in multiple settings, but may be more noticeable at home or at school. Five to 15% of all school-age children are diagnosed with oppositional defiant disorders. Before puberty, oppositional and defiant behavior is more frequently found in boys than in girls. In adolescence, boys and girls may be equally defiant and oppositional.

Behind the overt disruptiveness of oppositional children are feelings of demoralization, resentment, self-doubt, and self-hatred. Such youngsters almost always feel poorly understood. A dramatic and persistent state of hyperalertness, oriented toward guarding their self-worth, characterizes the *affective states* of these children. They are poised to feel put upon and righteously indignant. Their efforts to maintain their self-esteem may look more stimulating and euphoric than anxious. Problems with self-regulation are often present.

As to their *thoughts and fantasies,* most children with this diagnosis are unaware that they have a problem. In fact, from their perspective, the problem lies in the demands for conformity that others make on them. Their impulsivity leads to behaviors that adults find unacceptable, yet they seem oblivious to the consequences of those behaviors. Although expressions of remorse or contrition may follow some defiant actions, oppositional children more often feel justified in their behavior and see themselves as victims of injustice. Recurrent disapproval from others may erode the sense of self-cohesion in an oppositional child, making him or her more vulnerable to narcissistic injury and fragmentation. Their inability to demonstrate their competence leads such youngsters to feel especially vulnerable to criticism and to failure.

Social and family *relationships* are usually impaired because of the child's disruptiveness, bossiness, and oppositional behaviors. In a vicious cycle, the disapproval to which they are regularly subjected may lead oppositional children to be more rebellious and defiant. These responses, and their related tendency to associate with peers on the fringe, may crystallize into delinquent patterns.

Clinical Illustration

Six-year-old David personified the word negativism. Sensitive to sound, taste, touch, and movement in space (swinging), he tried to control every aspect of his life, from wearing only soft cotton to eating only selected foods. His somewhat authoritative parents tried to force their will on David, leading to more intensive power struggles, tantrums, and refusals to cooperate in school and at home. David also had difficulty asserting himself constructively or putting his feelings into words or pretend play, except for themes of dominance and anger. As David's parents were helped to be more flexible, to empathize with his concerns, and to be selective and gently firm in setting limits, David began improving. Finding ways for David to be the "boss" constructively was very helpful as well.

Related studies include: Farley, et al., 2005; Frick & Kimonis, 2005; Hinshaw & Lee, 2003; Keenan & Wakschlag, 2004; Maughan, Rowe, Messer, Goodman, & Meltzer, 2004; Scott 2005.

SCA311. Substance Abuse Related Disorders

These disorders are described on pp. 138-141 of the Adult Symptom Patterns section of this manual.

Substance abuse patterns are not infrequently found in children and, to a much greater extent, in adolescents. A variety of *affective states* may be involved, including excitement associated with experimentation, anxiety about developmental and social challenges, and attempts to counteract feelings of numbness, emptiness, embarrassment, humiliation, and rage. Feelings of belonging to a group may be pursued and achieved via substance abuse.

Thoughts and fantasies leading up to the substance abuse often relate to the motives inherent in the affective states just mentioned. Once the substance is used, resultant cognitive patterns reflect the effect of the substance on the nervous system. These range from agitated, fragmented, and paranoid thinking, to fantasies of specialness and brilliance, to wish-fulfilling convictions of desirability, potency, and invulnerability.

Somatic states accompany both the affects described above and the substances used. They range from arousal and agitation to numbness and tranquility. Use of alcohol and other drugs also has consequences, both immediate and long-term, for many organ systems and physiological processes.

Relationships range from active involvement in a social group where the substance abuse pattern is ritualized, to isolated, self-absorbed states of solitary withdrawal. Once a person is involved in regular substance abuse, relationships tend to be valued as a means of obtaining the desired substance and thus take on a very manipulative quality. Interestingly, many young adult males report that their first experiences with alcohol were with fathers, whom they describe as having offered infrequent opportunities for closeness. Some children report being "pulled in" to a pattern of drug use by a substance-abusing parent; in such instances, they tend to have had little or no experience with sincere and intimate relationships.

Clinical Illustrations

- An 18-year-old young man was brought for psychotherapy by his mother because of school performance far below his capacity. His father was hostile to the treatment. The parents had separated when the boy was 4 years old, after his father, who was heavily involved in drugs, had overdosed, attempted suicide, been hospitalized, and lost his driver's license. At age 14, the boy began using marijuana occasionally, escalating to daily use by tenth grade. During a four-year course of twice-a-week psychotherapy that was only partially successful, it became apparent that the boy's marijuana use constituted an effort to identify with his father. His escalation during high school reflected a determination to distract himself from emerging homosexual feelings.

- A very bright adolescent boy who had always been quite shy had difficulty attending regular school in ninth grade because of anxiety over social interactions. His parents began home schooling when he was in tenth grade, but by eleventh grade he was unable to complete any schoolwork, at which time his parents brought him for consultation. His history was remarkable for marijuana use beginning in seventh grade. By the end of ninth grade, he was using cocaine and hallucinogens. In tenth grade he overdosed on a cocktail of amphetamines and hallucinogens and was admitted to the emergency room of the local hospital. By the time of the consultation, he was almost constantly under the influence of some street drug. A prolonged residential drug treatment achieved detoxification, during which he began to reveal hallucinations and delusions. After a year in convalescence, he stabilized, but his extreme social anxiety and poor social skills reappeared with a vengeance. These deficiencies had evidently created anxiety so unbearable that he felt driven to use street drugs to reduce it. The use of the drugs had then seriously complicated his difficulties.

Related studies include: Shedler & Block, 1990; Wieder & Kaplan, 1969.

SCA312. Psychic Trauma and Posttraumatic Stress Disorder

For an overview of trauma and posttraumatic conditions, see pp. 100-104 of the section on Adult Symptom Patterns.

Psychological trauma in children and adolescents can create disturbances similar to those found in adults There is some evidence that adolescent females are more vulnerable to posttraumatic stress syndromes, while adolescent males are more disabled by their symptoms Regressive responses to trauma are particularly visible in childhood, especially in younger children. For example, a toilet-trained child may become incontinent, or a previously confident child may cling to a caregiver. Older children may withdraw from social contact. All traumatized children and adolescents may show hyperalertness, increased startle response, increased volatility, poor concentration, and more labile affect. There are frequently disturbances in eating, sleeping, and learning. Other common responses in children include the defensive use of super-heroes and attempts to avoid stimuli associated with the traumatic events.

Affective patterns range from anxiety and panic to obsessive preoccupation and fear, which may appear most vividly in nightmares. Exhaustion and depression may accompany these patterns.

Thoughts and fantasies involve the types of preoccupation described above, compulsive ruminations, fragmented thinking, "all-or-nothing" thinking, and escapist fantasies. In the play of children who have been traumatized, the drama may be compulsively re-enacted, often in a distorted form that seeks to prevent the return of traumatic memories.

Somatic states follow the affective patterns, most notably those associated with anxiety, such as rapid heart rate, tense muscles, gastrointestinal symptoms, headaches, and muscle aches. If the traumatic experience involved physical pain, this may be re-experienced in dissociated ways. Sexual trauma is particularly likely to trigger somatic symptoms. A variety of somatic complaints can come to be viewed as illnesses in their own right.

Relationships may be needy and dependent, characterized by seeking relief from the traumatic anxiety. In children whose somatic complaints become the vehicle for achieving closeness and support, relationships may come to have a manipulative cast. They may also be avoided by a child who has learned to regard new experiences as potentially traumatizing.

Clinical Illustrations

- A 12-year-old boy was walking in a city with his friend when the friend was suddenly killed by a gunman involved in a drug transaction twenty feet away. Evidently because he felt so vulnerable and helpless, the boy constructed a narrative in which he had time to save his friend but chose not to because he was angry at him for some slight.

- A 10-year-old boy followed his ball into the street and was hit by a car. When he recovered, he re-enacted this event in play over and over again.

- An adolescent who had seen his mother killed in a barroom brawl when he was 6 years old frequently incited fights with groups of other adolescents.

Related studies include: Gaensbauer, 1994, 2002; Hesse & Main, 1999; Kestenberg & Brenner, 1996; Schwartz & Kowalski 1991; Steele, 1994; Yovell 2000.

SCA313. Adjustment Disorders (other than developmental)

Adjustment disorders in children can be characterized by a wide range of subjective states. They may feel anxious or depressed, angry or impulsive, or bereft and defeated. Their thoughts and fantasies will reflect whatever emotional pattern is triggered by the loss, illness, family problem, or school problem to which they are reacting. Their relationships may become more dependent and clinging or more distant and aloof. They may experience a variety of somatic discomforts, sleeping problems, and eating difficulties. In short, the subjective states accompanying adjustment disorders are similar to those accompanying other childhood disorders. There is a critical difference, however. In adjustment disorders, the reaction is temporary and related to a specific situation or event. Helping the child understand the subjective reaction in relationship to the current challenge, along with providing extra support and opportunities for mastery, can favorably influences the child's subjective state.

No single pattern characterizes adjustment disorders, as children's affective states, thoughts and fantasies, somatic states, and relational patterns vary widely.

Clinical Illustration

An 8-year-old boy was brought for evaluation by his parents, who were concerned about his severe nightmares that had started nine months previously. They described his needing a parent to be with him while he fell asleep and his waking up in the middle of the night to crawl into their bed because he was too frightened to sleep by himself. The symptoms began when the family had invited a fire-alarm salesman to their apartment to give a demonstration of his product. The salesman gave a graphic video demonstration of a devastating fire. The boy was transfixed. About a week later, he developed the sleep disorder. Upon further exploration with the boy, the therapist became aware of an unresolved separation problem that had been reactivated by the incident.

Please Note: Many of the terms used in describing the following disorders are defined in the Selected Definitions Related to Attention, Regulation, and Learning section, pp. 196-201.

SCA314. Motor Skills Disorders

[Gross and/or fine motor problems; motor planning and sequencing (praxis), vestibular disorders]

To be diagnosed with a motor skills disorder, a child's performance in daily activities that require physical coordination must be substantially below that expected for the youngster's age and intelligence. Motor skills disorders may be manifested by marked delays in achieving milestones such as sitting, crawling, and walking; by a pattern of dropping things and general "clumsiness;" by poor performance in sports; and by poor handwriting. In infancy and early childhood, the problems may not be fully apparent but may become evident as the child moves on developmentally and as the demands for performance in areas of weakness intensify. Developmental coordination disorders have been estimated to be as high as 6% for children 5 to 11 years old.

No single pattern of affect, ideation, somatic involvement, or relationship characterizes the disorder, as children's responses to a motor problem vary widely. If the context requires or expects, for cultural or other reasons, high functioning in certain motor areas, the child may begin to avoid such activities. The avoidance may then generalize, invading the larger social context. If the child's context lacks such expectations, the child's motoric weaknesses may not constitute a felt psychological problem.

Clinical Illustration

A boy who was 3 years and 9 months old showed significant delays in both gross and fine motor skill development. He separated well from his mother and worked cooperatively at a table for fine motor testing. As items became difficult for him, he would throw the test objects. In the relatively unstructured setting for gross motor testing, he grew excited, running on his toes and flapping his arms. It was difficult to engage him in test items, but he did cooperate when reinforced by ball throwing, an activity he enjoyed. Consistent with his parents' report of tactile defensiveness, he did not like his clothes removed for neuromuscular testing. He also did not like having his feet off the ground and was hesitant to climb, but he appeared to enjoy activities that provided deep pressure and proprioceptive input.

His mother reported that his developmental delay did not present a problem at school. His neuromuscular skills were basically adequate, but his equilibrium responses were somewhat delayed. His fine motor skills were affected by an intention tremor, which appeared to reduce his manual dexterity. In addition to his tactile defensiveness, he appeared to be hypersensitive generally. This sensitivity and the resulting excited behaviors compromised his ability to follow directions and imitate another person's movements. Although he had normal muscle tone in his lower and upper extremities, his truncal tone appeared somewhat lower. He found it difficult to stand on one foot: He was able to stand for five seconds on his left foot, but he would not attempt to stand on his right. Despite his mother's report that he could gallop, he refused to do so. He could not yet hop on one foot. He could throw a tennis ball at least ten feet and hit a target from a distance of five feet, and he could throw a ten-inch lightweight ball at least eight feet. He failed in an attempt to throw a larger ball overhand to a target. In contrast to his ability to throw a ball, his skill at catching one was poor: He was unable to catch a ten-inch ball even when it was thrown lightly from a short distance. He would close his eyes as the ball approached and would protect his face with his arms.

He manipulated objects using both hands but appeared to prefer his right hand for most fine motor tasks. He had a fine pincer grasp bilaterally. In holding a marker, he used either a supinated palmar grasp or a pronated grasp, holding the marker at the end with his fingers. His tremor was particularly noticeable in his block-stacking. Although it was difficult for him, he was able to build a tower of seven blocks. He enjoyed using a marker and paper, was able to copy a horizontal and vertical line, and made circular motions on the paper. He did not appear to understand directions to copy pictures of a circle and a cross. Despite his difficulty in manipulating them, he was very interested in using scissors. He needed assistance in placing his fingers into the scissors, and he would also press on the blades to close them on the paper. He persisted at this task for a relatively long time. This child had the most difficulty with tasks requiring manual dexterity. He was unable to string beads, unscrew a small cap from a bottle, or unbutton buttons, and he had great difficulty winding up a toy. Items like these that frustrated him would be thrown.

SCA315. Tic Disorders

Tic disorders are neurological conditions involving stereotypic motor movements or vocalizations. They include Tourette's syndrome and transient tic disorders. Some children develop tics that remit spontaneously within a brief period of time, while others develop more permanent tics that wax and wane as the child matures but do not dissipate permanently. The latter children are often diagnosed with Tourette's Syndrome. Their tics may take the form of involuntary vocalization (often including swearing and other taboo utterances), eye movements, or more generalized movements involving the limbs or trunk.

The *affective states* of children with tic disorders are complex, as they involve both innate temperamental factors and social factors. Often the social factors dominate a child's responses of intense embarrassment, anxiety, and depression. School refusal may become a problem as a child tries to avoid teasing or ridicule. Parents confront the dilemma that some medications reduce the overt symptoms at the cost of diminished cognitive and emotional functioning.

With respect to their *thoughts and fantasies,* children with tic disorders express confusion about the reason for their problem. They may personalize others' responses to them and blame themselves for not being able to control symptoms that they are sometimes able to inhibit temporarily.

In terms of *somatic states*, beyond the motoric elements of the tic process, no somatic conditions have been associated with tic disorders.

In terms of *relationship patterns*, children with tic disorders may be so self-conscious that they withdraw and isolate themselves from peers.

Treatment goals with tic-disordered children include helping them accept their symptoms as they might accept any other handicap, diminishing their sense of shame, and helping them learn to advocate on their own behalf.

Clinical Illustration

A 7-year-old girl was diagnosed with Tourette's syndrome. She presented with severe facial tics and involuntary vocal swearing. Prior to her diagnosis, her parents considered her disrespectful and oppositional, since there were times when the symptoms subsided and she appeared to be in control of them. Following the diagnosis they insisted on medicating her even though the anti-psychotic drugs that helped to diminish the symptoms led to a severe deterioration in her ability to function cognitively. Formerly a good student, she began to fail many of her subjects. Since conditions at school were not optimal, she was the target of much teasing and bullying. Eventually she began to refuse to go to school and to avoid other settings in which she would be with other children. Psychotherapeutic intervention was geared toward helping the parents gain a better understanding of Tourette's and helping the patient gain self-esteem by framing her tics as a disability that required adaptation.

Related studies include: Apter, et al., 1993; Kurlan, Whitmore, Irvine, McDermott, & Como, 1994.

SCA316. Psychotic Disorders

Psychotic disorders are defined by loss of reality testing, specifically by delusions, hallucinations, and disordered thinking. Affect states may be disrupted, and executive functions may be impaired. The condition may be chronic, as in the case of schizophrenia, or transient, as in the case of severe depression, bipolar illness, and dissociative disorders. It is important to distinguish children who have poor reality testing from those whose reality sense is compromised as a result of severe trauma or narcissistic injury and consequent psychological fragmentation. The diagnosis of a psychotic condition in childhood includes positive symptoms (delusions, hallucinations, incoherent speech, paranoid ideation) and negative symptoms that are the result of such impairments. The latter may include disturbances of affect, inability to function in daily tasks, and inadequate self-care. From a psychodynamic perspective the positive symptoms, while expressing specific brain dysfunctions, may be understood as restitutive efforts to establish a sense of self-cohesion.

Because reality testing has its own developmental line, disruption in that function must be evaluated within the context of a child's maturation. The capacities to separate reality from fantasy and to organize thoughts into successively higher-level organizations develop gradually in children. Typically, children 4 years of age and older have a reasonably stable capacity to differentiate fantasy from reality and to appreciate increasingly subtle distinctions. A very healthy 10-year-old is capable of commenting, "I only think other kids are being unfair to me when I'm really upset." Not infrequently, however, children persist in confusing reality and fantasy, either during fairly circumscribed challenges or chronically, in which case the child may have highly organized and elaborate delusions (e.g., a 7-year-old child insisted that he was having conversations with creatures from outer space and that only he knew their plans for poisoning the planet).

It is often difficult to distinguish whether a child with a psychotic disorder has never developed age-expected reality testing or has developed this capacity and then lost it. The developmental histories of psychotic children vary considerably. Some children, for example, have a history of difficulty in modulating sensation and/or processing auditory or visual-spatial experiences, while other children have a history of severe emotional distress; still others have both. Thought disorder may not emerge fully until adolescence when the capacity for formal operational thought normally emerges.

The *affective states* of children with reality-testing problems vary considerably, based on the nature of their difficulties. Anxiety, depression, and combinations of the two are common. Such feelings can be intense and disorganizing.

Thoughts may reflect poor judgment, disorganized or illogical thinking, and unrealistic beliefs and experiences. *Fantasies*, especially those of specialness (both positive, as in grandiosity, and negative, as in delusions of persecution) may be experienced not as products of the imagination but as self-evident truths.

Somatic patterns consistent with these affective states are also often present.

Relationship patterns may be either excessively dependent or excessively aloof.

Clinical Illustration

An 11-year-old boy was in treatment for serious behavioral problems, some of which were related to his ADHD. During one session the therapist had to control him physically to prevent his injuring himself. The child responded to the intervention with rage, during which he accused the therapist of taping the sessions with the intention of reporting all that happened to his parents. He believed that the pen in the therapist's shirt pocket was a transmitter connected to a recording machine hidden in another room and insisted on seeing the tapes and having them destroyed. When the therapist tried to reason with him, the boy stated that a picture on the wall was looking at him angrily and was put there by the therapist to make him feel he was being watched. It took several weeks of supportive work before the child's former sense of self-cohesion and accompanying reality sense were restored.

Related studies include: Arboleda & Holzman, 1985; Caplan, Guthries, Fish, Tanguay, & David-Lando, 1989; Gartner, Weintraub, & Carlson, 1997.

SCA317. Neuropsychological Disorders

SCA317.1 Visual-Spatial Processing Disorders

When visual processing is a major area of weakness, the child shows deficits in visuospatial working memory and visual imagery, often signaled by difficulties recognizing people's faces, particularly those with whom the child has little familiarity. Visual-spatial processing is a set of functions mediated by the right brain hemisphere that include facial recognition, recognition of facial emotional expression, right-left orientation, mental rotation of shapes, and comprehension of nonverbal communication cues. Visual perception involves visual sequential memory, figure-ground discrimination, visual memory, visual closure, and visual form constancy.

No single pattern of affect, thought, somatic response, or relationship characterizes the visual-spatial processing disorders.

Clinical Illustration

A 9½-year-old child had a long history of difficulties for which he had been evaluated repeatedly, including articulation and speech problems, fine motor problems, occasional perseveration, and problems with peers. He also had a "social imperception" problem; he could not decode visual-spatial social cues. He was doing reasonably well academically in fourth grade, but the teacher reported that in groups he had trouble connecting with classmates. He did not know when to talk and when to listen, did not realize how he was coming across to others, and would miss the big picture while focusing on tangents. When attempts were made to correct him, he would stubbornly hold to his view.

At home, when his father would interrupt him to explain something, this boy would keep on talking, not even acknowledging that he was being addressed. The father described how, while he was helping his son with a Pinewood Derby project, the boy insisted on painting the car backwards. When father tried to point out the error, his son stubbornly insisted that he was correct. This child was described by his parents as having a stunning lack of insight into his behavior. He did not seem to worry about others' perceptions of him. He coped well on his own, enjoyed computers, took karate lessons, and participated in Cub Scouts. The fact that he had no friends did not appear to trouble him. His parents saw this attitude as a positive and were reluctant to interfere with it at the risk of "cracking his shell."

This boy also liked to stay up late at night, a preference that predated his being on medication. The parents also noted that their son seemed to suffer considerable anxiety: While sitting quietly, he would pick tissues apart; in bed he would shred his blanket. The boy was also not a good historian; he had trouble reporting on his experiences in sequence and would leave out important details.

Some children with Asperger's Syndrome evidence visual-spatial processing difficulties, but children with visual-spatial processing problems do not necessarily evidence Asperger's Syndrome. The quality of the child's intimacy, emotional interactions, and capacity for creative and abstract thought plays an important role in determining the proper diagnosis.

SCA317.2 Language and Auditory Processing Disorders

[Expressive Language Disorders, Mixed Receptive/Expressive Language Disorders, other Communication Disorders]

Expressive language disorders include markedly limited vocabulary, errors in tense, and difficulty recalling words or producing sentences with developmentally appropriate length or complexity. Receptive language disorders include symptoms such as difficulty with understanding words, sentences, or specific types of words, such as spatial terms. Language disorders typically emerge at fifteen to eighteen months, when language acquisition occurs. Because of individual differences in development, however (some children do not begin to speak until about age three), the judgment as to whether a child has a language problem cannot be made definitively until 3 or 4 years of age. Dyslexia, for example, may not be diagnosed until a child is in first grade. Because communicative competence is essential to social discourse, receptive or expressive language disorders may contribute to a child's relational problems. Without early remediation, these disorders become increasingly problematic as the child matures. It is estimated that between 3% and 5% of school-age children have a language or auditory processing disorder.

No single pattern of affect, cognition, somatic involvement, or relationship characterizes language and auditory processing disorders, as children's responses to them vary widely.

Clinical Illustration

A 14½-year-old boy was referred by the school social worker, who felt that he was underachieving. She described him as a kind, gentle young man who appeared much brighter than his school performance demonstrated. He was liked by peers and had one or two close friends, but he seemed to keep a certain distance from others. The educational psychologist who tested him concluded that although he was functioning at the lower limits of the superior range of intelligence, he had a problem in both auditory processing and expressive language. She noted that he had difficulty with word retrieval and could not grasp inferential language.

This child was unable to retain and integrate complete ideas. He would store them in fragmented form for future retrieval. Although his intelligence was potentially high, his deficit in sequencing and retaining language for functional use was sabotaging his success. His auditory problems and his receptive language deficit were undermining the coherence of information he would hear or read, thus limiting what was available for future retrieval. Children with auditory processing disorders are often unable to use context well in reading, and consequently may fail to build vocabulary or enhance their comprehension. The deficits of this young man interfered with his ability to develop a sound conceptual language foundation on which higher-level cognitive skills are based.

Related studies include: Baker & Cantwell, 1987; Lewis, 1977.

SCA317.3 Memory Impairments

Memory is constituted of working memory, declarative memory, and non-declarative memory. *Working memory* is a short-term memory buffer that retains auditory inputs and/or visual images. *Declarative memory,* which is for the most part conscious, consists of semantic memory and episodic memory. Semantic memory is memory for facts; it is our dictionary memory. Episodic memory refers to the memory of things personally experienced, as opposed to the knowledge of facts one has learned. *Non-declarative memory* contains non-conscious memories. It consists of procedural memory, priming, and associative and non-associative learning. Memory problems can result from brain damage, innate factors, or traumatic experiences. Depending on the type of memory function that is impaired, different symptoms may result. Memory dysfunctions caused by innate factors emerge early during development; those that result from trauma to the brain may be traced to the period when the trauma occurred. Although these dysfunctions are often irreversible, the patient may be able to compensate for the deficits.

No single pattern of affect, cognition, somatic state, or relationship characterizes memory impairments.

Clinical Illustration

A third-grade boy with a long history of school evaluations was referred by a teacher, who was concerned about his difficulty keeping up with classroom demands despite substantial individual assistance, especially in math and written language. Additionally, teachers expressed concern about his variable performance, distractibility, difficulty remaining on task, and poor comprehension of oral directions. He was noted to tire easily and to require one-to-one assistance to begin tasks and to follow through to completion. The therapist noted relative strengths in verbal reasoning, word knowledge and usage, social reasoning, attention to visual detail, and part-to-whole synthesis, and relative weaknesses in tasks involving manipulation of information in working memory, retrieval of factual information, attention, and visual-motor integration within a structured format. This boy's auditory memory was somewhat weak compared to other verbal areas. Visual-perceptual skills were variable, with visual sequential memory falling in the low-average range. He had a word retrieval problem, which inhibited his capacity to communicate fluidly.

SCA317.4 Attention Deficit/Hyperactivity Disorders

According to DSM-IV-TR, there are three components to attention deficit/hyperactivity disorders (ADHD): inattention, impulsivity, and hyperactivity. Three subtypes are identified: combined type, predominantly inattentive type, and predominantly hyperactive-impulsive type. Most developmental milestones are achieved on time by children diagnosed with ADHD; some children's level of activity is noticeably higher than average in infancy; frequently, a child's hyperactivity becomes evident around the time he or she begins to walk. Academic performance may be impaired, but the impairment is secondary to the impulsivity or inattentiveness.

Research suggests that there is a genetic/familial component to this disorder. There are other possible contributors as well, including overstimulation, traumatic experiences, and experiences that give rise to depression and anxiety. In addition, many children diagnosed with attentional problems have learning disabilities. Challenges with auditory-verbal processing, visual-spatial processing, sensory modulation (over- or underresponsivity to sensation such as touch or sound), and motor planning and action sequencing can contribute to problems with attention.

This syndrome is frequently diagnosed in some communities and relatively infrequently seen in others. Approximately twice as many boys as girls are diagnosed with ADHD. Estimates of its overall prevalence are as low as 3% and as high as 20% of school-aged children. The estimates seem to depend on various demographic factors, including socioeconomic status and urban versus rural residence.

The *affective states* of children with problems of attention and hyperactivity may come across as an overabundance of energy combined with an infectious excitability. The combination of impulsivity and a frequently agitated mood makes them feel often on the brink of being out of control. Hyperactive children appear to be in perpetual motion, with motor discharge being the favored means of dealing with most situations. Children with these tendencies can also have underlying anxieties, or reactive or intrinsic mood difficulties. For example, it is not uncommon to see a child who recently lost a parent to death or divorce having difficulty with attention.

Somatic states may include feelings described by comments such as "I have to move" or "My muscles are exploding." They may also involve a sense that the body has its own imperatives, in the face of which one is helpless ("My legs just do what they need to.").

The *thoughts and fantasies* of hyperactive children are notably unruly: They may jump from topic to topic or activity to activity with no apparent connecting thread. On the other hand, they may be capable of sustained attention if an object is sufficiently stimulating. Many children with ADHD are obsessed with video games.

In their *relationships*, themes of neediness, opportunism, or manipulation may occur.

Clinical Illustration

A 9-year-old fourth-grade boy whose pediatrician had diagnosed ADHD and prescribed Ritalin was referred to a therapist by his mother, who reported that he was preoccupied with fire and with being injured. He had nightmares, feared going to sleep, and was hard to get up in the mornings. He still had difficulties with separation. When anxious, he appeared clumsy, and he had been repeatedly hurt while playing with other children. His emotional reactions were always intense. He and his mother got into constant power struggles; when he lost, he would collapse and withdraw to his room for hours.

This boy had been an active infant who was difficult to comfort. He had also been a very active toddler, whose enthusiasm for exploring his environment had made it difficult for his mother to keep up with him. He walked at one year, swam well by age 3, and rode a two-wheeler by 4. He was developing into a superb athlete. He started in a developmental nursery at age $3\frac{1}{2}$. Both mother and father accompanied him and stayed with him there initially because of his problems with separation.

This boy's school troubles began in first grade. He had two teachers who he felt did not understand him, and he acted out a lot. Behavior problems had continued in school ever since. Teachers complained that he would not listen, was easily distracted, had problems concentrating, failed at tasks requiring sustained attention, and had difficulty sticking to a play activity. He would often act before thinking. Despite these attentional difficulties, his parents reported that he could sit and watch television for hours. They complained that he was negativistic to the point where "everything is a hassle." Getting him off to school in the morning was particularly troublesome; he had poor hygienic habits and did things hastily. They also noted his low frustration tolerance, overreaction to stimulation, and poor impulse control. He sometimes made self-deprecating comments such as "I hate myself!" or "I can't do it!" or "I am bad!"

This boy was seen for two diagnostic sessions, in which he struck the therapist as an exceedingly anxious, somewhat restless, but attractive 9-year-old. He was quite verbal and calmed down somewhat as he communicated his anxieties and fears. He expressed confusion about what was happening between him and his mother. He felt generally uncomfortable in the school setting, but he could not articulate why that was so.

Related studies include: Fowler, 1992; Gilmore, 2000, 2002; Hallowell & Ratney, 1994; Lerner, Lowenthal, & Lerner, 1995; Zabarenko, 2002.

SCA317.5 Executive Function Disorders

Executive function disorders involve a complex set of deficits that include difficulties in the initiation, conception, and implementation of a plan. These difficulties include the inability to manage time, organize resources, self-monitor, and self-regulate so as to translate a plan into productive activity that insures its completion. Generally, children with these disorders know what they have to do but cannot take the initiative or implement their knowledge. Academically, the child underachieves because homework assignments are lost or not turned in. The child has poor study skills, procrastinates, is inefficient in doing class assignments, and is scattered and disorganized. No distinctive emotional problems are associated with this disorder, although a pattern emerges of not being able to keep life occurrences straight and in order. Children with problematic executive function generally achieve developmental milestones on schedule. Problems do not begin to emerge until demands are made of them to undertake tasks whose complexity is greater than their capabilities. Because these demands increase with maturation, they encounter greater difficulties over time. As they get closer to young adulthood, they are generally ineffectual in adapting to social and life situations, perhaps reflecting an inadequacy of psychic structure.

No single pattern of affect, thought, somatic state, or relationship characterizes the executive function disorders.

Clinical Illustration

A boy of almost 13 was referred because despite notable intellectual gifts, he had a history of attentional, behavioral, and social difficulties since preschool that had interfered with his peer relations, general socio-emotional adjustment, and, at times, his schoolwork. His mother described him as having been a very active toddler, sometimes given to serious tantrums. He learned the alphabet by eighteen months. By age three, he liked to take risks such as climbing and jumping off the jungle gym. His elementary school teachers said he always rushed through his work, made careless mistakes, and was poorly organized. They also said he needed to show more control and not speak out so often in class. He was reported to be oppositional and aggressive with his peers, although not intentionally hurtful. His lockers and desks were unorganized and messy throughout his years at school. From grade school through high school, his mother would joke that she was going to tie him to his desk. When he would go to his room to study, he would stay ten minutes at most before leaving to watch television or tease his brother. He seldom brought his assignments home; he would procrastinate about getting to work on them; and even if he completed them, he would forget to take the work he had done back to school. His mother had to prod him constantly to do his schoolwork. This boy was described as "oblivious" to the teachers' instructions.

This adolescent appeared to have great difficulty adjusting his behavior to fit differing social situations, a problem that impeded his peer relationships and his making transitions between daily routines and tasks. Despite his demonstrated academic abilities, his motivational, organizational, and attentional difficulties were evidently preventing optimal learning and classroom performance. He exhibited much frustration and anxiety, and despite his attempts to appear confident, his self-esteem seemed quite fragile. He had very poor time management skills. In the mornings, his mother frequently found him lying in bed 15 to 20 minutes after she had awakened him. It was a daily battle to get him out of the house and to school on time. His bedroom and bathroom were cluttered with papers, clothes, and books. At home, he required repeated nagging before following through with his chores

---

Related studies include: Gillman, 1994; Tyson, 1996.

SCA317.6 Severe Cognitive Deficits

See also other categories in this section and in the Infant and Early Childhood section on Regulatory-Sensory Processing Disorders and Neurodevelopmental Disorders of Relating and Communicating.

Traditionally, IQ tests have been used to evaluate the extent of cognitive deficits, which are estimated to exist in 1% of the general population. A condition of severe cognitive deficits, or mental retardation, has been characterized as a significant sub-average intellectual function: the child's IQ is 70 or below on an individually administered test (for infants, clinical judgment infers significantly sub-average intellectual functioning). In children with such deficits, there are also impairments in communication, self-care, home living, social/interpersonal skills, use of community resources, self-direction, functional academic skills, leisure, health, and safety.

Current research is demonstrating, however, that mentally retarded children may have strengths of various kinds as well as deficits. Standard intelligence tests do not always pick up such nuances and may be erroneously interpreted as establishing a consistent pattern of deficits across, for example, verbal and nonverbal areas of functioning. It is therefore important to profile the unique features of each child. Often children classified with this disorder manifest a variety of learning, memory, language, and visual-spatial impairments with different degrees of impairment and capacity in different areas. A framework for describing the child's individual differences is presented in the Infancy and Early Childhood section of the PDM. A child's subjective experience of cognitive deficit depends on his or her level of self-awareness.

No single pattern of affect, thought, somatic state, or relationship characterizes the severe cognitive deficits.

Clinical Illustration

A 6-year-old girl was having a difficult time learning to read, do math, and communicate logically with peers. Her educators raised the question of a severe cognitive deficit after testing indicated an overall IQ of 65, with little differentiation between verbal and nonverbal areas of functioning. A more in-depth clinical evaluation, however, revealed that although she had severe difficulties in auditory processing, her level of conceptual understanding was higher when she was given instructions in a highly animated form that combined short verbal explanations with ample gesturing and visual information (pictures). Once she had information to work with, her verbal reasoning was considerably better than her IQ profile had suggested. This girl did demonstrate, however, a history of low muscle tone and severely compromised motor planning and sequencing capacities that made it difficult for her to follow through and complete tasks.

Both her auditory and visual memory capacities were weak relative to her ability to reason with verbal information. Interestingly, she could also reason with visual designs once she had enough exposure to them to be able to retain them. A highly individualized program was developed that focused on utilizing her relative strengths in conceptual reasoning to help her master her severe motor planning and sequencing and memory challenges. Her rapid progress with this program further confirmed the diagnostic profile constructed from a more in-depth clinical evaluation and functional assessment.

Related studies include: Ack, 1966; Arboleda & Holzman, 1985; Caplan, 1993, 1994; Caplan, et al., 1989; Ellison, van Os, & Murray, 1998.

SCA318. Learning Disorders

SCA318.1 Reading Disorders

Reading disorders are diagnosed when reading achievement, as measured by individually administered standardized tests of reading comprehension, is substantially below what is expected for the person's chronological age, measured intelligence, and age-appropriate education. To be considered a diagnosable disorder, a reading deficit must interfere significantly with academic achievement or activities of daily living that require reading skills. These disorders are diagnosed in roughly 4% of the population.

Development is usually unremarkable in children with reading problems, and no social problems are associated with this learning disorder until children are required to complete reading tasks. Their embarrassment at not being able to do what other children do easily may then interfere with peer relationships. No single set of emotional problems beyond this experience of shame is associated with this learning disability. The repeated embarrassment of children with reading difficulties may eventually lead to self-esteem problems.

No single pattern of affect, thought, somatic state, or relationship characterizes reading disorders.

Clinical Illustration

The parents of a 15½-year-old freshman in a large urban high school consulted a psychiatrist because their son had been arrested for driving without a license. They were also worried that a local gang was actively recruiting him. He had begun to dress like the gang members but had recently discontinued at his girlfriend's urging. He was skipping school and failing most of his academic classes.

This boy was born in a small southwestern town to first-generation immigrants who were fluent in English but spoke Spanish at home. They described his early years as unremarkable. A change occurred when he began first grade: He did not like school, and a pattern of misbehavior began. By the end of second grade, his teacher was regularly complaining about his "laziness" because he made no effort to do the schoolwork. The school psychologist found both a reading problem and a language-processing problem when she tested him, which she attributed to difficulties processing visual materials. He was also found to have difficulties in dealing with numbers. Because the school did not have the resources to provide special tutoring, no intervention was made. When the family relocated to a large city, the boy entered the third grade in a new school system, where his reading ability tested at the first-grade level. He was retained in third grade but not retested until fourth grade, at which point he received help from a tutor who tried to teach him keyboarding. His teachers, who were bilingual, were less harsh and more understanding of his problems than those in his prior school had been. Still, no remediation for his learning disability was instituted. In fourth grade, he was placed in a special education class with three girls. Instead of feeling helped, he felt humiliated, and he became more aggressive. In spite of these behavior problems at school, he remained affectionate and obedient at home. By this time he had lost interest in reading, complaining that the effort it took to read a single page quickly tired him. In sixth grade, he went to junior high school, where he was placed again in a special education class. Academically, he was far behind his peers. He felt isolated and escalated his aggressive behavior, announcing that he would rather be in a class of children with behavioral disorders than with the "dumb kids." The family tried to obtain some special help for him at a private learning center, but he hated to go there and soon refused.

By seventh grade, this boy insisted on being mainstreamed, but he was so far behind academically that he stopped going to school. Signs of depression emerged. He complained that he felt dumb and began talking about wishing he were dead. He made a suicidal gesture by taking half a bottle of aspirin, but his parents did not consider this a serious attempt. When he entered eighth grade, his being a year older than most of his classmates became an asset, and he became more socially outgoing, but his parents felt that he had "hooked up with the wrong kind of crowd." His best friend was a bully who was in a class for children with behavior disorders. He began to smoke, and they suspected that he was also on drugs. He developed a relationship with a girl in the class for children with behavioral disorders. His parents stated that he was a strong-willed, affectionate child, who now wanted to get back on track and improve his self-esteem. Testing revealed severe dyslexia.

When asked to describe the source of his academic problems, this young man related them directly to his dyslexia. He said that when he tried to read, the lines on the page ran into each other and he could not distinguish individual words. He and the therapist traced his difficulties in reading back to kindergarten. He was eager to drop out of school and work so that he could get a car. While elaborating on this theme, he noted that he had a terrible temper: He would become enraged and out of control, especially when required to perform academically. On occasion he had punched holes in the wall in his room. He felt it strange that often, after having one of those fits, he would feel exhausted and would fall asleep for a long time. On waking up, he would feel as though nothing had happened. He was aware that his inability to control his temper was a serious problem and said that he would like to do something about it.

Related studies include: Aaron, Phillips, & Larsen, 1988; Abrams, 1991; Arkowitz, 2000; Beitchman & Young, 1997; McNulty, 2003; Richards, 1999; Shaywitz, Pugh, & Fletcher, 2000.

SCA318.2 Mathematics Disorders

A mathematics disorder is diagnosed when mathematical ability, as measured by individually administered standardized tests, is substantially below what is expected for a person's chronological age, measured intelligence, and age-appropriate education. To be considered a diagnosable disorder, the deficit must interfere significantly with academic achievement or activities of daily living that require mathematical ability. Approximately 1% of the school-age population is diagnosed with this disorder.

Development is usually unremarkable in children with mathematics disorder, and as with reading disorders, no social problems are associated with this learning disorder until children are required to complete mathematical tasks. Their embarrassment at not being able to do what other children do easily may then interfere with peer relationships. No single set of emotional problems beyond this experience of shame is associated with this learning disability, although difficulties emerge when the child is faced with academic and life tasks requiring mathematical computation and reasoning. The repeated embarrassment of children with mathematics disorder may eventually lead to self-esteem problems.

No single pattern of affect, thought, somatic state, or relationship characterizes mathematics disorders.

Clinical Illustration

The parents and teacher of an 8-year-old girl reported that she was struggling with, and anxious about, quantitative reasoning and mathematical operations. In the past, she had been seen as having trouble making transitions in the classroom from topic to topic, especially when it shifted to math. She was described as a slow reader who required much repetition when completing mathematics problems. Although she had learned to compute well by rote, she would be defeated by mathematical problems requiring multiple steps, and more broadly, by any multi-step problem requiring hypothesis-testing and logic.

A psychoeducational evaluation showed weaker functioning in the realms of visual-perceptual and visual-spatial abilities, mathematical and other multi-step reasoning abilities, and cross-modal associative learning implemented in the reading process. Her mother said that she had performed well in mathematics until recently, when the focus shifted towards spatial concepts. With bi-weekly math tutoring, her performance began to improve.

SCA318.3 Disorders of Written Expression

A disorder of written expression is diagnosed when writing skills, as measured by individually administered standardized tests, are substantially below what is expected for the person's chronological age, measured intelligence, and age-appropriate education. To be considered a diagnosable disorder, the deficit must interfere significantly with academic achievement or activities in daily living that require written composition.

Development is usually unremarkable in children with disorders of written expression. No social problems are associated with this learning disorder until children are required to complete writing tasks. Their embarrassment at not being able to do what other children do easily may then interfere with peer relationships. No single set of emotional problems beyond this experience of shame is associated with this learning disability, although difficulties emerge when the child is faced with having to write an essay. The repeated embarrassment of children with this disorder may eventually lead to self-esteem problems.

No single pattern of affect, thought, somatic state, or relationship characterizes disorders of written expression.

Clinical Illustration

A seventh-grade boy of above-average intelligence was chronically late with written assignments and sometimes would not bother to hand them in. In sessions he described having particular difficulty with English assignments. When asked to write a brief essay, he would stare at his computer screen and have no idea about how to begin. After putting down a sentence, he would feel dissatisfied with how he expressed his thought. Efforts to improve it would keep failing until he would walk away from the task in frustration. At times, his mother would try to help him. They would make an outline, but that alone would not work. She would then suggest a sentence to begin the process, but then he would get stuck, having no idea of what should follow. When he and she would discuss what he wanted to say, in contrast, he would have no problem; in fact, he would have many ideas. When his mother would write down them down, he could begin to write, but he would then have a terrible time sequencing them and separating what is important from what is not important. Testing revealed an underlying language problem that impaired his ability to express his thoughts.

SCA318.4 Nonverbal Learning Disabilities

Children with nonverbal learning disabilities have a complex set of neurocognitive strengths and weaknesses: Strengths in rote verbal memory, in reading decoding, and in spelling; weaknesses in tactile and visual perception and attention, concept formation, reading comprehension of complex materials, problem solving, and dealing with novel materials. They tend to have problems in math and science, and they may show a pattern of socio-emotional difficulties involving the reception and expression of modulated affects and of nonverbal modes of communication. They typically have poor handwriting and are deficient in arithmetic skills. Their reading comprehension is not on a par with their verbal skills; although they are good readers, they have great difficulty with art assignments. They also have problems with attention, novel materials, and new situations.

As infants they are passive, fail to engage in exploratory play, and do not respond as expected. They appear clumsy and poorly coordinated. They have difficulties interacting with other children in groups. They are unable to form friendships or to be with other children even for brief periods without erupting. They usually interact well with adults but not with peers. They are unable to decode social cues, failing to "read" other people's body language, facial expressions, and vocal intonations. They are inept in social situations.

With respect to their *affective states*, children with NLD have difficulties in the reception, expression, and processing of affective states of communication. Their self-esteem is usually damaged by their recurrent failures to complete tasks that appear simple to others and by their lack of success in social relationships. They suffer from chronic anxiety and have difficulties in self-regulation.

Thoughts and fantasies may focus on being a failure, being different, or being lost. Thinking may be piecemeal or fragmented, especially in situations that require "big-picture" or synthetic thinking. As a result of efforts to reduce fragmentation, thinking can be narrow and rigid.

Somatic states may include a diffuse physical clumsiness, especially with respect to fine motor skills.

In their *relationship patterns*, children with this problem may appear out of step with those around them. They lack the ease and fluidity in social discourse that we associate with social competence. They may make people anxious or uncomfortable, yet they appear to have little awareness of the impact they have on others. Some such children appear socially disconnected and out of touch with what goes on around them. In group situations, they tend to withdraw into silence, or, if they attempt to engage others, speak in ways that show a lack of understanding of the subtleties of the group's interactions.

Clinical Illustration

A third-grade boy was referred for trouble with nonverbal communication. He did not make good eye contact or show emotions in his facial expression, and he seemed stiff and wooden. He could not process visual-spatial information, despite being highly verbal and capable of expressing himself at a level beyond his chronological age. Because of his visual-spatial processing problem, he had academic difficulties, especially in math and art. He was acutely aware of these difficulties and of his relative isolation in school. His fragile sense of self and low self-esteem provided a filter through which he understood interpersonal situations; he not only misinterpreted them but also presumed that the poorly understood pieces constituted negative commentary about him. In conversations, he could become easily confused, had a difficult time integrating ideas to develop a synthesized meaning, and when overwhelmed, would fall into a daydreaming, non-responsive wide-eyed gaze. He seemed unable to determine the relevant aspects of a situation and decode their meanings conventionally.

Stimulating situations disorganized his thinking, leading to heightened emotional arousal until he would explode in helpless anger. Although he seemed unaware of his contribution to interpersonal conflicts, he seemed to perceive at some level that most of his relationships were dysfunctional and unrewarding, a fact that undermined his self-esteem. His organizational difficulties were greatly exacerbated by anxiety, which tended to increase in proportion to his level of visual stimulation. His anxiety about relationships kept him more attentive to other people's feelings than are most children with nonverbal learning disability. He was often unhappy and anxious, prone to mood fluctuations, and in need of reassurance. While he was not good at understanding and responding to affective states in other children, he had some capacity to accommodate to adult emotional display, perhaps because such expression is more controlled, and at times more obvious. He also had trouble expressing his own feelings.

Related studies include: Little, 1993; Molenaar-Klumper, 2002; Pally, 2001; Palombo, 1996, 2006; Rourke, 1989; Rourke & Tsatsanis, 2000; Stein, et al., 2004; Tanguay 2001, 2002.

SCA318.5 Social-Emotional Learning Disabilities

Children with social and emotional learning disabilities have difficulties interacting with other children in groups. They are unable to be with other children even for brief periods of time without great distress; consequently they rarely make friends, though they may interact reasonably with adults. They fail to "read" other people's body language, facial expressions, and vocal intonations and are therefore socially inept. While they have many of the social features of children with nonverbal learning disabilities, they do not have the same cognitive or academic deficits.

These children appear unimpaired during their early development; it is only when they begin to interact with others that their problems emerge. Their self-help skills do not develop comparably to those of other children their age. Because they do not seem to know how to play with other children, they are eventually excluded from social groups. Their consequent isolation deprives them further of opportunities to develop socially and thus compounds their difficulties. Although they may have one or two individual friends, by adolescence they are rejected by peers and excluded from group activities.

With respect to their *affective states*, children with social-emotional learning difficulties understand the world of emotion only intellectually. Feelings are like a foreign language. Only when their feelings reach a threshold of explosive intensity can they experience their own affective states. Most often, those are frustration, rage, and terror.

With respect to their *thoughts and fantasies*, these children seem to have a diminished capacity to develop a theory of mind. They seem unaware that others have beliefs, desires, and intentions. Consequently, they appear to disregard others' thoughts and feelings. Their capacity for pretense, whether imaginative play or intentional deception, is greatly limited.

There are no typical *somatic states* that characterize children with social and emotional learning disabilities.

As to *relationships*, for these children the world is unrewarding, unpredictable, and unintelligible. They try to memorize rules that would explain how people are supposed to behave, but then they are mystified as to when rules apply and when they do not. They very much long for contact with others, yet when they occasionally make forays to befriend someone, they are disappointed at being met with indifference. For reasons inexplicable to them, their relationships fall apart. These children appear immature or inappropriate and are socially disconnected when with others. Their behavior may become socially dysfunctional, as they become argumentative, disruptive, or disrespectful. There are not successful in maintaining peer relationships, have no close friendships, and are rejected, teased, or bullied by peers.

Clinical Illustration

A 9-year-old boy was somewhat awkward with ordinary social interactions; although he apparently had learned rules for behavior, he applied them repeatedly and mechanically such that they lost their meaning. He showed little emotional responsivity to social cues and jokes. Because of his difficulty negotiating the reciprocal nature of play and other social interactions, he had few friends and was seldom included in games at school. His caregivers said that he was sometimes unresponsive when other children would speak to him: He talked mainly about his own interests, and had problems changing topics. In addition, he asked inappropriate personal questions, made people uncomfortable by standing too close or touching them, failed to grasp abstract ideas, and took jokes too literally.

At a basic level, this boy could not always perceive and interpret situations as most others would. Sometimes his perceptions were accurate, yet he would focus upon peripheral detail. Other times, especially in complex situations, he would develop idiosyncratic interpretations of an occurrence, the factors leading up to it, and its meaning. His marked difficulty reading other people's emotional expressions prevented his appreciating the impact of his behavior on other people, and he seemed to lack feelings such as guilt and empathy that are predicated upon knowledge of others' feelings towards oneself.

Related studies include: Adolphs, 2003a, 2003b; Bryan, 1991; Palombo 1996, 2006

Related studies for the general category of learning disorders include: Adelman & Adelman 1987; Bauminger, Edelsztein, & Morash, 2005; Palombo 1992, 1994, 2001a, 2001b; Pennington 1991; Rothstein, Benjamin, Crosby, & Eisenstadt, 1988; Rothstein & Glenn, 1999.

SCA319. Bulimia

Bulimia is described on pp. 119-122 of the Adult Symptom Patterns section of this manual.

Related studies on bulimia in children and adolescents include: Barth, 1988; Keck & Fiebert, 1986.

SCA320. Anorexia

Anorexia is described on pp. 119-122 of the Adult Symptom Patterns section of this manual.

Related studies on anorexia in children and adolescents include: Fischer, 1989; Gila, Castro, Cesena, & Toro, 2005; Goodsitt, 1977; Keck & Fiebert, 1986; Ritvo, 1984; Seiffge-Krenke, 1997.)

SCA321. Regulatory Disorders

Regulatory Disorders and SCA322 through SCA326.3 below are described in the Diagnostic Classification of Mental Health and Developmental Disorders of Infancy and Early Childhood, Revised—DC: 0-3R (Zero to Three, 2005). They generally begin in infancy or early childhood and may continue into latency or adolescence.

SCA322. Feeding Problems of Childhood

Feeding Problems in Childhood are described in IEC115, p. 341, and IEC207.4, p. 355.

SCA323. Elimination Disorders

Elimination Disorders are described in IEC116, p. 341, and IEC207.5, p. 355.

SCA323.1 Encopresis
SCA323.2 Enuresis

SCA324. Sleep Disorders

Sleep Disorders are described in IEC114, p. 339, and IEC207.3, p. 355.

SCA325. Attachment Disorders

Attachment Disorders are described in IEC109, p. 335.

SCA326. Pervasive Developmental Disorders

Pervasive Developmental Disorders are described in IEC301-304, pp. 360-368.

SCA326.1 Autism
SCA326.2 Asperger's Syndrome
SCA326.3 Pervasive Developmental Disorder (PDD) not otherwise specified

SCA327. Gender Identity Disorders

Children with gender identity disorders express, in the absence of chromosomal or hormonal abnormalities, an intense dislike of their gender and a determined wish to be the other gender. This may be expressed as a wish to be the other gender or a conviction that they *are* a girl rather than a boy, or vice versa. Boys are referred for evaluation for this disorder five times as frequently as girls, and the condition carries considerably more stigma for them. Cross-gender identification may be manifested by a persistent preference for cross-sex roles in make-believe play, persistent fantasies of being the other sex, an intense desire to participate in the stereotypical games and pastimes of the other sex, and a strong preference for playmates of the other sex. The disorder is defined by the persistence, pervasiveness, and duration of the cross-gender identity, as opposed to both normal, time-limited cross-gender interests and gender nonconformity (e.g., boys who prefer solitary or artistic activities, girls considered to be tomboys).

The developmental course is better understood for boys than girls. Gender identity disorder develops in a child who is temperamentally at risk during a critical period (18-36 months) when there is an awareness of gender difference but when self and object constancy are not fully established. Children with this disorder have been noted to be unusually sensitive and highly reactive to sensory stimuli from birth on. Such sensitivity may involve awareness of nuance in caregivers, including resonance to any ambivalence in a parent about the child's gender. Boys with cross-gender identification tend to be constitutionally shy, inhibited, and timid. It is possible that the lower incidence in girls reflects significantly greater tolerance for gender-atypical dress and behavior in females. Outside the child's preoccupation with gender issues there is no evidence of other psychological difficulties.

With respect to *affective states,* mood may fluctuate in response to teasing from others, but may otherwise be stable. Feelings of shame about being different may be painful; parental and peer discomfort, disapproval, ostracism, and teasing may intensify low self-esteem. Anger about having the wrong body for one's psychological gender may be mild and intermittent or intense and chronic.

With respect to *thoughts and fantasies,* there is recurrent preoccupation with the wish to be, or the feeling that one is, the other gender. Such thoughts vary in frequency and intensity from child to child and in some may be of obsessive proportions. The child's play may reflect this state of mind in becoming rigid, compulsive, and repetitive.

There are no characteristic *somatic states* associated with this disorder, beyond those related to the painful affects that can accompany it.

In terms of *relationships,* parental responses of anxiety, overinvolvement, and/ or withdrawal may complicate family interactions. Rejection from peers may increase social isolation in children who are already sensitive, thereby hampering their learning and social skills.

Clinical Illustration

A quiet, sad 4-year-old boy was unable to separate from his mother or to make friends. He would sometimes state that he wanted to be a girl; at other times he would say that he was a girl. He avoided rough play with boys, preferring to play house with girls. His play was repetitive and restricted. He cried easily and would quickly become overwhelmed with almost any feeling. He had recently been expressing displeasure with his penis.

This boy's maternal grandmother had died when he was 2, leaving his mother (a woman seen by the therapist as uncomfortable with closeness) depressed and unavailable to her son. She tended to hover anxiously over him. His father was described as very involved in his business.

Related studies include: Coates & Wolfe 1995; Frenkel, 1993; Gender identity disorder in boys, 1993; Parens, 1990, 2001; Parens, Pollock, Stern, & Kramer, 1976; Tyson 1982, 1986a, 1986b, 2001.

Concordance of PDM and DSM IV Axis I Diagnostic Caregories for Children and Adolescents

PDM Category		PDM Code	PDM Disorder	DSM-IV-R Disorder
Healthy Response			**Developmental Crises**	Disorder of Infancy, Childhood or Adolescence NOS
			Situational Crises	
Disorders of Affect	**Anxiety Disorder**	SCA301	**Anxiety Disorder**	Generalized Anxiety Disorder
		SCA302	**Phobias**	Specific Phobia
		SCA303	**Obsessive-Compulsive Disorders**	Obsessive-Compulsive Disorder
		SCA304	**Somatization (Somatoform) Disorders**	Somatization Disorder
	Affect/ Mood Disorder	SCA305	**Prolonged Mourning/ Grief Reaction**	Bereavement
		SCA306	**Depressive Disorders**	Major Depressive Disorder or Dysthymic Disorder
		SCA307	**Bipolar Disorders**	Bipolar I Disorder
		SCA308	**Suicidality**	
Disruptive Behavior Disorders		SCA309	**Conduct Disorders**	Conduct Disorder
		SCA310	**Oppositional-Defiant Disorders**	Oppositional-Defiant Disorder
		SCA311	**Substance Abuse Related Disorders**	Cannabis Dependence
Reactive Disorder		SCA312	**Psychic Trauma and Posttraumatic Stress Disorder**	Post-Traumatic Stress Disorder
		SCA313	**Adjustment Disorders**	Adjustment Disorder

(continued)

PDM Category	PDM Code	PDM Disorder	DSM-IV-R Disorder
Disorders of Mental Functioning	SCA314	**Motor Skills Disorders**	Motor Skills Disorder
	SCA315	**Tic Disorders**	Tic Disorders
	SCA316	**Psychotic Disorders**	Psychotic Disorders
	SCA317	**Neuropsychological Disorders** 317.1 Visual-Spatial Processing Disorders	
		317.2 Language and Auditory Processing Disorders	Expressive or Mixed Receptive-Expressive Language Disorder
		317.3 Memory Impairments	Amnestic Disorder NOS
		317.4 Attention Deficit/ Hyperactivity Disorder (AD/HD)	Attention Deficit/ Hyperactivity Disorder
		317.5 Executive Function Disorders	
		317.6 Severe Cognitive Deficits	Mental Retardation
	SCA318	**Learning Disorders** 318.1 Reading Disorders	Reading Disorder
		318.2 Mathematics Disorders	Mathematics Disorder
		318.3 Disorders of Written Expression	Disorder of Written Expression
		318.4 Nonverbal Learning Disabilities	Learning Disorder NOS
		318.5 Social-Emotional Learning Disabilities	Learning Disorder NOS
Psychophysiologic Disorders	SCA319	**Bulimia**	Bulimia Nervosa
	SCA320	**Anorexia**	Anorexia Nervosa

PDM Category	PDM Code	PDM Disorder	DSM-IV-R Disorder
Developmental Disorders	SCA321	Regulatory Disorders	Disorders of Infancy, Childhood, and Adolescence, NOS
	SCA322	Feeding Problems of Childhood	Feeding Disorder of Infancy or Early Childhood
	SCA323	Elimination Disorders 323.1 Encopresis	Encopresis Without Constipation and Overflow Incontinence
		323.2 Enuresis	Enuresis
	SCA324	Sleep Disorders	Primary Insomnia Nightmare Disorder
	SCA325	Attachment Disorders	Reactive Attachment Disorder of Infancy or Early Childhood
	SCA326	Pervasive Developmental Disorder 326.1 Autism	Autistic Disorder
		326.2 Asperger's Syndrome	Asperger's Disorder
		326.3 PDD-not otherwise specified	PDD-NOS
Other Disorders	SCA327	Gender Identity Disorders	Gender Identity Disorder

REFERENCES

Blos, P. (1967). The second individuation process of adolescence. *Psychoanalytic Study of the Child, 22,* 162-186.

Noshpitz, J. (1991). Disturbances in early adolescent development. In S. I. Greenspan & G. H. Pollock (Eds.), *The Course of Life, Vol. IV: Adolescence.* 119-180. Madison, CT: International Universities Press.

Offer, D. (1991). Adolescent development: A normative perspective. In S. I. Greenspan & G. H. Pollock (Eds.), *The Course of Life, Vol. IV: Adolescence.* 181-200. Madison, CT: International Universities Press.

Zero to Three (2005). *Diagnostic Classification of Mental Health and Developmental Disorders of Infancy and Early Childhood, Revised—DC: 0-3R.* Washington, DC: Zero to Three.

RELATED STUDIES

Aaron, P. G., Phillips, S., & Larsen, S. (1988). Specific reading disability in historically famous persons. *Journal of Learning Disabilities, 21,* 523-538.

Abrams, J. (1991) The affective component: Emotional needs of individuals with reading and related learning disorders. *Journal of Reading, Writing and Learning Disabilities International, 7,* 171-182.

Ack, M. (1966). Julie: The treatment of a case of developmental retardation, *Psychoanalytic Study of the Child, 21,* 127-149.

Adelman, K. A., & Adelman, H. S. (1987). Rodin, Patton, Edison, Wilson, Einstein: Were they really learning disabled? *Journal of Learning Disabilities, 20,* 270-279.

Adolphs, R. (2003a). Cognitive neuroscience of human social behaviour. *Nature Reviews: Neuroscience, 4,* 165–178.

Adolphs, R. (2003b). Investigating the cognitive neuroscience of social behavior. *Neuropsychologia, 41,* 119–126.

Allen-Meares, P. (1987). Depression in childhood and adolescence. *Social Work, 32,* 512-516.

Anthony, E. J. (1987). Risk, vulnerability, and resilience: An overview. In E. J. Anthony & B. J. Cohler (Eds.), *The invulnerable child* (pp. 3-48). New York: Guilford Press.

Apter, A., Pauls, D. L., Bleich, A., Zohar, A. H., Kron, S., Ratzoni, G., et al. (1993). An epidemiologic study of Gilles de la Tourette's syndrome in Israel. *Archives of General Psychiatry, 50,* 734-738.

Arboleda, C., & Holzman, P. S. (1985). Thought disorder in children at risk for psychosis. *Archives of General Psychiatry, 42,* 1004-1013.

Arkowitz, S. W. (2000). The overstimulated state of dyslexia: Perception, knowledge, and learning. *Journal of the American Psychoanalytic Association, 48,* 1491-1520.

Baker, L., & Cantwell, D. P. (1987). A prospective psychiatric follow-up of children with speech/language disorders. *Journal of the American Academy of Child and Adolescent Psychiatry, 26,* 546-554.

Barth, F. D. (1988). The treatment of bulimia from a self psychological perspective. *Clinical Social Work Journal, 16,* 270-281.

Bauminger, N., Edelsztein, H. S., & Morash, J. (2005). Social information processing and emotional understanding in children with LD. *Journal of Learning Disabilities, 38,* 45-61.

Beidel, D., & Turner, S. (1998). *Shy children, phobic adults: Nature and treatment of social phobia.* Washington, DC: American Psychological Association.

Beitchman, J. H., Young, A. R. (1997). Learning disorders with a special emphasis on reading disorders: A review of the past 10 years. *Journal of the American Academy of Child and Adolescent Psychiatry, 36,* 1020–1032.

Bernstein, G. A., Borchardt, C. M., & Perwien, A. R. (1996). Anxiety disorders in children and adolescents: A review of the past 10 years. *Journal of the American Academy of Child and Adolescent Psychiatry, 35,* 1110–1119.

Birman, B., Ryan, N. D., Williamson, D. E., Brent, D. A., Kaufman, J., Dahl, R. E., et al. (1996). Childhood and adolescent depression: A review of the past 10 years. Part I. *Journal of the American Academy of Child and Adolescent Psychiatry, 35,* 1427-1439.

Blair, R. J., Budhani, S., Colledge, E., & Scott, S. (2005). Deafness to fear in boys with psychopathic tendencies. *Journal of Child Psychology and Psychiatry, 46,* 327-336.

Bonnard, A. (1963). Impediments of speech: A special psychosomatic instance. *International Journal of Psycho-Analysis, 44,* 151-162.

Bostic, J. Q., Rubin, D. H., Prince, J., & Schlozman, S. (2005). Treatment of depression in children and adolescents. *Journal of Psychiatric Practice, 11,* 141-154.

Bowlby, J. (1961). Process of mourning. *International Journal of Psycho-Analysis, 42,* 317-340.

Bowlby, J. (1969). *Attachment and Loss: Vol. I. Attachment.* New York, Basic Books.

Brent, D., Johnson, B., Perper, J., Connolly, J., Bridge, J., Bartle, S., et al. (1994). Personality disorder, personality traits, impulsive violence, and completed suicide in adolescents. *Journal of the American Academy of Child and Adolescent Psychiatry, 33,* 1080-1086.

Brown, E. J., & Goodman, R. F. (2005). Childhood traumatic grief: An exploration of the construct in children bereaved on September 11. *Journal of Clinical Child and Adolescent Psychology, 34,* 248-259.

Bryan, T. (1991). Assessment of social cognition: Review of research in learning disabilities. In H. L. Swanson (Ed.), *Handbook on the assessment of learning disabilities: Theory, research, and practice* (pp. 285–312). Austin, TX: Pro-ed.

Caplan, R. (1993). Childhood schizophrenia assessment and treatment: A developmental approach. *Child and Adolescent Psychiatric Clinics of North America, 3,* 15-30.

Caplan, R. (1994). Thought disorder in childhood. *Journal of the American Academy of Child and Adolescent Psychiatry, 33,* 605-615.

Caplan, R., Guthries, D., Fish, B., Tanguay, P. E., & David-Lando, G. (1989). The Kiddie Formal Thought Disorder Rating Scale: Clinical assessment, reliability, and validity. *Journal of the American Academy of Child and Adolescent Psychiatry, 38,* 408-416.

Chused, J. (1999). Obsessional manifestations in children. *Psychoanalytic Study of the Child, 54,* 219–232.

Clark, D., & Bolton, D. (1985). Obsessive-compulsive adolescents and their parents: A psychometric study. *Journal of Child Psychology and Psychiatry, 26,* 267-276.

Coates, S., & Wolfe, S. (1995). Gender identity disorder in boys: The interface of constitution and early experience. *Psychoanalytic Inquiry, 15,* 6-38.

Diller, L. (2005). Antidepressants and children's depression. *American Journal of Psychiatry, 162,* 1226–1227.

Dilsaver, S. Benazzi, C., F., Rihmer, Z., Akiskal, K. K., & Akiskal, H. S. (2005). Gender, suicidality and bipolar mixed states in adolescents. *Journal of Affective Disorders, 87,* 11-16.

Doka, K. J. (Ed.) (1995). *Children mourning, mourning children.* Washington, DC: Hospice Foundation of America.

Ellison, Z., van Os, J., & Murray, R. (1998). Special feature: Childhood personality characteristics of schizophrenia: Manifestations of, or risk factors for, the disorder? *Journal of Personality Disorder, 12,* 247-261.

Evans, R. (1975). "Hysterical materialization" in the analysis of a latency girl. Psychoanalytic Study of the Child, 30, 307-339.

Faedda, G. L., Baldessarini, R. J., Glovinsky, I. P., & Austin, N. B. (2004). Pediatric bipolar disorder: Phenomenology and course of illness. *Bipolar Disorders, 6,* 305-313.

Farley, S. E., Adams, J. S., Lutton, M. E., Scoville, C., Fulkerson, R. C., & Webb, A. R. (2005). Clinical inquiries: What are effective treatments for oppositional and defiant behaviors in preadolescents? *Journal of Family Practice, 54,* 162-165.

Fischer, N. (1989). Anorexia nervosa and unresolved rapprochement conflicts. *International Journal of Psycho-Analysis, 70,* 41-54.

Flament, M. F., Koby, E., Rapoport, J. L., Berg, C. J., Zahn, T., Cox, C., et al. (1990). Childhood obsessive-compulsive disorder: A prospective follow-up study. *Journal of Child Psychology and Psychiatry, 31,* 363-380.

Fleming, J., & Altschul, S. (1963). Activation of mourning and growth by psycho-analysis. *International Journal of Psycho-Analysis, 44,* 419-431.

Fowler, M. C. (1992). *CHADD educators manual: An in-depth look at attention deficit disorders from an educational perspective.* Fairfax, VA: CHADD National Education Committee.

Francis, G., & Gragg, R. A. (1996). *Childhood obsessive compulsive disorder*. Thousand Oaks, CA: Sage Publications.

Francis, G., Last, C., & Strauss, C. C. (1992). Avoidant disorder and social phobia in children and adolescents. *Journal of the American Academy of Child and Adolescent Psychiatry, 31,* 1086-1089.

Frankiel, R. V. (1994). *Essential papers on object loss*. New York: New York University Press.

Frenkel, R. (1993). Problems in female development. Comments on the analysis of an early latency-aged girl. *Psychoanalytic Study of the Child, 48,* 171-192.

Freud, S. (1917). Mourning and melancholia. *Standard Edition, 14,* 239-258.

Frick, P. J., & Kimonis, E. R. (2005). Externalizing disorders of childhood and adolescence. In J. E. Maddux & B. A. Winstead (Eds.), *Psychopathology: Foundations for a contemporary understanding* (pp. 325-351). Mahwah, NJ: Lawrence Erlbaum.

Frick, P. J., O'Brien, B. S., Wootton, J. M., & McBurnett, K. (1994). Psychopathy and conduct problems in children. *Journal of Abnormal Psychology, 103,* 700-707.

Furman, E. (1974). *A child's parent dies: Studies in childhood bereavement*. New Haven, CT: Yale University Press.

Furman, R. A. (1994). A child's capacity for mourning. In R. V. Frankiel (Ed.), *Essential papers on object loss* (pp. 376-381). New York: New York University Press.

Gaensbauer, T. J. (1994). Therapeutic work with a traumatized toddler. *Psychoanalytic Study of the Child, 49,* 412-433.

Gaensbauer, T. J. (2002). Representations of trauma in infancy: Clinical and theoretical implications for the understanding of early memory. *Infant Mental Health Journal, 23,* 259-277.

Galatzer-Levy, R. M. (1987). Manic-depressive illness: Analytic experience and a hypothesis. In A. Goldberg (Ed.), *Progress in self psychology: Vol. 3. Frontiers in self psychology* (pp. 87-102). Hillsdale, NJ: Analytic Press.

Gartner, J., Weintraub, S., & Carlson, G. A. (1997). Childhood-onset psychosis: Evolution and comorbidity. *American Journal of Psychiatry, 154,* 256-261.

Gender identity disorder in boys: Panel report (1993). *Journal of the American Psychoanalytic Association, 41,* 729-742.

Gila, A., Castro, J., Cesena, J., & Toro, J. (2005). Anorexia nervosa in male adolescents: Body image, eating attitudes and psychological traits. *Journal of Adolescent Health, 36,* 221-226.

Gillman, R. D. (1994). Narcissistic defense and learning inhibition. *Psychoanalytic Study of the Child, 49,* 175-189.

Gilmore, K. (2000). A psychoanalytic perspective on attention deficit/hyperactivity disorder. *Journal of the American Psychoanalytic Association, 48,* 1259-1293.

Gilmore, K. (2002). Diagnosis, dynamics, and development: Considerations in the psychoanalytic assessment of children with AD/HD. *Psychoanalytic Inquiry, 22,* 372-390.

González-Tejera, G., Canino, G., Ramirez, R., Chavez, L., Shrout, P., Bird, H., et al. (2005). Examining minor and major depression in adolescents. *Journal of Child Psychology and Psychiatry, 46,* 888-899.

Goodsitt, A. (1977). Narcissistic disturbances in anorexia nervosa. In S. C. Feinstein & P. L. Giovacchini (Eds.), *Adolescent Psychiatry* (pp. 304-312). New York: Jason Aronson.

Goodwin, R. D., Brook, J. S., & Cohen, P. (2005). Panic attacks and the risk of personality disorder. *Psychological Medicine, 35,* 227-235.

Hallowell, E. M., & Ratney, J. J. (1994). *Driven to distraction: Recognizing and coping with attention deficit disorder from childhood through adulthood*. New York: Simon & Schuster.

Harrington, R. C. (2001). Childhood depression and conduct disorder: Different routes to the same outcome? *Archives of General Psychiatry, 58,* 237-238.

Hesse, E., & Main, M. (1999). Second-generation effects of unresolved trauma in nonmaltreating parents: Dissociated, frightened, and threatening parental behavior. *Psychoanalytic Inquiry, 19,* 481-540.

Hinshaw, S. P., & Lee, S. S. (2003). Conduct and oppositional defiant disorders. In E. J. Mash & R. A. Barkley (Eds.), *Child psychopathology* (pp. 144-198). New York: Guilford Press.

Hofer, M. (1984). Relationships as regulators: A psychobiologic perspective on bereavement. *Psychosomatic Medicine, 46,* 183-197.

Hofer, M. (1995a). An evolutionary perspective on anxiety. In S. P. Roose & R. A. Glick (Eds.), *Anxiety as symptom and signal* (pp. 17-38). Hillsdale, NJ: Analytic Press.

Hofer, M. (1995b). Hidden regulators: Implication for a new understanding of attachment, separation, and loss. In S. Goldberg, R. Muir, & J. Kerr (Eds.), *Attachment theory: Social, developmental, and clinical perspectives* (pp. 203-230). Hillsdale, NJ, Analytic Press.

Keck, J. N., & Fiebert, M. S. (1986). Avoidance of anxiety and eating disorders. *Psychological Reports, 58,* 432-434.

Keenan, K., & Wakschlag, L. S. (2004). Are oppositional defiant and conduct disorder symptoms normative behaviors in preschoolers? A comparison of referred and nonreferred children. *American Journal of Psychiatry, 161,* 356-358.

Kernberg, P. F., & Chazen, S. (1991). *Children with conduct disorders: A psychotherapy manual.* New York: Basic Books.

Kestenberg, J.S., & Brenner, I. (1996). *The last witness: The child survivor of the holocaust.* Washington DC: American Psychiatric Press.

King, R. A., & Apter, A. (1996). Psychoanalytic perspectives on adolescent suicide. *Psychoanalytic Study of the Child, 51,* 491-512.

Kochman, F. J., Hantouche, E. G., Ferrari, P., Lancrenon, S., Bayart, D., & Akiskal, H. S. (2005). Cyclothymia temperament as a prospective predictor of bipolarity and suicidality in children and adolescents with major depressive disorder. *Journal of Affective Disorders, 85,* 181-189.

Kurlan, R., Whitmore, B. A., Irvine, C., McDermott, M. P., & Como, P. G. (1994). Tourette's syndrome in a special education population: A pilot study involving a single school district. *Neurology, 44,* 699-702.

Lerner, J., Lowenthal, B, & Lerner, S. (1995). *Attention deficit disorders: Assessment and teaching.* Pacific Grove, CA: Brooks/Cole Publishing.

Lewis, M. (1977). Language, cognitive development, and personality: A synthesis. *Journal of the American Academy of Child Psychiatry, 16,* 646-661.

Little, M. I. (1990). *Psychotic anxieties and containment: A personal record of an analysis with Winnicott.* Northvale, NJ: Jason Aronson.

Little, S. S. (1993). Nonverbal learning disabilities and socioemotional functioning: A review of the recent literature. *Journal of Learning Disabilities, 26,* 653-665.

March, J. S., & Leonard, H. L. (1996). Obsessive-compulsive disorder in children and adolescents: A review of the past 10 years. *Journal of the American Academy of Child and Adolescent Psychiatry, 34,* 1265-1273.

Maughan, B., Rowe, R., Messer, J., Goodman, R., & Meltzer, H. (2004). Conduct disorder and oppositional defiant disorder in a national sample: Developmental epidemiology. *Journal of Child Psychology and Psychiatry, 45,* 609-621.

McClowry, S. G., Davies, E. B., May, K. A., Kulenkamp, E. J., & Martinson, I. M. (1995). The empty space phenomenon: The process of grief in the bereaved family. In K. J. Doka (Ed.), *Children mourning, mourning children* (pp. 149-162). Washington, DC: Hospice Foundation of America.

McNulty, M. A. (2003). Dyslexia and the life course. *Journal of Learning Disabilities, 36,* 363-381.

Michael, K. D., Huelsman, T. J., & Crowley, S. L. (2005). Interventions for child and adolescent depression: Do professional therapists produce better results? *Journal of Child and Family Studies, 14,* 223-236.

Milrod, B. (2002). A 9 year-old girl with conversion disorder, successfully treated with psycho-analysis. *International Journal of Psycho-Analysis, 83*, 623-631.

Moffitt, T. E. (1993). Adolescence-limited and life-course-persistent antisocial behavior: A developmental view. *Psychological Review, 100*, 674-701.

Moffitt, T., Caspi, A., Dickson, N., Silva, P., & Stanton, W.(1996). Childhood-onset versus adolescent-onset antisocial conduct problems in males: Natural history from ages 3 to 18 years. *Development and Psychopathology, 8*, 399-424.

Molenaar-Klumper, M. (2002). *Non-verbal learning disabilities: Characteristics, diagnosis and treatment within an educational setting.* London: Jessica Kingsley Publishers.

Najman, J. M., Hallam, D., Bor, W. B., O'Callaghan, M., Williams, G. M., & Shuttlewood, G. (2005). Predictors of depression in very young children: A prospective study. *Social Psychiatry and Psychiatric Epidemiology, 40*, 5 367-374.

Ollendick, T. H., Shortt, A. L., & Sanders, J. B. (2005). Internalizing disorders of childhood and adolescence. In J. E. Maddux & B. A. Winstead (Eds.), *Psychopathology: Foundations for a contemporary understanding* (pp. 353-376). Mahwah, NJ: Lawrence Erlbaum.

Pajer, K. A. (1998). What happens to "bad" girls: A review of the adult outcome of antisocial adolescent girls. *American Journal of Psychiatry, 155*, 862-870.

Pally, R. (2001). A primary role for nonverbal communication in psychoanalysis. *Psychoanalytic Inquiry, 21*, 71-93.

Palombo, J. (1981). Parent loss and childhood bereavement: Some theoretical considerations. *Clinical Social Work Journal, 9*, 3-33.

Palombo, J. (1992, April). Learning disabilities in children: Developmental, diagnostic and treatment considerations. In *Proceedings: Fourth National Health Policy Forum, Healthy children 2000: Obstacles and Opportunities.* Washington, DC: National Academies of Practice.

Palombo, J. (1994). Incoherent self-narratives and disorders of the self in children with learning disabilities. *Smith College Studies in Social Work, 64*, 129-152.

Palombo, J. (1996). The diagnosis and treatment of children with nonverbal learning disabilities. *Child and Adolescent Social Work Journal, 13*, 311-332.

Palombo, J. (2001a). *Learning disorders and disorders of the self in children and adolescents.* New York: W.W. Norton.

Palombo, J. (2001b). The therapeutic process with children with learning disorders. *Psychoanalytic Social Work 8*, 143-168.

Palombo, J. (2006). *Nonverbal learning disabilities: A clinical perspective.* New York: W. W. Norton.

Parens, H. (1979). *The development of aggression in early childhood.* New York: Jason Aronson.

Parens, H., (1987), *Aggression in our children: Coping with it constructively.* New York: Jason Aronson.

Parens, H. (1988). Siblings in early childhood: Some direct observational findings. *Psychoanaltyic Inquiry, 8*, 31-50.

Parens, H. (1989a). Toward a reformulation of the psychoanalytic theory of aggression. In S. I. Greenspan & G. H. Pollock (Eds.), *The course of life: Vol. 2. Early childhood* (pp. 83-121). New York: International Universities Press.

Parens, H. (1989b). Toward an epigenesis of aggression in early childhood. In S. I. Greenspan & G. H. Pollock (Eds.), *The course of life: Vol. 2. Early childhood* (pp. 129-161). New York: International Universities Press.

Parens, H. (1990). On the girl's psychosexual development: Reconsiderations suggested from direct observation. *Journal of the American Psychoanalytic Association, 38*, 743-772.

Parens, H. (1991). A view of the development of hostility in early life. *Journal of the American Psychoanalytic Association, 39(Suppl.)*, 75-108.

Parens, H. (1997). The unique pathogenicity of sexual abuse. *Psychoanalytic Inquiry, 17*, 250-266.

Parens, H. (2001). The analysis of a four-and-a-half-year-old boy with a feminine identification. In R. L. Tyson (Ed.), *Analysis of the under-five child* (pp. 71-98). New Haven, CT: Yale University Press.

Parens, H. (2002a). An obstacle to the child's coping with object loss. In S. Akhtar (Ed.), *Three faces of mourning: Melancholia, manic defense, and moving on* (pp. 157-183). Northvale, NJ: Jason Aronson.

Parens, H. (2002b). We all mourn: C'est la condition humane. In S. Akhtar (Ed.), *Three faces of mourning: Melancholia, manic defense, and moving on.* Northvale, NJ: Jason Aronson.

Parens, H., Pollock, L., Stern, J., & Kramer, S. (1976). On the girl's entry into the Oedipus complex. *Journal of the American Psychoanalytic Association, 24,* 79-107.

Pennington, B. F. (1991). *Diagnosing learning disorders: A neuropsychological framework.* New York: Guilford Press.

Pfeffer, C. R. (1982). Clinical observations of suicidal behavior in a neurotic, a borderline, and a psychotic child: Common processes of symptom formation. *Child Psychiatry and Human Development, 13,* 120–134.

Pollock, G. H. (1961). Mourning and adaptation. *International Journal of Psycho-Analysis, 42,* 341-361.

Rapoport, J. L. (1991). *The boy who couldn't stop washing: The experience and treatment of obsessive-compulsive disorder.* New York: Signet.

Richards, R. G. (1999). *The source for dyslexia and dysgraphia.* East Moline, IL: LinguiSystems.

Ritvo, S. (1984). The image and uses of the body in psychic conflict: With special reference to eating disorders in adolescence. *Psychoanalytic Study of the Child, 52,* 449-469.

Rothstein, A., Benjamin, L., Crosby, M., & Eisenstadt, K. (1988). *Learning disorders: An integration of neuropsychological and psychoanalytic considerations.* Madison, CT: International Universities Press.

Rothstein, A. & Glenn, J. (1999). *Learning disabilities and psychic conflict: A psychoanalytic casebook.* Madison, CT: International Universities Press.

Rourke, B. P. (1989). *Nonverbal learning disabilities: The syndrome and the model.* New York: Guilford Press.

Rourke, B. P., & Tsatsanis, K. D. (2000). Nonverbal learning disabilities and Asperger syndrome. In A. Klin, F. R. Volkmar, & S. S. Sparrow (Eds.), *Asperger syndrome* (pp. 231-253). New York: Guilford Press.

Schneider, F. R., Blanco, C., Antia, S. X., & Liebowitz, M. R. (2002). The social anxiety spectrum. *Psychiatric Clinics of North America, 25,* 757-774.

Schwartz, E. D., & Kowalski, J. M. (1991). Malignant memories: PTSD in children and adults after a school shooting. *Journal of the American Academy of Child and Adolescent Psychiatry, 30,* 936-944.

Scott, S. S. (2005). Conduct and oppositional defiant disorders: Epidemiology, risk factors and treatment. *Child and Adolescent Mental Health, 10,* 106-107.

Seiffge-Krenke, I. (1997). One body or two. *Psychoanalytic Study of the Child, 52,* 340-355.

Shaywitz, B. A., Pugh, K. R., Fletcher, J. M., & Shaywitz, S. E. (2000). What cognitive and neurobiological studies have taught us about dyslexia. In L. L. Greenhill (Ed.), *Learning Disabilities: Implications for psychiatric treatment* (pp. 59-95). Washington, DC: American Psychiatric Press.

Shedler, J., & Block, J. (1990). Adolescent drug use and psychological health: A longitudinal inquiry. *American Psychologist, 45,* 612-630.

Spitz, R. (1946). Anaclitic depression: An inquiry into the genesis of psychiatric conditions in early childhood. *The Psychoanalytic Study of the Child, 2,* 313-342.

Steele, B. F. (1994). Psychoanalysis and the maltreatment of children. *Journal of the American Psychoanalytic Association, 42,* 1001-1025.

Stein, M. T., Klin, A., Miller, K., Goulden, K., Coolman, R., & Coolman, D. M. (2004). When Aperger's syndrome and a nonverbal learning disability look alike. *Journal of Developmental and Behavioral Pediatrics, 25,* 190-195.

Strauss, C. C. (1990). Overanxious disorder in childhood. In M. Hersen & C. G. Last (Eds.), *Handbook of child and adult psychopathology* (p. 237).New York: Pergamon Press.

Tanguay, P. B. (2001). *Nonverbal learning disabilities at home: A parent's guide.* London/Philadelphia: Jessica Kingsley Publishers.

Tanguay, P. B. (2002). *Nonverbal learning disabilities at school: Educating students with NLD, Asperger syndrome, and related conditions.* London/Philadelphia: Jessica Kingsley Publishers.

Tyson, P. (1982). A developmental line of gender identity, gender role, and choice of love object. *Journal of the American Psychoanalytic Association, 30,* 61-86.

Tyson, P. (1986a). Female psychological development. *The Annual of Psychoanalysis, 14,* 357-373.

Tyson, P. (1986b). Male gender identity: Early developmental roots. *Psychoanalytic Review, 73,* 405-425.

Tyson, R. L. (1996). The good boy syndrome and malignant academic failure in early adolescence. *Psychoanalytic Study of the Child, 51,* 386-408.

Tyson, R. L. (Ed.). (2001). *Analysis of the under-five child.* New Haven, CT: Yale University Press.

Wallerstein, J. S., Lewis, J. M., Blakeslee, S. (2000). *The unexpected legacy of divorce: A 25 year landmark study.* New York: Hyperion.

Warren, S. L., Emde, R. N., & Sroufe, L. A. (2000). Internal representations: Predicting anxiety from children's play narratives. *Journal of the American Academy of Child and Adolescent Psychiatry, 39,* 100–107.

Wieder, H., & Kaplan, E. (1969). Drug use in adolescents: Psychodynamic meaning and pharmacogenic effect. *Psychoanalytic Study of the Child, 24,* 399-431.

Wilcox, H. C., & Anthony, J. C. (2004). Child and adolescent clinical features as forerunners of adult-onset major depressive disorder: Retrospective evidence from an epidemiological sample. *Journal of Affective Disorders, 82,* 9-20.

Yovell, Y. (2000). From hysteria to posttraumatic stress disorder: Psychoanalysis and the neurobiology of traumatic memories. *Neuro-Psychoanalysis, 2,* 171-181.

Zabarenko, L. M. (2002). ADHD, psychoanalysis, and neuroscience: A survey of recent findings and their applications. *Psychoanalytic Inquiry, 22,* 413-432.

Zetzel, E. R. (1965). Depression and the incapacity to bear it. In M. Schur (Ed.), *Drives, affects, behavior* (Vol. 2, pp. 243-274). New York: International Universities Press.

ADDITIONAL GENERAL REFERENCES

Ainsworth, M. D. S., Blehar, M., Waters, E., & Wall, S. (1978). *Patterns of attachment: A psychological study of the strange situation.* Hillsdale, NJ: Lawrence Erlbaum.

Asperger, H. (1991). *Autistic psychoapthy in childhood* (U. Firth, Trans.). Cambridge: Cambridge University Press. (Original work published in 1944)

Atwood, T. (1998). *Asperger's syndrome: A guide for parents and professionals.* London: Jessica Kingsley Publishers.

Baron-Cohen, S. (1997). *Mindblindness: An essay on autism and theory of mind.* Cambridge, MA: MIT Press.

Baron-Cohen, S., & Swettenham, J. (1997). Theory of mind in autism: Its relationship to executive function and central coherence. In D. J. Cohen & R. R. Volkmar (Eds.), *Handbook of autism and pervasive developmental disorders* (pp. 880-893). New York: John Wiley & Sons.

Baron-Cohen, S., Tager-Flusberg, H., & Cohen, D. J. Eds. (1993). *Understanding other minds: Perspectives from autism*. Oxford: Oxford University Press.

Baron-Cohen, S., Wheelwright, S., Cox, A., Baird, G., Charman, T., Swettenham, J., et al. (2000). The early identification of autism by the Checklist for Autism in Toddlers (CHAT). *Journal of the Royal Society of Medicine, 93*, 521-525.

Beebe, B., Lachmann, F. M., & Jaffe, J. (1997). Mother-infant structures and presymbolic self and object representations. *Psychoanalytic Dialogues, 7*, 133-182.

Blanchard, P. (1946). Psychoanalytic contributions to the problems of reading disabilities. *Psychoanalytic Study of the Child, 2*, 163-187.

Broussard, E. R., & Hartmer, M. S. S. (1971). Further considerations regarding maternal perception of the first born. In J. Hellmuth (Ed.), *Exceptional infant: Vol. 2. Studies in Abnormalities* (pp. 432-449). New York: Brunner/Mazel.

Cicchetti, D., & Toth, S. (1995). Child maltreatment and attachment organization. In S. Goldberg, R. Muir, & J. Kerr (Eds.), *Attachment theory: Social, developmental, and clinical perspectives* (pp. 279-308). Hillsdale, NJ: The Analytic Press.

Crowell, J., Keener, M., Ginsberg, N., & Anders, T. (1987). Sleep habits in toddlers 18 to 36 months old. *Journal of the American Academy of Child and Adolescent Psychiatry, 26*, 510-515.

Fonagy, P. (2001). *Attachment theory and psychoanalysis*. New York: Other Press.

Gergely G. (2000). Reapproaching Mahler: New perspectives on normal autism, symbiosis, splitting and libidinal object constancy from cognitive developmental theory. *Journal of the American Psychoanalytic Association, 48*, 1197-1228.

Goldberg, S. (1990). Attachment in infants at risk: Theory, research, and practice. *Infants and Young Children, 2*, 11-20.

Green, A. H., & Kocijan-Hercigonja, D. (1998). Stress and coping in children traumatized by war. *Journal of the American Psychoanalytic Association, 26*, 585-597.

Haddon, M. (2003). *The curious incident of the dog in the night-time*. New York: Vintage Books.

Happe, F., & Frith, U. (1996). The neuropsychology of autism. *Brain, 119*, 1377-1400.

Hardin H., & Hardin, D. (2000). On the vicissitudes of early primary surrogate mothering: Loss of the surrogate mother and the arrest of mourning. *Journal of the American Psychoanalytic Association, 48*, 1229–1258.

Harlow, H. F., Harlow, M. K., Dodsworth, R. D., & Arling, G. L. (1966). Maternal behavior of rhesus monkeys deprived of mothering and peer associations in infancy. *Proceedings of the American Philosophical Society, 110*, 58-66.

Hofer, M. (1996). On the nature and consequences of early loss. *Psychosomatic Medicine, 58*, 570-581.

Hofer, M. (2003). The emerging neurobiology of attachment and separation: How parents shape their infant's brain and behavior. In S. W. Coates, J. L. Rosenthal, & D. S. Schechter (Eds.), *Trauma and human bonds* (191–209). Hillsdale, NJ: Analytic Press.

Kanner, L. (1943). Autistic disturbances of affective contact. *The Nervous Child, 2*, 217-250.

Klein, M. (1981). On Mahler's autistic and symbiotic phases. *Psychoanalysis and Contemporary Thought, 4*, 69–105.

Klin, A. (1994). Asperger syndrome. *Child and Adolescent Psychiatric Clinics of North America, 3*, 131.

Klin, A., & Volkmar, F. (2003). Asperger syndrome: diagnosis and external validity. *Child and Adolescent Psychiatric Clinics of North America, 12*, 1-13.

Kobayashi, R. (2000). Affective communication of infants with autistic spectrum disorder and internal representation of their mother. *Psychiatry and Clinical Neurosciences, 54*, 235-243.

Lorenz, K. (1935). Companionship in bird life. In C. H. Schiller (Ed.), *Instinctive Behavior* (pp. 83-175). New York: International Universities Press.

Lorenz, K. (1953). Comparative behaviorology. In J. M. Tanner & B. Inhelder (Eds.), *Discussions on child development* (Vol. 1, pp. 108-117). New York: International Universities Press.

Mahler, M. S., Pine, F., & Bergman, A. (1975). *Psychological birth of the human infant.* New York: Basic Books.

Main, M. (2000). The organized categories of infant, child, and adult attachment: Flexible vs. inflexible attention under attachment-related stress. *Journal of the American Psychoanalytic Association, 48,* 1055-1096.

Marans, S. (2000)."That's what my imagination says": A study of antisocial behavior in two boys. Psychoanalytic Study of the Child, 55, 61-86.

Parens, H., & Saul, L. J. (1971). *Dependence in man.* New York: International Universities Press.

Pine, F. (2004). Mahler's concepts of "symbiosis" and separation-individuation: Revisited, reevaluated, and redefined. *Journal of the American Psychoanalytic Association, 52,* 513-533

Post, R. M. (1992). Transduction of psychosocial stress into the neurobiology of recurrent affective disorders. *American Journal of Psychiatry, 149,* 999-1010.

Prince-Hughes, D. (2004). *Songs of the gorilla nation: My journey through autism.* New York: Harmony Books.

Sachs, L. J. (1969). Mental retardation and emotion acrescentsim (deprivation). Psychoanalytic Quarterly, 38, 287-315.

Sacks, O. (1994, January 3). An anthropologist on Mars. *The New Yorker.*

Sander, L. (1964). Adaptive relationships in early mother-child interaction. *Journal of the American Academy of Child and Adolescent Psychiatry, 3,* 231-264.

Schmidt, E., & Eldridge, A. (1986). The attachment relationship & child maltreatment. *Infant Mental Health Journal, 7,* 264-273.

Schore, A. N. (2001). Effects of a secure attachment relationship on right brain development, affect regulation, and infant mental health. *Infant Mental Health Journal, 22,* 7-66.

Schore, A. N. (2003). Attachment and the regulation of the right brain. *Attachment and Human Development, 2,* 23-47.

Slade, A. (1999) Representation, symbolization and affect regulation in the concomitant treatment of a mother and child: Attachment theory and child psychotherapy. *Psychoanalytic Inquiry, 19,* 797-830.

Spitz, R., & Cobliner, W.G. (1965). *The First Year of Life.* New York: International Universities Press.

Stanford, A. (2003). *Asperger syndrome and long-term relationships.* London/Philadelphia: Jessica Kingsley Publishers.

Stern, D. (1985). *The interpersonal world of the human infant.* New York: Basic Books.

Tanguay, P. E. (2000). Pervasive developmental disorders: A 10-year review. *Journal of the American Academy of Child and Adolescent Psychiatry, 39,* 1079-1095.

Tronick, E. Z. (2002) A model of infant mood states and Sandarian affective waves. *Psychoanalytic Dialogues, 12,* 73-99.

Volkmar, F. R., Klin, A., Schultz, R. T., Rubin, E., & Bronen, R. (2000). Asperger's disorder. *American Journal of Psychiatry, 157,* 262-267.

Volkmar, F. R., Klin, A., Siegel, B., Szatmari, P., Lord, C., Campbell, M., et al. (1994). Field trial for autistic disorder in DSM-IV. *American Journal of Psychiatry, 151,* 1361-1367.

Willock, B. (1987). The devalued (unloved, repugnant) self: A second facet of narcissistic vulnerability in the aggressive, conduct-disordered child. Psychoanalytic Psychology, 4, 219-240.

Case Illustrations of the PDM Profile with Child and Adolescent Mental Health Disorders

As in the Case Illustrations of the PDM Profile with Adult Mental Health Disorders (p. 157), we include here three sample psychological assessments of individual children. Again, the personal styles and degrees of detail of the different writers are evident in these examples of case formulations for treatment planning.

CASE ILLUSTRATION I

Janice presented as a frail-looking, shy, sweet 15½-year-old. When I went to greet her and her parents in the waiting room, she was complaining bitterly about how cold she was. In fact, with the air conditioner turned on high, it was realistically very cold. She asked to go sit outside where it was warmer, but her parents were concerned that if they permitted her to do so, she would wander off and get lost.

I started with the parents, leaving her in the waiting room. I was soon called by the secretary, however, who said that Janice had indeed gone out and could not be stopped. After a couple of attempts to have her stay in the waiting room, I eventually took the decorative rug off the wall in the hallway and wrapped her with it, having found nothing else to cover her to keep her warm. At the end of the session with the parents, we found her asleep on the floor of the waiting room.

When she came into my office, she chose to sit facing away from me, quietly eating from a bag of potato chips while I struggled to engage her in conversation. She gave brief, cursory responses while playing with the potato chips. She struck me as detached and unrelated.

I asked her to tell me about school. Janice responded that "School sucks!" She said that she didn't care about school. She had no concerns for her grades, for what her teachers thought—nothing seemed to matter. I mentioned her parents' concern, but that did not seem to matter to her, either. After 15 minutes (which seemed more like an hour) of my working very hard to find something around which we could connect, I was prepared to give up. But at that point she turned toward me, looked at me directly and asked what I was. I told her I was a clinical social worker. She asked my specialty, I said I specialized in understanding the problems of children with learning disabilities.

She looked directly at me and said "Do you know what pisses me off? It is when people label me!" I said that I was not interested in labeling her, but rather in helping her. Could she tell me what she meant? She went on to say that she had been labeled autistic, Asperger's, schizophrenic, depressed, ADD. One person had told her she had a split personality. She doesn't care what others think about her. I said I knew that Dr. X thought she had Asperger's. She insisted that she was not. I said that she was probably right, but wondered if she could help me figure out what went wrong that she developed this attitude. She agreed that her problem was her "attitude." She had been told that.

I asked what she thought was the problem. She said she had been depressed since third grade, but now she has stopped caring about anything. She simply does whatever she wants regardless of what others think. At school she wanders in and out of class; it does not matter to her that teachers object. I asked if she had gotten any help from speaking to the psychiatrist. She laughed, saying she had seen a dozen people. In elementary school she was put into a group that was supposed to help her with her relationships with other kids. Instead, she was kicked out of the group. She laughed, saying, "Can you imagine getting kicked out of a group that's supposed to help you?" In seventh grade she saw a school counselor. In eighth grade she saw a psychologist. He was "a dork;" he kept referring to her in the third person, asking "How is Janice today?!" She hated him. She saw him for six months. She was sure he hated her also, because she gave him such a hard time. In eighth grade she saw another school counselor, but he did not do much, either.

As a freshman she saw "a stupid lady" for drug problems because she was caught with some marijuana. She was mad at her brother for turning her in to her parents when she bought the marijuana from her friend. I said that I knew about that and that I also knew that she was caught drinking in school. I asked if she liked drugs because they made her feel good. She said it made no difference. She asked if what she shared with me was confidential, and I said it was. She related that she had tried lots of drugs, including acid. I felt that she was exaggerating to test my response. I continued, saying that sometimes kids take drugs to help their depression. She did not respond to that.

By this time, I felt fully engaged with her and was empathizing with her sense of emptiness. I asked her whether she was concerned about herself and her future. What is to become of her? She said she didn't care. She has never been a people person. As far back as she could remember, kids didn't like her. She had no interest in them, either. They only made her feel bad. She could not articulate why that was. When I tried to pin down when those feelings started, all she could say was "sometime in third grade," but she could not recall any specific incidents. It was obvious that she had detached herself from people as well as activities long ago.

I then turned to question her as to whether there was anything that was important to her; anything that she cared about. She responded by saying: Music, reading, and sleeping. I expressed concern that her life was so limited and said that I would worry about her having no interest in doing well in life. At one point I said something about trying to understand her. She smiled and said, "You can't!" People have tried to understand her, some have even thought they could, but no one has. I said that I could see why.

I then asked if she could help me figure out what would help. She said "nothing." We went through a list: Medication is not helping, therapists haven't helped, and no one in school does anything for her, so there is nothing! She looked at me directly and said, "Yes! A lobotomy!" There was a moment of stunned silence until I caught a glimmer of a smile on her face, at which point I said, trying to defuse the tension, "Well, maybe a brain transplant!" She laughed and said that one of her teachers has been saying to her that she should get a lobotomy. But then she became serious and lapsed back into her totally demoralized state. I asked how she would feel about a boarding school. She was surprised by that suggestion and quickly asked if that was why she was here. I said it was not.

Presenting Problems and Current Functioning

Janice, a 15½-year-old high school sophomore in special education, was referred for evaluation. Her behavior has deteriorated since entry into adolescence. She has become rebellious. She spends a lot of time lying on her bed, listening to CDs. She picks friends who are fringe characters and into drugs, although her mother believes that Janice is not on drugs. She was caught drinking in school once, but that appears to have been an isolated incident. Last spring she ran away from home after she was forbidden to associate with a friend. She was found at the home of another friend.

Emotionally, Janice does not appear to exhibit much depth. She was thought to be depressed and placed on Prozac last November. She often talks about suicide, and has cut herself on one occasion. She has low self-esteem. She has had a chronic sleep problem; she seems to need little sleep.

From a social perspective, she has poor social skills: She has been disruptive in some classes and truant from many classes. At times, she has had hostile relations with some teachers, administration officials, and other students. Her mother reported that she never seemed to understand people as having intentions or motives. She would ask her mother, "Why are you smiling at me?" She could react with appropriate empathy to situations that were magnified and obvious, but not to more subtle situations. When in Brownies, she was minimally involved and then only because her mother was the troop leader. If her mother tapped her affectionately and gently on the leg, she would ask, "Why are you hitting me?" If a child accidentally bumped into her seat, she would react as if it were done intentionally. Other inappropriate behaviors include tackling a kid and beating him up because he said something to her.

Last year was Janice's first year in high school. She seemed more determined to figure out relationships with other children. She appeared to want to find a group to which she could belong. She latched onto a child from a minority group but then seemed to gravitate to kids who were "losers" and who acted outrageously. She followed them in their flamboyant style—dyed hair and piercings in various body parts. This year she has hung out with kids from troubled families, who use drugs. She walks in and out of class whenever she feels like it; she walks into an ongoing class to speak to a friend, and she feels free to walk into the teachers' lounge to get a soda from their machine. It seems as if she wants to identify herself as rebellious. She also wishes to present an image that says, "If you screw with me, I'll get you!" Last spring, she went to a school where a friend was taking a class. Since she was not a student there, she was asked to leave. She returned in spite of that. Finally, the police were called. It took considerable effort on the part of the Janice's mother to explain to the police that the child was disturbed and should not be taken to detention.

Two months ago, she was found cutting herself at school with the blade of a safety razor. The parents found out that a friend had been doing that and assumed that Janice was imitating her. There has been no recurrence of that. When she and mother were in a bookstore, she decided she wanted to buy the autobiography of Courtney Love. When her mother forbade her from doing so, she threatened to steal the book, but did not. Then in the car she refused to put on her seat belt and threatened to jump out of the car on the expressway. When they got home, she went into a kitchen drawer and took a knife, threatening to kill herself. Her mother took the knife away with no difficulty.

At a cognitive level, she obsesses on topics, dwelling on things for an inordinately long time. She does not understand directions. This year she passed only the courses in the self-contained classes. Organization is a tremendous problem for Janice. She tends to lose assignments and seems unable to pull all the pieces together in order to complete major assignments. Her teacher reports that she does not pay attention fully in class activities, whether with the whole group or a small group. According to this teacher, when Janice is confronted with her behavior, she usually denies it. She often turns in tasks with less than 10% of the answers completed. She has difficulty completing work and often loses it. During cooperative group work, other students complain that Janice does not contribute. On field trips, chaperoning parents have noted that she did not pay attention to the leader. In class, she often fiddles with papers and other things in her desk, rather than making eye contact with the speaker. At times she talks with other students and at other times she stares into space.

Overall, Janice's difficulties with organization and integration seem to be significantly affecting her learning, information processing, and social functioning. She has considerable trouble putting disparate pieces of information together into a meaningful, coherent whole. For Janice, this seems to result in being able to manage only small portions of the information at a time and subsequently not fully understanding what is happening, whether it is learning a lesson at school or watching a television show at home.

Her approach to learning tasks indicates that she seems to get overwhelmed by too much information and anchors herself by understanding or memorizing some specific details, while losing the overall gestalt of the task. Janice's current problems, such as losing assignments because there is too much for her to keep track of, or not understanding certain academic subjects that require putting together complex ideas, suggest that she feels overwhelmed without having effective organizing and integrating strategies. She performs better on tasks that are broken down into more manageable pieces of information so that she can integrate and internalize the overall structure piece by piece. She needs specific help with developing strategies, such as categorizing pieces of information, clustering like items, and using mnemonic cues to help her organize and remember.

Because Janice does not readily integrate different kinds of information or appreciate the whole of interpersonal situations, she has difficulties with understanding the meaning of social experiences. Being able to take into account a person's intonation, content of speech, and facial and body gestures, as well as the overall context of an interpersonal interaction requires putting many different kinds of information together. This is hard for Janice. She also struggles with accessing her own feelings and expressing herself emotionally.

Staff in the Student Center have found Janice extremely difficult to assist. She typically refuses offers of help. She comes to the Student Center at her scheduled time, but with no materials. When sent back to her locker for work, she generally returns without any material. She does not sit in a seat to work. She frequently makes hostile comments to staff when they speak to her. For example, when asked to find a place to sit, her reply was, "Don't give me the teacher stare, that doesn't work on me." Another time her teacher asked her to find a place to sit, whereupon she lined up four chairs, sat down, and then scooted around from chair to chair, announcing, "You didn't say I had to stay in one place." Many times when the Student Center staff has been busy with other students, she has walked out. On one occasion, when a Student Center staff member told her very firmly to have a seat, she replied, "Since you asked me so nicely, I will sit down." Within moments, she was on the move again. She continually talks to students when tests are in progress, and many times she has kicked or hit other students.

Janice infrequently looks at people when she is speaking to them. If she does look at them while speaking, she does not maintain eye contact. She has a difficult time with peer relationships. She alienates herself from her peers physically, and she makes inappropriate comments that turn students away. Janice had a problem at one time during the year of staring at students in her classes. Her teachers addressed this situation and eventually it subsided.

Profile of Mental Functioning

Capacity for Regulation, Attention, and Learning

Janice evidences cognitive deficits in visual-spatial processing, nonverbal communication, and executive function. Her primary strengths are in the verbal modalities, in particular, reading. The deficits severely impair her learning capacity because of multiple "processing" difficulties.

Capacity for Relationships

Her capacity for relationships is superficial and need-oriented, lacking intimacy and empathy.

Quality of Internal Experience

Janice's internal experience includes feelings of depletion, emptiness, incompleteness, and self-involvement.

Affective Experience, Expression, and Communication

Her affective experience indicates some need-oriented, purposeful islands of behavior and emotional expressions. There are no cohesive larger integrated emotional patterns. In selected relationships, she can read basic intentions of others (such as acceptance or rejection), but she is unable to read subtle cues (e.g., respect, pride, or partial anger).

Defensive Patterns and Capacities

In order to deal with internal and external stressors and to keep disturbing feelings and thoughts out of awareness, Janine makes extensive use of defenses that distort experience and/or limit the experience of relationships. These include disavowal, denial, projection, and acting out.

Capacity to Form Internal Representations

Janice uses representations or ideas in a concrete way to convey desire for action or to get basic needs met. She does not elaborate on a feeling in its own right and often puts wishes and feelings into action.

Capacity for Differentiation and Integration

Her capacity for differentiation and integration is limited to just a few emotional realms. Challenges outside these limited areas often lead to the fragmentation or polarization (all-or-nothing extremes) of internal experience.

Self-Observing Capacities

Janice has limited self-observing capacities. She is unable to reflect genuinely on feelings or experiences, even in the present. Her self-awareness is often of polarized feeling states or simple basic feelings without an appreciation of subtle variations in feelings.

Capacity for Internal Standards and Ideals

Her internal standards and ideals tend to be rigid. They are not sufficiently sensitive to her own capacities and social contexts. She experiences guilt more as self-criticism than as a signal for reappraising her behavior.

Summary of Profile of Mental Functioning

Janice evidences major constrictions in her mental functioning. **PDM Code: MCA206**.

Personality Patterns

Janice presents with a profile of moderately to severely dysfunctional personality patterns. These patterns are self-defeating and include elements of dysregulation with depressive features. **PDM Codes: PCA106 and PCA114**

Symptom Patterns

- Disorder of Mental Functioning: Neuropsychological Disorder: Executive Function Disorder. **PDM Code: SCA317.5**
- Disorder of Mental Functioning: Learning Disorder: Nonverbal Learning Disability. **PDM Code: SCA318.4**
- Developmental Disorder: Regulatory Disorder. **PDM Code: SCA321**
- Conduct Disorder. **PDM Code: SCA309**

Case Illustration II

Ten-year-old Danny came into the office on his own and was extremely friendly, almost as if he had known me for many, many years. He had a big smile, sat down right away, looked me in the eyes, and radiated warmth. He started chatting about his life, mostly about school. His concentration and focus were good as he looked at me. He stayed on the subject of school and sat in one spot for most of the session, except for when he switched from the chair to the floor, sitting with his legs crossed. His impulse control was excellent as he followed the implicit rules of the playroom, talking rather than throwing things or breaking things. His mood was on the excitable side, with a great deal of anxiety and sense of exasperation about things that were not going exactly his way. There was more a "how dare they do this to me" quality than a sense of sadness, depression, or emptiness. He showed a mixture of outrage, worry, anxiety, impatience, and a flighty hyperactiveness and tension.

As he sat down smiling warmly, he immediately said, as though he had been primed by his mother or had been waiting to see a psychiatrist for many years, "I have too many enemies in school. I don't know what to do about them. They tease me." When I inquired in what way they teased him, he said, "They talk behind my back, spreading rumors about me." He readily gave an example, saying, "One time I came in with new sneakers on and was very proud of them, and someone started making fun of the style, saying they looked yucky. Then that person started giggling with the other kids behind my back. Then they spread rumors. I can't figure out exactly what they were."

Danny then went on listing other things that embarrassed him. "I'm sort of between toy cars and big-kid stuff, not quite there yet. One time I hit another kid, just sort of friendly not to really hurt him, but he was getting mean, and I sort of pushed him a little bit, and then his friends all became my enemies. What I really need are friends I can count on, but there's this kid I read with—he's real cool, and I worry about losing friends to him. Every time I have someone I think I can count on, he seems to make friends with them and takes them away from me."

I inquired as to how he felt about this state of affairs, and he said, "I feel so angry. I'm enraged. I get this feeling in my head, it goes to my chest. I want to cry. I feel tight. It's not just a physical feeling; it's like I'm upset, and I want to cry and I feel too emotional, and yet I also feel like my heart isn't working right."

When I inquired further about what the feelings were like, he said, "I feel so mad sometimes I feel so mad I get sad." I wondered about the difference between the sad feeling and feeling sort of frenzied, overwhelmed, and angry, and he said, "Well, I feel sad when my middle brother acts up, when we can't go out, like if we're supposed to go to the movies or something on a nasty day, or sometimes, even worse, my little brother, who tends to be the aggressive one in the family, if he has been bad, we all get punished for him. Then I feel disappointed. But that's different from when I feel angry and cornered by one of the kids at school."

As I summarized some of the feelings he was telling me about—how sometimes he feels disappointed and other times he feels cornered, overwhelmed and angry—he smiled. I commented on his pleasure in my comment, and he said, "Well, I may be smiling, but actually when these situations happen, I feel furious inside." He went on, "Often, I try to put on a nice face. I smile in class; I smile at other kids. I want to be friendly, but I might be feeling cornered and overwhelmed and really enraged at them inside, but I keep those thoughts private." I wondered that he must feel it is best to keep all his feelings private, and he said, "If people would know how angry and furious I get, no one would be my friend." I said, "No one?" He said, "No one." I wondered whether these were just people at school or even his family, or the world in general, and he said, "Well, the only one who might be my friend would be my little brother because he's mean, and he might understand how mean I feel. But my mother and father do not like me to be angry or mean, although I've seen my mother be mean to me—she has quite a temper—she can yell and scream. And certainly the teachers and the kids at school, some of them would just start teasing me, and I couldn't take that. And I think the teacher thinks of me as a nice boy and kind of her pet, and she wouldn't like it either."

I commented on his dilemma. He then went on to say, "After a fight, when Joey gets other kids after me and they kind of pick on me, I often feel very alone. I feel like I'll never have a friend again. I feel like crying. It's an empty feeling inside me. I feel very alone." When I commented that this "alone" feeling seemed to be very upsetting and very painful, he went on to say, "I hate that feeling. It's the feeling I dread the most, to have no friends." He further elaborated, "At home, my mother tends to be very busy, often grading papers and things for school. My father works hard. I hate my two brothers. I feel very much alone some of the time. I have some kids around the block I could play with, but I feel like sometimes there's no one I can be close to. Other times, I might like my mother, and we might be really talking."

Danny then went on to associate—quite on his own—about how angry he gets. "I can't stand it when I get cornered and then people aren't proud of me. I get so mad." (He was hinting at a relationship between the mean part of himself that no one but his little brother can understand and the lonely feeling he gets when worrying that he cannot be close to anyone, hinting, perhaps, that his meanness and embarrassment over it make him feel very much alone.)

It was then getting near the end of the session, and I suggested that he might like to draw a picture. He drew a picture of a house with lots of detail, including windows and doors. There were clouds and trees around it, but there were no people. It was a detailed house without life or richness to it. He said, "I added a clubhouse to the house for my friends. I can get away to the clubhouse, especially to get away from my dad because he bugs me, wanting me to study harder and get better grades. My mom bugs me too and my two brothers; I really need to get away from them. But Dad screams the most; he really makes me feel like I can't think when he screams so loud. My mother bears down on me, not screaming like my father does, but she just creates pressure. I don't know what to do to get away from her. I have no peace. Even the housekeeper bugs me."

I expressed sympathy with his dilemma, commenting that he likes to have lots of friends and does not like to feel alone. He often wants to be in the middle of things, but at the same time, people bug him and he wants to be back in the clubhouse all by himself (even though it is a clubhouse for friends). At this point, he gave a big smile and said, "You seem to know how I feel. I can't stand it when anyone else is getting attention other than me. I mean, I get A's, and I have the best ideas, and I can sing, and I'm a better musician than a lot of the kids, but I don't get the credit in school. I mean, I should be the most popular kid, but I'm not. Joey is, and he seems to have it in for me. He always wants to put me down and I don't know what I could do to win out over the other kids." He then went on to describe how, "Even though I can do everything better than everyone else, I get confused easily, and I get real mad so that my thoughts don't seem to work."

Comments

My impression at the end of this first interview was that Danny was a youngster who could attend and engage very warmly. He was capable of nice give-and-take communication, with appropriate gestures. He used ideas (representational thinking) to communicate his feelings and thoughts in an organized and intentional way. He was obviously quite verbal and very bright. It was also evident, however, that he could easily get overloaded and feel fragmented and that in interacting with others, he was very sensitive to every subtle emotional nuance. When he got overloaded, he would feel fragmented and disorganized ("like a thousand thoughts all at once").

Danny's mood was intense and at times frenzied. He evidenced many affects, mostly around anxiety over competition and neediness, and fear of humiliation and loss. Themes were represented and sometimes organized, but they also could become fragmented. There were indications that he was in conflict: He wanted to be in the middle of everything, but became easily overwhelmed; he wanted to compete, but he feared disappointment and loss.

Though he was engaged and attentive, and related interactively in gestures, concepts, and words, he was limited in his ability to apply these capacities to certain realms of emotion. The emotions related to competition, anger, and loss were especially difficult for him. His conflict between wishes and fears to compete seemed relevant to possible emerging difficulties feeling good about himself as a male. Experiencing his father as distant and critical, he seemed to lack both admirable male role models and close male friends. This would be an important area to explore in a subsequent interview.

Danny had a marked constriction in the flexibility of his personality, even though, for the most part, he had mastered aspects of engagement, two-way communication, using ideas to label and conceptualize emotions, and organizing emotions into categories. When he was anxious, he lost this last ability and felt overwhelmed and confused. In addition, when anxious, he quickly felt that he was treated unfairly by "enemies" (an all-or-nothing concept), rather than being able to see competition as an integral part of complex relationship patterns. He was unable to maintain a broad range of affects and also unable to consider a range of possible explanations for other people's actions. Inflexibly, he replayed the same "drama" ("They are my enemies") over and over. My subjective reaction was to feel a bit overloaded, much as Danny did, and at times not very drawn into the seemingly dramatic content.

Danny was at age expectations in some categories (relating, organization of themes) but was below age expectations in others (mood, affects, anxiety, and thematic range and content).

Profile of Mental Functioning

Capacity for Regulation, Attention, and Learning

When not overwhelmed by anxiety, Danny's basic capacities to process and regulate experience functioned reasonably well. He did evidence a general tendency to be over-responsive to sensations, and he was relatively stronger in his auditory processing and language than his visual-spatial processing and motor planning and sequencing. When he was anxious, his capacity to attend and learn could be compromised by the many feelings and thoughts that flooded his consciousness.

Capacity for Relationships

Danny was a warm, trusting, and very open youngster, who had a capacity for intimacy and many deep emotions. When he became overwhelmed with anxiety or fragmented thinking, however, his relationship patterns became more need-oriented and easily polarized (i.e., different feeling states could quickly color a given relationship).

Quality of Internal Experience

Danny's internal experiences were characterized by vacillations between feeling flooded with anxiety and the associated conflicts and themes that are described in more detail below, and attaining states of well-being, where he could feel a sense of mastery and self-worth. In his anxious states, self-doubt, embarrassment, and feelings of being out of control were not uncommon.

Affective Experience, Expression, and Communication

He showed a capacity for warmth and could elaborate on some affects and themes but not others. In his difficulty with feelings of competition and anger, he often felt overloaded and paralyzed. He felt devastated by feelings of loss and emptiness. He also had a tendency to feel dominated by his need to be the center of everything and had difficulty finding a synthesis between that need and the tendency to feel overwhelmed and alone. Feelings of fragmentation and global anxiety and the sense that everyone was his enemy repeated themselves in many situations. There were, therefore, constrictions in the flexibility of age-appropriate experience of affective patterns.

Defensive Patterns and Capacities

Danny's defensive patterns were characteristic of a younger child (a 4- to 7-year-old), rather than a 10-year-old. He had not yet found a cohesive synthesis for his conflicts and associated affective states. Most 10-year-olds are better able to balance the need to be the center with the need also to have a supporting role in the peer group. They are also better able to integrate being competitive with being fearful of loss or disappointment. Competition for Danny was a life-and-death struggle rather than one in which there can be momentary and relative winners and losers in each contest. His unusual gift for being alert to even the most subtle emotional nuances in interactions further overwhelmed him, suggesting the possibility of sensory over-responsiveness.

There were hints of internal conflicts that were contributing to his character pattern and limitations. Within the family, he saw his mother as someone who cannot accept his mean and competitive side, even though he perceived these traits in his mother. He perceived his father as unavailable, critical, and demanding. He certainly presented as a child who wants to be in the middle of the oedipal drama, but he acted as if he could not bear to put too many "toes in the water" before he would get scared and feel overwhelmed and fearful of the competition and loss. He seemed to be in some conflict about his emerging identity as a young man.

Capacity to Form Internal Representations

Danny showed a capacity to represent affects and wishes, but when anxious, his representational world tended to operate in rapidly fluctuating "islands" of experience, rather than in a cohesive, well-integrated pattern of internal representation.

Capacity for Differentiation and Integration

Danny's basic capacity for reality testing was intact. He had a partially stable mood, relationship capacity, impulse control, and the ability, when not anxious, to focus and concentrate. Under pressure or stress, however, he lacked the capacity for age-expected differentiation and integration. He was able, however, to describe this process.

Self-Observing Capacities

When not intensely anxious, he had the ability to describe his feelings and thoughts and even explore the reasons why he felt a certain way. His self-observations indicated that the fragmentation is probably only a transient phenomenon associated with intense anxiety.

Capacity for Internal Standards and Ideals

Danny was in the process of forming internal standards and ideals. At the time of this interview, however, the emerging content of his inner standards was characterized by fluctuating images of his caregivers, many of them shaded with punitive and hostile characteristics. If this pattern were to continue, one would expect Danny to develop a harsh and rigid internal system of values and ideals, which would tend to maintain states of anxiety, perhaps coupled with a growing tendency toward depression.

Summary of Profile of Mental Functioning

Danny evidenced moderate constrictions in mental functioning characterized by limitations in the full range of age-expected feelings, thoughts, self-esteem modulation, and ability to integrate polarities of experience. **PDM Code: MCA205**

Emerging Personality Patterns

While Danny showed features of several personality styles, the anxious personality pattern best captures the majority of his ongoing ways of engaging the world. **PDM Code: PCA111.**

Symptom Patterns

Danny was a very anxious child, flooded with conflicting ideas and affects, resulting in many symptoms of anxiety. His internal experience is characteristic of many late-latency children who have not resolved significant early issues and consequently become flooded with anxiety when those conflicts are reactivated. **PDM Code: SCA301.**

CASE ILLUSTRATION III

Presenting Picture

With the birth of a brother when he was 3 years, 8 months old, and the family's move a month later, Jeremiah became constipated and developed obsessive worries about things being lost. He animated his feces, food, and urine. He wanted the toilet from his old house, believed that the urine got lonely, wondered about the fate of his feces after being flushed, feared winds, refused to allow garbage to be thrown away, and compulsively engaged in a toilet ritual as a prerequisite to moving his bowels in a diaper. After his sitter left when he had just turned 4, he did not want to be alone and occasionally spoke of suicide.

Two weeks before Jeremiah's fourth birthday, the referring physician had instructed the parents to deanimate the food, feces, and urine, and to reassure the boy that it is okay to feel angry about losses. In three weeks, he was able to eat at a restaurant, and he dropped the animation of food and toilet products, but he was still constipated, fearful of the toilet and wind, and preoccupied with toilet rituals.

Developmental History

Jeremiah was born at full term after an uncomplicated pregnancy, labor, and delivery. He was initially breast-fed but always received supplementary bottles of formula or breast milk, and within a month was switched to bottle feeding because his mother felt her milk supply was insufficient. He ate voraciously and gained weight quickly. From 3 months on, he was always above the 90th percentile for height and weight.

Starting at a few weeks of age, he had episodes of colic, for which he was treated with Mylicon for about three months. His first tooth erupted at 8 months, and he had six teeth by the time he was a year old. He started solid foods at 6 months with cereal and then ate a variety of foods with no evidence of any intolerance.

Although Jeremiah was a happy baby, almost from birth he seemed to need constant holding. He startled easily and would wake up from naps almost immediately if he were not being held. While he was sleeping through the night at 3 months, it was not until 4 months that he found it easier to nap and be amused without being held.

He first sat with support at 3 months and preferred being held in that position from then on. By 6 months he was able to sit for short periods without support. Between 11 and 12 months he could get into a crawling position, and he crawled for the first time one week before his first birthday. He first pulled himself up to a standing position at 14½ months and began cruising one month later. As his mother described how Jeremiah could cross a room holding his parents' hands at 16 months, and could walk alone by 17 months, she seemed unaware that this is quite late, an attitude suggesting that the parents had inadvertently interfered with their son's autonomous functioning.

Jeremiah began making repetitive sounds at 6 months and said several words by 1 year of age. His vocabulary increased rapidly, and by 2 years he was using phrases and sentences. Except for three or four ear and throat infections, he had had no illnesses.

At 1 year old he was switched from formula to cow's milk, at which point he first developed constipation. His pediatrician prescribed a fiber supplement that was usually helpful, but he continued to have occasional hard stools. He had to eat large amounts of fruit or other fiber to maintain regular bowel functioning. Toward the end of the first year, Jeremiah began wearing disposable diapers, but he had developed an attachment to a cloth diaper that he called "Ma," which he usually wanted with him at bedtime or outside the home. When first seen, he still took it with him occasionally, generally just to sleep with it. Around the time his brother was born, he was using his quilted pillow, receiving blanket, and "Ma" to get to sleep.

The development of his concerns about separation did not seem unusual. His mother emphasized that she began staying home full-time after Jeremiah's birth and noted that for the first two years he had less experience with separation than many children his age. After Jeremiah turned 2, a college student began sitting for him.

When he was 22 months old, the family moved. Jeremiah seemed to tolerate it well, though he got more attached to his bottle, which he had begun to give up. He stopped daytime bottles at 30 to 32 months and continued taking a bottle (usually water) to bed until shortly after his third birthday, at which time he agreed to give it up in favor of a bedtime snack.

The potty was introduced during the first half of his second year, but he had little interest in it. Bladder training was completed easily during the second half of the second year, but there were some problems with bowel training. He began using the potty for this, but at 2 years, 10 months, he began insisting on wearing a diaper to defecate. He was allowed to do so but was encouraged to use the toilet. Constipation continued to be an episodic problem. When the daytime bottles were stopped, he no longer wanted to take the fiber supplement. Mineral oil was tried, but he did not take it regularly, and he continued to have periods of hard, painful stools. Several times between ages 2 and 3 he was given glycerin suppositories, which seemed to help.

Around 3 years of age (when his mother got pregnant), he became fearful of bathing, shampooing, and hearing the heater noises in the night. The latter fears improved when he was allowed to sleep with the light on. He also worried about losing his teeth.

Jeremiah began nursery school at age 3. After initially being very reserved around the other children, he made a good adjustment. His mother gradually separated from him over several days with little stress.

He showed some curiosity about male and female genitalia around 2 years, an interest that seemed to recede and reappear at intervals from then on. Recently, he had been especially affectionate toward his mother and more aggressive toward his father than previously, but this did not last very long.

Jeremiah was told about the pregnancy at about three months of gestation. He had various questions and concerns, including not wanting his mother to look "fat," wondering how the baby would get out, and wondering how long the baby would be staying. The parents tried to give brief, honest answers. During this time, in preparation for the expected child, they switched him from a crib to a bed.

There were other changes during the pregnancy. Four months prior to delivery, Jeremiah's father lost his job. He stayed home full-time until a month postpartum, when he accepted a new position with a large corporation. The parents sold their home and made many trips (with Jeremiah) to another area to buy a new home. Mother and father tried to answer all Jeremiah's questions about the move but did not always have answers immediately. Just before his brother was born, Jeremiah decided by himself to stop using diapers. He began using a potty when moving his bowels, though he expressed some concern about flushing the feces.

When the family moved to their new home six weeks before the brother's birth, their regular babysitter, to whom Jeremiah was deeply attached, moved with them for the summer. After her departure for college, he became reluctant to throw anything away, even trash (paper cups, empty bags, straw wrappers, leftover foods at restaurants). He became upset about flushing anything down the toilet or sink. He began to ask about the urine: "Will it make new friends down the pipes?" He had to be told "yes" before he would flush it. Before moving his bowels in his diaper, he would insist on his mother's leaving the bathroom. Then he would place the wastepaper basket outside the bathroom door and throw all the towels on the floor between the toilet and the closed door.

His brother, Robbie, was born two weeks before the due date. Jeremiah had known for several months that the baby was a boy and knew his name. He went to the hospital to help bring his brother home. A few days later he began asking for a diaper for his bowel movements. Because he seemed more worried about flushing them, his mother usually did it after he had left the bathroom.

The mother and father talked with the referring doctor when Robbie was 10 weeks old and Jeremiah was almost 4. Jeremiah seemed miserable and was fleetingly ruminating about suicide. (The month before the delivery, he was asking why his grandfather, his tadpole, and the dinosaurs had died.) His parents were advised to emphasize that trash, urine, and feces are not alive and to throw trash away even if Jeremiah were to get upset. They were also encouraged to spend more time talking with Jeremiah about all the losses and changes he had experienced, and to connect them with his concern about throwing things away. After three weeks of their following this advice, Jeremiah became more able to allow the disposal of food. His parents also related his concern about losing his teeth to his wish to bite, which they told him was a natural expression of upset over the move. In discussing his anger about things left behind, Jeremiah emphasized how much he had wanted to bring along the toilets from the old house and how much he wanted to find a toy dinosaur that had been lost there.

He stopped asking about his waste products making friends, but he would still say "See you later, pee!" before flushing. As Robbie approached 12 weeks old, however, his parents insisted that Jeremiah flush his feces as well. He balked at this idea, insisting that they were alive. He described a "big drain dance" in which they would come back out of the pipes and dance around. At this point he vigorously began withholding his own feces. He had no bowel movements for close to two weeks before beginning school. The problem continued despite occasionally remitting when he was given mineral oil.

Family History

Jeremiah's mother presented as a soft-spoken, concerned, articulate, intelligent homemaker who was dumb-struck by her son's worries and constipation problems. While acknowledging the impact of the move, the loss of the babysitter, and the birth of a sibling, she worried that she was partly to blame. She cried as she wondered if reverberations from the trauma of the birth of her own younger brother were making their presence known in her adult life.

The mother's mother had been 22 years old when she gave birth to the mother, who believes she was an unplanned baby and then a disappointment because she was not a boy. She had been toilet trained by 1 year of age. Her own younger brother had taken her place in her parents' bed, where she had slept every night until his birth. Food dyscrasias, constipation, procrastination, and sloppiness were persistent habits that she related to this history.

She had many difficulties after her father died of melanoma when she was 8. She started therapy at age 25 for a longstanding depression, switching therapists after several years because the doctor reminded her of her depressed mother. After five years with a second therapist, she had temporarily discontinued her own treatment because of the family move.

Jeremiah's father presented as a highly moral, well spoken, scholarly individual with more equanimity about his son's difficulties. Even though somewhat resentful of the cost of his wife's therapy, he participated readily in the evaluation. He frankly accepted responsibility for Jeremiah's animating things. He felt he and his wife had been too indecisive in managing Jeremiah's bottle feeding, bowel training, and learning to walk. His wife would make him feel guilty when he would set limits, and he would generally defer to her judgment in childrearing matters. Because of the challenges he had been facing at work, he was unaware of Jeremiah's rituals until they had become firmly established.

Being careful not to denigrate his wife, Jeremiah's father revealed that she had constipation difficulties and mentioned that her mother had irritable bowel problems. Although not sure that Jeremiah required treatment, he emphasized his appreciation of his wife's analysis, which had helped her get over her fear of having children.

Two Evaluation Interviews with Jeremiah

After I had several evaluation sessions with his parents, Jeremiah came to see me when he was 4 years, 1 month old. He stood approximately three feet tall and resembled his mother. On greeting me in the waiting room, he announced, "I have a BM problem." Jeremiah left his mother without hesitation and made eye contact easily. In this first session he was responsive to my probing for his level of knowledge about coming to see me.

He had a pinched look as he reported his mother's comment that he was coming because of his "BM problem." His belly was protrusive, and he was squeezing his buttocks. When I told him where the bathroom was, he denied the need to go. When I pointed out the pinched look on his face, he said, in a reserved, sad matter, "I just have an ache in my bottom." I asked, "Is that the ache you get when you feel you have to go to the bathroom, don't want to go, or feel you can't go?" He nodded soberly. He spent the rest of the session walking around the ottoman with magic markers and paper I had put out for him, holding his hands across his belly, and obviously feeling intermittent pressure to move his bowels. As he thoughtfully concentrated on answering my questions, he occasionally played with the toy bedroom furniture and assorted characters in nonspecific themes. As much as he seemed to want to confide in me, he also seemed amnestic and unable to expand on each subject I brought up.

We did get to touch on his "Mummy" (his belly), his "Naughty Dog" (transitional play dog and imaginary companion, assigned sinister meanings), his fears of the toilet and wind, his toilet ritual, his scary ideas about alligators eating the feces in the pipes of the toilet during the "BM dance," his ideas about hurting himself and the tissue that is "afraid of blowing," and his finicky eating habits. During the first session, his affect was limited to a serious, workman-like tone with little creative flair, joy, or playful assertiveness or anger.

The second session was spent reviewing the mothers' notes from the prior weekend. She described Jeremiah's rituals associated with piecemeal defecating, and mentioned his preoccupations with his "Mummy," "baby-eating bugs," and "pumping up people to blow them out the window." She mentioned his mild agoraphobia (tearful clinging to her and overly reserved attitude in school) and noted the relative absence of any direct expression of anger about Robbie since his birth. Sibling rivalry seemed to be expressed only in symbolic language, fantasy talk, dreams, and enactments. For example, whenever she was attending to Robbie, Jeremiah would pretend to be Dracula, sucking blood from her leg. When she did not play along, Jeremiah imagined aloud pumping his mother up to blow her away. When I tried to discuss the latter incidents with him, he was, not surprisingly, amnestic. It was hard to revive his memories about these recent events in the absence of his mother. What he did say was, "Dr. F., I know that I bother Mommy with acting like Dracula sucking her blood, but I don't remember doing it for mean reasons, especially this past weekend." During this session his emotional range was as constricted as previously, and his tone was similarly grave. For example, as he was scribbling for a moment, he said, without elaborating, "I am trying to answer your questions, but I can't remember things."

Profile of Mental Functioning

Capacity for Regulation, Attention, and Learning

Despite his conflicts around his excretory function, Jeremiah's poise and forethought revealed capacities to process and regulate experience. He was verbal and attentive, and he learned easily. He tended to be overly sensitive about getting what he saw as his just due. Although his not playing much with things was probably due to my questioning him, it could suggest his being relatively stronger in auditory processing and language than in visual-spatial processing and motor planning and sequencing.

Capacity for Relationships

Jeremiah's warmth and openness in the evaluation sessions indicated a capacity for intimacy, caring, and many deeply felt feelings, even under the stress of working with an unfamiliar doctor. Mother's notes in the second interview indicate that Jeremiah's empathy can be disrupted by defensive symptomatic measures directed against angry rivalrous feelings, resulting in his becoming clingy and more need-oriented at home, and overly reserved in school.

Quality of Internal Experience

His confidence and realistic self-esteem were often depleted by his "BM problem," indicated by his sad affect when stating, "I just have an ache in my bottom."

Affective Experience, Expression, and Communication

Despite being all too fragmented for a 4-year-old with preoccupations about constipation, toilet rituals, things being lost, fears of the wind, and occasional suicidal thoughts, he was capable of give-and-take communication, using a relatively wide range of appropriate language to describe subtle emotions and wishes in a purposeful manner; for example, "I know that I bother mommy with acting like Dracula sucking her blood, but I don't remember doing it for mean reasons, especially this past weekend." Yet, he also showed significant constrictions in his affective range; for example, there were few to no expressions of joy, anger, or curiosity with gestures, play, or words.

Defensive Patterns and Capacities

Jeremiah seemed to express readily his strong sense that he did not remember being intrusive "for mean reasons," suggesting that he may be working hard to defend against angry feelings about his mother and brother. The history suggested a reluctance to move his focus from the "BM problem" to affect-laden issues behind the symptom (rage about the baby and the move, with imagery focused on oral expressions of aggression). Jeremiah's fears of the wind and the toilet defend against sadism. His blatant sibling rivalry was normal but was pathologically handled. His heightened pressure to hoard and his constipation problems suggested emerging reaction formations. Jeremiah may have identified with the fantasized/misperceived rejecting mother (manifested by his swollen belly that he called "his mummy") to contain his rage towards his sibling and parents, especially mother. Animating objects and declaring flying insects "baby-eating bugs" may respectively reflect reaction formation and projective defenses against his angry death wishes.

His animation of things showed an extraordinary capacity to symbolize, perhaps in identification with the father's imagination. The history suggests a developmental arrest abetted by the mother's difficulties in setting limits, yet his symptoms suggest neurotic-level conflicts, in that Jeremiah uses defenses to keep threatening themes out of awareness without significantly distorting experiences beyond age-appropriate magical thinking.

Capacity to Form Internal Representations

Jeremiah's capacity to represent the full range of age-expected affects and wishes was constricted, as shown in his limited expressions of joy, pleasure, assertiveness, and zestful anger. With the affect limitations just described, he could represent a sense of self and others. In the second interview, he symptomatically masked basic wishes and affects having to do with anger, competition, loss, and disappointment.

Capacity for Differentiation and Integration

Jeremiah's basic capacity for reality testing was intact. He clearly differentiated his sense of self from his sense of his mother (e.g., "I know I bother mommy . . . "). He had a partially stable mood. He showed capacities for relationships, impulse control, and concentration; he was learning to use ideas to label, conceptualize, and master emotions; and he was becoming able to organize emotions into categories. Still, he was unable, consciously, to connect his constipation, rituals, and obsessions with his fears about his rivalries and his anger over his losses and his mother's infantilizations.

Self-Observing Capacities

Initially, I could observe only what Jeremiah did and said, noting that he was limited in his capacity to observe connections between his feelings and ideas. But Jeremiah's comments to me in the second interview about his Dracula attacks, along with the changes he had made when his parents followed the referring physician's advice, suggest that his self-observation is intact and age-expected.

Capacity for Internal Standards and Ideals

Jeremiah is in the process of forming internal standards and ideals. His history suggests that the emerging content of his inner standards is characterized by fluctuating images of his loving parents infantilizing and overpowering him on one hand, and, on the other hand, undermining his confidence by acting as if they feel he cannot handle the stress that comes with walking alone, weaning, toilet training, and short separations. In reaction, he may be developing a harsh, rigid system of values and ideals, which could lead to anxiety and depression.

Summary of Profile of Mental Functioning

Jeremiah evidenced mild to moderate constrictions and alterations in mental functioning associated with encapsulated symptom formations (e.g., constipation, obsessions, compulsions, and phobias), tendencies toward fragmentation of self-object differentiation, and limitations in experience of feelings and thoughts. **PDM Code: MCA204-MCA205**

Emerging Personality Patterns

Jeremiah's symptoms and constrictions in expressing age-expected expansive joy, assertiveness, and zestful anger, coupled with his anxiety about angry wishes and feelings, suggest that he is heading toward an anxious personality pattern, with many normal or healthy features. The goal of treatment would be to enable him to move toward healthier adaptive patterns. **PDM Code: PCA111**

Symptom Patterns

Jeremiah is best understood as having recurrent constipation and an obsessive-compulsive disorder with depressive features. **PDM Codes: SCA303, with some features of SCA306**

The Classification of Mental Health and Developmental Disorders in Infancy and Early Childhood

IEC Axis

Mental development during infancy and early childhood reflects dynamic relationships between many dimensions of human functioning, including emotional, social, language, cognitive, regulatory-sensory processing, and motor capacities. Many pioneers have contributed to this field, especially to our understanding of early emotional development and sensory processing, including Jean Ayers, John Bowlby, Berry Brazelton, Sibylle Escalona, Selma Fraiberg, Anna Freud, Margaret Mahler, Lois Murphy, Sally Province, René Spitz, D. W. Winnicott, and many contemporary infant researchers and clinicians.[1]

A biopsychosocial model of early development includes the infant's (1) developmental level of emotional, social, and intellectual functioning; (2) biologically based individual processing differences (the way the baby reacts to and comprehends different sensations (e.g., auditory, visual-spatial, tactile), and the way in which the child plans, sequences, and executes actions); and (3) relationships, including child/caregiver/family and other relationship patterns. Infant experiences (as well as those throughout the course of life) can only be understood in the context of a relational, social, and cultural framework (Greenspan, 1989; 1992; Greenspan & Lourie, 1981; Greenspan & Shanker, 2004).

The classification presented below is more fully described in the new diagnostic classification manual—*The Interdisciplinary Council on Developmental and Learning Disorders Diagnostic Manual for Infancy and Early Childhood Mental Health Disorders, Developmental Disorders, Regulatory-Sensory Processing Disorders, Language Disorders, and Learning Challenges—ICDL-DMIC* (ICDL-DMIC Work Groups, 2005). The ICDL-DMIC builds on earlier efforts (see Greenspan & Lourie, 1981; Greenspan, 1992; Diagnostic Classification Task Force, 1994; ICDL Clinical Practice Guidelines Workgroup, 2000). Three broad categories of mental health disorders are considered:

1. **Interactive Disorders**, involving symptom patterns such as anxiety, depression, and disruptive behaviors;

2. **Regulatory-Sensory Processing Disorders**, involving symptom patterns such as inattention, overreactivity, sensory seeking; and

---

[1] See Greenspan and Lourie (1981), Greenspan (1989, 1992, 1997), and Greenspan and Shanker (2004) for fuller descriptions. Also see selected references at the end of this section.

3. **Neurodevelopmental Disorders of Relating and Communicating**, involving symptom patterns such as self-absorption, perseveration, and dysfunctional communication (e.g., autism spectrum disorders and patterns).

These categories include problems that the DSM-IV-TR describes, but not in a sufficiently developmental or comprehensive manner.

The ICDL-DMIC includes not only these three primary diagnoses, but language and learning disorders. It also includes a number of axes that provide a comprehensive picture of the infant/young child and his or her family. The Psychodynamic Diagnostic Manual (PDM) includes these elements of this comprehensive approach that are relevant to mental health professionals with an interest in infancy and early childhood.

The developmental biopsychosocial perspective evident in the previous section is particularly critical to the diagnosis of problems that occur in infancy and early childhood. Readers who have worked with infants and young children may find many of the developmental observations and concepts familiar; those readers who have worked predominantly with older children and adolescents may find the descriptions clear, but may not have an immediate reference point in their clinical experience.

The format for infant and early childhood mental health disorders is unique to this age group and does not mirror the one used for older children and adults.

OVERVIEW OF PRIMARY MENTAL HEALTH DIAGNOSES IN INFANCY AND EARLY CHILDHOOD

Interactive Disorders, such as anxiety and depression, refer to challenges in which infant- or child-caregiver interaction patterns and/or related family and environmental patterns play the major role. **Regulatory-Sensory Processing Disorders** refer to those challenges in which the child's constitutional and maturational variations, in terms of sensory over- or underresponsivity, visual-spatial, auditory processing, or motor planning difficulties, are a primary contributor. **Neurodevelopmental Disorders of Relating and Communicating** refer to developmental disorders, including autism spectrum disorders, in which there are significant difficulties with the fundamental capacities to relate, communicate, and think.

Neurodevelopmental disorders of relating and communicating often include regulatory and interactive difficulties. Even in such instances, if a child's basic relating, communicating, and thinking are disrupted, the problem should be considered a neurodevelopmental disorder of relating and communicating. Regulatory-sensory processing disorders may also involve interactive difficulties, but if constitutional-maturational variations make a significant contribution, they should be diagnosed as regulatory-sensory processing disorders. The diagnosis of interactive disorder should be reserved for instances in which, despite some constitutional and maturational aspects, the caregiver-child interaction and related family and environmental patterns play the dominant role in pathogenesis.

In addition to the primary diagnosis, the unique qualities of each young child and family should be captured on a multi-axial developmental profile. This profile should include descriptions of (1) six basic functional, emotional, developmental capacities; (2) constitutional and maturational variations (regulatory-sensory processing patterns); (3) caregiver-infant or caregiver-child and family interaction patterns; and (4) other medical or neurological diagnoses (see Figure 1).

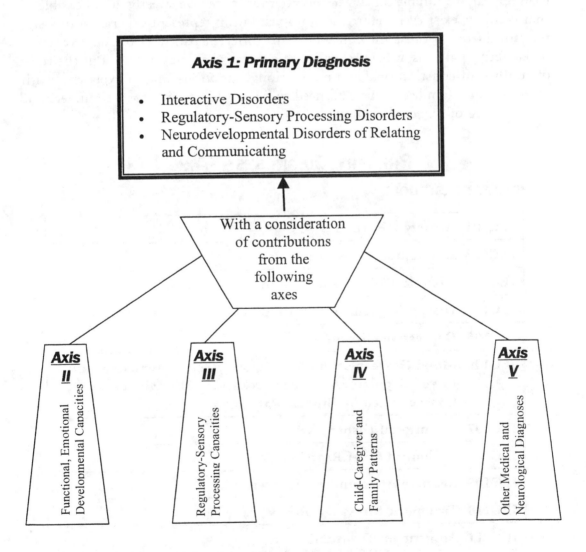

Figure 1 Multi-Axial Approach.

During early emotional development, infants and young children continually organize their experience of the world at higher and higher levels. As experience is represented or symbolized, the young child is able to comprehend gradually the connections between different wishes, feelings, and thoughts. As these are discerned, it becomes possible for the child to experience conflicts. This capacity emerges around 18 months of age and develops through about age 4. Even before a young child is able to represent experience to a significant degree, however, he or she can organize affects and behaviors into tendencies that are differentiated, such as those associated with warmth and dependency and those associated with assertiveness and anger. Although we cannot confidently determine what the preverbal (and presymbolic playing) toddler is experiencing, we can observe conflicting tendencies as a 16-month-old begins acting angrily and then appears to inhibit the anger and attempt to behave sweetly. It is possible that conflicts exist even before the young child can represent experience to a significant degree. Because there may be many different pathways to adaptive and maladaptive patterns, we are reluctant to generalize about etiology. But the roles of conflict, of constitutional and maturational variations, and of experience with caregivers and family members all need to be considered in efforts to understand the meaning of one of these observed patterns in a particular child.

PRIMARY DIAGNOSES—AXIS I

Interactive Disorders

IEC101. Anxiety Disorders
IEC102. Developmental Anxiety Disorders
IEC103. Disorders of Emotional Range and Stability
IEC104. Disruptive Behavior and Oppositional Disorders
IEC105. Depressive Disorders
IEC106. Mood Dysregulation: A Unique Type of Interactive and Mixed Regulatory-Sensory Processing Disorder Characterized by Bipolar Patterns
IEC107. Attentional Disorders
IEC108. Prolonged Grief Reaction
IEC109. Reactive Attachment Disorders
IEC110. Traumatic Stress Disorders
IEC111. Adjustment Disorders

| IEC112. Gender Identity Disorders |
| IEC113. Selective Mutism |
| IEC114 – 116 Sleep, Eating, and Elimination Behavior Disorders |
| IEC114. Sleep Disorders |
| IEC115. Eating Disorders |
| IEC116. Elimination Disorders |

Interactive disorders are characterized by the problematic way a child perceives and experiences his or her emotional world and/or by a particular maladaptive child-caregiver interaction pattern (Greenspan, 1992). The caregiver's personality, fantasies, and intentions; the child's emerging organization of experience; and the way these come together through child-caregiver interactions are important components; all must be taken into account in an effort to understand the nature of the difficulty and to devise an effective intervention plan. As with all infant and early childhood disorders, it is also important to consider the contributions of the child's regulatory-sensory processing capacities and the current environmental stresses on the child and family. The goal of treatment is not only to alleviate the presenting symptoms, but also to facilitate the child's progress toward an age-appropriate developmental level and an age-appropriate degree of stability and range of thematic experience.

Symptoms that can reflect an interactive disorder include anxiety, fears, behavior control problems, and sleeping and eating difficulties. That the same symptoms can be reflective of any number of challenges is understandable in light of the limited number of behaviors of which infants and young children are capable. This category also includes transient situational adjustment reactions, such as a child's response to the mother's return to work, as well as reactions to trauma that do not involve multiple aspects of development.

IEC101. Anxiety Disorders

Infants and young children may experience persistent levels of anxiety and fear which impede the attainment of an age-expected range of emotions and functioning. Anxiety can take the form of specific fears or verbalized worries, obsessions or preoccupations, excessive tantrums, distress and agitation, and avoidance behaviors. The primary source of the anxiety may not always be clear.

PRESENTING PATTERN

Depending on the age of the child, the expression of anxiety takes different forms. Infants and very young children who cannot yet communicate or elaborate verbally show anxiety of a more generalized nature in which symptoms—such as excessive fearfulness, tantrums, agitation, avoidance, panic reactions, and worries—are in evidence on a persistent basis, even when the child is not threatened by separation from a primary caregiver. The older child may talk about his fears but not respond to reassurances, or may have a freeze, fight, or flight reaction. In some cases children may even have counterphobic reactions in which they approach or provoke what they fear to alleviate the anxiety they cannot control and "get it over with!" The pathogenically anxious child is clearly distressed and fearful and cannot carry on usual routines and activities without significant disruptions during the day or night.

We also observe, even in very young infants (3 to 4 months of age), hypervigilant behavior. The child appears frightened, overly reactive, and overly focused, as if there were imminent danger. Infants who are abused may show this reaction quite early in their development, although it can manifest itself at any time.

Most typically, anxiety is manifested in a moderate level of apprehensiveness and fear in relationship to many age-expected experiences, such as playing with peers, going into a new social setting, attending a birthday party, performing in school, or trying new foods. These behaviors may be accompanied by whining, crying, withdrawal, and refusal. Not infrequently, difficulties with sleeping or eating, and, in older children, difficulties with toilet training and comfortable patterns of elimination, can arise from the child's anxiety even when they are not the source of the anxiety. It should be noted, however, that difficulties with sleeping, eating, toilet training, and elimination can also be related to Regulatory-Sensory Processing Disorders, depending on whether the primary contributing factors lie in infant-caregiver interactions or constitutional-maturational variations.

We can see an interactive disorder when the child's anxieties and fears are related to the primary caregiver(s)' insufficient provision of regulating, comforting relationship patterns. For example, the caregiver may be unable to use various strategies to help the child, anticipating what might be anxiety-producing through problem-solving conversations, initiating practice via pretend play, preparing the child for what will occur, and planning strategies to reduce anxiety.

Often, the caregiver is also anxious and distressed. The caregiver's anxiety may stem, in part, from anticipating the child's anxiety and feeling ill-equipped to help or feeling annoyed or overly worried. The caregiver may also be bringing his or her own anxieties to the situation at hand; a caregiver's social inhibition or phobia, for example, may impede the process of helping an anxious child. A caregiver's overidentification with a child may overwhelm the caregiver with unresolved childhood issues. In either case, the interaction between the child and caregiver increases the anxiety and distress.

IEC102. Developmental Anxiety Disorders

Development itself can induce significant anxiety in children who have difficulty negotiating emotional milestones and making developmental transitions. As their maturation launches children into uncharted territory, some apprehension or mild anxiety is inevitable, until the child begins to feel safe and develops an emotional understanding of his or her experience. For example, a stranger may evoke anxiety initially, but with repeated and sensitive interactions, the infant begins to experience the new person as safe and enjoyable, and is able to adapt to the generic situation of dealing with strangers. Similarly, as the infant or toddler recognizes the experience of separation and feels the associated anxiety, a sensitive caregiver can help the child find comfort in a transitional object (a teddy bear or blanket, for example) and thereby adapt to future separations.

As the child continues to develop, other emerging emotional experiences may challenge his or her sense of security and competence. Fears of bodily injury, of imagined pursuers (monsters or ghosts), of aggression, and related worries may develop. With supportive interactions, the child develops an understanding of these experiences through regulating interactions, conversations, and symbolic play, thereby learning to meet security needs through using words and play, exercising good judgment, and seeking support when needed.

In some cases, however, the anxiety is very intense and highly disruptive. For example, the child may be extremely fearful of separation from the primary caregiver and may consequently shrink from venturing out into new situations. Overt behaviors include desperate clinging, crying, and tantrums. A child's anxiety about possible separation may interfere with his or her functioning, even when separation is not involved, causing the child to avoid age-appropriate experiences with toys, peers, or new physical settings. Anxiety in some children persists far beyond the developmental stage in which it originates and may generalize to later situations.

The child may be vulnerable as a result of other health matters in the past. The caregiver may have conflicts or fears related to the child's growing up, or may be reminded of his or her own past separation challenges. In some cases, the child's anxiety masks problems in the parental relationship or the family's environment. The child may sense some threat or danger related to the caregiver and therefore want to cling. Or the child may be overwhelmed by the unexpected impact of touch and sounds in a new busy environment and may become anxious in the absence of a protective caregiver.

While stranger and separation anxieties are very familiar, other developmental anxieties exist. For example, the toddler becomes aware, usually after mastering some motor activity, that the body can be hurt. This awareness is not yet discriminated, in that the child cannot yet distinguish between serious and trivial injury:

Each bodily insult may be experienced as a potential catastrophe with attendant kisses and band-aids for the boo-boos. With developmental maturation and adequate sensory-motor capacities, these concerns typically resolve over a year or two, such that the child seeks help if really hurt, takes appropriate risks during physical activities, and copes with doctor visits or medical procedures. When the expected developmental anxiety does not resolve, and the child continues to be excessively anxious, avoids physical risks, tends to panic, and is fearful of bodily injury, even in the absence of experiencing real injury or trauma, developmental anxiety disorder may be diagnosed.

Caregiver interactions play a critical role here, as they do in situations of stranger anxiety and separation anxiety. On the one hand, if they are also anxious about bodily injury, they may find it hard to provide the reassurance and support their children need to master body competence. On the other hand, if they are embarrassed by or ashamed of their child's timidity, they may transmit these feelings either covertly or overtly. Interactions with a shaming caregiver exacerbate the child's anxiety and need to be carefully examined to understand the caregiver's experiences.

As development moves forward, additional emotional milestones can generate anxiety. Negative affects such as jealousy, competition, resentment, wishes to retaliate, and other emerging emotional states may feel frightening. As children become aware of these affects, they may insist on being the "good guy," claim only positive feelings, deny negative motives and feelings, have frightening dreams, and avoid conflict or competition lest they lose. Anxiety may be palpable as the child shows alarm, fear, impulsivity, and even panic in the face of threats related to internal aggressive feelings. The child may even become aggressive towards others.

Typically, these heightened emotions are accompanied by the development of symbolic solutions as the child begins the process of differentiating reality and fantasy. When children begin to report dreams and worries about ghosts and monsters, they are beginning to imagine the first symbols of danger and vulnerability. Those who can, counter their fears with fantasies of magical power (wands, wizards, superpowers), and symbolic play. They may construct dramas in which they and their playmates "fight back" and outwit their imagined "enemy." Some children willingly take the role of the enemy or bad guy just to be sure they are in charge of the danger. Eventually, children can explore both the "good guy and bad guy" sides of themselves and abstract the reasons for their fighting. These symbolic experiences lay the foundation for higher- level abstract thinking and personal standards.

When a child is not prepared to deal with the broader range of affects, anxiety can increase significantly. Some children try to keep safe by avoiding all negative emotions, protesting vehemently, getting angry, or throwing objects if approached with these themes by other children. The anxiety can escalate into panic as the child feels genuinely endangered, or can drive the child into avoidance of anxiety-provoking experiences, or even trigger regressions as the child tries to escape into the safety of dependency. Other children embrace new emotions more slowly, tempering their anxiety through over-reliance on magical solutions, and attempts to control the environment. Such children are unable to move forward into logical reasoning and may be handicapped in the task of building the boundary between reality and fantasy.

As with the other developmentally based anxieties, caregiver interactions can have a crucial impact on the child's emotional development. Here, too, the caregiver's comfort or discomfort with certain emotions can support or impede the child. If the caregiver is loving only when the child is "good" (rejecting of anger, jealousy, meanness, and aggression), the child may not get sufficient support to experience the full range of emotions safely and learn that both positive and negative feelings are involved in relationships. If the child does not have encouragement to experiment and practice with feelings in safe symbolic ways, the developmental process can be derailed.

PRESENTING PATTERN

Children with developmental anxieties present with similar patterns as children with other anxieties and trauma reactions. Some children cling, cry, lash out, hit, bite, or tantrum, often in panic-stricken proportions. Others may appear very apprehensive and subdued, and may withdraw from their usual interests and refuse activities. The verbal child may protest, express more worries, show mood shifts, and withdraw from anxiety-inducing situations. In some cases, the child is afraid to go to sleep or wakes up frequently from frightening dreams that are either reported or indicated by sweaty, anxious awakenings. Eating may be disrupted, with changes in appetite and choices of foods or even with difficulty holding food down. Anxiety can be readily transmitted back-and-forth from child to caregiver and caregiver to child. In some cases, the child's development may have been proceeding smoothly until the anxiety becomes obvious. In others, it is preceded by struggles to master earlier developmental transitions. The anxiety may also be an intense but transient symptom of a child's determined effort to move forward developmentally; anxious, disorganized, and even regressive behavior can be the step taken backwards before moving forward. All children with this diagnosis show more intense or prolonged reactions than expected at developmental crossroads and are not readily soothed or reassured.

IEC103. Disorders of Emotional Range and Stability

From early infancy into the preschool years, children experience a gradual increase in their emotional range and stability. A 2- to 3-month-old infant shows a limited number of global emotions (joy, distress, range, fear) and shifts rapidly from one to another. In contrast, a 16-month-old toddler may evidence warmth and security, pleasure and delight, curiosity, excitement, caution, fear, annoyance, assertiveness, irritation, sympathy, sadness, and other more nuanced emotional states. The adaptive toddler experiences and expresses emotions in a relatively stable manner in relationship to expectable experiences; for example, happiness when a parent appears, smiling and ready to play, and anger when a favorite toy is put back on the shelf because it is bedtime.

Although difficulties with age-expected emotional range and stability may be subtle and less obvious than states of anxiety, these kinds of difficulties are important to recognize because of their potential long-term consequences. A child's capacity to experience the full range of age-expected emotions and to regulate them in stable ways is an important foundation of that child's future social and intellectual development.

To determine if a child has difficulty with age-appropriate emotional range and stability, a clinician must have a roadmap of expected emotional development in infants and young children, as it can be observed in their interactions with others and in their play. While the rudiments of most emotions are present from infancy, emotions get more and more differentiated as the child develops in the first five years of life and is able to describe more complex feelings, including ambivalence and conflicting emotions and the reasons for them. A 2-year-old boy may first bop his baby sister and then hug and kiss her. At 3, he may pout and grab her toy. At 4, he may protest verbally that mommy never spends time with him and the baby always comes first, while acknowledging his love for the baby. Between 5 and 6, he may be protective and helpful but also able to talk about his jealousy.

It is the lack of differentiation, range, and stability of emotions that characterizes this disorder. In contrast to children with developmental anxieties, children who are appropriately given this diagnosis present with a narrow range of affects or interests, and their experience lacks the full-blown intensity of anxiety reactions.

PRESENTING PATTERN

Many infants and toddlers do not evidence the increasing range and stability of emotions just described. As toddlers and preschoolers, they may persist in showing only a few global emotional states, such as joy and rage. The lack of stability may be seen in rapid fluctuations from one emotional state to another or in variations in the intensity of the same emotion. The functioning of such children is disrupted by their limited capacity to tolerate frustration in an age-expectable manner. They may even confuse or reverse emotions inappropriately. They have trouble answering questions about feelings and seem unable to reflect on the connection between thoughts, feelings, and behavior. Their interests tend to be limited to a few areas (e.g., construction, vehicles, transformer toys), and the emotional drama that could accompany such interests seems absent. Play with other children may also be affected, as the child has fewer emotionally based ideas and is less interested in the symbolic play of others.

IEC104. Disruptive Behavior and Oppositional Disorders

Disruptive behaviors are a common challenge in infancy and early childhood. Problems with impulse control often emerge as a toddler begins to walk. Very young children may hit, bite, or scratch instead of using interactive gestures and emotional signals to convey intentions. In some cases, even very young children behave aggressively and destructively, hurting others, setting fires, destroying property, or torturing animals with little remorse.

PRESENTING PATTERN

When a child behaves disruptively enough to be considered a problem, there is often a related problem of insufficient limit-setting and structure by a parent. Some constitutionally intense children can easily exhaust a caregiver who is alone for long stretches with the child. Some caregivers read and respond to an infant's signal of pleasure or fear with appropriate reciprocal gestures (smiles beget smiles, fear begets comfort, and so forth), but become either nonreactive or overreactive, often because of temporary anxiety, when the child begins to show annoyance and anger. Sometimes caregivers appear almost "stone-faced" as a child becomes increasingly angry and impelled to push or bite. Others quickly become too punitive. Not infrequently, one caregiver "freezes" while the other is overly punitive, leaving the child without sensitive reciprocal regulating and limit-setting responses. If a child's immediate environment provides neither warmth nor firm, consistent limits, or if limits are imposed capriciously and abusively, a child's sensation-seeking can take on an enraged quality, with indiscriminate, aggressive acting out[2] (Lewis, 1992; Yeager & Lewis, 2000).

---

[2] In a classic study of institutionalized children deprived of affection in infancy, Spitz (1945) noted two responses. One group of children became withdrawn, depressed, or apathetic; some stopped developing physically, failed to gain weight, and even became quite ill; some did not survive. Others sought out sensation, becoming aggressive, promiscuous, and indifferent to others, relating to them only as need-satisfying objective. Other early researchers found a higher than expected degree of subtle difficulties in the functioning of the nervous system among antisocial children and adults, with problems in perception, information processing, and motor functioning (Bowlby, 1944). These early findings have been confirmed and reconfirmed over the years with many additional studies (see Greenspan, 1997 and Greenspan and Pollock, 1991 for overviews).

During the preschool years, children may have difficulties with both attention and disruptiveness. Some young children have both a high activity level and
poor frustration tolerance and consequently react to frustration with pushing,
hitting, throwing things, being oppositional, and shifting rapidly from one activity to another. Often, when assessing children's relative mastery of functional
emotional developmental capacities, we observe that those with a disruptive
behavior pattern have some mastery but also some constriction at each level.
These constrictions can impede self-regulation and social problem solving. Disruptive behavior tends to derail maturation toward using language, negotiation,
and pretend play to express needs and feelings, resolve conflicts, and delay
gratification.

IEC105. Depressive Disorders

In healthy development, infants and young children gradually expand their
capacities for emotional experience and expression within a secure infant-caregiver relationship. Adaptive interactive patterns enable the infant to negotiate
each of the functional emotional developmental capacities, and thereby experience, by age two or so, a large range of emotions, from joy, pleasure, and enthusiasm to transient sadness and fear. Emotionally healthy toddlers are curious,
exploratory, and assertive.

PRESENTING PATTERN

Depressed infants and young children show a consistent mood pattern,
rather than the range of emotional states expected for their age and developmental stage. Some toddlers and preschoolers display a persistent sadness
(Cytryn & McKnew, 1974) evidenced by mournful expressions, statements of sadness, and readiness to well up with tears. They show little pleasure or interest in
activities they have previously enjoyed and do not initiate "fun" activities. Some
children have difficulty showing or verbalizing sadness in situations that would
normally elicit sad feelings; they may insist they are "happy" even as they cry or
look pained. As they become symbolic, they may play out depressive themes. Preschoolers may, for example, enact in play and/or verbalize persistent feelings of
being "bad," while slightly older children may talk about wishing they were not
alive or explore themes of death in their play, whether or not they have been
bereaved.

Some depressed infants and young children show persistent agitation, and
inability to be soothed, while others move slowly, show little energy, and turn
down activities they once enjoyed. Difficulties with sleeping, eating, and weight
regulation may signal depression in infants and toddlers as well as in older
children.

Infant-caregiver interaction patterns often play a major role in a child's difficulties regulating mood. The child may experience the loss of love or support when a parent cannot accept his or her full range of behavior and feelings. A caregiver who behaves lovingly when the child is compliant but rejects him or her when the child is angry may inadvertently contribute to a depressive response. Some parents are unresponsive to children when their own conflicts are triggered; others may be too depressed or distracted themselves to maintain a warm connection to a child through his or her range of mood states.

Infantile depression may contribute to problems later, when the child experiences some loss or conflict and is unable to rely on an internalized, nurturing image for support and solace. Such difficulties can, if left unaddressed, persist into adulthood.

IEC106. Mood Dysregulation: A Unique Type of Interactive and Mixed Regulatory-Sensory Processing Disorder Characterized by Bipolar Patterns

In recent years, there has been growing interest in early identification and treatment of bipolar-type mood dysregulation in children (Carlson & Weintraub, 1993; Cytryn & McKnew, 1974; Egland, Blumenthal, Nee, Sharp, & Endicott, 1987; Geller, Zimmerman, Williams, Bolhofner, & Craney, 2001; Lish, Dime-Meenan, Whybrow, Arlen-Price, & Hirschfeld, 1994; Radke-Yarrow, Nottelmann, Martinez, Fox, & Belmont, 1992). In children, manic or hypomanic states often manifest themselves in aggressive behavior or agitation rather than in the frantic, grandiose thinking commonly seen in adults. Diagnosing bipolar patterns in children is therefore difficult (Harrington, Fudge, Rutter, Pickles, & Hill, 1991; Strober, Morrell, Burroughs, Lampert, Danforth, & Freeman, 1988). We do not have a clear understanding of the antecedent variables leading to bipolar disorder in children, although a host of neuropsychological vulnerabilities and deficits has been suggested, including problems in language, motor development, perception, executive functioning, and social functioning (Castillo, Kwock, Courvorisie, & Hooper, 2000; Sigurdsson, Fombonne, Sayal, & Checkley, 1999). Furthermore, a comprehensive intervention program that addresses not only biochemical phenomena but also family interactions and educational issues has not yet been formulated.

PRESENTING PATTERN

We propose a novel hypothesis: bipolar patterns in children can be understood as arising from a unique configuration of antecedents involving sensory processing and motor functioning, early child-caregiver interaction patterns, and early states of personality organization. Specifically, we suggest that children at risk for developing bipolar-type mood dysregulation share the following characteristics (Greenspan & Glovinsky, 2002):

1. An unusual processing pattern in which over-responsivity to sound, touch, or both coexists with a craving of sensory stimulation, particularly movement (most overresponsive children are more fearful and cautious). Sensory craving is usually associated with high activity and aggressive, agitated, or impulsive behavior. Therefore, when they are overloaded with stimuli, children with this unusual combination of processing differences cannot self-regulate by withdrawing, as a cautious child might. Instead, they become agitated, aggressive, and impulsive, thereby overloading themselves even more.

2. An early pattern of interaction, continuing into childhood, characterized by a lack of fully co-regulated reciprocal affective exchanges. In particular, caregivers are unable to interact with the infant or child in ways that help him or her "up-regulate" and "down-regulate" moods to modulate states of despondency and agitation.

3. A personality organization in which the fifth and sixth functional emotional levels of development have not been mastered. Emotions either are not addressed at the symbolic level, instead remaining at the level of behavior or somatic experience, or are represented as global, polarized affect states rather than in integrated form.

IEC107. Attentional Disorders

One of the most complicated mental health disorders in infants and young children is a problem with sustained attention. It is complicated because while certain shared symptoms, such as inattentiveness, characterize a large number of children who receive the diagnosis of ADD or ADHD, there may very well be many different patterns (i.e., many different pathways) leading to these symptoms, and many different reasons for inattentiveness. A comprehensive approach to understanding attentional problems must take into account children's processing patterns, separately and in combination, and their variable developmental organizations and interactive patterns.

A child's current developmental tasks should first be examined. Clinicians should consider whether developmental anxieties or social challenges or the child's environment may be disrupting the child's attention, and whether such conditions can be addressed or modified.

Regulatory-sensory processing differences to look for include: hypo- or hyper-responsivity to different sensations, patterns of sensory craving, motor planning and sequencing, auditory processing, and visual-spatial processing. Interactive patterns that may be relevant include caregiver-infant interactions characterized by short bursts (rather than long chains) back-and-forth gestural and emotional signaling. Family or physical environments that are overwhelming, chaotic, negligent, or abusive should be noted. Each of the patterns just described, individually or in various combinations, may lead to the common symptoms involved in inattentiveness (also see regulatory-sensory processing disorders).

In both interactive and regulatory-sensory processing attention problems, the same developmental pathways are involved. Interactions can be more challenging. Based on a complete profile, the clinician can determine which developmental pathway is contributing to the symptom choice.

Presenting Pattern

Variations in attention can be expected in early development. Difficulties sustaining attention can be observed as early as 2 to 4 months when the infant becomes more capable of turning and focusing to look and listen and coo responsively. By 8 to 12 months, an attention-disordered infant may attend only fleetingly, rather than in the sustained manner needed for two-way interactions such as peek-a-boo or pat-a-cake. In the second year of life, many toddlers with attentional problems move from toy to toy and appear highly distracted even when playing with an object of choice. Slightly older children with this problem may always be on the move, always changing "topics," unable to stick with a conversation or a game. One common pattern involves spurts or intermittent stop-and-go interactions. Some children with attention deficits, in contrast, become overly self-absorbed or over-focused on special interests that make it hard to shift their attention, even when others ask them to do so.

Variations in attention can also be related to what is available to claim a child's attention. Some young children are attentive to books and videos but not to activities chosen by others or activities that involve minimal interaction. Often, the tolerance or expectations of those in the environment affect perceptions of the problem. A child who plays alone for long periods may be valued as self-propelled rather than labeled self-absorbed; or adults in the environment may change activities every few minutes because they assume very short attention spans in young children. Despite all these variations, attention difficulties are readily identified. Determining the primary contributants based on the child's individual profile is the next step.

IEC108. Prolonged Grief Reaction

The loss of a parent or primary caregiver is such a profound calamity for young children that it always requires clinical attention.

PRESENTING PATTERN

Reactions to significant loss can take many forms and may progress over time. Most often, when infants and young children lose a primary caregiver, their initial grief is characterized by searching for the lost person and protesting the caregiver's absence. The child may also withdraw, become more passive and self-absorbed, and avoid expected or pleasurable activities. Anxiety, agitation, despondency, and self-absorption may follow. In other cases, the child gives the appearance of not reacting and may take on the role of comforting or distracting other family members from their grief, either by being entertaining or by becoming demanding.

Reactions to major loss can also take the form of increased separation anxiety. Some children cling to the remaining caregiver and cannot tolerate separation. Some express their anger and aggression at the parent who is still there, and may idealize the missing parent. In some cases, children appear to carry on in one environment (e.g., at pre-school or daycare) but not in another (e.g., at home). Many suffer sleep and eating disruptions, weight loss, weight gain, illness and somatic symptoms, reduced frustration tolerance, or regression in recently mastered developmental tasks. Prolonged grief reaction is distinguished from normal mourning by the persistence and/or multiplicity of these symptoms.

Even though very young children have not yet developed the concept of the permanence of the loss, they may be nevertheless severely affected by it. Infants, toddlers, and children with significant developmental delays who may have many of the reactions described above are frequently misunderstood as too young to remember the loss and therefore not devastated by it. It is not unusual for the verbal child to express expectations of the parent's return, assumptions that a dead caregiver is alive elsewhere, or fantasies of reunion. Some children show marked distress at reminders of their missing caregiver, while others seek reminders to the extent that they want nothing changed or moved.

Whatever the reaction of the child to the loss of a parent or primary caregiver, and however they try to comprehend its meaning, it is important to help the child in age-appropriate ways, to understand the reasons for and the finality of the loss. The child's age and developmental profile determine the length of normal mourning and thus the temporal criteria for regarding the child's emotional state as a prolonged grief reaction or disorder.[3] Therapeutic factors include the availability of a nurturing substitute caregiver who provides extra security and emotional warmth, the opportunity to express feelings, and, in pre-schoolers, the opportunity to play out emerging fears as well as feelings of loss.

---

[3] Bowlby described and the Robertsons filmed very young children evidencing such a grief reaction when separated from their primary caregivers during a hospitalization. These famous films are available at the New York University film library (Bowlby & Robertson, 1953).

IEC109. Reactive Attachment Disorders

Forming an attachment or, more broadly, an emotionally trusting relationship, is a well-established critical dimension of healthy emotional development. We can observe, however, many compromises in forming or sustaining healthy relationship patterns.

PRESENTING PATTERN

Attachment problems include a wide range of difficulties. Some infants and young children are not able to engage in any type of intimacy, do not seek or respond to comfort, and seem despondent, withdrawn or self-absorbed; others are diffusely aggressive, impersonal and promiscuous in their relationships. Still others show more subtle variations in degrees and qualities of intimacy, empathy, and the capacities for negotiating and sustaining relationships.

When extreme, disruptions in early attachment may be associated with compromises in growth and weight gain (failure to thrive) and with language, cognitive, and social difficulties. The most severe versions of these reactions are seen in children who grow up in orphanages that do not provide sufficient emotional nurturance and in children who experience extensive neglect or abuse within their families. If attachment problems have significantly disrupted the fundamental capacities of relating, communicating, and thinking, the child may appear to have neurodevelopmental disorders of relating and communicating, such as autism. Children with little capacity for shared attention, social reciprocity, or social problem-solving require the same type of treatment program as children with derailed development.

In many cases, however, attachment and relationship problems in infancy and early childhood are not extreme. There are many subtle variations within which the early relationship lacks emotional depth, range, and optimal levels of trust and security. In looking at the more subtle attachment and relationship problems of infants and young children, the clinician should consider the implications of infant-caregiver relationships in light of the infant's capacity to master each of the functional emotional developmental capacities. The attachment relationship needs to be viewed from the perspective of the full range and stability of age-expected feelings. Progression through the functional developmental capacities may be difficult to negotiate with parents who have experienced severe deprivation themselves, as seen in multi-problem families, and who are consequently unable to form intimate attachments with their own infants. Child-caregiver interactions may be infused with anxiety, despair, ambivalence and other outcomes of a parent's experience and current relationships.

The clinician also needs to consider the contributions of the child's regulatory-sensory processing capacities. For example, infants who are unusually responsive to sensations such as touch and sound may show far more insecurity in their early relationship patterns than less highly sensitive infants. On the other hand, challenges in forming relationships can lead to challenges in sensory modulation, sensory processing, and motor planning. Such difficulties may appear to have a biological origin despite being secondary to interactive challenges. Infants born with excellent nervous systems, who have good muscle tone, and the ability to focus, attend, and respond to visual and auditory sensations can lose these competencies during the first 3 months of life if their environments are either chaotic or non-nurturing (Greenspan, Wieder, Lieberman, Nover, Lourie, & Robinson, 1987). Such infants can develop low muscle tone, under-responsivity to touch and sound, and difficulties in auditory and visual-spatial processing, or (especially in chaotic, overstimulating environments) sensory hypersensitivity and patterns of avoidance. Even when these patterns are secondary to interactive difficulties, they may be indistinguishable from those in infants who are born with comparable processing challenges.

IEC110. Traumatic Stress Disorder

We prefer the term "traumatic stress disorder," rather than "posttraumatic stress disorder" because infants and young children may respond to severe trauma or stress immediately. The reaction may then continue, depending on factors discussed below.

PRESENTING PATTERN

Traumatic stress can severely disrupt children's emotional, social, language, and intellectual development. Such stresses include the witnessing of terrifying events (e.g., accidents, animal attacks, fires, war, natural disasters) or overwhelmingly frightening interpersonal events (e.g., severe abuse of self or loved one, witnessing the murder of a parent, witnessing rape of a caregiver, or sexual activity of a drug-addicted parent).

Traumatized children may suffer disruption in basic capacities such as sleep, eating, elimination, attention, impulse control, and mood. Physiological disruption, which is common in traumatized children, reflects the powerful impact of the traumatic stress on the young child's autonomic functions and regulation of basic states (as evidenced in startle responses, increased heart rate, heavy breathing, shaking, or sweating). Some children become sick and needy after a traumatic experience. They may also find it difficult to focus and may be so vigilant, anxious, or avoidant that typical routines and activities become impossible for them.

Fears that were not present before the trauma may emerge as a child becomes more worried in general and displaces fears of recurrence of the traumatic event onto other objects. These fears may be accompanied by night-mares. Some children ask relentless questions about the event, repeating questions to which they already know the answer. Children who play symbolically may re-enact the trauma in their play over and over, in an unchanging, ritualized manner.

Whenever a known trauma or series of traumatic events is associated with disruption (immediate or delayed) in a child's age-expected emotional, social, language, and/or cognitive capacities, the diagnosis of traumatic stress disorder should be considered. Even when a child's initial reactions to trauma are tempered by a parent's ability to help the child quickly feel safe again, posttraumatic reactions may surface later on. For example, there may be a disruption in ongoing mastery of the functional emotional developmental capacities. Difficulties with concentration and/or hyper-vigilance may make it difficult for the child to attend and engage in the aftermath of trauma and subsequent insecurity. Engagement may be disrupted; the child may feel either distrustful or angry about not having been protected, or may become more clingy, frightened, or sad. Some traumatized children slowly become less communicative and more helpless, unable to sustain the longer back-and-forth problem-solving interactions of ongoing development. Children who are able to play symbolically may reenact a version of the trauma with themselves as the victim or the perpetrator. Reality testing can get derailed as the child resorts to denial, becomes confused about what is remembered, or regresses to magical thinking.

IEC111. Adjustment Disorders

Like older children and adults, infants and young children may have difficulty adapting to change, loss, and developmental challenges. Experiences such as a change of caregiver, the beginning of school, conflicts with peers, illness of a family member, birth of a sibling, separation and divorce of parents, or moving from one home to another may trigger an adjustment reaction. In infants and young children, adjustment disorders are inferred from behaviors that are notably at variance with their prior adaptation.

PRESENTING PATTERN

In addition to easy-to-observe temporary shifts in sleeping and eating, minor regressions in language and behavior, mood shifts, poor frustration tolerance, increased anxiety or fears, oppositional behaviors, or impulse control patterns, one must look for subtle changes in the child's ongoing mastery of each of the functional emotional developmental capacities. Does the child who was fully engaged withdraw even a little? Does the child begin to object to going to pre-school or leaving the house? Does symbolic play get restricted to earthquakes or battles?

IEC112. Gender Identity Disorders

In infants and young children, a sense of gender is beginning to form. In most children one can see gender-specific behaviors throughout infancy and early childhood. These become more pronounced in the latter part of the second year and into the third and fourth years of life.

PRESENTING PATTERN

There is an enormous range of patterns that are part of a healthy exploration of gender roles. These may be related to constitutional, maturational and cultural differences.

Children's difficulties with their biological gender are most frequently identified when a preschooler goes beyond healthy exploration and insists on dressing up as the other gender, not simply as part of playful exploration and experimentation but as a persistent pattern. In play, there may be a strong preference for opposite-gender roles, dolls, and so on. There may also be a strong preference for opposite-gender playmates as well as for activities associated with the opposite gender. Verbal preschool children may express a clear dislike for their own anatomy and a wish to change their genitals. This reaction can be particularly strong and associated with a great deal of anxiety as the preschool child becomes more aware of the anatomical differences between boys and girls. The patterns of preference for the opposite gender and rejection of one's own gender can begin in early childhood. If not addressed, the patterns can persist and intensify as the child develops. These patterns can emerge at older ages as well.

Unique constitutional-maturational variations as well as caregiver-child interactions and family patterns may contribute to a child's gender identity difficulties. A parent's wish for a child of the opposite sex or perceptions of one parent as weak and devalued, for example, may fuel gender dysphoria. Underlying concerns with separation from the primary caregiver, conflicts over aggression and assertiveness, conflicts identifying with the parent of the same gender or the absence of a positive relationship with that parent may contribute to the child's difficulties (Coates, Friedman, & Wolfe, 1991).

IEC113. Selective Mutism

Selective mutism refers to a continuing difficulty in talking in social situations coupled with an ability to comprehend language and to speak in other settings (e.g., at home). While this pattern is reported to be found in less than one percent of children, it is nonetheless challenging for parents, educators, and the child.

PRESENTING PATTERN

Children with selective mutism tend to be anxious and are often highly reactive to new environments, especially those that are crowded and noisy, in which sounds and movements can be surprising and unpredictable. The inability to speak may be symptomatic of a subjective state of overwhelming fear and vigilance. Often the child attempts to retreat in a selective manner. In play or conversation with a child with selective mutism, one often observes content having to do with fear, worry, and danger. One may also see patterns of avoidance, e.g., the insistent representation of safe, non-emotional scenes such as very friendly tea parties. Relationships may be characterized by an anxious dependent pattern with a reluctance to take initiative and be assertive. While the child appears most anxious and becomes selectively mute and hyper-vigilant in selected settings, constrictions of the functional emotional developmental capacities are evident even where the child is comfortable speaking. Unresolved developmental anxieties related to fears of body damage, aggression, and other negative emotions are evident with constricted capacities to symbolize and express feelings safely in play or conversation. Although related to anxiety disorders, the highly specific symptom of selective mutism warrants a separate diagnostic category.

IEC114.–116. Sleep, Eating, and Elimination Behavior Disorders

Difficulties with sleeping or eating and, in older children, difficulties with toilet training and comfortable patterns of elimination are very common in infancy and early childhood. In some cases, they initially appear to be the only challenge the child experiences. Often, these difficulties arise in response to various interactive challenges, including trauma, anxiety, and adjustment reactions to transitions, illness, and psychosocial stress. The choice of the symptoms is often determined by the underlying sensory-motor vulnerability in combination with the developmental anxiety and/or interactive patterns. Difficulties with sleeping, eating, toilet training, and elimination can also be related to regulatory-sensory processing disorders.

The contributing factors may lie in infant-caregiver interactions or constitutional-maturational variations. The child's developmental profile always reflects the relative contributions of constitutional-maturational variations, child-caregiver interactions, and family and environmental factors.

IEC114. Sleep Disorders

Establishing sleep-wake cycles is one of the first tasks of infancy. Most children establish sleep-wake routines within the first few months or the first year of life. Many factors may contribute to problems in this area. Disruptions in sleep patterns can occur naturally with illness, changes in location, transitions in development, and other stress, but the patterns usually get re-established with the resumption of security and soothing relationships. In some cases, healthy sleep routines have not been established in the first place, via inconsistent times or settings for sleep, or parental difficulties in helping children learn to fall asleep on their own. Some infants rely on nursing or sucking a bottle to initiate sleep. Parents do not always learn other techniques for helping the child calm and fall asleep independently. Some infants maintain disorganized tendencies that originated in fussy, irritable periods of early infancy, even after maturation appears to have resolved these periods. In other cases, the environment is too chaotic to sustain routines and security, with resulting disorganized sleep patterns.

Another factor to consider is the culture of the family. Sleep disorders are to some extent in the eye of the beholder. Complaints of a sleep disorder can be subject to the perceptions and feelings of caregivers, who may have varying tolerance for irregular or disrupted sleep patterns, or who may have similar patterns themselves. In cultures where sleeping with children is acceptable or desired, it may be an alien idea to help a child learn to go to sleep separately. What presents as a sleep disturbance for one parent may not be a sleep disturbance for another.

Since sleep disorders are such a common pathway for conveying distress, they can signify any of the primary interactive disorders described earlier, or they can be rooted in constitutionally based regulatory-sensory processing disorders associated with other regulatory challenges described below.

PRESENTING PATTERN

Infants and young children may have difficulty settling into sleep when they first go to bed, or they may wake up and be unable to fall asleep again on their own. Some restless, sensitive sleepers wake frequently throughout the night. Others may sleep too much and be hard to arouse. Sleep disruption can also occur when a child who is becoming more symbolic awakens from a nightmare and is not sure what is real and not real.

Interactions between caregivers and children may contribute heavily to a sleep disorder. The relationships of children with this problem are often characterized by neediness, negativism, and impulsivity, with different parts of this pattern dominating in different children and families. Some parents feel very inadequate on learning that their child can fall asleep with others but not with them. They may, especially if there are preexisting marital conflicts, blame each other for not being able to get the baby to sleep. Marital conflict may also maintain a sleep disorder, as the child picks up the tension between the caregivers.

IEC115. Eating Disorders

Eating disorders, like sleep disorders, can be symptomatic of many of the interactive disorders. Or they may represent a regulatory disorder with sensory hypersensitivities and oral motor difficulties, as described below. They may reflect the residual anxiety from resolved biological problems, such as gastrointestinal difficulties, reflux, and other illnesses that created anxiety and lack of pleasure around eating.

The interactions between caregivers and children may contribute significantly to an eating disorder. For example, in the absence of appropriate nurturance, eating can become an over-relied-on source of comfort and self-soothing. In the absence of symbolic expression, fear, anger, or rejection can be expressed in food refusal.

PRESENTING PATTERN

The eating disorder may involve poor or irregular intake, food refusal, vomiting, restricted eating or insatiable eating. Since eating is essential for survival, eating disorders cannot be overlooked for long. Because the health and weight of a baby is often seen as indicative of "good" parenting, problems in a child's eating can become an enormous source of worry, stress, and inadequacy to the caregiver. The interaction between caregiver and infant can involve vacillations between neediness, negativism, and anxiety, with different parts of this pattern dominating in different children and families. Even simpler feeding challenges can undermine the confidence of infant and caregiver when coincidental with family disruptions, transitions, or inconsistencies. The absence of routine and timely eating patterns in a family may derail a child, and an eating disorder in a caregiver can create an eating disorder in a child.

IEC116. Elimination Disorders

Elimination disorders include functional encopresis and enuresis. There is a primary type, in which expected urinary or bowel control has not been reached by an age-expected outer limit of normal development, and a secondary type in which it has been reached but has been subsequently lost. Children who withhold their stool or urine are also considered to have elimination disorders.

PRESENTING PATTERN

Children with elimination disorders may experience a range of affective states. Fear, shame, and embarrassment over the "accident" are readily observed.

At a deeper subjective level, the child often feels unsure about his or her body. There is a pervasive sense of insecurity about bodily functioning with significant anxiety over "not being in control" of unexpected urges. Because of this apprehensiveness, some children defend against perceiving the bodily signals to eliminate and may hide or deny their bodily needs. They may compensate by trying to "control" everyone else. Some children are not sufficiently aware of needing to urinate or defecate until "too late." They may have poor sensory registration of their bodies' signals, coupled with reduced muscle tone, leaving them confused and embarrassed. For others, mastery of toileting implies demanding expectations of being "big" which conflict with wishes to remain the baby. This conflict may originally be either the child's or the parent's, but it usually becomes a mutual theme as caregiver and child struggle with fears of loss and separation, incompetence, changes in alliances, (e.g., babies belong to mom but big boys go to daddy), or other conflicts.

The child's mental content in play and conversation tends to mirror the affective patterns described above. Play themes may be characterized by avoidance of strong affect, explosive bursts of affective content, and alternations between the two. The child often verbalizes a wish to "do better" and please the caregivers, coupled with less conscious negativism and intermittent impulsivity. In the content of the child's play, one sees shame, embarrassment, avoidance, impulsivity, and fragmentation. An examination of functional developmental capacities can help identify the constrictions contributing to these problems and the specific dynamic formulation which may be relevant.

REGULATORY-SENSORY PROCESSING DISORDERS (RSPD)

Sensory Modulation Difficulties (Type I)
IEC201. Overresponsive, Fearful, Anxious Pattern
IEC202. Overresponsive, Negative, Stubborn Pattern
IEC203. Underresponsive, Self-Absorbed Pattern IEC203.1 Self-Absorbed and Difficult-to-Engage Type IEC203.2 Self-Absorbed and Creative Type
IEC204. Active, Sensory-Seeking Pattern
Sensory Discrimination Difficulties (Type II) and Sensory-Based Motor Difficulties (Type III)
IEC205. Inattentive, Disorganized Pattern IEC205.1 With Sensory Discrimination Difficulties IEC205.2 With Postural Control Difficulties IEC205.3 With Dyspraxia IEC205.4 With Combinations of All Three
IEC206. Compromised School and/or Academic Performance Pattern IEC206.1 With Sensory Discrimination Difficulties IEC206.2 With Postural Control Difficulties IEC206.3 With Dyspraxia IEC206.4 With Combinations of All Three
Contributing Sensory Discrimination and Sensory-Based Motor Difficulties
IEC207. Mixed Regulatory-Sensory Processing Patterns IEC207.1 Attentional Problems IEC207.2 Disruptive Behavioral Problems IEC207.3 Sleep Problems IEC207.4 Eating Problems IEC207.5 Elimination Problems IEC207.6 Selective Mutism IEC207.7 Mood Dysregulation, including Bipolar Patterns IEC207.8 Other Emotional and Behavioral Problems Related to Mixed Regulatory-Sensory Processing Difficulties IEC207.9 Mixed Regulatory-Sensory Processing Difficulties where Behavioral or Emotional Problems Are Not Yet in Evidence

Regulatory-sensory processing disorders (RSPD) should be viewed as being on a continuum. The regulatory-sensory profile of each child is unique. Children vary in the ways they respond to different sensations (such as touch and sound), comprehend these sensations, and plan actions. Some children have processing differences that are extreme enough to interfere with daily functioning at home, in school, in other interactions with peers or adults, and with routine functions such as self-care, sleeping, and eating. As we describe regulatory-sensory processing patterns below, note that while we focus on the disorders end of the continuum, the same patterns in more minor versions can characterize children without diagnosable disorders. Understanding individual differences in regulatory-sensory processing can help therapists and families find ways to promote healthy emotional, social, and intellectual functioning in any child.

Although researchers have long noted variations in motor and sensory functioning in infants and young children, the concept of RSPD arose in the 1980s and early 1990s with Greenspan's concept of Regulatory Disorders (Greenspan, et al., 1987; Greenspan, 1992). Ayers' (1964, 1972) concept of Sensory Processing Disorders has been developing along parallel lines for several decades. In 2004, a framework describing a new taxonomy of classic patterns and subtypes of sensory processing problems was presented (Miller, Cermak, Lane, Anzalone, & Koomar, 2004).

Regulatory Disorder as a diagnostic entity was subsequently incorporated into the classification system of Zero to Three: National Center for Infants, Toddlers, and Families. More recently, the Regulatory-Sensory Processing Work Group of the Interdisciplinary Council on Developmental and Learning Disorders (ICDL) has brought together the occupational therapy literature and the Developmental, Individual-Difference, Relationship-Based (DIR) model of Infant and Early Childhood Mental Health (Greenspan, 1992) and has reformulated and expanded the description of Regulatory-Sensory Processing Disorders.[4]

All children have individual regulatory-sensory processing patterns. Personal variations are important to consider when constructing a developmental profile for a specific infant or child and family. An RSPD should be considered when the child's motor and sensory patterns interfere with age-expected emotional, social, language, cognitive (including attention), motor, or sensory functioning. RSPD gives rise to some of the same symptoms and behaviors as interactive disorders, including nightmares, withdrawal, aggressiveness, fearfulness and anxiety, sleeping and eating disturbances, and difficulty in peer relationships. In contrast to interactive disorders, however, RSPD involves clearly identifiable constitutional-maturational factors in the child.

---

[4] See the Interdisciplinary Council on Developmental and Learning Disorders' Diagnostic Manual for Infancy and Early Childhood (ICDL-DMIC) for a fuller description of these disorders (ICDL-DMIC Diagnostic Classification Task Force, 2005).

Clinical Evidence and Prevalence of Regulatory-Sensory Processing Differences

There is now considerable evidence for the existence of regulatory-sensory processing differences in children with a range of mental health, developmental, and learning Difficulties and disorders. For an overview of this research, please see the ICDL-DMIC (ICDL-DMIC Diagnostic Classification Task Force, 2005) section on regulatory-sensory processing disorders. To understand the contributions of regulatory-sensory processing differences to children's functioning, one must discriminate between research which includes attention to these processes as part of a comprehensive, developmental, biopsychosocial intervention program (Greenspan & Wieder, 2003) and studies that focus only on interventions for specific sensory processing dimensions.

Diagnosis of Regulatory-Sensory Processing Disorders

RSPD involves a distinct behavior pattern *and* a sensory modulation, sensory-motor, sensory discrimination or attentional processing difficulty. When a behavioral and a sensory pattern are not both present, other diagnoses may be more appropriate. For example, an infant who is irritable and withdrawn after being abandoned may be suffering a relationship or attachment difficulty. An infant who is irritable and overly responsive to routine interpersonal experiences, in the absence of a clearly identified sensory, sensory-motor or processing difficulty, may have an anxiety or mood disorder.

General terms such as "overly sensitive," "difficult temperament," or "reactive" have commonly been used to describe infants and children with atypical motor and sensory processing. But clinicians have tended to use such terms without specifying the sensory system or motor functions involved. There is growing evidence that constitutional and early maturational patterns contribute to the difficulties of such infants, but it is also clear that early care-giving patterns can exert considerable influence on how constitutional-maturational patterns develop and become part of a child's evolving personality. As interest in these children increases, it is important to systematize descriptions of the sensory, motor, and integrative patterns, as well as the care giving patterns presumed to be involved.

For a Regulatory-Sensory Processing Disorder to be appropriately diagnosed in an infant or young child, the clinician must observe one or more behavioral difficulties *and* a sensory processing difficulty, such as a problem with sensory modulation, sensory-motor functioning, sensory discrimination or attention.

SENSORY MODULATION DIFFICULTIES (TYPE I)

The first group of regulatory-sensory processing disorders involves difficulties in *sensory modulation,* characterized by an inability to grade the degree, intensity, and nature of responses to sensory input. Often the child's responses do not fit the demands of the situation. The child therefore has trouble achieving and maintaining an optimal range of performance and adaptation to ordinary challenges. There are three subtypes of sensory modulation problems.

IEC201. Overresponsive, Fearful, Anxious Pattern

Some children have responses to sensory stimuli that are more intense, quicker in onset, or longer-lasting than those of most children facing the same conditions. Their responses are particularly pronounced when the stimulus is not anticipated. They may demonstrate over-responsivity in only one sensory system (e.g., "auditory defensiveness" or "tactile defensiveness") or they may demonstrate it in multiple sensory systems. Over-responsivity to sensory stimuli in multiple modalities is often referred to as sensory defensiveness. Children with this problem are usually particularly reactive to specific types of stimuli within a sensory domain (e.g., in the tactile domain they respond defensively to light touch but not to deep pressure), rather than to all stimuli within a domain.

Responses to sensory stimuli occur along a spectrum. Some children manage their tendency towards over-responsivity most of the time, while other children are overresponsive almost continuously. Responses may appear inconsistent because over-responsivity is highly dependent on context. While children may generally attempt to avoid particular sensory experiences, sensitivities may vary throughout the day, and from day to day. Since sensory input tends to have a cumulative effect, a child's efforts to control responses to sensory stimuli may build up and result in a sudden behavioral disruption in response to a seemingly trivial stimulus.

A child's behavioral characteristics when faced with uncomfortable stimuli can fall within a broad range. At one end, the child shows fearfulness and anxiety, often avoiding many sensory experiences. At the other end, the child shows negativity and stubbornness, or obstinacy exemplified by attempts to control the environment. This latter tendency is described as a separate type below. This range of reactions is often termed the "fight, flight, fright, or freeze" response, and is attributed to sympathetic nervous system activation. Secondary behavioral characteristics include irritability, fussiness, poor adaptability, moodiness, inconsolability, and poor socialization. In general, children who are overresponsive to sensation have difficulty with transitions and unexpected changes.

Sensory over-responsivity is often seen with other sensory reaction patterns. For example, children may show overresponsiveness to tactile stimuli while seeking proprioceptive stimuli. Sensory over-responsivity also may be observed concomitantly with sensory discrimination problems and dyspraxia.

Associated behavior patterns include excessive cautiousness, inhibition, and fearfulness. The child avoids sensation in an effort to control unexpected incoming stimuli. In early infancy, one sees a restricted range of exploration and assertiveness, dislike of changes in routine, and a tendency to be frightened and to cling. The behavior of toddlers and older preschoolers with sensory over-responsivity is characterized by excessive worrying and shyness in new experiences, such as forming peer relationships or engaging with new adults. Occasionally, the child behaves impulsively when overloaded or frightened, becoming easily upset, hard to soothe, and slow to recover from frustration or disappointment, especially in environments with multiple or intense sensory stimuli. The fearful and cautious child may have a fragmented, rather than an integrated, internal representational world, and may therefore be easily distracted by different stimuli.

Caregiver patterns that are characterized by soothing, regulating interactions; that respect the child's sensitivities; and that do not convey that the child has "bad behaviors" are helpful. Supportive parents anticipate noxious environments and minimize them or prepare the child for them. Enhancing flexibility and assertiveness in fearful and cautious children requires empathy, especially for the child's sensory and affective experience. Caregivers who give low-key support to explore new experiences and also set gentle but firm limits do well with these children. Inconsistent caregiver patterns intensify their difficulties, as when caregivers are overindulgent or overprotective some of the time and punitive or intrusive at other times.

IEC202. Overresponsive, Negative, Stubborn Pattern

Children with an overresponsive, negative, stubborn pattern may show evidence of the same physiologic responses described above for the overresponsive, fearful and anxious child. These children, however, seek to control their sensory environments and thus may prefer repetition and the absence of change or, at most, change at a slow, predictable pace. Rather than becoming fearful, anxious, and cautious, they attempt to control their environments to minimize fear and anxiety.

Behavior patterns may appear negative, stubborn, and controlling. The child can become aggressive and impulsive in response to sensory stimulation, often doing the opposite of what is requested or expected. Infants with this pattern tend to be fussy, difficult, and resistant to transitions and changes. Preschoolers tend to be negative, angry, and stubborn, as well as compulsive and perfectionistic. However, these children can display joyful, flexible behavior in certain situations.

In contrast to the fearful or cautious child, the negative and stubborn child does not become fragmented but organizes an integrated sense of self around negative patterns. In contrast to the impulsive, sensation-seeking child (described below) the negative and stubborn child is more controlling, tends to be avoidant of, or slow to engage in, new experiences rather than to crave them, and is not generally aggressive unless provoked.

Caregiver patterns that enhance flexibility involve soothing, empathetic support of slow, gradual change and avoidance of power struggles. (Caregivers can avoid power struggles by offering the child choices and opportunities for negotiation whenever possible.) Caregivers' warmth, coupled with gentle, firm guidance and limits—even in the face of negative or impulsive responses that may feel like rejection—is critical to helping an oppositional child. Encouragement of symbolic representation of affects (especially dependency, anger, and annoyance) also helps children with this pattern to become more flexible. In contrast, caregiver patterns that are intrusive, excessively demanding, over-stimulating, or punitive tend to intensify negative patterns.

IEC203. Underresponsive, Self-Absorbed Pattern

Children who are underresponsive to sensory stimuli are often quiet and passive, disregarding or not responding to available sensory information. Alternatively, they may be so enthralled by a world of their own imagination that they have trouble engaging in the here and now. They may appear withdrawn, difficult to engage, and/or self-absorbed because they have not registered the sensory input in their environment. The term "poor registration" is often used to describe their behavior, as they do not seem to detect or "register" incoming sensory information. They may also appear apathetic and lethargic, giving the impression of lacking the inner drive that most children have for socialization and motor exploration. Actually, they do not notice the possibilities for action that are around them. Their under-responsivity to tactile and proprioceptive inputs may lead to poorly developed body schemata, clumsiness, or poorly modulated movement. These children may fail to respond to bumps, falls, cuts, scrapes, or objects that may burn or chill them, as they may not notice pain. This aspect of their sensory problem presents a significant danger. Children with sensory under-responsivity also may have sensory discrimination problems and dyspraxia.

Children who are underresponsive to sensation often do not seek greater intensity in sensory input even though they may require it for optimal maturation. Because they fail to make demands on people and things in the environment, children with this pattern may be overlooked as the "good baby" or "easy child." They often need high intensity and highly salient input in order to become actively involved in the environment, the task, or the interaction.

Some children who are easily overloaded by sensory stimulation may appear to be underresponsive when in fact they are extremely overresponsive. The observable behavior is one that suggests withdrawal and shutdown, perhaps as a defense mechanism.

Some children with an underresponsive pattern are self-absorbed, unaware, and disengaged, while others, equally self-absorbed, are very creative and overly focused on their own fantasy lives. Therefore, we describe two subtypes for the underresponsive self-absorbed pattern.

IEC203.1 Self-Absorbed and Difficult-to-Engage Type

Behavior patterns in the self-absorbed, difficult-to-engage child include seeming disinterest in exploring relationships or engaging with challenging games or objects. These children may appear apathetic, easily exhausted, and remote. High affective tone and saliency are required to attract their interest, attention, and emotional engagement. Infants may appear delayed or depressed, lacking in motor exploration and social overtures. In addition to continuing the above patterns, preschoolers may evidence diminished verbal dialogue. Their behavior and play may present a limited range of ideas and fantasies. Sometimes, children seek out desired sensory input by engaging in repetitive sensory activities, such as spinning, swinging, or jumping up and down on a bed. The child needs the intensity or repetition of these activities in order to experience them fully.

Caregiver patterns that provide high-energy interactive input help engage the child in activities and relationships and foster initiative. These involve energized wooing and robust responses to the child's cues, however faint. In contrast, caregiver patters that are low-key, "laid back," or depressive in tone and rhythm tend to intensify these children's patterns of withdrawal.

IEC203.2 Self-Absorbed and Creative Type

Behavior patterns of some self-absorbed children, many of whom are also creative, include a tendency to tune into their own sensations, thoughts, and emotions rather than communications from others. Infants may become interested in objects through solitary exploration rather than in the context of interaction. They may appear inattentive, easily distracted, or preoccupied, especially when they are not pulled into a task or interaction. Preschoolers with this pattern tend to escape into fantasy when faced with external challenges, such as a demanding activity or competition from a peer. They may prefer to play by themselves if others do not actively join into imaginative play as they have scripted it. In their fantasy life, they may show enormous imagination and creativity.

Caregiver patterns that are beneficial include efforts to help the child engage in genuine dialogue; that is, to "open and close circles of communication." Caregivers should also encourage a good balance between fantasy and reality and help a child who is attempting to escape into fantasy stay grounded in external reality (e.g., by showing sensitivity to the child's interests and feelings; by promoting engagement and discussion of daily events, feelings, and other real-world topics; and by making fantasy play a collaborative endeavor between parent and child rather than a solitary activity). In contrast, a caregiver's self-absorption or preoccupation tends to intensify the child's difficulties, as does any pattern of confusing family communications.

IEC204. Active, Sensory-Seeking Pattern

Some children actively seek sensory stimulation and seem to have an almost insatiable desire for sensory input. They energetically engage in activities geared toward adding more intense "feelings" to satisfy this craving. They tend to be constantly moving, crashing, bumping, and jumping; they may want to touch everything and have difficulty inhibiting this behavior; they may play music or television at loud volumes, fixate on visually stimulating objects or events, or seek out unusual smells and tastes. Their sensory experiences are more intense and longer lasting than those of children with typical sensory responsivity.

Atypical responses occur along a spectrum; some sensory-seeking behavior is normal. Children at the sensation-seeking end of the continuum prefer a higher level of arousal than adults usually feel is appropriate in a given situation. For individuals with reduced awareness of sensation, sensory seeking may be a means to obtain enhanced input – that is, to increase their level of arousal. For children who are sensory seekers, the need for constant stimulation is difficult to fulfill and may be particularly problematic in environments (e.g., schools, performances, movies, libraries) where children are expected to sit quietly. When it is unstructured, the sought-after additional sensory stimulation may increase the child's overall state of arousal and result in disorganized behavior. If directed, however, it can have an organizing effect.

When their sensory needs are not met, these children tend to become demanding and insistent. They may be impulsive, almost explosive, in their attempts to fill their quota for sensation. Adjectives that describe the secondary behavioral characteristics of these children include overly active or aggressive, impulsive, intense, demanding, hard to calm, restless, overly affectionate, and attention-craving. Constant or extreme craving of sensory input can disrupt children's ability to maintain attention and learn. Activities of daily living are frequently disrupted. Children with this pattern may have trouble in school because their drive to obtain extra sensory stimulation interferes with their focusing on tasks.

Behavior patterns involve high activity and the seeking of physical contact and stimulation; for example, through deep pressure and intense movement. The motorically disorganized child who craves stimulation is notable for disruptive behavior (e.g., breaking things, unprovoked hitting, intruding into other people's physical space). Behavior that begins as a result of craving sensations may be interpreted by others as aggression rather than excitability. Once others react aggressively, the child's own behavior may become aggressive in response.

Infants in this group are most satisfied when provided with strong sensation in the form of movement, sound, touch, or visual stimulation. They may be content only when held or rocked. Toddlers may be very active. Preschoolers often show aggressive, intrusive behavior and a daredevil, risk-taking style, as well as preoccupation with aggressive themes in pretend play. Young children who are anxious or unsure of themselves may use counterphobic behaviors such as hitting another child first, in anticipation of being hit, or repeating unacceptable behavior after being asked to stop. When older and capable of self-reflection, the child may describe the need for stimulation as a way to feel alive, vibrant, and powerful. Children with this pattern have a tendency to "get in trouble" as they create situations that others perceive as bad or dangerous.

Caregiver patterns characterized by continuous, warm relating, a great deal of nurturing, and empathy, together with clear structure and limits, enhance flexibility and adaptivity. Caregivers should understand the need for extra stimulation and give the child many opportunities to acquire more stimulation, preferably through interactive, modulated play. Encouraging the use of imagination and verbal dialogue to explore the environment and elaborate feelings further enhances the child's flexibility. Advocacy in settings outside the home is required so that others understand the child's behavior, adapt these constructive caregiver patterns, and avoid labeling the child a "behavior problem." In contrast, caregiver patterns that lack warm, continuous engagement (e.g., frequent changing of caregivers); that over- or underestimate the child; that are overly punitive; or that vacillate between harsh consequences and insufficient limit-setting may intensify the child's difficulties.

SENSORY DISCRIMINATION DIFFICULTIES (TYPE II) AND SENSORY-BASED MOTOR DIFFICULTIES (TYPE III)

As indicated earlier, in addition to problems related to sensory modulation, there are regulatory-sensory processing disorders related to difficulties in sensory discrimination and sensory-based motor skills (e.g., postural control problems and dyspraxia). For example, children with sensory discrimination difficulties may find it difficult to determine what they are touching or how close to stand to someone else. Children with dyspraxia (motor planning and sequencing problems) may find it difficult to carry out a multi-step task.

These two regulatory-sensory processing disorders are associated with inattentive, disorganized behavior patterns and problems in school performance. They may involve various combinations of difficulties in either sensory discrimination or sensory-based motor performance, or both.

IEC205. Inattentive, Disorganized Pattern
IEC205.1 With Sensory Discrimination Difficulties
IEC205.2 With Postural Control Difficulties
IEC205.3 With Dyspraxia
IEC205.4 With Combinations of All Three

Behavior patterns related to sensory discrimination, motor planning and/or postural control include a tendency to be inattentive and disorganized. For example, the child may have difficulty following through on tasks or school assignments. In the middle of a homework assignment or household chore, he or she may wander off to some other activity, seemingly unmindful of the original goal. In the extreme, the child's behavior may appear fragmented. As others put more pressure on these children, they may become more disorganized. When these challenges continue over a period of time, they can easily become demoralized, depressed, and/or angry. Impulsive or defiant behavior is not uncommon, nor are passivity, avoidance, and preference for activities, such as video games, that are experienced as less demanding in terms of sequencing and organizing complex plans of action.

When such children are expected to attempt difficult tasks, one often sees increasing avoidance, fragmentation, and disorganization, as well as "inattentiveness." It is not unusual for parents to describe a child as "organized" and "attentive" when getting ready to go to the ice cream shop or the video arcade, and yet "fragmented," "inattentive," and "disorganized," when attempting a multi-step math problem. Clinicians as well as caregivers often ask whether such patterns differ from attentional problems or Attention Deficit Disorder. Attention to this type of behavior pattern help clinicians observe the relationship between specific regulatory-sensory processing patterns and more general attentional and organizational problems.

Caregiver patterns that recognize the underlying challenges can help the child strengthen the processing areas that are contributing to his difficulties. In addition, while the child is working to improve underlying processing skills, caregivers and educators who can help break down complex tasks into manageable steps and provide patient, multi-sensory support (visual, auditory, and motor cues) can help the child make progress. On the other hand, care-giving patterns that characterize the child as "unmotivated," "bad," or "lazy," and that pressure and punish the child, rather than helping to set up achievable goals that foster a sense of mastery, inevitably intensify the child's problems. The key to constructive caregiver patterns is to understand and strengthen the contributing processing functions that are described in some detail below.

IEC206. Compromised School and/or Academic Performance Pattern

IEC206.1 With Sensory Discrimination Difficulties
IEC206.2 With Postural Control Difficulties
IEC206.3 With Dyspraxia
IEC206.4 With Combinations of All Three

Behavior patterns associated with dyspraxia, postural control problems, and sensory discrimination difficulties may include problematic school performance in circumscribed areas. For example, difficulties with motor planning and postural control can make handwriting very difficult. Sensory discrimination difficulties may make distinguishing shapes or letters difficult. Visual-spatial problems may make lining up columns in math or in understanding concepts involving graphs or diagrams difficult. Motor planning and sequencing difficulties may also contribute to problems with sequencing ideas into sentences. If the contributing processing contributions to these types of compromises at school are not addressed, the child may become avoidant, disinterested, and/or demoralized. School itself can become viewed as a place of failure and school activities, or school as a whole, may be avoided.

Caregiver patterns that recognize the processing contributions to the child's school performance and provide supportive, step-wise help tend to improve the child's overall functioning. Caregivers who can break the challenge down into small enough steps for the child to experience a sense of mastery 70 to 80% of the time are likely to be especially helpful. Caregivers who are punitive, rejecting, or overly expectant often increase the difficulties. In contrast to a child with natural gifts in an activity, a child who has difficulty with a particular motor or sensory discrimination task has little pleasure in performing it. Therefore, support, guidance, incentives, and breaking the challenge down into easily-mastered steps are essential to helping the child overcome his limitations and feel a sense of pride and accomplishment.

IEC207. Mixed Regulatory-Sensory Processing Patterns

Many children have mixed regulatory-sensory processing patterns. Combinations of subtypes in one child are common, as are differences among various sensory domains in the same child. For example, it is not uncommon for a child to experience sensory over-responsivity in the tactile system and sensory-seeking in the vestibular and proprioceptive systems. In addition, atypical response patterns to sensation can vary as a function of time of day, environmental context, stress, fatigue, level of arousal and many other factors.

COMMON BEHAVIORAL DIFFICULTIES RELATED TO MIXED REGULATORY-SENSORY PROCESSING PATTERNS

These mixed regulatory-sensory processing patterns can occur with and without concomitant behavioral and emotional complications. A number of well-known symptom patterns are associated with mixed types of regulatory-sensory processing problems, of which a few are briefly described below. First, however, we should note that they may, instead or in addition, be related to interactive difficulties and/or unique motor and sensory processing problems. Where caregiver-child relational patterns seem to be the predominant contributor, an interactive disorder may be diagnosed; where the predominant contributor seems to be a unique motor or sensory processing pattern, RSPD should be considered. Once a diagnosis of RSPD seems warranted, the clinician should determine whether it constitutes a specific pattern, such as sensory over-responsivity, or a mixed pattern.

As with all mental health and developmental disorders in infancy and early childhood, there are always regulatory-sensory processing and interactive dimensions. The very common problems listed below are included in both the interactive and regulatory-sensory processing categories because for different children, one or the other feature may predominate. It would, therefore, be an oversimplification to list them arbitrarily in only one or the other category.

IEC207.1 Attentional Problems

Children with problems in attending and sustaining their focus may have a number of regulatory-sensory processing problems. Most have difficulties with motor planning and sequencing. Unless there is a great deal of structure guiding them, it is hard for them to carry out a planned series of actions to solve a problem. Many children with attentional problems also evidence sensory discrimination difficulties; for example, in figuring out complex visual-spatial patterns and solving visual-spatial problems (e.g., searching systematically for a hidden object in all parts of a room). In addition, some children with attentional problems are sensory-craving and are consequently very active and sometimes aggressive. A small percentage of children with attentional problems are sensory overresponsive and hence highly distractible. They easily become overloaded and fragmented in a noisy or busy setting. Contrastingly, some children with attentional problems are sensory underresponsive to the extent that ordinary sensations such as the human voice, which can usually orient a child, fails to draw their attention. Some very bright children with this pattern spend a considerable amount of time daydreaming. Clearly, many children with attentional problems evidence combinations of the above, such as motor planning problems and sensory under-responsivity.

IEC207.2 Disruptive Behavioral Problems

Many toddlers and preschoolers with sensory craving act destructively without necessarily intending to do so. Some of these children also have areas of sensory under-responsivity, for example, they may be relatively insensitive to pain, with the result that their disruptive, stimulation-seeking behavior becomes even more intense. Children with sensory discrimination difficulties, such as difficulty sorting out stimuli in the auditory realm, may find it harder to understand limits and guidelines. Each or any combination of these patterns can contribute to disruptive behaviors.

IEC207.3 Sleep Problems

Many children with difficulties falling asleep or sustaining sleep evidence some degree of sensory overresponsivity. Some also show sensory discrimination difficulties. Those with a great deal of sensory craving may resist sleep. These sensory problems may be compounded by a variety of environmental and relational factors that further undermine healthy sleep patterns.

IEC207.4 Eating Problems

Many children with eating difficulties evidence sensory overresponsivity, especially in their oral cavity. Some also have low muscle tone, including low tone in their oral-motor area, as well as motor planning and sequencing problems. Their oral-motor functioning difficulties can make eating a difficult task. Other children are underresponsive to sensation in the oral cavity, a condition that may make eating difficult because expectable sensations from food are not occurring. Environmental and caregiving patterns may exacerbate such problems.

IEC207.5 Elimination Problems

Many children with elimination problems have combinations of sensory under-responsivity, low muscle tone, and difficulty with motor planning and sequencing. Some, however, are sensory craving and still others are sensory overresponsive. For example, the child who is unable to sense when his or her bladder is full and who has a hard time regulating motor actions is more prone to "accidents."

IEC207.6 Selective Mutism

Children with selective mutism are often sensory overresponsive and consequently highly anxious. Typically, a school environment is a challenging setting because of noise and other stimuli. Although over-responsivity is the predominant contributor, children with selective mutism may also have dyspraxia. Attention to these differences, coupled with increasing the child's level of security and attending to the gradualness with which the child enters unfamiliar settings, can be very helpful.

IEC207.7 Mood Dysregulation, including Bipolar Patterns

Infants and young children with fluctuating moods often have underlying sensory over-responsivity coupled with sensory-seeking. When overloaded, instead of retreating and becoming cautious, they become more agitated and impulsive. As they become symbolic, their mood dysregulation can take the form of shifting from themes of anxiety and depression to those of anger and power. See the Interactive Disorder section for a fuller description of infants and young children with mood fluctuations, including bipolar patterns.

IEC207.8 Other Emotional and Behavioral Problems Related to Mixed Regulatory-Sensory Processing Difficulties

Children with mixed regulatory-sensory processing problems may evidence emotional or behavioral problems or symptoms not listed above, including anxiety, fearfulness, and negativism. When these patterns are related to mixed regulatory-sensory processing difficulties, they should be diagnosed as such.

IEC207.9 Mixed Regulatory-Sensory Processing Patterns Where Behavioral or Emotional Problems Are Not Yet In Evidence

In the early years of life, many children with mixed regulatory-sensory processing problems do not yet evidence clear emotional, social, and/or behavioral problems. Their difficulties may be noted by their parent, early childhood educators, or primary healthcare provider who may, for example, see that they are overresponsive to touch and have difficulty sequencing motor responses. The recognition of these challenges provides an opportunity for family guidance geared to improving functioning in such areas, thus preventing the emergence of emotional, social, and/or behavioral problems. Many parents and educators already implement such preventive strategies intuitively. Identifying these patterns, however, can help systematize these efforts and increase the number of children who are helped.

NEURODEVELOPMENTAL DISORDERS OF RELATING AND COMMUNICATING

IEC301. Type I: Early Symbolic, with Constrictions
IEC302. Type II: Purposeful Problem Solving, with Constrictions
IEC303. Type III: Intermittently Engaged and Purposeful
IEC304. Type IV: Aimless and Unpurposeful Other Neurodevelopmental Disorders (Including Genetic and Metabolic Syndromes)

Neurodevelopmental Disorders of Relating and Communicating (NDRC) involve problems in multiple aspects of a child's development, including social relationships, language, cognitive functioning, and sensory and motor processing. This category includes earlier conceptualizations of multisystem developmental disorders (MSDD), as characterized in *Infancy and Early Childhood* (Greenspan, 1992) and *Diagnostic Classification: 0-3* (DC 0-3) (Diagnostic Classification Task Force, 1994). Additionally, it includes the DSM-IV category of pervasive developmental disorders (PDD), also referred to as autism spectrum disorders (ASD), which includes autism, Asperger's Syndrome, and PDD-NOS. The main distinction between NDRC and the earlier conceptualizations is that the NDRC framework enables a clinician to subtype disorders of relating and communicating more accurately, in terms of the child's level of social, intellectual, and emotional functioning and associated regulatory and sensory-motor processing profile. The framework thus helps to differentiate children commonly considered on the autism spectrum from children with other conditions. It also helps to define the variations seen among children with the same diagnosis. Such discriminations are important for both intervention planning and research purposes.

Since the descriptions of MSDD in 1992, and later in DC:0-3, and the description of PDD in DSM-IV, the ICDL Work Group has developed a broader framework to allow consideration of the full range of problems in relating, communicating, and thinking.[5]

---

[5] For a fuller discussion of neurodevelopmental disorders or relating and communicating, see the *Interdisciplinary Council on Developmental and Learning Disorders' Diagnostic Manual for Infancy and Early Childhood Mental Disorders, Developmental Disorders, Regulatory-Sensory Processing Disorders, Language Disorders, and Learning Challenges* (ICDL-DMIC Diagnostic Classification Task Force, 2005). The work group included Lois Black, Griffin Doyle, Barbara Dunbar, Stanley Greenspan, Barbara Kalmanson, Lori-Jean Peloquin, Ricki Robinson, Ruby Salazar, Rick Solomon, Rosemary White, Serena Wieder, and Molly Romer Witten.

As we look at individual variation and subtypes of disorders of relating and communicating, we discover that there are numerous biological and overall developmental pathways associated with them. For example, difficulty in connecting affect to perception and motor action, and subsequent difficulty in relating, communicating, and thinking, may be the result of several neurodevelopmental pathways, each with its own genetic or constitutional-maturational variations (Greenspan & Shanker, 2004). Therefore, we suggest a broad category of neurodevelopmental disorders of relating and communicating to facilitate advances in research, evaluation strategies, and clinical intervention programs.

Neurodevelopmental disorders of relating and communicating (NDRC) may be viewed as part of the broad neurological category of non-progressive central nervous system disorders. The technical term in ICD-10 is "static" (non-progressive) "encephalopathy" (a disorder of the central nervous system).

But developmental impairments may also result from severe environmental stress and trauma. For example, in failure-to-thrive syndrome and with severe deprivation patterns, an infant's motor, cognitive, language, affective, and/or physical growth may slow down or cease altogether. Persistent abuse or neglect can produce a similar global disruption in development and functioning.

The Developmental, Individual-Difference, Relationship-Based (DIR) approach helps us understand the development of adaptive capacities and pathologic symptoms in each infant or child. For example, an infant's impairments in auditory-verbal, visual-spatial, or perceptual-motor processing can make ordinary relating and communicating extremely difficult. Even reasonably stable, supportive, and empathic parents may be unable to find ingenious ways to engage and interact with a child with these difficulties. The resulting lack of appropriate human interaction may prevent vital social learning during key periods of development. Between 12 and 24 months of age, for example, most children develop several critical skills at an especially rapid rate—reciprocal affective and motor gesturing, comprehending the "rules" that govern complex social interactions, pattern recognition, a sense of self, and early forms of thinking. A deficit in these skills can easily be misunderstood as a primary deficit rather than a consequence of underlying biologically-based processing impairments.

A new hypothesis to understand the biological and experiential relationships in the developmental pathway leading to autism spectrum disorders has recently been formulated. According to the affect-diathesis hypothesis (Greenspan & Wieder, 1999; Greenspan & Shanker, 2004; ICDL Clinical Practice Guidelines Workgroup, 2000), the core biological deficit expresses itself as a difficulty in connecting emerging affects to sensation or perception, and to emerging sensory-motor patterns to form sensory-affect-motor patterns. Later on, this same difficulty compromises the toddler's capacity to connect affect to complex, problem-solving motor patterns and emerging symbols or language.

Normally, infants make sensory-affect-motor connections as they begin to attend to the world. For example, turning toward mother's smiling face and voice requires perception, pleasurable affect, and motor action. This sensory-affect-motor connection becomes especially important in the second half of the first year of life as the infant increasingly engages in reciprocal social and emotional communications. In these interchanges, affect clearly guides purposeful motor actions, such as exchanging vocalizations, trading funny little grins, reaching for the piece of banana in mommy's mouth, and so forth.

By the early part of the second year, the child's ability to connect sensation, affect, and motor action becomes even more vital as the toddler engages in shared social problem solving—for example, taking a caregiver by the hand, gesturing to the toy area, pointing to a toy on a shelf and making back-and-forth gestures to be picked up to reach the desired toy. In such interactions, as in earlier developmental stages, the child's purposeful or intentional behavior is clearly fueled by affect – in this example, desire for the toy. Yet now the child's affect is involved in many successive back-and-forth interactions. Affect thus guides the relationship between perception and a complex, multi-step social and motor action. The vast majority of children with autism spectrum disorders, even when these disorders are diagnosed at later ages, are reported by their parents to have had difficulty in mastering this early capacity (i.e., a flow of back-and-forth affective signals) for shared social problem-solving (Greenspan & Wieder, 1997).

Therefore, it is hypothesized that in the autism spectrum disorders, a biologically based difficulty forming an early sensory-affect-motor connection lays the groundwork for subsequent difficulties connecting affect to complex motor patterns and shared social problem-solving. As the capacity to repeat words emerges, this same difficulty compromises the child's learning to connect affect to words to give them meaning (e.g., the child repeats words without clear affective intent).

Children vary, however, in the degree to which this fundamental capacity is disrupted. They also differ in basic motor, sensory modulation, visual-spatial, auditory processing, and language capacities. Without the capacity to connect affect or intent to these fundamental capacities, especially the initial motor capacities, these related capacities are not properly developed. For example, children with relatively strong auditory processing and verbal capacities may, because of their strong auditory memory, repeat whole books but at the same time be unable to use language meaningfully. Similarly, children with relatively strong motor capacities may line up their toys but be unable to engage in motor-based interactive problem solving.

Children with weaknesses in these related developmental capacities may evidence little or no verbal behavior at all and only simple repetitive or aimless motor behavior. Children with relative strengths in the developmental capacities tend to make progress more rapidly once engaged in a comprehensive intervention program that works with their core difficulty connecting affect to sensations and movements. Such an intervention program must take into account the child's unique developmental profile. Children appear to have the flexibility to develop side-roads even when the main highway is fairly obstructed (Greenspan & Wieder, 1997, 1998, 1999).

Four general types of NDRC have been observed in children with significant difficulties in relating, communicating, and thinking (ICDL-DMIC Diagnostic Classification Task Force, 2005). These types exist on a continuum and often overlap. As children make progress in treatment, one sees movement within each type as well as movement from one type to another. Each type is described below, along with a brief clinical illustration.

IEC301. Type I: Early Symbolic, with Constrictions

Children with Type I disorders have constricted capacities for shared attention, engagement, initiation of two-way affective communication, and shared social problem-solving. Without intervention, they have difficulty maintaining a continuous flow of affective interactions and can open and close only four to ten consecutive circles of communication (a circle of communication is a back-and-forth interaction in which the infant or child both initiate engagement and respond to the caregiver's gestures). Perseveration and some degree of self-absorption are common in children with this type of disorder. At initial evaluation, one sees islands of memory-based symbol use, such as labeling pictures or repeating memorized scripts, but the child does not display an age-expected range of affect and has difficulty integrating symbol use with other core developmental capacities and engaging in all processes simultaneously.

With an intervention program that addresses individual processing differences and promotes shared attention and reciprocal affective communication, children with Type I difficulties tend to make rapid progress. Often, one sees such a child move from constricted relational patterns, perseveration, self-stimulation, and self-absorption toward warm, pleasurable engagement and a continuous flow of affective interactions. The child begins initiating such interactions by spontaneous use of language and maintains the flow of interactions at the level of two-way problem-solving communication, creating ideas and building bridges between ideas. Even when language is delayed, the child is able to sequence complex gestures (signs) and use toys to symbolize ideas until language is strengthened. Thus, such children move toward abstract and reflective levels of symbolic thinking. Their more robust capacities enable them to develop healthy peer relationships and participate in typical activities.

Eventually, with appropriate intervention, most children with Type I difficulties can participate fully in a regular academic program. An aide may be required for a period of time to help with regulatory-sensory processing and related attentional problems. In addition, because academic skills and abstract thinking depend on processing abilities, educational interventions to address specific learning difficulties may be required.

CLINICAL ILLUSTRATION OF TYPE I

David, age 2½ years, was self-absorbed, perseverative, and given to self-stimulation. He did not make eye contact with his parents or show much pleasure in relating to them, nor did he play with other children. During his evaluation, David spent most of his time reciting numbers or letters in a rote sequence, spinning and jumping around randomly, and lining up toys and cars while making self-stimulatory sounds. When he was extremely motivated, he could blurt out what he wanted. He occasionally showed affection by hugging his parents and although he never looked at them, he tolerated their hugs. He could imitate actions, sounds, and words, and he recognized pictures and shapes.

David's regulatory and sensory processing profile showed both weaknesses and strengths. He was a highly active child, interested in learning about the world, even though he could do so only in a fragmented and fleeting way as he flitted around the room, flapping his arms, searching for something familiar. His intense movement also served to increase his muscle tone and energy. When an object captured his attention, he would explore it briefly and sometimes blurt out its label with no evident communicative intent. He could recite memorized letters and numbers, but he could not process (comprehend) what others said to him. By his third year he was becoming increasingly self-absorbed and would resort to exciting himself with his recitations, but he was unable to respond to his name, much less engage in any two-way communication. David also demonstrated some visual-spatial strength, in that he could discriminate objects in his environment and later locate them again. As he could not process incoming auditory feedback from others, he sought out mirrors to reflect what he was doing and used them for visual feedback. He also manipulated toys and could use them in simple sequences that showed understanding of what they represented (e.g., he would pretend to eat the toy food or push the toy car), indicating he had the rudiments of connecting purposeful intent to motor planning. This was also seen in his ability to initiate new actions with toys and make ritualized movements to songs. It was also evident that David had strong affect. He showed great pleasure when happy—even in his self-absorbing pursuits—and intense anger or avoidance when thwarted. His ability to initiate and connect affect to intent was his strongest asset. While his auditory and visual processing capacities were significantly compromised, these relative strengths boded well.

With a comprehensive intervention program, David quickly became more engaged. He entered into a continuous flow of affective interactions, began initiating long pretend sequences, and gradually began using language purposefully and creatively. His early perseverative interest in cars transformed into a capacity to use them in elaborate symbolic dramas. Cars remained a special interest for several years, during which he became the resident "expert" on brands and models. This preoccupation gave way as he expanded his emotional range and interests and improved his motor planning abilities. In the highly interactive sessions he had with his parents and therapist, he spontaneously explored and rehearsed new emotional themes, and he eventually became an abstract thinker. He could also reflect on his feelings and became highly empathic with others.

In the pattern of progress described above, David's developing capacities enabled him to begin relating more to both parents and peers. At present, as a teenager, David attends a regular school, where he excels in English and math. He continues to have some difficulty with fine motor sequencing (e.g., with penmanship). Although he did not become an athlete, he enjoys shooting baskets or playing tennis with friends, and he writes the sports feature in his school paper. He is still quite active and enterprising; currently he is looking for opportunities to do "business." While he tends to become somewhat argumentative in competitive situations, he enjoys close friendships, has a good sense of humor, and shows insight into other people's feelings.

IEC302. Type II: Purposeful Problem Solving, with Constrictions

When seen initially (often between ages 2 and 4 years), children with Type II disorder have significant constrictions in the third and fourth core developmental capacities: purposeful, two-way presymbolic communication and social problem-solving communication. They engage in only intermittent interactions at these levels, completing at most two to five circles of communication in a row. Other than repeating a few memorized scripts from favorite shows, they exhibit few islands of true symbolic activity. Many of these children show some capacity for engagement, but their engagement has a global, need-oriented, on-their-own-terms emotional quality. They often have moderate processing dysfunctions in multiple areas.

Children in this group face greater challenges than those in Type I. In treatment, their progress is typically consistent yet slow. Overcoming each hurdle requires a great deal of work. Over time, they can learn to engage with real warmth and pleasure. They steadily improve their capacities for purposeful inter-action and shared social problem solving, learning to initiate and sustain a con-tinuous flow of affective interactions. The slow development of this continuous flow prevents a more robust development of symbolic capacities; these also improve, but tend to rely on imitation of books and videos as a basis for lan-guage and imaginative play. As these children gradually progress through each new capacity, they begin creating ideas and may even start to build bridges between ideas in circumscribed areas of interest. However, they do not display an age-appropriate depth and range of affect, and their abstract thinking is limited and focused on real-life needs.

Although many children in this group make continuous progress, most can-not participate in all the activities of a regular classroom, especially one with a large number of children. They can, however, benefit from appropriately staffed inclusion or integrated programs, or from special needs classrooms, providing that language development is emphasized and the other children are interactive and verbal.

CLINICAL ILLUSTRATION OF TYPE II

Three-year-old Joey was extremely avoidant, always moving away from his caregivers and making only fleeting eye contact with them. He displayed consider-able perseverative and self-stimulatory behavior, such as rapidly turning the pages of preferred books or pushing his toy train around and around the track. He also chose books and figures from his favorite shows, such as Barney or Win-nie the Pooh, and had them board his trains. No one dared to touch his figures because he would tantrum instantly when he thought they would be taken away. He could purposefully reach for his juice, put out his arms to get dressed, give his parents an object or take one from them, but despite some vocalizing, he could neither negotiate complex preverbal interactions nor imitate sounds. He showed pleasure with his parents only during roughhousing or tickle games and when his mother sang to him as he fell asleep.

Joey relied on visual information to deal with his environment. He had a remarkable memory for things and places. He was underresponsive to words spo-ken to him, but overresponsive to sudden, high-pitched or vibrating sounds, which distracted or alarmed him and kept him vigilant. He relied on ritualized patterns in daily life and protested changes he could not understand. While he seemed to find his favorite books or figures somehow, he did not search for things in any planned way, and was easily subject to frustration and tantrums. Obstacle courses were beyond him; rather than follow the other children in the preschool gym, he would collapse on the floor and watch them. These patterns reflect the multiple sensory and motor processing difficulties (auditory, visual-spatial and motor planning), compounded by over- and underresponsiveness and low tone. Life was becoming more and more challenging for Joey and for his family, as he pulled away from relationships and frustrated the expectations that went along with his getting older.

Joey's intervention program addressed each of the processing areas in individual therapies and a home program. The emphasis was on expanding pleasurable relating and establishing a continuous flow of interactions through affect cueing and problem solving. As he became more engaged and began to expand his play, it became evident that Joey had islands of receptive symbolic understanding as suggested by his early interest in Barney riding his train. He began to use figures from various books and shows, first scripting and then recreating real-life experiences such as birthday parties. Visual strategies and oral motor treatment, involving exercises to enable him to use his tongue and mouth muscles more effectively, helped reduce his frustration.

Now, at age 6½, after nearly four years of intensive intervention, Joey can relate with real pleasure and joy. He uses complex gestures and words to negotiate with his parents. He can describe what he wants in sentences ("Give me juice now, I'm thirsty!") and respond to simple questions ("What do you want to do?" "Go to Disneyworld on my trains!"). He can have conversations involving four or five exchanges of short phrases. He enjoys listening to story books and is beginning to read words. He also engages in early and joyful imaginative play, throwing grand birthday parties or dressing up and making his action figures fly around the room. Joey insists on being the superhero but does not always have a motive (e.g., to get the bad guy) even when he has a destination.

Although he cannot yet consistently answer abstract "why" questions, Joey can do basic, real-life reasoning about safety. With some adult involvement, he is able to play with peers in the context of action or structured games. He is now in an inclusion kindergarten program, and he participates in pre-academic activities, with relative strengths in visual thinking and math. He also enjoys play dates with his classmates. Joey continues to make progress at a slow but consistent pace. Interestingly, Joey's perseverative, self-stimulatory patterns have largely abated.

IEC303. Type III: Intermittently Engaged and Purposeful

Children in this group are highly self-absorbed. Their engagement with others is extremely intermittent, having an "in and out" quality. They display very limited purposeful two-way communication, usually in pursuit of concrete needs or basic sensorimotor experiences (e.g., jumping, tickling). They may be able to imitate or even initiate some rote problem-solving actions, but they usually evidence little or no capacity for shared social problem-solving or for a continuous flow of affective exchange.

With affect-based intervention, children with Type III difficulties can become more robustly engaged in pleasurable activities, but their capacity for a continuous flow of affective interactions improves only very slowly. They can learn to convey simple feelings ("happy," "sad," and "mad"), but the "in and out" quality of their relatedness constricts the range and depth of affect they can negotiate. Over time, they can learn islands of presymbolic purposeful and problem-solving behavior. These islands may, at times, also involve the use of words, pictures, signs, or two- to three-step actions or gestures to communicate basic needs. Receptive understanding of often-used phrases, in routines or when coupled with visual cues or gestures, can become a relative strength.

Some children in this group use toys as if they are real, for example, they try to eat pretend foods or feed a life-size baby doll, or put their feet into a pretend swimming pool as if they could go swimming. They do not usually reach the level of truly representing themselves using toys or dolls. Multiple severe processing dysfunctions, including severe auditory processing and visual-spatial processing difficulties and moderate-to-severe motor planning problems, impede the continuous flow of purposeful communication, thus preventing problem-solving interactions.

Some children in this group have severe oral-motor dyspraxia and speak only a few words if they speak at all; they may, however, learn to use a few signs or to communicate using pictures or a favorite toy.

Children in this group require very individualized educational approaches. They may eventually learn to read words and to understand visual-spatial concepts through motor pathways. It is important that they be included in hybrid programs to encourage social activities, ritualized learning, and the development of friendships.

CLINICAL ILLUSTRATION OF TYPE III

Sarah, age 3 years, ran into the playroom looking for Winnie the Pooh. She climbed up on the stool in front of the shelves but could not move the little figures in the basket around to search for her beloved character. She inadvertently pulled the basket off the shelf, causing all the figures to fall out. Without bothering to look on the floor, Sarah began searching in the next basket. Her mother ran over to prevent the second basket from being dropped and offered to help. Sarah echoed "Help!" and grabbed her mother's hands and put them in the basket. Her mother had to point to the Pooh figure before Sarah could see it. She grabbed it and ran off to lie on the couch. Her mother then brought Tigger over to say hello; Sarah grabbed Tigger and ran to the other side of the room. She held her figures tightly and turned away when her mother joined her. Her mother then took the Eeyore figure and started to sing "Ring around the Rosie..." while moving Eeyore up and down. This time, Sarah looked, and joined in singing "down" to the lyric "all fall down." She then moved rapidly away and went over to the mirror. This pattern of flight and avoidance after getting what she wanted, followed by not knowing what to do next, was typical of Sarah.

With a comprehensive intervention program, Sarah slowly learned the labels for things she wanted. She learned how to protest rather than scream. She recognized and could say familiar phrases like "come and eat," "go out," and "bath time." She became quite engaged when involved in sensorimotor play and loved to be swung and tickled. She even began to play with toys, first dipping her toes into the water of the play pool and then letting Winnie jump in. She began to imitate more words and actions. She would try to initiate problem-solving interactions to get her figures, but only when she was very motivated or angry, and usually only after energetic sensorimotor play had pulled her in. Her expressive language expanded to include more and more phrases indicating what she wanted, but because her weak receptive processing made it difficult for her to answer any questions, she relied on visual and affect cues to understand what was said to her. This achievement transferred to puppet play and even simple role-playing in which she took the part of a cook or doctor. Because of Sarah's very poor motor planning, problem-solving progressed only glacially, but she became more easily engaged and more responsive to semi-structured and structured approaches to learning. Between ages 4 and 5, she learned to count and to identify colors, and she loved to paint and cut with scissors.

At age 6½, Sarah demonstrates some pre-academic abilities, including reading some words. She attends a special education class which integrates activities with less limited peers. She enjoys being with other children and joins the crowd in running around, hiding, and chasing, but she does not yet play interactively. She has, however, learned various social rituals of greeting, sharing, protesting, and so on. Sarah can also spontaneously communicate, with a big smile, "Feel happy!" or, with a frown, "Feel mad!"

IEC304. Type IV: Aimless and Unpurposeful

Children in this group are passive and self-absorbed or active and stimulus-seeking; some exhibit both patterns. They have severe difficulties with shared attention and engagement unless they are involved in sensorimotor play. They tend to make very slow progress. Developing expressive language is extremely challenging.

With intervention, children with Type IV difficulties can become warmly engaged and intermittently interactive through use of gestures and action games. Through their ability to relate and interact, they can learn to solve problems. The goal is to challenge them to open and close many consecutive circles of communication so that they can progress as much as possible in their problem-solving ability.

Some children with Type IV profiles learn to complete organized sequences of the sort needed to play semi-structured games or carry out self-help tasks, such as dressing and brushing teeth. Many such children can share with others the pleasure they experience when they use their bodies purposefully to skate, swim, ride bikes, play ball, or engage in other motor accomplishments. These meaningful activities can be used to encourage shared attention, engagement, and purposeful problem-solving.

Children in this group have the most severe challenges in all processing areas. Many have significant motoric deficits, including oral-motor dyspraxia. As a consequence, their progress is very uneven. They have the most difficulty with complex problem-solving interactions, expressive language, and motor planning. Their progress tends to be periodically interrupted by periods of regression, the causes of which are hard to discern. Sometimes, regressions appear to occur because the environment is not sufficiently tailored to the child's processing profile.

To engage a Type IV child, an educational approach must be highly meaningful to that child. Both visual and motor pathways must be found to help the child focus and learn.

CLINICAL ILLUSTRATION OF TYPE IV

Harold progressed only very slowly to imitating sounds and words, even with an intensive program to facilitate imitation. He could say one or two words spontaneously when he felt mad or insistent on getting something, but otherwise he had to be prompted and pushed to speak. Every utterance seemed to defeat him, and he would sometimes stare at a caregiver's mouth to try to form the same movements. His severe dyspraxia interfered with his engaging in pretend play, although from his facial expressions, especially the gleam in his eye during playful interactions with his parents, one could infer that he was playing little "tricks." He sometimes used toy objects such as a soft sword or magic wand in ritualized ways, but he could not use toys to sequence new ideas. He could become engaged and even initiated sensorimotor interactions involving the expression of pleasure and affection.

Although games with his brother had to be orchestrated, Harold enjoyed running around the schoolyard and the pool with other children. At age 5, in the second year of intervention, he was able to communicate with three or four back-and-forth exchanges about what he wanted (e.g., pulling his dad over to the refrigerator and finding the hot dogs). He could even retrieve a few words at such moments: "Hot dog." "What else?" "French fries." Harold became more consistently engaged over time, developed islands of presymbolic ability, and tuned in to more of what was going on around him. He no longer wandered aimlessly and could be observed picking up trucks to push, putting together simple puzzles, or engaging in other cause-and-effect play. He let others join him but invariably turned the interaction into sensorimotor play, which brought him great pleasure.

In addition to being characterized by its functional emotional developmental capacity, each subtype should be described in terms of its regulatory-sensory processing profile. For research purposes, the regulatory-sensory processing profile can be simplified. For example, most children with NDRC, including autism spectrum disorders, have deficits in language and visual-spatial thinking, but they differ enormously in their capacities for auditory memory, visual-spatial memory, motor planning, and sensory modulation. These features that capture important clinical and, most likely, etiological pathway differences should therefore be highlighted. The form at the end of this section summarizes both the subtypes and the regulatory-sensory processing profile in terms of these dimensions.

Other Neurodevelopmental Disorders (Including Genetic and Metabolic Syndromes)

The four subtypes described above can be used to describe children with any type of non-progressive developmental disorder, including many of the well-known genetic syndromes. These syndromes involve problems with language, cognition, sensory and motor processing, and sometimes relating. Children born with these syndromes, including Down, Rett, Angelman, Prader-Willi, Turner, Fragile X, and others, may have relative strengths in relating, but often have compromises to different degrees in various developmental capacities. As with the other NDRC disorders, it is important to evaluate auditory processing and language capacities; motor planning and sequencing, including oral motor; visual-spatial processing; and sensory modulation. Only such a comprehensive evaluation permits the construction of an optimal intervention program. When a child's symptoms denote a known genetic or metabolic syndrome, both the syndrome and subtype of NDRC that best describes the child's functioning should be identified. In this way, the child can be described from the perspectives of both the etiology of his or her disorder *and* the developmental profile that characterizes it.

As with all infant and early childhood disorders, attempts at categorization should not substitute for constructing a developmental profile that includes the perspective of each axis of the multi-axial framework described earlier. This emphasis is especially important for many of the syndromes described in this category because despite significant difficulties in motor functioning, communication, and cognition, some children with these neurodevelopmental disorders can be warm and engaged and have a real strength in their capacity for intimacy.

In addition, while many children are best described, in addition to their etiologically based diagnoses, in terms of NDRC, others are better depicted in terms of their regulatory-sensory processing patterns.

SUMMARY TABLES OF NEURODEVELOPMENTAL DISORDERS OF RELATING AND COMMUNICATING (NDRC)

Below is a very brief overview of the types of NDRC, along with motor and sensory processing patterns that are also helpful in profiling a child. This summary may facilitate the use of this framework in a variety of clinical and research settings.

Overview of Clinical Subtypes of NDRC and Related Motor and Sensory-Processing Profile

IEC301. **Type I**	Intermittent capacities for attending and relating; reciprocal interaction; and, with support, shared social problem-solving and the beginning use of meaningful ideas (i.e., with help, the child can relate and interact and even use a few words, but not in a continuous and stable age-expected manner). Children with this pattern tend to show rapid progress in a comprehensive program that tailors meaningful emotional interactions to their unique motor and sensory-processing profile.
IEC302. **Type II**	Intermittent capacities for attention, relating, and a few reciprocal interactions, with only fleeting capacities for shared social problem-solving and repeating some words. Children with this pattern tend to make steady, methodical progress.
IEC303. **Type III**	Only fleeting capacities for attention and engagement. With considerable support, occasionally a few reciprocal interactions. Often no capacity for repeating words or using ideas, although the child may be able to repeat a few words in a memory-based (rather than meaningful) manner. Children with this pattern tend to make very slow but steady progress, especially in the basics of relating with warmth and learning to engage in longer sequences of reciprocal interaction. Over long periods of time, they may gradually master some words and phrases.
IEC304. **Type IV**	Similar to Type III above, but with a pattern of multiple regressions (loss of capacities). May also evidence a greater number of associated neurological difficulties, such as seizures, marked hypotonia, etc. Children with this pattern tend to make exceedingly slow progress, which can be enhanced if the sources of the regressive tendencies can be identified.

Overview of Motor and Sensory-Processing Profile

Children with NDRC tend to evidence very different biologically based patterns of sensory reactivity, processing, and motor planning. These differences may have diagnostic and prognostic value, and therefore it may be helpful to describe them. The child's tendencies can be briefly summarized in the framework outlined below.

Note: Almost all the children with an NDRC diagnosis have significant difficulties with language and visual-spatial thinking.

The patterns below are those that tend to differ among children. Please check all boxes that apply and, if sufficient clinical information is available, also use the box to indicate the degree to which that characteristic applies on a 1-to-3 scale (with 1 indicating minimum and 3 indicating the maximum degree).

Sensory Modulation

☐ Tends to be overresponsive to sensations, such as sound or touch (e.g., covers ears in response to mild sounds or gets dysregulated with light touch)

☐ Tends to crave sensory experience (e.g., actively seeks touch, sound, and different movement patterns)

☐ Tends to be underresponsive to sensations (e.g., requires highly energized vocal or tactile support to be alert and attentive)

Motor Planning and Sequencing

☐ Relative strength in motor planning and sequencing (e.g., carries out multiple-step action patterns, such as negotiating obstacle courses or building complex block designs)

☐ Relative weakness in motor planning and sequencing (e.g., can barely carry out simple movements; may simply bang blocks or do other one- to two-step action patterns)

Auditory Memory

☐ Relative strength in auditory memory (remembers or repeats long statements or materials from books, TV, songs)

☐ Relative weakness in auditory memory (difficulty remembering even simple sounds or words)

Visual Memory

☐ Relative strength in visual memory (tends to remember what is seen, such as book covers, pictures, and eventually words)

☐ Relative weakness in visual memory (difficulty remembering even simple pictures or objects)

Overview of the Multi-Axial Approach to Infant and Early Childhood Mental Health and Developmental Disorders

A multi-axial approach that describes the infant's unique profile includes:

- *Axis I – Primary diagnosis as described.*

- *Axis II – Functional Emotional Developmental Levels mastered and the degrees to which mastered (see Table 3 below).* For each level it should be noted whether that level is:

  - fully mastered in an age-appropriate manner
  - constricted (partially mastered, in that selected emotional themes or areas of sensory and motor processing are not operational at that level)
  - deficient (level is not at all reached)

Functional Emotional Developmental Level[6]	Emotional, Social and Intellectual Capacities
Shared attention and regulation (0-3 months and beyond)	Experiencing affective interest in sights, sound, touch, movement and other sensory experiences. Modulating affects (i.e., calming down).
Engagement and relating (3-6 months and beyond)	Experiencing pleasurable affects and growing feelings of intimacy in the context of primary relationships.
Two-way intentional, affective signaling and communication (6-9 months and beyond)	Using a range of affects in back-and-forth affective signaling to convey intentions (i.e., reading and responding to affective signals).
Long chains of co-regulated emotional signaling and shared social problem-solving (9-18 months and beyond)	Organizing affective interactions into action or behavior patterns to express wishes and needs and to solve problems (e.g., showing someone what one wants). Fragmented level: little islands of intentional problem-solving behavior. Polarized level: organized patterns of behavior expressing only one or another feeling state; e.g., organized aggression and impulsivity or organized clinging, needy, dependent behavior, or organized fearful patterns.

---

[6] Greenspan, DeGangi, & Wieder, 2001

Functional Emotional Developmental Level	Emotional, Social and Intellectual Capacities
	Integrated level: different emotional patterns—dependency, assertiveness, pleasure, etc.—organized into integrated, problem-solving affective interactions (e.g., flirting, seeking closeness, and then getting help to find a needed object).
Creating representations (or ideas) (18-30 months and beyond)	1. Using words and actions together (ideas are acted out in action, but words are also used to signify the action). 2. Using somatic or physical words to convey feeling states ("My muscles are exploding," "Head is aching"). 3. Using action words instead of actions to convey intent ("Hit you!"). 4. Conveying feelings as real rather than as signals ("I'm mad" "Hungry," "Need a hug" as compared with "I feel mad" or "I feel hungry" or "I feel like I need a hug"). In the first instance, the feeling state demands action and is very close to action; in the second, it is more a signal for something going on inside that leads to a consideration of many possible thoughts and actions. 5. Expressing global feeling states ("I feel awful," "I feel OK," etc.). 6. Expressing polarized feeling states (feelings tend to be characterized as all good or all bad).
Building bridges between ideas: Logical thinking (30-48 months and beyond)	1. Expressing differentiated feelings (gradually there are more and more subtle descriptions of feeling states, such as loneliness, sadness, annoyance, anger, delight, and happiness). 2. Creating connections between differentiated feeling states ("I feel angry when you are mad at me").

- *Axis III describes the regulatory-sensory processing profile of the child.* There are a number of constitutional-maturational differences in the way in which infants and young children respond to and comprehend sensory experiences and plan actions. The different observed patterns exist on a continuum from relatively normal variations to disorders. Disorders occur when the individual differences are sufficiently severe to interfere with age-expected emotional, social, cognitive, or learning capacities. The clinician should indicate in this axis the presence or absence of regulatory differences in the categories. It should be noted, however, that if the primary diagnosis is a regulatory-sensory processing disorder, these patterns will already be described and this axis need not be addressed. To summarize the range of these regulatory-sensory processing differences, the clinician may use the following demarcations to indicate the degree to which the pattern represents normal variations versus severe impairments. For each category the clinician can indicate:

- not present

- present, but within a range of normal variation

- mild impairment(s)

- moderate impairment(s) (e.g., makes it difficult for the child to get dressed or remain calm in noisy settings), and

- severe impairment(s) (makes it difficult for the child to engage in relationships, form basic patterns of communication, or learn to think).

- *Axis IV characterizes caregiver, family, and environmental patterns.* These are obviously complex dynamic patterns that can only be captured with a detailed narrative. However, for the purpose of this axis it should be noted whether the caregiver, family, and environmental patterns are supportive or undermining of the child's functioning. Therefore, caregiver, family, and environmental patterns should be characterized in terms of:

  - fully supporting the child's age-expected functional capacities

  - evidencing minor interferences, such as difficulty in engaging a child in one area of emotional functioning while supporting others (e.g., family conflicts over aggression),

  - moderate interferences, such as inability to support whole domains of functioning (e.g., assertiveness or autonomy), and

  - major impairments, such as the serious undermining of the foundation of healthy functioning (e.g., the capacity for intimacy).

- *Axis V describes other medical or neurologic diagnoses.* While the multi-axial approach summarizes the child's functioning, it does not replace the narrative developmental formulation depicting in more detail each of the factors outlined in these axes.

CONCLUSION

This special section has described infant and early childhood mental health and developmental disorders, including interactive, regulatory-sensory processing, and neurodevelopmental disorders of relating and communicating. It presented a developmental, biopsychosocial framework to capture individual variations and common patterns evidenced by infants, young children, and their families. Infant and early childhood mental health and developmental disorders is a growing field, which builds on many of the core principles at the foundation of psychodynamic frames of reference.

REFERENCES

Ayres, J. (1964). Tactile functions: Their relation to hyperactive and perceptual motor behavior. *The American Journal of Occupational Therapy, 18,* 6-11.

Ayres, J. (1972). *Sensory integration and learning disabilities.* Los Angeles: Western Psychological Services.

Bowlby, J. (1944). Forty-four juvenile thieves: Their characters and home life. *International Journal of Psychoanalysis, 25,* 19-52; 107-127.

Bowlby, J., & Robertson, J. (1953). A two year old goes to hospital. *Proceedings of the Royal Society of Medicine, 46,* 425-427.

Carlson, G. A., & Weintraub, S. (1993). Childhood behavior problems and bipolar disorder: Relationship or coincidence? *Journal of Affective Disorders, 28,* 143-153.

Castillo, M., Kwock, L., Courvorisie, H., & Hooper, S. R. (2000). Proton MR spectroscopy in children with bipolar affective disorder: Preliminary observations. *American Journal of Neuroradiology, 21,* 832-838.

Coates, S., Friedman, R., & Wolfe, S. (1991) The etiology of boyhood gender identity disorder: A model for integrating temperament, development, and psychodynamics. *Psychoanalytic Dialogues, 1,* 481-523.

Cytryn, L., & McKnew, D. H. (1974). Factors influencing the changing clinical expression of depressive process in children. *American Journal of Psychiatry, 131,* 879-881.

Diagnostic Classification Task Force (1994). *Diagnostic classification: 0-3. Diagnostic classification of mental health and developmental disorders of infancy and early childhood.* Arlington, VA: Zero to Three, National Center for Clinical Infant Programs.

Egland, J. A., Blumenthal, R. L., Nee, J., Sharp, L., & Endicott, J. (1987). Reliability and relationship of various ages of onset criteria for major affective disorder. *Journal of Affective Disorders, 12,* 159-165.

Geller, B., Zimmerman, B., Williams, M., Bolhofner, K., & Craney, J. (2001). Bipolar disorder at prospective follow-up of adults who had prepubertal major depressive disorder. *American Journal of Psychiatry, 158,* 125–127.

Greenspan, S. I. (1989). The development of the ego: Biological and environmental specificity and the psychopathological developmental process. *Journal of the American Psychoanalytic Association, 37,* 605-638.

Greenspan, S. I. (1992). *Infancy and early childhood: The practice of clinical assessment and intervention with emotional and developmental challenges.* Madison, CT: International Universities Press.

Greenspan, S. I. (1997). *The growth of the mind and the endangered origins of intelligence.* Reading, MA: Addison Wesley Longman.

Greenspan, S. I., DeGangi, G. A., & Wieder, S. (2001). *The functional emotional assessment scale (FEAS) for infancy and early childhood: Clinical & research applications.* Bethesda, MD: Interdisciplinary Council on Developmental and Learning Disorders.

Greenspan, S. I., & Glovinsky, I. (2002). *Children with bipolar patterns of dysregulation: New perspectives on developmental pathways and a comprehensive approach to prevention and treatment.* Bethesda, MD: The Interdisciplinary Council on Developmental and Learning Disorders.

Greenspan, S. I., & Lourie, R. S. (1981). Developmental structuralist approach to the classification of adaptive and pathologic personality organizations: Infancy and early childhood. *American Journal of Psychiatry, 138,* 725–735.

Greenspan, S. I., Pollock, G. H., (Eds.) (1991). *The course of life: Vol. I Infancy.* Madison, CT: International Universities Press.

Greenspan, S. I., & Shanker, S. (2004). *The first idea: How symbols, language, and intelligence evolved from our primate ancestors to modern humans.* Cambridge, MA: Da Capo Press.

Greenspan, S. I., & Wieder, S. (1997). Developmental patterns and outcomes in infants and children with disorders in relating and communicating: A chart review of 200 cases of children with autistic spectrum diagnoses. *Journal of Developmental and Learning Disorders, 1,* 87-141.

Greenspan, S. I., & Wieder, S. (1998). *The child with special needs: Encouraging intellectual and emotional growth.* Reading, MA: Perseus Books.

Greenspan, S. I., & Wieder, S. (1999). A functional developmental approach to autism spectrum disorders. *Journal of the Association for Persons with Severe Handicaps, 24,* 147-161.

Greenspan, S. I., & Wieder, S. (2003). Infant and early childhood mental health: A comprehensive developmental approach to assessment and intervention. *Zero to Three, 24,* 6-13.

Greenspan, S. I., Wieder, S., Lieberman, A., Nover, R., Lourie, R., & Robinson, M. (1987). *Infants in multirisk families: Case studies in preventive intervention.* (Clinical Infant Reports No. 3). New York: International Universities Press.

Harrington, R., Fudge, H., Rutter, M., Pickles, A., & Hill, J. (1991). Adult outcomes of child and adolescent depression: II. Links with antisocial disorders. *Journal of the American Academy of Child and Adolescent Psychiatry, 30,* 434-439.

ICDL Clinical Practice Guidelines Workgroup, (2000). *Interdisciplinary Council on Developmental and Learning Disorders' Clinical practice guidelines: Redefining the standards of care for infants, children, and families with special needs.* Bethesda, MD: Interdisciplinary Council on Developmental and Learning Disorders.

ICDL-DMIC Diagnostic Classification Task Force, (2005). *Interdisciplinary Council on Developmental and Learning Disorders Diagnostic manual for infancy and early childhood mental health disorders, developmental disorders, regulatory-sensory processing disorders, language disorders, and learning challenges—ICDL-DMIC.* Bethesda, MD: Interdisciplinary Council on Developmental and Learning Disorders.

Lewis, D. O. (1992). From abuse to violence: Psychophysiological consequences of maltreatment. *Journal of the American Academy of Child and Adolescent Psychiatry, 31,* 383-391.

Lish, J., Dime-Meenan, S., Whybrow, P., Arlen-Price, R., & Hirschfeld, R. (1994). The National Depressive and Manic-Depressive Association (DMDA) survey of bipolar members. *Journal of Affective Disorders, 31,* 281-294.

Miller, L.J., Cermak, S., Lane, S., Anzalone, M., & Koomar, J. (2004). Position statement on terminology related to sensory integration dysfunction. *S.I. Focus,* 6-8.

Radke-Yarrow, M., Nottelmann, E., Martinez, P., Fox, M. B., & Belmont, B. (1992). Young children of affectively ill parents: A longitudinal study of psychosocial development. *Journal of the American Academy of Child and Adolescent Psychiatry, 31,* 68-77.

Sigurdsson, E., Fombonne, E., Sayal, K., & Checkley, S. (1999). Neurodevelopmental antecedents of early-onset bipolar affective disorder. *British Journal of Psychiatry, 174,* 121-127.

Spitz, R. A. (1945). Hospitalism: An inquiry into the genesis of psychiatric conditions in early childhood. *The Psychoanalytic Study of the Child, 1,* 53-74.

Strober, M., Morrell, W., Burroughs, J., Lampert, C., Danforth, H., & Freeman, R. (1988). A family study of bipolar I disorder in adolescents: Early onset of symptoms linked to increased familial loading and lithium resistance. *Journal of Affective Disorders, 15,* 255-268.

Yeager, C. A., & Lewis, D. O. (2000). Mental illness, neuropsychologic deficits, child abuse, and violence. *Child and Adolescent Psychiatric Clinics of North America, 9,* 793-813.

SELECTED REFERENCES

Ainsworth, M., Bell, S. M., & Stayton, D. (1974). Infant-mother attachment and social development: Socialization as a product of reciprocal responsiveness to signals. In M. Richards (Ed.), *The integration of the child into a social world* (pp. 99-135). Cambridge, England: Cambridge University Press.

Boas, F. (1982). *A Frans Boas Reader: The shaping of American anthropology, 1883-1911.* Chicago: University of Chicago Press.

Bowlby, J. (1951). Maternal care and mental health. *Monographs of the World Health Organization (No. 51).* Geneva: World Health Organization.

Brazelton, T. B., & Cramer, B. (1990). *The earliest relationship: Parents, infants, and the drama of early attachment.* Reading, MA: Addison-Wesley Publishing Co.

Brazelton, T. B., Koslowski, B., & Main, M. (1974). The origins of reciprocity; the early mother-infant interaction. In M. Lewis & L. Rosenblum (Eds.), *The effect of the infant on its caregiver.* New York: John Wiley & Sons.

Bromfield, R. (2000). It's the tortoise race: Long term psychodynamic psychotherapy with a high functioning autistic adolescent. *Psychoanalytic Inquiry, 20,* 732-745.

Bruner, J. S. (1982). *Child's talk: Learning to use language.* New York: Norton.

Damasio, A. (1994). *Descartes' error: Emotion, reason, and the human brain.* New York: Putnam.

Descartes, R. (1637). *Discours de la methode: Pour bien conduire sa raison et character veinte dans la sciences.* Leyde: Ian Maire.

Dickson, K. L., Fogel, A., & Messinger, D. (1998). The development of emotion from a social process view. In F. Mascolo & S. Griffen (Eds.), *What develops in emotional development?* (pp. 253-271). New York: Plenum Press.

Ekman, P. (1992). Facial expression of emotion: New findings, new questions. *Psychological Science, 3,* 34–38.

Ekman, P., Friesen, W., & Ellsworth, P. (1972). *Emotions in the human face.* Elmsford, NY: Pergamon.

Ekman, P., Friesen, W., O'Sullivan, M., & Scherer, K. (1980). Relative importance of face, body, and speech in judgments of personality and affect. *Journal of Personality and Social Psychology, 38,* 270-277.

Emde, R. N., Gaensbauer, T. J., & Harmon, R. J. (1976). Emotional expression in infancy: A biobehavioral study. *Psychological Issues Monograph*(No. 37). New York: International Universities Press.

Erikson, E. H. (1940). Studies in interpretation of play: I. Clinical observation of child disruption in young children. Genetic Psychology. Monograph 22.

Erikson, E. H. (1959). *Identity and the life cycle.* New York: International Universities Press.

Erikson, E. H. (1963). *Childhood and society.* New York: W. W. Norton.

Erikson, E. H. (1964). *Insight and responsibility.* New York: W. W. Norton.

Erikson, E. H. (1968). *Identity: Youth and crisis.* New York: W. W. Norton.

Escalona, S. (1968). *The roots of individuality.* Chicago: Aldine.

Fogel, A., Nelson-Goens, G. C., Hsu, H. C., & Shapiro, A. F. (2000). Do different infant smiles reflect different positive emotions? *Social Development, 9,* 497-520

Fonagy, P., Steele, M., Moran, G., Steele, H., & Higgitt, A. (1993). Measuring the ghost in the nursery: An empirical study of the relation between parents' mental representations of childhood experiences and their infants' security attachment. *Journal of the American Psycho-analytic Association, 41,* 957-989.

Fraiberg, S. (1979, December). *Treatment modalities in an infant mental health program.* Paper presented at the National Center for Clinical Infant Programs, Washington, DC.

Fraiberg, L. (Ed.). (1987). Selected writings of Selma Fraiberg. Columbus, OH: Ohio State University Press.

Freud, A. (1965). *Normality and pathology in childhood; assessments of development.* New York: International Universities Press.

Freud, S. (1911). Formulations on the two principles of mental functioning. *Standard Edition, 12,* 216-226.

Gaddini, R. D. B. (1993). On autism. *Psychoanalytic Inquiry, 13,* 134-143.

Greenspan, S. I. (2001). The affect diathesis hypothesis: The role of emotions in the core deficit in autism and the development of intelligence and social skills. *Journal of Developmental and Learning Disorders, 5,* 1–45.

Greenspan, S. I., & Press, B. K. (1985). The toddler group: A setting for adaptive social/emotional development of disadvantaged 1- and 2-year-olds in a peer group. *Zero to Three, 5,* 6-8.

Greenspan, S. I. (1979). Intelligence and adaptation: An integration of psychoanalytic and Piagetian developmental psychology. *Psychological Issues Monograph* (No. 47-48). New York: International Universities Press.

Greenspan, S. I. (1999). *Building healthy minds: The six experiences that create intelligence and emotional growth in babies and young children.* Cambridge, MA: Perseus Publishing.

Hofer, M. A. (1988). On the nature and function of prenatal behavior. In W. Smotherman & S. Robinson (Eds.), *Behavior of the fetus.* Caldwell, NJ: Telford.

Hunt, J. M. (1941). Infants in an orphanage. *Journal of Abnormal and Social Psychology, 36,* 338.

Izard, C. E. (1977). *Human emotions.* New York: Plenum Press.

Izard, C. E. (1978). Emotions as motivation: An evolutionary-developmental perspective. In R. A. Dienstbier (Eds.), *Nebraska symposium on motivation* (pp. 163-200). Lincoln, NE: University of Nebraska Press.

Izard, C. E. (1993). Four systems for emotion activation: Cognitive and noncognitive processes. *Psychological Review, 100,* 68-90.

Izard, C. E. (1997). Emotions and facial expressions: A perspective from differential emotions theory. In J. Russell & J. Fernández-Dols (Eds.), *The psychology of facial expression.* Cambridge: Cambridge University Press.

Klaus, M., & Kennell, J. (1976). *Maternal-infant bonding: The impact of early separation or loss on family development.* St. Louis, MO: C. V. Mosby.

Klaus, M. H., & Klaus, P. H. (2000). *Your amazing newborn.* Cambridge, MA, Perseus.

Klinnert, M. D., Campos, J., Sorce, F. J., Emde, R. N., & Svejda, M. J. (1983). Emotions as behavior regulators: Social referencing in infancy. In R. Plutchik & H. Kellerman (Eds.), *Emotion: Theory, research, and experience* (pp. 57-86). New York: Academic Press.

LeDoux, J. E. (1996). *The Emotional Brain.* New York: Simon & Schuster.

Lutz, C. (1988). *Unnatural emotions: Everyday sentiments on a Micronesian atoll and their challenge to Western theory.* Chicago: University of Chicago Press.

Mahler, M. S., Pine, F., & Bergman, A. (1975). *The psychological birth of the human infant: Symbiosis and individuation.* New York: Basic Books.

Messinger, D., Fogel, A., & Dickson, L. (1997). A dynamic systems approach to infant facial action. In J. A. Russell & F. M. Dols (Eds.), *The psychology of facial expression* (pp. 205-226). New York: Cambridge University Press.

Messinger, D. S., Fogel, A., & Dickson, K. L. (1999). What's in a smile? *Developmental Psychology, 35,* 701–708.

Murphy, L. B. (1974). The individual child. Publication No. OCD 74-1032. Washington, DC, US Government Printing Office, Department of Health, Education and Welfare.

Piaget, J. (1952). *The origins of intelligence in children.* New York: International Universities Press.

Provence, S., & Lipton, R. C. (1962). *Infants in institutions.* New York: International Universities Press.

Sander, L. (1962). Issues in early mother-child interaction. *Journal of the American Academy of Child Psychiatry, 1,* 141-166.

Schacter, D. L. (1997). The neuropsychology of false recognition. *Current Directions in Psychological Science, 6,* 65-70.

Sroufe, L. A. (1979). Socioemotional development. In J. Osofsky (Ed.), *Handbook of Infant Development* (pp. 462–515). New York: John Wiley & Sons.

Sroufe, L. A., Waters, E., & Matas, L. (1974). Contextual determinants of infant affective response. In M. Lewis & L. Rosenblum (Eds.), *The Origins of Fear* (pp. 49-72). New York: Wiley & Sons.

Stern, D. N. (1974). The goal and structure of mother-infant play. *Journal of the American Academy of Child Psychiatry, 13,* 402-421.

Stern D.N. (1985). *The interpersonal world of the infant: A view from psychoanalysis and developmental psychology.* New York: Basic Books.

Thomas, A., Chess, S., & Birch, H. G. (1968). *Temperament and behavior disorders in children.* New York: New York University Press.

Tomkins, S. (1962). *Affect, imagery, consciousness: Vol. 1. The positive effects.* New York: Springer Publishing.

Tomkins, S. (1963). *Affect, imagery, consciousness: Vol. 2. The negative effects.* New York: Springer Publishing.

Tronick, E., Ricks, M., & Cohn, J. (1982). Maternal and infant affective exchange: patterns of adaptation. In T. Field & A. Fogel (Eds.), *Emotion and early interaction* (pp. 83-100). New Jersey: Lawrence Erlbaum Associates.

Witherington, D. C., Campos, J. J., & Hertenstein, M. J. (2001). Principles of emotion and its development. In G. Bremmer & A. Fogel (Eds.), *Blackwell handbook of infant development* (pp. 427-464). Oxford, UK: Blackwell Publishing Ltd.

Yanof, J. A. (1996a). Language, communication, and transference in child analysis: I. Selective mutism: The medium is the message. *Journal of the American Psychoanalytic Assocation, 44,* 79-100.

Yanof, J. A. (1996b). Language, communication, and transference in child analysis: II. Is child analysis really analysis? *Journal of the American Psychoanalytic Association, 44,* 100-116.

Yarrow, L. J. (1975). *Infant and environment: Early cognitive and motivational development.* New York: John Wiley and Sons, Inc.

Part III

Conceptual and Research Foundations for a Psychodynamically Based Classification System For Mental Health Disorders

Introduction to Research Section

Part III of this volume is an illustrative, but far from exhaustive, overview of the conceptual and empirical research literature that supports the underlying premises of our effort, (1) that the view of human functioning that takes into account the full depth and range of relationships, feelings, ideas, wishes, defensive and coping strategies, etc., can be systematically substantiated by available research on how human beings develop (see the article by Greenspan and Shanker), and on neural science research on the nature and the functioning of unconscious mental processes (see the paper by Shevrin); (2) that the concepts that characterize this complex, depth psychological, view of mental functioning can be operationalized and assessed in ways useful for psychological case formulation and treatment planning (see the differently conceptualized articles by Shedler and Westen, by Blatt, Auerbach, Zuroff, and Shahar, and by Dahlbender, Rudolf, and the OPD Task Force); (3) that the factors that are associated with therapeutic change and outcome can be specified to a very significant extent (see Wallerstein's article on the historical unfolding of process and outcome research, as well as the article by Blatt, Auerbach, Zuroff, and Shahar); and (4) that there is a substantial accumulating literature on the effectiveness and efficacy of psychodynamic approaches in relation both to changes in symptoms and manifest behaviors, as well as, beyond that, demonstrable changes in underlying personality structure and functioning (see Wallerstein's paper on process and outcome research, as well as the articles by Herzig and Licht, by Westen, Novotny, and Thompson-Brenner, by Fonagy, and by Leichsenring).

Preceding these articles just mentioned, this part of the volume begins with a historical overview, by Wallerstein, of the development of a psychoanalytically based nosology for mental disorders centered around Freud's own considerable efforts in the earlier parts of his psychoanalytic career, and then pointing to significant additions, post-Freud, in further developing these ramifying conceptions. This is followed by a contribution by six French authors (Braconnier, Guedeney, Hanin, Sauvagnat, Thurin, and Widlöcher) offering a distinctively French view of suitability and indications for psychoanalytic therapy, with greater focus on the conceptual contributions of Bowlby and Lacan to these issues than is usually offered in the English speaking psychoanalytic world.

Taken together, the articles in this section provide significant support for a depth psychological approach to diagnostic assessment and treatment planning, and thus for the construction of this *Psychodynamic Diagnostic Manual* (PDM). Clearly, as with all such efforts, this is very much a work in progress. This section shows, however, that taking into account the full complexity of human mental functioning need not be compromised in order to conduct reliable, and ever more valid, systematic study and research. In fact, emergent conceptions and empirical findings, as presented in these papers, strongly suggest that all those who work in the field of mental health and illness should best embrace the full range and depth of human mental functioning within their conceptual purview.

Editorial Note: The papers in Part III were solicited from a (geographically dispersed) range of contributors, in an effort to demonstrate, from multiple perspectives, the degree of current conceptual and empirical support for the PDM's conceptions of an individualized, dimensional depth-psychological approach to complement the symptom-based DSM system. The individually-authored presentations in this section inevitably contain, in ensemble, differing emphases and, at times, some redundancy. We felt it was important for each author's individual voice to be available to the reader along with the basic consensual perspective that has united the PDM effort.

Psychoanalytically Based Nosology: Historic Origins

Robert S. Wallerstein, MD[1]

Editor's Note: This first paper details Sigmund Freud's own very early efforts to differentially categorize the complex clinical phenomena with which he was confronted when he undertook to listen to his psychiatric patients in order to understand them in ways that he could then use to influence them in the direction of cure. At first these were distinctions between what he called the actual neuroses and the symptom neuroses, and among the latter, the distinctions between the hysterical and the obsessional symptom pictures, as well as what he called the narcissistic neuroses, which we know today as the psychoses.

It was only after Freud that the conception of the borderline states was developed, leading quite naturally into our modern-day concerns with the borderline personality disorders and the narcissistic neuroses, conceptualized very differently than Freud's using that designation to describe psychotic disorders. And although begun by Freud, the concern with character, both character style and character neuroses, has been vastly elaborated since Freud's early conceptions. And along with character neuroses, the impulse neuroses (addictions, perversions, etc.).

What the whole chapter demonstrates is the constantly fluid and continuously evolving nature of our nosological conceptions as accumulating clinical experience and conceptual theorizing constantly interact in spiraling dialectical interchange. This makes all classification effort, such as in this volume, a creature of its time and place in human history and context, and makes regular revision a scientific requirement.

Conceptions of nosology represent an uneasy interface in the relationship between psychoanalysis as a theory of mind (and also a therapy for the disorders of mind) and the array of mental illnesses encompassed within psychiatry as a medical discipline. This was less so during the days of DSM-I and -II which originated out of the experiences of military psychiatry in World War II and were guided by the psychodynamic (psychoanalytic) framework applied to the understanding and treatment of combat stress. It was the adoption of the much more descriptive, precise, research-oriented, and (at least in intention) atheoretical, DSM-III, that brought into sharp focus all the problems that psychoanalysis has

---

[1] Emeritus Professor and Former Chair, Department of Psychiatry, University of California, San Francisco School of Medicine

in fitting its formulations and its methods into the framework of mental disorders determined by the classificatory and research needs of organized psychiatry.

In essaying to assess the conceptual and clinical complexities that DSM-III introduced into psychoanalytic work around issues of diagnosis, prognosis, research classification, peer review, and eligibility for third party reimbursement, to name the most salient, it is worthwhile, for much more than the usual reasons of historical obeisance, to review the evolution of psychoanalytic nosological conceptions about mental illness starting of course with Freud's own evolving conceptions over his clinical lifetime. Two especially useful, quite psychoanalytic, perspectives are highlighted by such a review. The first is a dynamic conception of nosology as a living, ever-changing, and constructed corpus, in a constant state of flux and growth as our clinical and theoretical knowledge base grows, rather than as a static classificatory reality that somehow exists out there in nature and that we think we discover rather than create. The second, equally psychoanalytic, perspective is that nosology and diagnosis derive their relevance from their full imbrication with issues of overall case formulation and understanding, of prognosis, of treatability and treatment indications, and then of differential treatment planning. In isolation from these, nosology becomes indeed a static, almost meaningless, enterprise. I essay to demonstrate both of these perspectives through the chronological tracing of our major psychoanalytic conceptions of nosology and diagnosis, with my fuller focus on the original contributions of Freud.

As we know so well, Freud's earliest psychoanalytic writings were about the phenomena of hysteria, and in his paper on "The Neuro-Psychoses of Defence" he began with an effort to distinguish three varieties of hysteria, hypnoid, retention, and defence hysteria (Freud, 1894, p. 47). Hypnoid hysteria results, he said, when "the ideas which emerge in hypnoid states [i.e. states of altered or hypnoid consciousness] are cut off from associative communication with the rest of the content of consciousness" (p. 46). In retention hysterias, on the other hand, "the splitting of consciousness plays an insignificant part . . . . They are those cases in which what has happened is only that the reaction to traumatic stimuli has failed to occur, and which can . . . accordingly, be resolved and cured by 'abreaction'" (p. 47). Whereas in defence hysteria, "the splitting of consciousness is the result of an act of will on the part of the patient; that is to say, it is initiated by an effort of will whose motive can be specified [p. 46] . . . an occurrence of *incompatibility* took place in their ideational life" (p. 47, ital. added). Though Freud made use of these distinctions of hypnoid and retention hysteria at a number of places in the "Studies on Hysteria" (Breuer & Freud, 1893-1895), thereafter they dropped from his vocabulary and his conceptualizing completely except for a single isolated reference to hypnoid hysteria in "An Autobiographical Study" (1925, p. 23). The three categories were simply very early collapsed together as a "neurosis of defence." This was the early delineation by Freud of hysteria as a diagnostic entity within what he came to call the broad category of the psychoneuroses.

In that same earliest of his nosological papers (1894), Freud pursued additional diagnostic distinctions. He said, "In hysteria, the incompatible idea is rendered innocuous by its *sum of excitation* being *transformed into something somatic*. For this I should like to propose the name of *conversion* .... It [the conversion] proceeds along the line of the motor or sensory innervation which is related—whether intimately or more loosely—to the traumatic experience" (p. 49). Then he went on to say "If someone with a disposition [to neurosis] lacks the aptitude for conversion ... then *that affect is obliged to remain in the psychical sphere ... affect, which has become free, attaches itself to other ideas which are not in themselves incompatible; and thanks to this 'false connection,' those ideas turn into obsessional ideas*" (p. 51-52, ital. added). Which means that "the obsession represents a substitute or surrogate for the incompatible sexual idea and has taken its place in consciousness" (p. 53). To complete the diagnostic array proposed in that same paper, Freud set out another category of "hallucinatory confusion" (p. 58) or "*psychosis of defence*" (p. 60, ital. added). This was characterized as "*the accentuation of the idea* which was threatened by the precipitating cause of the onset of the illness. One is ... justified in saying that the ego has fended off the incompatible idea through a flight into psychosis" (p. 59, ital. added). That is, in this first nosological paper of Freud's (1894), conversion hysteria, obsessional neurosis, and hallucinatory psychosis represented varying ways to cope with or to defend against, an incompatible idea, or set of ideas.

At the same time during which Freud was working out his first categorization of these defence neuroses (later psychoneuroses), he was also occupied with another different grouping that seemed to him fundamentally different in etiology and in the kind of treatment that would then be indicated. Within this other grouping he was separating out anxiety neurosis from neurasthenia (Freud, 1895a). Of anxiety neurosis he said that there is "a quantum of anxiety in a freely floating state" (p. 93) and that this "affect [of anxiety] does *not* originate in a repressed idea, but turns out to be not further reducible by psychological analysis, nor amenable to psychotherapy" (p. 97, ital. added). Here, rather, "careful enquiry directed to that end reveals that a set of noxae and influences from [current] sexual life are the operative aetiological factors" (p. 99). Among these noxae Freud listed virginal anxiety, the sexual anxiety of newlyweds, the anxiety of widows, of intentionally abstinent women, of senescent men, and mostly the anxieties of men and women in the face of premature ejaculation, of coitus interruptus, and other varieties of incompletely consummated excitation (p. 99-101). What these all have in common is an "accumulation of excitation" with "insufficient satisfaction" and "no psychical origin" (p. 107). Since Freud was from the very start mindful of the relationship between diagnosis and therapeutic consequence, this etiologic hypothesis could of course be put to a proper therapeutic test. In this instance, this would not be psychotherapy; rather "If, as a physician who understands this aetiology, one arranges ... for coitus interruptus to be replaced by normal intercourse, one obtains a therapeutic proof of the assertion I have made. The anxiety is removed, and—unless there is fresh cause for it of the same sort—it does not return" (p. 104).

Alongside anxiety neurosis based thus on accumulated and undischarged excitation, in that same paper (1895a) Freud delineated neurasthenia as based on opposite noxious sexual practices related to what he called impoverishment of excitation (p. 114). Of this Freud said, "Neurasthenia develops whenever the adequate unloading is replaced by a less adequate one—thus, when normal coition, carried out in the most favorable conditions, is replaced by masturbation or spontaneous emission" (p. 109). But the two, anxiety neurosis and neurasthenia, share an important common distinction from the defence neuroses. In Freud's language "It [anxiety neurosis] shares with neurasthenia one main characteristic—namely that the source of excitation, the precipitating cause of the disturbance, lies in the somatic field instead of the psychical one, as in the case of hysteria and obsessional neurosis" (p. 114).[2]

Thus, in two very early papers written within one year, Freud laid much of the groundwork for the nosological structure he was in later years to continue to elaborate but also to modify. It encompassed the distinction between what Freud came to call the 'actual neuroses' (without psychic causation) and the "psycho-neuroses" (based on psychic causation). Though Freud held to this distinction for many years, the concept of the actual neuroses later fell into disuse with the growing conviction in the psychoanalytic community that no psychological symptoms could be devoid of psychic instigation and psychic meaning—though the concept of actual neuroses can be felt to have been revived, in significantly altered form, in recent years, with the growing recognition of severe trauma as a major precipitant of psychic distress, under the rubric of traumatic neurosis (called in prior times neurocircularity asthenia in the U.S. Civil War, shell shock in World War I, battle fatigue or war neuroses in World War II, and post-traumatic stress disorder [PTSD] since Vietnam).

These same distinctions were further elaborated in another sequence of papers, published very soon after, in 1896. In the first of these (1896a), Freud reviewed what he called all the "major neuroses ... functional pathological modifications [that] have as their common source the subject's sexual life, whether they lie in a disorder of his *contemporary* sexual life [as in neurasthenia, the

---

[2] In another paper within the year (1895b), titled "A Reply to Criticisms of my paper on Anxiety Neuroses," Freud repeated this statement even more categorically, "anxiety neurosis is created by everything which keeps *somatic* sexual tension *away* from the psychical sphere, which interferes with its being worked over psychically ... [sexual] abstinence whether voluntary or involuntary, sexual intercourse with incomplete satisfaction, coitus interruptus, deflection of psychical interest from sexuality and similar things, are the specific aetiological factors of the states to which I have given the name of anxiety neuroses" (p. 124, ital. added).

tension depletion syndrome based on excessive masturbation, or anxiety neurosis, the tension accumulation syndrome based on coitus interruptus and comparable practices] or in important events in his *past* life [hysteria and obsessional neurosis]" (p. 149, ital. added). In addition to this distinction between present and past sexual perturbations as marking off etiologically these two classes of neuroses, Freud further now distinguished within the defence neuroses (hysteria and obsessional neurosis) on a different etiological basis than he had two years earlier. Hysteria he now said stemmed from a "*passive* sexual experience before puberty" (p. 151, ital. added). This he called "the specific aetiology of hysteria" (p. 151).

Obsessional neurosis was also declared to be rooted in the infantile past but on a different etiological basis than the presumed causative passive sexual experiences of the hysteric. Freud explained it thus:

> The obsessional neurosis . . . arises from a specific cause very analogous to that of hysteria. Here too we find a precocious sexual event, occurring before puberty . . . . There is only one difference which seems capital. At the basis of the aetiology of hysteria we found an event of passive sexuality, an experience submitted to with indifference or . . . annoyance or fright. In obsessional neurosis it is a question on the other hand, of an event which has given pleasure [i.e. an active experience] . . . . The obsessional ideas . . . are nothing other than *reproaches addressed by the subject to himself on account of this anticipated sexual enjoyment*, but reproaches distorted by an unconscious psychical work of transformation and substitution (p. 155).

This distinction between passivity in the genesis of hysteria and activity in the genesis of obsessional illness Freud thought gave him in turn a clue to another etiological puzzle. To quote, "The importance of the active element in sexual life as a cause of obsessions, and of sexual passivity for the pathogenesis of hysteria, even seems to unveil the reason for the more intimate connection of hysteria with the female sex and the preference of men for obsessional neurosis" (p. 156).

In the second of the 1896 papers, Freud (1896b) reiterated these distinctions between past and present causative events and between passive and active infantile sexual traumata. He put the past-present distinction a little differently however, now in terms of indirect or direct sexual noxae. To quote:

> The aetiology of the two neuro-psychoses of defence [psychoneuroses] is related as follows to the aetiology of the two simple neuroses, neurasthenia and anxiety neurosis. Both the latter disorders are *direct* effects of the sexual noxae themselves, as I have shown in my paper on anxiety neurosis . . . both the defence neuroses are *indirect* consequences of sexual noxae which have occurred before the advent of sexual maturity—are consequences, that is, of the psychical memory-traces of those noxae" (p. 167-168, ital. added).

And further in this paper, Freud took his second foray into trying to encompass a psychotic disturbance in his etiological scheme of things, again as a "psychosis of defence." He said here "For a considerable time I have harboured a suspicion that paranoia too . . . is a psychosis of defence; that is to say, that, like hysteria and obsessions, it proceeds from the repression of distressing memories and that its symptoms are determined in their form by the content of what has been repressed" (p. 174-175). It is this germinal idea that of course Freud developed much more fully in the etiological formulae he subsequently constructed to explain the paranoid dementia of Daniel Paul Schreber (Freud, 1911). In an article reviewing these basic distinctions amongst the various neuroses, Freud first used the term "actual neuroses" (1898, p. 279) to describe what up to then he had called "simple neuroses."

Over the subsequent years this overall nosological schema of psychoneuroses and actual neuroses, the former amenable to psychoanalysis, the latter only requiring corrected sexual behaviors, was both further filled out and also very substantially modified, even in major ways undone. In a 1906 article, Freud retreated from his passive-active formulation, "I believed *at that time* [i.e. in the period of the original formulations] . . . that a passive attitude in these scenes produced a predisposition to hysteria and, on the other hand, an active one a predisposition to obsessional neurosis Later on I was obliged to abandon this view entirely" (1906, p. 275, ital. added).

Much more consequentially, it was in this 1906 paper that Freud explicitly declared that he had previously much overestimated the frequency of "cases in which sexual seduction by an adult or by older children played the chief part in the history of the patient's childhood" (p. 274). He was

> . . . at that [earlier] period unable to distinguish with certainty between falsifications made by hysterics in their memories of childhood and traces of real events. Since then [he said] I have learned to explain a number of phantasies of seduction as attempts at fending off memories of the subjects' *own* sexual activity . . . . When this point had been clarified, the 'traumatic' element in the sexual experiences of childhood lost its importance and what was left was the realization that infantile sexual activity (whether spontaneous or provoked) prescribes the direction that will be taken by later sexual life after maturity (p. 274).

This led to the statement that "infantile sexual traumas" were in a sense replaced by the "infantilism of sexuality" (p. 275). Here, Freud has incorporated into his nosological framework the fateful turn of psychoanalysis—based so much on the discoveries of his own self-analysis—from the original traumatic theory of the neuroses in which the outer reality was the locus of the pathogenic impact in the form of the adult sexual seductions of the unformed child, to an inner psychology of the vicissitude of drive, and subsequently of ego development, in the genesis of neurosis.

In his next nosological expansion, in the Little Hans case (1909), Freud placed phobias within his explanatory scheme as one of the psychoneuroses, alongside conversion hysteria and obsessional neuroses. Of this he said,

> In the classificatory system of the neuroses no definite position has hitherto been assigned to 'phobias' . . . . For phobias of the kind of which little Hans's belongs, and which are in fact the most common, the name of 'anxiety hysteria' seems to me not inappropriate . . . . It finds its justification in the similarity between the psychological structure of these phobias and that of hysteria—a similarity which is complete except upon a single point. That point, however, is a decisive one and well adapted for purposes of differentiation. For in anxiety-hysteria the libido which has been liberated from the pathogenic material by repression is not *converted* (that is, diverted from the mental sphere into a somatic innervation), but is set free in the shape of anxiety . . . (p. 115).

Symmetrically, three years later, Freud (1912) added a third member as well, hypochondria, to the category of the actual neuroses (p. 248) though he adduced no special diagnostic or etiologic criteria to demarcate this state from the other actual neuroses.[3] More importantly in this paper, Freud clearly undertook to link the actual neuroses *dynamically* to the psychoneuroses. He said that the three actual neuroses

> . . . provide the psychoneuroses with the necessary 'somatic compliance;' they provide the excitatory material, which is then psychically selected and given a 'psychical coating,' so that, speaking generally, the nucleus of the psychoneurotic symptom—the grain of sand at the centre of the pearl—is formed of a somatic sexual manifestation (p. 248).

This linkage led Freud then to modify his previous more absolute therapeutic dictum. Though he still held that the symptoms of actual neuroses, unlike psychoneurotic symptoms, could not be analysed, he did say,

> I will grant today what I was unable to believe formerly—that an analytic treatment can have an indirect curative effect on 'actual' symptoms. It can do so either by enabling the current noxae to be better tolerated, or by enabling the sick person to escape from the current noxae by making a change in his sexual regime (p. 249–250).

---

[3] Freud repeated this new distinction in 1914 ("I have said before that I am inclined to class hypochondria with neurasthenia and anxiety-neurosis as a third 'actual' neurosis." p. 83); and in 1917 ("we distinguish three pure forms of 'actual' neurosis: neurasthenia, anxiety neurosis and hypochondria." p. 390). But again, Freud did not specify the basis for the distinction at these subsequent times either. He seems to have felt that it was either common knowledge or self-evident; both why hypochondria should be classed with the actual neuroses, and how it differed, descriptively and etiologically, from the others in that class.

In making this linkage and this concession, Freud, of course, moved his therapeutic thinking closer to the more modern position in which this sharp separation of so-called actual neuroses from so-called psychoneuroses on the basis of their presumed differential causation and differential accessibility to psychoanalytic therapy is simply no longer adhered to. I will return to this later.

Though Freud on a number of subsequent occasions (1917, p. 387-390; 1923a, p. 243; 1925, p. 25-26) reaffirmed these same distinctions between the actual neuroses and the psychoneuroses, his major diagnostic preoccupations shifted rather abruptly with his paper "On Narcissism" (Freud, 1914) towards the distinctions between the neuroses and the psychoses. A main demarcating line that he drew here was around the issue of proneness to transference formations. Although he had alternatively designated the psychoneuroses as transference neuroses on a number of scattered occasions as far back as 1905 (1905, p. 217-218; 1910, p. 214; 1913a, p. 125; 1913b, p. 319), it was in the paper "On Narcissism" that transference neuroses became his common usage. The distinction of course was to be from the psychotic afflictions that he was calling narcissistic neuroses.

This distinction was drawn sharply in Freud's paper on "The Unconscious" (1915). There, he said

> ... we have tried to base our characterization of Kraepelin's 'dementia praecox' (Bleuler's 'schizophrenia') on its position with reference to the antithesis between ego and object. In the transference neuroses ... there was nothing to give special prominence to this antithesis ... neurosis involves a renunciation of the real object ... libido that is withdrawn from the real object reverts first to a phantasied object and then to one that has been repressed .... But in these disorders object-cathexis in general is retained with great energy .... Indeed, the capacity for transference, of which we make use for therapeutic purposes in these affections, presupposes an unimpaired object-cathexis. In the case of schizophrenia, on the other hand, we have been driven to the assumption that after the process of repression the libido that has been withdrawn does not seek a new object, but retreats into the ego; that is to say, that here the object-cathexes are given up and a primitive objectless condition of narcissism is re-established. The incapacity of these patients for transference ... their consequent inaccessibility to therapeutic efforts, their characteristic repudiation of the external world, the appearance of signs of a hypercathexis of their own ego, the final outcome in complete apathy—all these clinical features seem to agree excellently with the assumption that their object-cathexes have been given up. (p. 196-197)

Here, Freud has clearly made his cardinal distinctions. In the psychoneuroses or the transference *neuroses,* object cathexes, though distorted, are maintained, transferences form, and therefore a *transference neurosis,* the declared sine qua non for analyzability, will eventuate. By contrast in the narcissistic neuroses (the psychoses), object-cathexes are declared to be abandoned (ego-libido is withdrawn back into the ego), transferences cannot form, and the patient is felt to be untreatable by analytic means. This dichotomy Freud adhered to throughout his lifetime, and he repeated this description of it a number of times subsequently (1917, p. 423, 447; 1919, p. 209; 1923a, p. 249; 1924b, p. 203).[4] However, he did refine it after a while by making a special accommodation for the case of psychotic depression, or as it was then called, melancholia. At first (1919, p. 209; 1923a, p. 249) he had put melancholia on a par with dementia praecox and paranoia, among what he called the "narcissistic disorders."[5] In his 1924 paper on "Neurosis and Psychosis" (Freud, 1924a) written after the crystallization of the structural theory in "The Ego and the Id" (1923b), Freud introduced the super-ego as the conception that provided a distinctive nosological position for melancholia. He said there

> We may provisionally assume that there must also be illnesses which are based on a conflict between the ego and the super-ego. Analysis gives us a right to suppose that melancholia is a typical example of this group. Nor will it clash with our impressions if we find reasons for separating states like melancholia from the other psychoses. We now see that we have been able to make our simple genetic formula more complete, without dropping it. Transference neuroses correspond to a conflict between the ego and the id; narcissistic neuroses [i.e. melancholia], to a conflict between the ego and the super-ego; and psychoses [the former 'narcissistic neuroses'], to one between the ego and the external world (p. 152).

In addition to this refinement of his conceptions, the better to place melancholia in relation to the (transference) neuroses and also the psychoses, Freud in that same year (1924b) also modified and (properly) blurred the sharpness of the boundaries of his entire nosological conceptual scheme. He put it this way,

---

[4] The description in the Introductory Lectures (1917) is a most colorful one. There Freud said, "The Narcissistic neuroses can scarcely be attacked with the technique that has served us with the transference neuroses . . . . What always happens with them is that, after proceeding for a short distance, we come up against a wall which brings us to a stop. Even with the transference neuroses, as you know, we met with barriers of resistance, but we were able to demolish them bit by bit. In the narcissistic neuroses the resistance is unconquerable; at the most, we are able to cast an inquisitive glance over the top of the wall and spy out what is going on the other side of it. Our technical methods must accordingly be replaced by others; and we do not know yet whether we shall succeed in finding a substitute" (p. 423). Further on in this lecture series he continued the same theme. "I promised to make you understand by the help of the fact of transference why our therapeutic efforts have no success with the narcissistic neuroses. I can do so in a few words, and you will see how simply the riddle can be solved and how well everything fits together. Observation shows that sufferers from narcissistic neuroses have no capacity for transference or only insufficient residues of it. They reject the doctor, not with hostility but with indifference. For that reason they cannot be influenced by him either . . . . They manifest no transference and for that reason are inaccessible to our efforts and cannot be cured by us" (p. 447).

[5] It should go without saying that Freud's usage of narcissistic disorders (as meaning psychoses, "narcissistic neuroses") is quite distinct from our common current conceptions of narcissistic characters or narcissistic disorders as expounded and defined by Kohut (1971), Kernberg (1975), and, of course, a host of others.

It could not be doubted that neuroses and psychoses *are not separated by a hard and fast line,* any more than health and neurosis; and it was plausible to explain the mysterious psychotic phenomena by the discoveries achieved on the neuroses, which had hitherto been equally incomprehensible. The present writer had himself . . . made a case of paranoid illness [the Schreber case] partly intelligible by an analytic investigation and had pointed out in this unquestionable psychosis the same contents (complexes) and a similar interplay of forces as in the simple neuroses (p. 204).

This conceptual modification (and blurring) notwithstanding, Freud's focus on the capacity (or presumed incapacity) to form transferences and therefore to be accessible to therapeutic influence as a major criterion clearly separating off psychotic from neurotic manifestations, proved to be one of his signal theoretical and clinical errors. It took a whole subsequent psychoanalytic generation, spearheaded by Frieda Fromm-Reichmann (1960), but including a goodly number of other as well (Rosen, 1953; Schwing, 1954; Sechehaye, 1951; and Sullivan, 1956), to demonstrate that psychotics did establish intense transferences, that they were at least in some instances, and albeit with far greater difficulty, reachable by psychoanalytic treatment approaches,[6] and that their considerable refractoriness to psychoanalytic interventions stemmed not from the failure to establish transference involvements but rather from (among many other things of course) the far greater difficulty in coping with their explosively turbulent and wildly fluctuating transferences in the absence of a stabilizing and reliable therapeutic alliance.

This has not been the only point on which Freud's nosological categories have been substantially modified, and even undone, in the light of subsequent theoretical and clinical advances. The conception of the actual neuroses, and of course their sharp distinctness from the psychoneuroses, has, as already indicated, likewise fallen into almost total neglect, though here too, Gediman (1984) tellingly reminded us that though the designation, actual neurosis, has fallen into disrepute, these states themselves have nonetheless been acknowledged all along by other names: she mentioned terror, traumatic neuroses, anxiety neurosis, visceral anxiety neurosis, psychophysiological reactions, somatizations, etc. (p. 182).

In fact, drawing on contemporary sources as diverse as Rangell (1968) and Kohut (1977), Gediman tried to refocus our conceptions of the actual neurotic state as not an entity but a dimension of experience, a tension buildup with

---

[6] Actually, Melanie Klein (1948), and her followers, importantly Herbert Rosenfeld (1965), espoused this same position: the amenability, albeit more difficult, of psychotic states to psychoanalytic intervention, a whole generation earlier, as far back as 1930 (see Klein, 1948), but given the near universal American rejection of the entire Kleinian corpus at the time, these Kleinian views were mostly, then, ignored. See, for example, Rapaport's famous scathing commentary on Klienianism: "The 'theory' of object relations evolved by Melanie Klein and her followers is not an ego psychology but an id mythology" (in Erikson, 1959, p. 11).

attributes of intensity, of quantity, and of threshold, cutting across all conditions in all people. That is, she views it as a quantitative dimension of experience for which there are developmentally acquired differential individual pronenesses. In this she sided with Rangell's (1968) efforts to synthesize Freud's two anxiety theories, the (second) theory of signal anxiety elaborated in "Inhibitions, Symptoms, and Anxiety" (1926), with the (first) theory of anxiety elaborated in the whole sequence of early papers on the actual neuroses, to synthesize these into a comprehensive and unitary psychoanalytic theory of anxiety. Pari passu, she took sharp issue with Kohut's (1977) continued dichotomization in which he talks about actual neurotic clinical states as "contentless mental states" and therefore different from drive and fantasy motivated anxiety phenomena. She said "one must take issue with Kohut's failure to appreciate fully the ramifications of the ways that fantasy content can be linked to these [actual neurotic] states" (p. 195).

My own point here is the one with which I began this review, that psychological nosology, like all else psychological, is a dynamic, evolving enterprise, subject to change and growth as the needs for it and the uses of it correspondingly change with growing knowledge of psychological functioning and malfunctioning, and of our ways of influencing and ameliorating it. Before concluding this overview of Freud's basic nosological placements, I do want to also set in place his inconclusive struggles with another kind of entity, the so-called traumatic neuroses (or war neuroses) that he sought to relate in various ways to his emerging three-fold conceptualization of actual neuroses, psychoneuroses or transference neuroses, and narcissistic neuroses or psychoses.

In his three earliest statements on the traumatic neuroses (1895a, p.107; 1895b, p. 125; 1905, p. 202), Freud made nearly identical statements—that hysteria *or* a traumatic neurosis (but never an anxiety neurosis) could be acquired from a single fright, though the mechanism is "not yet understood" (1905, p. 202). Thus, he originally put the traumatic neuroses together with the psychoneuroses (like hysteria) and apart from the so-called actual neuroses.[7] Freud's continued thinking in this arena was stimulated sharply under the impact of the World War I experiences. He expressed his concern, and his puzzlement, in this area as follows,

> The closest analogy to this behaviour of our neurotics is afforded by illnesses which are being produced with special frequency precisely at the present time by the war—what are described as traumatic neuroses. Similar cases, of course, appeared before the war as well, after railway collisions and other alarming accidents involving fatal risks. Traumatic neuroses are not in

---

[7] In subsequent years this of course has shifted oppositely so that today when we think in terms of actual neurotic states, we think of traumatic anxiety states as one of their form variants. (See my quotation from Gediman, 1984, p. 182).

their essence the same thing as the spontaneous neuroses which we are in the habit of investigating and treating by analysis; *nor have we yet succeeded in bringing them into harmony with our view* . . . (1917, p. 274, ital. added).

Freud's most intensive treatment of this subject was in his very short "Introduction to Psycho-Analysis and the War Neuroses" (1919). There he began with the disclaimer, "If the investigation of the war neuroses (and a very superficial one at that)[8] has *not shown* that the sexual theory of the neuroses is *correct,* that is something very different from its *showing* that that theory is incorrect" (p. 208). From there he went on to say that it was clear that the war neuroses have been "promoted by a *conflict in the ego* . . . The conflict is between the soldier's old peaceful ego and his new warlike one, and it becomes acute as soon as the peace-ego realizes what danger it runs of losing its life owing to the rashness of its new formed parasitic double" (p. 209, ital. added). Freud then sought to reconcile this statement with his conceptualizations of neurosis in terms of conflict over instinctual impulses as follows,

In traumatic and war neuroses the human ego is defending itself from a danger which threatens it from without . . . In the transference neuroses of peace the enemy from which the ego is defending itself is actually the libido, whose demands seem to it to be menacing. In both cases the ego is afraid of being damaged—in the latter case by the libido and in the former by external violence. It might, indeed, be said that in the case of the war neuroses . . . what is feared is nevertheless an internal enemy. The theoretical difficulties standing in the way of a unifying hypothesis of this kind do not seem insuperable: after all, we have a perfect right to describe repression, which lies at the basis of every [psycho]neurosis, as a reaction to a trauma—as an elementary traumatic neurosis (p. 210).

Clearly, this is a forced and unconvincing formulation, and Freud really did not take this thinking much further. The major question of the existence of sources of the traumatic neuroses in underlying infantile sexual conflicts remained unresolved in Freud's mind, as did then the nature of the exact relationship of the traumatic neuroses to the actual neuroses on the one hand and

[8] What Freud specifically meant by this he made clear in a discussion in Inhibitions, Symptoms, and Anxiety (1926) on this selfsame subject. There in the context of making the point that "Most of those who observed the traumatic neuroses that occurred during the last war took this line [that the anxiety is solely a reaction of the ego to danger], and triumphantly announced that proof was forthcoming that a threat to the instinct of self-preservation could by itself produce a neurosis without any admixture of sexual factors and without requiring any of the complicated hypotheses of psycho-analysis" (p. 129), Freud immediately went on to say, "It is in fact greatly to be regretted that *not a single analysis* of a traumatic neurosis of any value is extant" (p. 129, ital. added). This same point had also been made a year earlier in An Autobiographical Study (1925). "After the war our opponents were pleased to announce that events had produced a conclusive argument against the validity of the theses of analysis. The war neuroses, they said, had proved that sexual factors were unnecessary to the aetiology of neurotic disorders. But their triumph was frivolous and premature . . . . no one had been able to carry out a thorough analysis of a case of war neurosis, so that in fact nothing whatever was known for certain as to their motivation and no conclusions could be drawn from this uncertainty" (p. 54).

the psychoneuroses on the other. We can refer to the book, *Psychic Trauma* (Furst, 1967), for an update, as of that time, of the continuing evolution of psychoanalytic theorizing in this murky area. Of course, the growing body of work over the most recent decades with concentration camp survivors, and with their children as well, has expanded in painful direction our knowledge of the nature of extreme trauma coming at any point in the life cycle, of its long enduring effects and of its intergenerational transmission, and of the complex problems it creates for efforts at psychotherapeutic intervention.

To this point, I have indicated three familiar modern psychoanalytic modifications (actually more transformations) of Freud's original nosologic categorizations:

1. The modification and major blurring now of Freud's originally proclaimed unbridgeable divide between neurosis and psychosis on the basis of the presumed ability or inability to form transferences and the consequent presumed amenability—or absolute lack of it—to psychotherapeutic mitigation;

2. The current revival of concern with the *phenomenon* of the actual neurotic anxiety state—though not with Freud's original conceptualization nor with his proclaimed distinctive etiology in compromised current sexual practices—its revival rather in the preoccupation from many perspectives (cf. Kohut, Rangell, and Gediman and a host of others) with the nature of traumatic anxiety and its relationship to the conception of signal anxiety; and

3. The fuller evolution—born of the horrors of the World War II, the concentration camp experiences, the emerging narratives of individuals who have suffered childhood sexual trauma, and currently, the newest worldwide genocidal outbreaks, and terrorism and suicide bombings as political instruments—of our knowledge of the genesis and of the indefinitely enduring nature, once established, of the traumatic neuroses, at least in their severer forms.

I have not yet mentioned three other very major conceptual alterations in psychoanalytic nosology that more fully postdate Freud. These are, again by listing:

1. The major shift in psychoanalytic clinical and therapeutic concern from the symptom neuroses that were the prototypical illnesses of Freud's day to current concern with the varieties of character, character problems and character neuroses, inaugurated in modern form with Wilhelm Reich's landmark book, *Character Analysis* (1933);

2. The emergence into awareness of a major diagnostic grouping lying between the neuroses and the psychoses, designated by Knight as borderline states (1953); and

3. Drawing conceptually on both these developments, the distinctive delineation by Kohut (1971, 1977) and his adherents of the Narcissistic Personality Disorders or Narcissistic Character Disorders, marked by specific characteristic

transferences (designated self-object transferences), and by declared specific therapeutic intervention requirements.[9]

Because of our shared familiarity with these nosological, diagnostic, and therapeutic issues which form so much of the fabric of our current daily practice, I will make for our specific purposes here only a single nosological point about each of these three major diagnostic groupings. In regard to the character neuroses that have essentially supplanted the symptom neuroses of earlier days as the commonest presenting pictures in our "best" (i.e., most analyzable) patients, what needs to be emphasized is the to-this-point still very unsystematic, and even haphazard, construction of our psychoanalytic conceptions of character diagnosis. Baudry (1984) stated this most sharply as follows:

> The multiple points of view contributed by psychoanalysis to the study of character is reflected in the confused classification of character according to libidinal type (e.g. anal), neurotic organization (e.g. phobic, hysterical), or mode of relating (e.g. passive, feminine character). Study of the superego indirectly led to the description of certain types, but with no attempt at setting up a classification—e.g. the 'exceptions' or 'those wrecked by success' (Freud, 1916); the 'fate neuroses' belong here. Interest in the partial instincts also contributed its own nomenclature, e.g. sadistic or masochistic character. Concern with affects and object relations led to further types—the depressive character and the 'as-if' character. Clearly, not all of these 'types' are on the same level of abstraction (p. 467).

Incidentally, this is exactly the same kind of classification problem that the makers of DSM-III and IV have encountered in the construction of their so-called Axis II disorders. It is also the same problem that we deal with in this volume in the construction of our classification of Personality Disorders.

At this point, a necessary related diagnostic clarification is the distinction between the varieties of these character neuroses, conceived in this way as the neurotic exaggeration of trait or style or configuration, from the impulse neuroses, or the so-called character *disorders*, the addicted, the sexually disordered, the compulsive gambler, the kleptomaniac, the pyromaniac, etc., all the varieties of disorder where the presenting symptoms yield specific drive gratifications, unlike the symptom neuroses, where the symptoms are painful and ego-alien, and also unlike the character *neuroses* where there may be no symptoms as such,

---

[9] The growing shift over the past few decades of (at least American) psychoanalysis away from the primarily intrapsychic focus upon unconscious conflict (dubbed a 'one-person psychology'), towards a more central focus upon interpersonal, object-relational, and intersubjective perspectives (called collectively 'two-person psychology' or the 'relational turn') has not altered, or added to, the currently existing array of psychoanalytic nosological considerations. It has, however, shifted emphases somewhat within existing categorizations, away from conceptions built centrally around repression (for example, Freud's conceptualizations of hysterical and obsessional disorders), towards conceptions built centrally around dissociative phenomena. An outstanding exemplar is Philip Bromberg's 1998 book, *Standing in the Spaces*.

only character traits and configurations that are problematic for the patient or for others. These impulse neuroses (or character *disorders*) seem best grouped as among the borderline states or the narcissistic disorders to which I turn next.

About the all-too-familiar borderline and narcissistic states, I want only, with each, to call attention to a comparable caveat. We are all aware of how much the multiple contributions and the many-faceted formulations of Otto Kernberg (1975) have illuminated and given modern form to our understandings of the psychogenesis, the psychopathology, and the psychoanalytic therapy of the borderline states—albeit we are mindful that there are a host of other significant contributors to this realm (for example, Gunderson, 1984, Masterson, 1981, and Rinsley, 1982, to mention some of the best known). The caveat here is that of a beguiling pseudo-precision in the elaboration of nosological distinctions and of the boundaries from the neuroses on the one side and from the psychoses on the other side, a pseudo-precision that can be—but should not be—drawn from Kernberg's formulations. The proper psychoanalytic conception here is rather of the same continuum along a spectrum from the neurotic to the borderline to the psychotic that Freud first made familiar to us with his blurring of the distinctions along the spectrum from the normal to the abnormal or neurotic.

Similarly with the narcissistic disorders, we are equally familiar with the many contributions of the self-psychology school within psychoanalysis to the elaboration of the genesis, the pathology, and the analytic treatment of these narcissistic problems and narcissistic states. But again, I want to insert a caveat, that of an equally beguiling pseudo-ubiquity in being able to see narcissistic pathology everywhere, with a concomitant minimizing or even ignoring of object-cathected pathology, a pseudo-ubiquity that can be readily enough—but again I would say, should not be—drawn from the writings of Kohut and his followers.

This, then, is the modern kaleidoscope of our working psychoanalytic nosology and its developmental unfolding. It has been a clinically and heuristically remarkably useful, albeit untidy, array of diagnostic and prognostic categories, devised initially by Freud and subsequently both systematically altered and added to, both by him and by the psychoanalytic generations after him, as our clinical experience has grown and our predictive and therapeutic capacities have enlarged. It is from this nosological platform that we today face the challenges posed to our conceptions by the new and far more precise and reliable psychiatric nomenclature of DSM-III and IV, which, however, no longer has room for the most central of psychoanalytic diagnostic categorizations, that of neuroses or psychoneuroses, at least not in a psychoanalytically meaningful sense. Nonetheless, it should be said in this connection that even DSM-III and IV have maintained some basically psychoanalytic conceptualizations, at least implicitly, for example in creating Axis II, Personality Disorders, albeit in a more categorical than dimensional manner, and in Axis V, Highest Level of Adaptive Functioning Past Year, with its tacit acknowledgment of the continuum that Freud originally enunciated from healthy to the typically neurotic, and onto the more severely dysfunctional, the psychotic, level of functioning.

To summarize: I have tried to portray clearly not only the evolution of the nosological classifications created by Freud, and then amplified by his successors, to help order and deal with the phenomena uncovered by psychoanalysis, but also to convey the ever changing and developing nature of that nosology, both in the hands of Freud and of those who came after. The ready fit of this evolving psychoanalytic nosology with the psychiatric nomenclature of DSM-II, which was our official guide for so many earlier years is, I think, equally clear without specific spelling out. That this is so is of course no accident since DSM-II was created largely by psychoanalytic psychiatrists trying to accommodate the psycho-dynamic formulations of psychoanalysis to the classification requirements of the established psychiatric syndromes, and Freud's nosological conceptions represented the original base from which this was done.

However, there is now a many-decade time span between Freud's day and its immediate World War II aftermath out of which DSM-II emerged, and the time today in which we are faced with the new challenges posed by DSM-III and IV and all the related clinical and research, as well as socio-economic and socio-political, issues that converge on today's nosological tasks. Much happened in psychiatry, the explosion in neurobiological knowledge, and all the implications for differential diagnosis, prognosis, and therapeutics, of the ever burgeoning knowledge of neurotransmitters and receptors, of central nervous system facilitations and inhibitions. Equally so, much has happened in psychoanalysis with all the shift in focus to the newer categories of the borderline (a word never used by Freud in our modern sense of a specifiable category of patients) and the narcissistic (a grouping used by Freud in a very different way than its modern sense); and the major and more encompassing shift as well to our preoccupation today with the character neuroses and character diagnoses, of which the borderline and narcissistic disorders are but particular examples—also concepts which were only rudimentarily (and mostly by implication) developed in Freud's writings.

All of this represents a plethora of new and still not fully resolved issues within the realm of psychoanalytic nosological formulation, which burdens our effort to link our distinctive nosological conceptions to the now almost universally deployed DSM system—almost universally, that is, within the clinical realm of disorders of mental health, within the constraints of mental health research, within insurance and third party reimbursement requirements, within the categorizations of the judicial system and the educational system, etc. This volume is an effort to present a psychoanalytic nosological conceptualization of the range of personality (character) disorders, of the degrees of mental illness, and of the distinctive psychiatric symptom complexes, that articulates with the standardized

DSM formulations and that enhances them in a manner that aids in psychodynamic case formulation, in treatment planning and prognostication, and in psychotherapeutic implementation.

REFERENCES

Baudry, F. (1984). Character: A concept in search of an identity. *Journal of the American Psychoanalytic Association, 32,* 455-477.

Breuer, J., & Freud, S. (1893-1895). Studies on hysteria. *Standard Edition, 2:7,* 319.

Bromberg, P. M. (1998). *Standing in the spaces. Essays on clinical process, trauma, and dissociation.* (pp. 365). Hillsdale, NJ: The Analytic Press.

Erikson, E. H. (1959). Identity and the life cycle. *Psychological Issues, Mono. 1,* (pp. 171). New York: International Universities Press.

Freud, S. (1894). The neuro-psychoses of defence. *Standard Edition, 3,* 41-68.

Freud, S. (1895). On the grounds for detaching a particular syndrome from neurasthenia under the description 'Anxiety Neurosis.' *Standard Edition, 3,* 85-117.

Freud, S. (1895). A reply to criticisms of my paper on anxiety neuroses. *Standard Edition, 3,* 119-139.

Freud, S. (1896a). Heredity and the aetiology of the neuroses. *Standard Edition, 3,* 141-156.

Freud, S. (1896b). Further remarks on the neuropsychoses of defence. *Standard Edition, 3,* 157-185.

Freud, S. (1898). Sexuality in the aetiology of the neuroses. *Standard Edition, 3,* 259-285.

Freud, S. (1905). Three essays on the theory of sexuality. *Standard Edition, 7,* 135-243.

Freud, S. (1906). My views on the part played by sexuality in the aetiology of the neuroses. *Standard Edition, 7,* 269-279.

Freud, S. (1909). Analysis of a phobia in a five-year-old boy. *Standard Edition, 10,* 1-149.

Freud, S. (1910). The psycho-analytic view of psychogenic disturbance of vision. *Standard Edition, 11,* 209-218.

Freud, S. (1911). Notes on an autobiographical account of a case of paranoia (dementia paranoides). *Standard Edition, 12,* 9-82.

Freud, S. (1912). Contributions to a discussion on masturbation. *Standard Edition, 12,* 239-254.

Freud, S. (1913a). On beginning the treatment (further recommendations on the technique of psycho-analysis, I). *Standard Edition, 12,* 121-144.

Freud, S. (1913b). The disposition to obsessional neuroses. *Standard Edition, 12,* 311-326.

Freud, S. (1914). On narcissism: An introduction. *Standard Edition, 14,* 67-102.

Freud, S. (1915). The unconscious. *Standard Edition, 14,* 159-215.

Freud, S. (1916). Some character-types met with in psychoanalytic work. *Standard Edition, 14,* 311-333.

Freud, S. (1917). Introductory lectures on psycho-analysis. (Part III). General theory of the neuroses. *Standard Edition, 16,* 241-496.

Freud, S. (1919). Introduction to psycho-analysis and the war neuroses. *Standard Edition, 17,* 205-210.

Freud, S. (1923a). Two encyclopedia articles. *Standard Edition, 18,* 233-259.

Freud, S. (1923b). The ego and the id. *Standard Edition, 19,* 1-66.

Freud, S. (1924a). Neurosis and psychosis. *Standard Edition, 19,* 147-153.

Freud, S. (1924b). A short account of psychoanalysis. *Standard Edition, 19,* 189-209.

Freud, S. (1925). An autobiographical study. *Standard Edition, 20,* 1-76.

Freud, S. (1926). Inhibitions, symptoms and anxiety. *Standard Edition, 20,* 77-174.

Fromm-Reichmann, F. (1960). *Principles of intensive psychotherapy.* Chicago: University of Chicago Press.

Furst, S. S. (Ed.) (1967). *Psychic trauma.* New York: Basic Books.

Gediman, H. K. (1984). Actual neurosis and psychoneurosis. *International Journal of Psychoanalysis, 65,* 191–202.

Gunderson, J. G. (1984). *Borderline personality disorder.* (pp. 204). Washington, DC: American Psychiatric Press, Inc.

Kernberg, O. (1975). *Borderline conditions and pathological narcissism.* (pp. 361). New York: Jason Aronson, Inc.

Klein, M. (1948). *Contributions to psycho-analysis, 1921-1945.* (pp. 416). London: Hogarth Press.

Knight, R. P. (1953). Borderline states. *Bulletin of the Menninger Clinic, 17,* 1-12.

Kohut, H. (1971). *The analysis of the self.* (pp. 368). New York: International Universities Press.

Kohut, H. (1977). *The restoration of the self.* (pp. 345). New York: International Universities Press.

Masterson, J. F. (1981). *The narcissistic and borderline disorders: An integrated, developmental approach.* (pp. 264). New York: Brunner/Mazel.

Rangell, L. (1968). A further attempt to resolve the "problem of anxiety." *Journal of the American Psychoanalytic Association, 16,* 371-404.

Reich, W. (1933). *Charakteranalyse.* (pp. 288). Germany: Sexpol Verlagpp. Reprinted as *Character Analysis.* (pp. 328). New York: Orgone Institute Press, 1945.

Rinsley, D. B. (1982). *Borderline and other self disorders: A developmental and object-relations perspective.* (pp. 322). New York: Jason Aronson.

Rosen, J. N. (1953). *Direct analysis: Selected paper.* (pp. 184). New York: Grune & Stratton.

Rosenfeld, H. A. (1965). *Psychotic states: A psychoanalytical approach.* (pp. 263). New York: International Universities Press.

Schwing, G. (1954). *A way to the soul of the mentally ill.* (pp. 155). New York: International Universities Press.

Sechehaye, M. A. (1951). *Symbolic realization.* (pp. 184). New York: International Universities Press.

Sullivan, H. S. (1956). *Clinical studies in psychiatry.* (pp. 386). New York: Norton.

Suitability and Indications for Psychoanalytic Psychotherapy

Alain Braconnier, MD,[1] Nicole Guedeney, MD,[2] Bertrand Hanin, MD,[3] François Sauvagnat, PhD,[4] Jean-Michel Thurin,[5] MD, Daniel Widlöcher, MD[6]

Editor's Note: The second paper presents a French perspective on these important planning and treatment issues that highlights the contributions to them of John Bowlby, and even more, of Jacques Lacan, that are simply not accorded such attention in the Anglo-American psychoanalytic world. Though French psychoanalytic theorizing is now sharply split into Lacanian and anti-Lacanian camps—with, for example, Daniel Widlöcher, one of this chapter's authors, once a follower of Lacan, and now, a past-president of the International Psychoanalytical Association, and a firm anti-Lacanian—they all agree on the enormous formative influence that Lacan's ideas have had on the development of French psychoanalytic thought, and with extension, to some degree, into other romance language areas.

By contrast, Lacanian thinking has had little influence throughout the much larger Anglophone psychoanalytic world or in the Central and North European areas like Germany, the Low Countries, Scandinavia, etc.—though, at least in America, Lacanian perspectives have found significant place in psychoanalytic scholarship in academia, in the humanities, especially in language areas, literary criticism, rhetoric, and philosophy. This chapter provides some insight into the influence of Lacanian perspectives in psychoanalytic theorizing.

INTRODUCTION

An indication for psychoanalytical treatment implies not only that the doctor judges this treatment to be the most appropriate for the patient's condition, but also that the patient is considered able to follow this treatment. Compliance with treatment is a widespread problem in all fields of medicine, but particularly in psychiatry. In this case, compliance involves the taking of any medication prescribed, making recommended lifestyle changes, and the following of

---

[1] Psychiatrist, Praticien Hospitalier, Centre De Santé Mentale Philippe Paumelle, Paris 13è
[2] Psychiatrist Praticien Hospitalier, Centre Médico-Psychologique, Paris 5è
[3] Psychiatrist, Private Practice
[4] Professor of Psychology, Rennes 2 University
[5] Psychiatrist, Private Practice
[6] Psychiatrist, Private Practice; Emeritus Professor, Paris 6 University, Past Chief of the Department of Psychiatry, Salpêtrière Hospital, Paris

recommended therapeutic methods, such as case work, group therapy, family therapy and cognitive-behavioral therapy. However, the issue of compliance is most important in the domain of psychoanalysis, due to the specific nature of this type of treatment (e.g., duration of treatment, development of capacity for insight, and focus on the transference). Therefore, we need to specify the criteria for which psychotherapy, for a given patient at a given time, may be considered to have a reasonable chance of success, with the processes specific to this treatment having a chance to develop in a satisfactory manner.

Suitability for treatment has always been the subject of considerable clinical reflection. Progressively, objective evaluative studies have been carried out based on an empirical and quantitative methodology, which will be described below. The major difficulty associated with empirical evaluation lies in the large number of variables to be considered and the importance of individual factors related to the particular patient, the particular clinician and their interaction.

Therefore, it is currently difficult to define a list of criteria reflecting a consensus among clinicians that comes from the data from empirical research. The list presented here includes a number of items that may be considered redundant, with considerable overlap. This may be due to the state of development of our clinical and empirical research and the demands of specific methodologies.

A principal empirical constraint concerns the interference between the different therapeutic solutions that can be applied in each clinical instance. Methods other than psychoanalytic psychotherapy are often feasible and potentially useful for cases that could also be treated by psychoanalytical methods. The problem is thus to determine whether the suitability for psychoanalytical treatment is sufficiently high for priority to be given to this treatment or whether it is more prudent to renounce this treatment and to give more immediate priority to another therapeutic strategy. Therefore, it is always necessary to compare the expected benefits of this treatment and other treatments.

Another difficulty concerns the variety of methods used in psychoanalytic psychotherapy. Without considering brief therapy and therapeutic consultations, which are associated with very specific problems, it is clear that the criteria for suitability are not the same for psychoanalysis in the strict sense of the word and for psychotherapies, in which one or more technical parameters have been modified. As pointed out by Tyson and Sandler (1971), analysts currently practice both psychoanalysis and other forms of therapy. Therefore, for a given patient, even if that patient is considered suitable for analytic psychotherapy, they may take into account other criteria and decide to treat the patient with, or advise the patient to follow, another psychotherapeutic method, that they consider more appropriate in the given state of illness. We should also not forget that the therapeutic aims of psychoanalysis are only indirectly concerned with the symptoms, and are therefore compatible with more flexible strategies than other therapeutic modalities.

Finally, there is a semantic problem. We have used the term "suitability" ("convenance" in French), which seems to us to be the term most widely used in opposition to "indication" in the sense in which it is used here. Other terms, such as "accessibility" and "feasibility" could also be used as synonyms. The term "analyzability" is more ambiguous because it could encompass the results of treatment as well as the suitability of such treatment.

CLINICAL REFLECTION

Preliminary Interviews and Analyzability

The place of preliminary interviews and their function in assessment of the potential of a patient to undergo psychoanalytic psychotherapy has been very little considered in psychoanalytic literature. Other than therapy for a trial period, this question has been dealt with mostly by works devoted to the techniques of psychoanalysis. The most well known are those of Etchegoyen (1991), Glover (1958), D. Greenson (1992), and R. Greenson (1992). The first work specifically devoted to preliminary interviews did not appear until 1954 (Gill, Newman, Redlich, & Sommers, 1954).

This may appear surprising, particularly as another question—that of the termination of analysis—has been the subject of many more specific studies. It is true that Freud's article "Analysis terminable and interminable" (1937), one of his major texts during the latter part of his career, focuses much more on theoretical than on technical aspects. Should we deduce from this that preliminary interviews are no more than a marginal point in the technique? Nothing could be less certain. Indeed, most analysts agree that all the elements to be developed during the treatment are identified during the preliminary interviews. It is also clear that the interventions of the analyst during these interviews can have effects that manifest themselves years later. However, the identification of these elements may be difficult, if not impossible, because these elements generally come to the fore towards the end of the process, or after therapy has ended. Taking up this image of the condensation or clustering of elements, it could be suggested that the preliminary interviews cover a large number of fundamental questions.

It is during these interviews that the following subjects are dealt with: diagnosis, indications, analyzability, choice of psychotherapeutic method, establishment of a contract or the search for criteria predictive of the response to treatment. This extension has not only enlarged the perspectives of theoretical research, but has also led to changes in the techniques used in patient management. A reconsideration of the techniques used in preliminary interviews is therefore clearly required, to evaluate these "new" indications, as the strictly psychoanalytic model proposed by Freud does not always seem appropriate for many patients. This has led to the development over the last several decades of the notions of psychodynamic evaluation, structural interviews or case formulation. All these notions raise the same question concerning whether interviews should be directed and the potentially more fundamental question concerning what differentiates the standard treatment from other forms of psychoanalytic psychotherapy.

This part will deal with the viewpoints of Freud, Etchegoyen, Glover, Greenson, and Zetzel on the role of preliminary interviews in psychoanalytic technique. We will then deal with the more specific aspects developed in the approaches of Bowlby and Lacan and their successors. In considering these viewpoints, we aim to identify landmarks in reflection and practice relating to the question of preliminary interviews, while trying to identify the currently most important issues, rather than attempting to cover the subject exhaustively, which is beyond the scope of this work.

Freud

General Principles

In his article "On psychotherapy" (1905), Freud briefly touched on the issue of indications and contraindications for his method of treatment. Rather than delivering a list of the diseases for which psychoanalysis was or was not an appropriate treatment, he laid down a certain number of principles governing the choice of patients to be treated. According to Freud (1905), the patient needed to have a reasonable level of education and a character pattern that indicated reliability. He preferred to consider the notion of "educability" of the patient, which would clearly be subject to argument today. However, what Freud actually meant by "educability" was the accessibility to treatment of the patient, or the patient's analyzability. Freud also specified that treatment should be limited to people in a "normal state" because, in psychoanalysis, it is by starting from the normal state that we manage to control the pathological state. He stated clearly that psychoses, confusional states, and profound melancholy, are not appropriate for treatment by psychoanalysis, at least as practiced at the time. However, he pointed out that these contraindications might cease to exist if the method was modified appropriately to constitute a "psychotherapy of psychoses." It is remarkable that Freud anticipated the possibility of developing psychoanalytic psychotherapies, requiring the modification of techniques and enlarging the field of indications, as early as 1905.

Freud also suggested that his method should be used only for patients under the age of 50, as he feared that older patients would no longer display the plasticity of psychic processes on which the therapy is based and that the quantity of material to be analyzed would be too great. By means of this notion of age, Freud highlighted the importance of mechanisms for the defense of self, their rigidity or plasticity, as criteria for accessibility to psychoanalysis. This question stimulated considerable subsequent debate, particularly in the work of Anna Freud (1936/1967). As a result, the notion of an upper age limit for beginning analysis actually no longer seems relevant. Instead, emphasis is now placed on the capacity of the subject to enter the process. The continual increase in life expectancy throughout the 20th Century also resulted in a displacement of the upper age limit for treatment. Myers (1990), taking into account elements such as somatic health status, and the need for psychotropic drug treatment, indicated that there was no reason not to propose analysis to older patients. He cited examples of therapeutic cures initiated after the age of 65 and pointed out that reticence with respect to counter-transference more frequently inhibits these indications. It should be noted that even if indications for the standard method are limited in this age group, it is unfortunate that the resources provided by psychoanalytic psychotherapy remain poorly explored and exploited for them.

In terms of the minimum age for psychoanalysis, Freud indicated that it depended above all on the individual concerned, and that children are too easily influenced before adolescence. However, this did not prevent him from taking an interest in the phobia of a five-year-old boy, Hans, four years later. Psychoanalysis for children has developed considerably following the pioneering work of Anna Freud and Melanie Klein.

Therapy for a Trial Period and Preliminary Interviews

In Freud's article "On beginning the treatment (technique of psychoanalysis I)" (1913) and the additional details concerning the preliminary phase given in this text may be considered complementary to the article in which he first dealt with the indications (Freud, 1905). In his text, he explained that for patients that he did not know very well, he began with a trial period of one to two weeks of therapy. If he decided to stop the treatment at this point, the patient was not left with the impression that the treatment had failed. This made it possible to get to know the case better and therefore to decide whether indeed psychoanalysis was suitable. Freud felt that no other sort of test was possible and that interviews, even if frequent and long, and discussions during ordinary consultations, could not replace this trial period. However, he understood that this trial period constituted the start of analysis, and should therefore conform to the rules governing analysis, including the fundamental notion of abstinence. The only difference was that the psychoanalyst let the patient speak without making any comment unless absolutely necessary. Freud felt that this short period of preliminary treatment made diagnosis easier. Thus, in only a few lines of text, Freud laid down the basis of the reference model for preliminary interviews that is still used by most analysts today before psychoanalysis really begins.

Freud clearly challenged the principle of interviews, or at least of classical medical interviews, with the reporting of antecedents and the taking of the patient's illness history. The only way to determine whether a patient can be treated by psychoanalysis is to apply the method itself, in routine conditions, taking care to interfere as little as possible, and only intervening when necessary, in order to encourage the patient to continue speaking. This process makes it possible to narrow the diagnosis down, and to identify possible contraindications not detected on first contact. In fact, what Freud was seeking to test was not the validity of a diagnostic category, but the possibility of a patient entering the analytic process. For Freud, this preliminary phase already constituted a treatment, with the cure constituting a natural development if the treatment was to be continued. This provides a clearer idea of why the exchange that takes place during the preliminary interviews is as essential as exchanges during and towards the end of therapy.

Freud's model was subsequently modified, with trial periods being replaced by preliminary interviews, which are generally carried out face-to-face rather than with the patient on the couch. The retention of the term "interview" could be called into question, given that these preliminary interviews are totally different from classical medical interviews and their aim, by means of their non-directive nature, and the lack of intervention by the analyst, is to resemble the analytic situation as closely as possible. Furthermore, although this reference model was created for the evaluation of requests for psychoanalysis from neurotic patients, the same cannot be said for evaluations of the indications for psychoanalytic psychotherapy in patients with a borderline organization. For this reason, alongside Freud's initial model, a number of other preliminary interview models have been developed. Many of these models are more structured and directive and focus much more on personality diagnosis, with the aim of taking into account the indications for the different forms of psychoanalytic psychotherapy.

Glover

The work of Glover on the technique of psychoanalysis (1958) dates from 1954. Although this work is still cited in recent contributions, it is more as a historical document than as a realistic reference work of interest in current discussion. However, Glover dealt in a very concrete manner with technical questions relating to the preliminary interviews that are still posed today, and that analysts are often little inclined to discuss, in writing at least. It is for this reason that the work of Glover merits special attention. Glover differed from Freud in providing many more indications and prescriptions concerning the manner in which the preliminary interviews should be conducted. He explained that what distinguished an analytic consultation from other forms of examination was the encouragement given to the patient to recount his or her own history. During an analytic consultation, with the exception of things said out of non-committal politeness, the real initiative belongs to the patient. A number of useful deductions can be made from the behavior and attitudes of the patient, and the sequence in which his or her confidences are given. However, the consultation also involves a certain degree of intervention, especially in regard to the formulation of an immediate, approximate diagnosis. The patient unconsciously begins to regret his rashness from the moment at which he rings the analyst's doorbell. It is therefore only to be expected that the patient will use mechanisms of condensation, displacement, or secondary development, when relating his history. A few relevant questions are generally enough, however, to identify symptoms, specific features and conflicts, when possible and necessary.

It is clear that Glover's view of the preliminary interview contains a much larger diagnostic element than that of Freud, who was more concerned with testing the suitability of the patient for the process of analysis. Freud proposed identifying the defense mechanisms, symptoms and conflicts where possible. By contrast, the idea of producing a list or anything else systematically is absent from Glover's model. Although Glover proposed some intervention, that intervention remained minimal. Glover felt that the preliminary interview should have two principal objectives, in addition to providing a brief diagnostic summary. First, it should confirm the conscious motivation of the patient to undergo analytic therapy. Second, it should identify various practical details essential to the smooth-running of the therapy. According to Glover, careful attention should be paid to these details, as any negligence in this domain may subsequently lead to violent transference reactions, preventing the analysis from advancing. These details include decisions about the number of sessions per week, the duration of the sessions, whether sessions occur at regular or variable times, the number and duration of interruptions due to holidays, fees, the method and time of payment, the problem of "cancelled" sessions, and the establishment of an urgent means of communication between the analyst and the patient when this is necessary. Glover felt that it was essential to have a well-defined line of conduct for all these points and for other similar points, and to make sure that the patient was fully aware of all these arrangements. He pointed out that being reasonable in the organization of these details avoided many later problems.

Freud initially recommended six sessions per week, each lasting one hour. Glover pointed out that the British custom of having a weekend had necessitated certain modifications in this regime. He nonetheless suggested that an analysis comprising anything less than five 45-minute sessions per week should be considered suspect.

The debate concerning the number and duration of sessions has been extremely vigorous, with Lacan's position concerning short sessions even leading to his exclusion from the International Psychoanalytical Association. The question is still far from resolved because practices do differ widely from one country to another. According to Glover, if the analysis is interrupted by periods of longer than 48 hours due to there being too few sessions, then the treatment should be classified as a psychotherapy, and cannot be considered an analysis in the strict sense of the word. It is up to the analyst (and here Glover referred to the notion of honesty) to determine when an analysis is not an analysis and to assume the weight of his own economic necessities in his practice. Glover stressed that when dealing with the practicalities concerning interruptions of treatment due to holidays and cancelled sessions, the analyst must take his own needs into account, every bit as much as the ideal reference conditions for analysis that he has made clear to the patient. Glover was essentially flexible and recommended rigor and honesty rather than rigidity. The same was true for Glover's view of fees. Whilst accepting that some financial sacrifice encouraged the progress of an analysis, Glover stated that if the analyst could not afford to carry out an analysis at a price that the patient could reasonably pay, then he should not attempt that analysis.

Invariably linked to the question of fees, the question of the predicted duration of the analysis imposes great caution in the response given to the patient. A significant error could have deleterious effects on the subsequent analysis, and Glover felt that if the circumstances demanded more precise indications, then the analyst should determine what sum the patient could afford to pay per year and adapt his fees accordingly.

Glover suggested that hard-and-fast rules concerning abstinence should be avoided and that it was better to wait until the analytic situation demanded it. Glover also felt that the manner in which the patient was received was important. He recommended adopting a natural conduct, with tact and respect and to follow the patient's example in cases of doubt.

As far as the formulation of the fundamental rule given to patients at the end of the preliminary interviews, or at the start of analysis, was concerned, Glover paid particular attention to the affective element, asking patients to describe their feelings as well as their thoughts and to highlight the uncomfortable or euphoric sensations evoked by particular associations. Freud placed much more emphasis on resistance and censure than on affect.

Greenson

Ralph Greenson died in 1979, before completing the second volume of his work on the technique and practice of psychoanalysis (R. Greenson, 1992; Sugarman, Nemiroff, & D. Greenson, 1992). It was in this volume that he intended to include chapters devoted to preliminary interviews, analyzability and the start of analysis. Greenson explained in the introduction to this volume why he did not follow chronological order in his exposure of the technical and practical problems arising in the course of psychoanalytic therapy. He felt that it was impossible to write in an intelligible manner and to deal in depth with the most detailed technical and tactical aspects without first having discussed resistance, transference, working relationships, and the analytic situation.

Greenson was more of a clinician than a theorist, as demonstrated by the large number of examples and clinical illustrations he provided for each technical point dealt with. His aims were above all pedagogical. He wanted to provide trainee analysts with the bases required to understand fundamental aspects of the technique, to enable them to be at least partly prepared to face the problems arising during analysis, which, even when typical, may be complex and unexpected. Greenson wrote that not even the most complete and well-written manual could replace the interaction with the patient. This is why the many criticisms of Greenson, especially in France, should be seen in perspective. Greenson never claimed to have written a manual of psychoanalytic practice codifying or reducing the work of the analyst to the giving of certain advice or certain precepts.

Greenson dealt with technical problems in his own way, by matching them with clinical illustrations. It is perfectly legitimate to think that the particular example provided by Greenson might better illustrate another technical point or practice. However, this does not diminish the validity of the clinical example. At best, there is plenty to discuss, and that is important in itself. The incomplete chapter concerning preliminary contact with the patient shows that Greenson saw psychoanalysis as an appropriate treatment for only a restricted number of patients. From the start, he tried to create a context in which he could evaluate the suitability of the patient for treatment and the value of psychoanalytic treatment for that patient. He felt that the quality of the patient-analyst relationship was a key element of the treatment, and he made efforts to establish an analytic environment favoring the establishment of an effective working relationship from the first contact with a new patient. To this end, he developed certain rules concerning, for example, the first telephone call. He felt that it was important to take these calls directly only when he had sufficient time to devote to them, ruling out the possibility of taking a call during a session. He even tried to interpret resistance when a patient seemed to be ambivalent.

Greenson structured his preliminary interviews with the aim of determining whether the case was suitable for analysis. The classic psychiatric categories—based on signs, symptoms and diagnosis—were not, in his opinion, very useful in this respect. Instead, he tried to determine the capacities and qualities of the patient required for a productive working relationship during analysis. He identified three types of criteria governing analyzability: (1) the patient's motivation, (2) the patient's capacities and (3) the patient's personality traits and character.

Greenson was unable to complete the development of these criteria and we will see how his son, Daniel Greenson, dealt with the evaluation of analyzability. In the last few lines of his text, evoking his motivations as an analyst, Greenson said that he did not feel that he could successfully treat a patient by analysis unless he felt some real interest in that patient, emphasizing the availability of the analyst, rather than just the patient.

Daniel Greenson's (1992) work pursues the reflections begun by his father and builds on the assessment of the strengths and weaknesses of the ego. His views, although less categorical, illustrate one of the ways of considering analyzability. He does not structure interviews, and although he often remains silent for some time, he feels free to ask questions, perhaps more so during the preliminary interview than during the analysis. He tries to ensure that interviews do not turn into a series of questions and answers, and instead tries to see how the patient will react to particular questions and points. Indeed, for Daniel Greenson, part of the assessment of the patient involves the patient's reaction to the analyst. Those who feel that the analyst should remain absolutely silent are unlikely to recognize themselves in this approach. For other analysts, Daniel Greenson's attitude may be not so far from their own, when dealing with patients requesting psychotherapy rather than psychoanalysis.

Daniel Greenson pays particular attention to the following elements:

1. *The functioning of the patient in his own environment.* This involves an evaluation of difficulties and conflicts, the patient's capacities and strengths, and sectors that do not provoke conflict. The aim is to understand the patient's relationship to his work (type, professional success etc.), personal relationships, the patient's capacity to differentiate between objective and subjective reality, symptom severity, and the type and quality of defense mechanisms.

2. *Objective relationships*, which are likely to indicate the patient's ability to develop an analyzable transference, an essential condition for analyzability. They are evaluated in terms of their significance, relationships to parents, experiences of losses and separations, blocking points in previous therapies, and the objective investment of the analyst.

3. *Emotions*: Degree of tolerance and capacity to modulate anxiety, depression, frustration, anger and excitement.

4. *Character traits*: Interest in psychological functioning, ability to fantasize, to dream and to be interested in the meaning of dreams, ability to establish links between past and present events, ability to observe oneself, and to ensure that conflicts are dealt with internally rather than externally, good control over impulsiveness, ability to face adversity.

5. *Motivation*: Taking into account unrealistic expectations and the determination to change the other rather than the self.

6. *Superego*: Evaluation of masochistic tendencies, to take into account the risk of a negative therapeutic reaction, and lacunae in the superego, of which dishonesty is one example.

Daniel Greenson's list was not produced with the aim of structuring the interview. However, if used in this way, the determination to explore every point could hinder monitoring, and render the interview too directive.

Zetzel

Zetzel (1968) produced a list of indices of pathological severity compromising the prognosis of cases of hysteria, usually thought to be the ideal indication for psychoanalysis:

1. Parental separation or absence of one or both parents during the first four years of life

2. Severe psychological problems in one or both parents, frequently associated with an unhappy marriage or divorce

3. Serious and/or prolonged physical disease during childhood

4. Persistence of a hostile relationship and dependence upon the mother, who is seen as rejecting and deprecating.

As pointed out by Etchegoyen (1991), Zetzel's criteria are based on the theory of autonomous functioning of the ego, which can reduce the field of analysis to such an extent that it leads one to wonder whether there would still be patients to analyze. Etchegoyen pointed out that he uses these criteria for analyzability based on the principles of ego-psychology to establish a prognosis rather than to select his patients.

Bowlby

The Contributions of Attachment Theory

Attachment theory shows how early interpersonal experiences with figures to whom the subject is particularly attached give the subject the experience that there are people who are both a base and a haven of security. A second aspect is that negative emotions (anger, sadness and fear) are valorized and considered important as precious indicators of communication both for oneself, providing the subject with information about his own internal state, and for others. These negative emotions are controllable, if they are not disorganizing, thanks to the actions of those who are there, or whom the subject finds to help him. This interaction enables the subject to develop a model of others as worthy of trust and dependable in cases of need, and to develop a model of self as worthy of interest and valuable, even in times of distress. This basis of security has significant advantages for subsequent development. It encourages the subject to communicate openly about negative emotions, to develop a sense of partnership in joint construction in cases of conflict, and to cope better with negative emotions, whatever their cause. The inevitable conflicts in development (intrapersonal and interpersonal) are less easily overcome in cases of insecure attachment. In cases of insecurity, the self-protective strategies developed by the young child are likely to re-emerge in situations of stress, or in situations involving the attachment system (loss of love, conflict, aggressiveness, assertiveness etc.), making it more likely that the subject will not manage to come through the conflict in a satisfactory manner. The conflicts usually targeted in psychoanalysis are now seen in a chronological perspective at two levels: the basis of interpersonal relations, and an intrapsychic problem, interacting with a balance that depends on the subject.

According to Bowlby (1969/1982, 1988), secure attachment enables the individual to face up to the challenges of life with as little discomfort as possible, because the individual has confidence in others, which gives him a sense of personal worth, and because the development of his capacities of emotional regulation and subtle cognitive strategies enables him to develop a choice of adaptive strategies in all situations where he is confronted with unsettling negative emotions. This is the difference between primary and conditional strategies (Main & Hesse, 1990).

A Recap of the Key Points of Attachment Theory for Application to the Evaluation of Suitability for Psychoanalysis

What "idea of assistance" does the subject have?

The representational system of attachment in adults can only be seen as a complex system of different representational levels. The attachment system can be seen as being organized into a representational metasystem. The representations, in the form of operating internal models, are organized and made available in various forms, according to different dimensions: storage in different memory systems, their link to different successive vital experiences, their availability and their accessibility according to the level of stress or the context in which the subject finds himself. As there is probably metacommunication between the adult subject and his system of attachment and metaknowledge concerning what he can expect from others, each subject also has metaknowledge concerning the help seeking situation.

In terms of attachment, what representation is given to the meeting with the psychoanalyst?

According to Bowlby (1988), a subject seeking psychotherapy is in a situation of distress: this individual is requesting help from a professional who is supposed to be able to, and wants to, help him. This could be seen as a model of the contexts activating the attachment system because the primary motivation of this act is to do just that (Bowlby, 1969/1982). The expectations placed on the relationship developed during psychotherapy are influenced by the same Internal Operating Models (IOM) of self and others applied by the subject to his near relations. These conditional strategies (Main & Hesse, 1990) are developed by the subject as the best adaptive solutions for the specific environment that he faces. They make it possible for the subject to satisfy his own needs for protection, and to adapt to the responses of his figures of attachment to the expression of his needs.

What attachment needs are expressed in a therapeutic relationship?

According to Kivlighan, Patton, and Foote (1998), the needs expressed by the patient in a therapeutic relationship are those of intimacy, the ability to trust others, and freedom from the fear of abandonment. West and Keller (1994) summed the situation up elegantly, based on this general process of care in the light of attachment. They explained that their therapeutic response to this desire/fear of attachment crisis, involves separating the desire and fear elements. They allow the desire for attachment, the primary expression of the need for attachment, to remain in the background whereas they examine the secondary strategy of fear in detail with the patient.

According to Bowlby (1988), childhood relationships play a key role in determining whether a client is capable of entering into a therapeutic relationship. He raised two important points. He pointed out that the psychotherapeutic situation, due to the usual methods of working (speaking about one's dissatisfaction, uneasiness, or depression, and exposing one's inner self to the therapist) may conflict with the general rules imprinted in the patient's semantic memory: does the patient have the right to complain, to ask for help or to pay attention to his emotions? He explained that resistance could be seen as a deep reticence to disobey parental orders in the past concerning what can and cannot be said. He recommended that this type of prohibition should be investigated if the patient is not willing to speak at the start of psychotherapy.

His second point concerned transference, in the classical sense of the word. Adults seeking psychotherapy have developed their own emotional and interpersonal relationships in the context of other relationships, before entering into the therapeutic relationship (Tyrrell, Dozier, Teague, & Fallot, 1999). They will use these habitual strategies when establishing new interpersonal relationships. Thus, given the complex structure of IOM, it seems likely, depending on the context, the type of material brought up and the reaction of the therapist, that some IOM may be activated and the corresponding conditional strategies aroused (Mallinckrodt, 2000). This insight into transference differs fundamentally from transference as it is usually defined in psychoanalysis. In psychotherapy, we go over lasting impressions, elements that have been interiorized, and the response from the environment as well as the adaptive strategy used by the patient to deal with this environmental response.

Value of the patient's biography and of real events in the patient's life

Bowlby overdeveloped the role of reality in reaction to the lack of consideration for the reality of traumas. He felt that this denial of reality added insult to injury and placed the blame on the victim (Bowlby, 1988). If a patient talks about what happened during his childhood, in his interactions with figures of attachment, we should believe that his account is real, rather than simply reflecting his fantasies. This position remains fundamental as the first step in the psychotherapeutic process. As highlighted by Dornes (2000), fantasies are placed in an interpersonal reality that is experienced and inscribed in procedural scenarios that cannot be readily evoked by the patient. The events brought up by the patient, particularly if they relate to the system of attachment, provide a glimpse of the patient's model of others and of himself.

Reactions to the therapist's interventions

The reactions of patients to the interventions of the therapist are re-examined in the light of attachment theory. For example, Farber, Lippert, and Nevas (1995) pointed out that patients may feel threatened and/or criticized by incisive interpretations, particularly if they believe that they can only maintain relationships by maintaining the constant approval of the therapist.

Different memories. Consistency or inconsistency?

Discords may be observed between experiences linked to episodic memory and those linked to semantic memory, concerning the mechanisms of defensive exclusion and the multiple internal operating models (Liotti, 2004).

The capacity to integrate information from different memories has important implications for treatment (Bowlby, 1988; Bretherton, 1990; Dornes, 2000). In all cases, the semantic memory is of particular importance in allowing or refusing access to the multiple memory systems and facilitating interpretation. It acts as a kind of guide, determining the importance of or the manner of dealing with specific information (Bretherton, 1990). It may include prohibitions acquired from the speeches of attachment figures concerning the access to certain types of memories, or based on the subject's own cognitive procedures for avoiding uncomfortable or painful situations (Bowlby, 1988).

Slade (1999) carried out research into symptoms reflecting the integration of generalizations into the episodic memory, and of episodic and non-episodic memories. In particular, she asked whether adults could recall specific memories illustrating general descriptions of their primary relationships. By asking the patient to describe specific memories, or his early interactions and relationships in detail, the clinician has the opportunity to hear descriptions of clear abandonment and of ruptures linked to the loss of something precious, to separations, or to traumas. These are significant histories (Bowlby, 1988).

Meeting the psychoanalyst leads to the activation of different memories in the subject, particularly those relating to his different models of the world in relevant attachment situations: procedural (automatic, unconscious, behavioral and emotional), semantic (rules of functioning of the world and of the self in relevant attachment situations not linked to particular events) and episodic (memories, the access to which, will depend on the representational cognitive filters linked to the previous levels of memory).

This speech semiology is taken from the Adult Attachment Interview (Main, Kaplan, & Cassidy, 1985) and identifies consistency, collaboration and attitudes concerning the importance of attachment. It is now being generalized for psychotherapeutic applications (Brisch, 2002; Cassidy & Kobak, 1988; Crowell, 2003).

Which systems are likely to assist or damage the working relationship?

Affiliative strategies are useful as a subdimension of the working relationship. The pleasure of exploring one's autonomy in the presence of another is one aspect: "What would I have done all by myself, with what resources and what benefits?" Neurotic subjects, whose pleasure in autonomic functioning is reactivated by the psychotherapeutic situation (being alone in the presence of the other) may, after treatment, discover interpersonal strategies of various degrees of suitability and this may complicate the working relationship. Dozier, Cue, and Barnett (1994) noted that preoccupied subjects were those most at risk of subsequent problems within the interpersonal transference situation. According to Lichtenberg, Lachmann, and Fosshage (1992), the patient's own resource systems plays a role in maintaining the assistance process—when the relationship with the professional becomes aversive, for example—with the strength of the motivation to explore the rupture determining whether the patient progresses successfully.

Lacan

Lacanian theory has undergone diverse and contradictory transformations, and each of these transformations has its supporters. We will therefore consider the issue of suitability for each of these models.

1. *The first theory, from 1936 to the end of the 1940s* (Lacan, 1936, 1956, 1966, 1967/2001, 1975/2005), tried to reconcile Anna Freud's theory of defense mechanisms (Freud, 1936/1967) and Melanie Klein's concept of inner objects and primitive anxieties (Klein, 1948), using the concept of "imagos." These imagos are a series of prototypes including both drive-fixations and intersubjective elements (determined by social and familial conflicts), which in the course of time give rise to symptoms, which are thought to be consubstantial with character and ego traits. Lacan rejected the ego-psychological view that a non-conflictual core (Hartmann, 1939/1958) could be used as the basis of a possible therapeutic alliance. The suitability of the patient for therapy was predicted from the preliminary interview, based on the intensity and primitive nature of imago-fixations. Few accounts of Lacan's practice are available (Roudinesco, 1994), but various documents show the following:

   - Psychotic cases were generally considered unsuitable, unless the patient was found to be particularly good at limiting the effects of the delusional experiences.

   - Cases with strong character rigidity were considered to be unsuitable.

   - The early development of modes of transference involving strong narcissistic characteristics was seen as the forerunner of possible negative therapeutic reactions, with the patients "refusing to be cured by someone else."

   - Neuroses and perversions were generally seen as suitable for psychoanalytical treatment, provided they remained moderate.

2. *The second theory,1950-1961* (Lacan, 1962, 1966), corresponding to the "structuralist period" is characterized by six dimensions:

   - Development of the concept of transgeneration and symbolic (intersubjective) unconscious determining symptoms, influenced by structuralist linguistics (Jakobson & Halle, 1956), structural anthropology (Lévi-Strauss, 1963), Alexander and French's (1946) views of the "mechanicity" of the "sadistic superego" and contemporary cybernetics research (Lacan, 1966; Sauvagnat, 1994).

   - Development of the idea that transference and counter-transference are irrevocably joined and marred by imaginary and narcissistic traits, and that they should therefore not be directly interpreted.

   - Differentiation between the "empty discourse" taking place at the start of treatment and the "full discourse" at the end of the cure, when the subject analyzed has gained insight into the significant elements determining his destiny.

   - Development of the idea that the analyst's interventions should focus on what Lacan came to see as "core interpretations" from the unconscious.

- Development of a specific theory of perversion focusing on the "phallus destruction" fantasy as a specific determinant of this fetish.

- Description of strict structural differences between neurosis and psychosis and an attempt to develop a possible treatment for psychosis based on Federn's (1952) concept of "re-repression" rather than the "heroic" modes of treatment developed by others, such Sechehaye (1951), Rosenfeld (1965) and Rosen (1953).

Thus, in this period, suitability remained dependent on psychiatric diagnosis. An attempt was made to differentiate between the parts of unconscious symptom determination to be tackled (some resistances, some of them dependent on the "other," generally referred to as "the other's demand") and that which is to be encouraged (desire). The limit between the two is referred to as the "coat of arms," the basic defenses making up desire, with which the patient is encouraged to reconcile himself as much as possible.

3. *The third theory, 1961-1970* (Lacan, 1936, 1967/2001, 1975/2005), has probably considered the issue of suitability in the most detail. It rehabilitated the concept of transference, defining it as the result of a "supposition of knowledge." The core position of the patient was defined as dependent on a specific object (object a), derived from Winnicott's (1953) "transitional object," which was subsequently renamed the object of anxiety (Lacan, 1962) and then the object of desire (Lacan, 1966). This object was endowed with specific formal qualities, providing a framework for the individual's perception of the world. It was also described as the "fundamental fantasy framework," derived from the theory of perspective, and was presented as an alternative to the concept of "session framework" developed by various French IPA analysts (notably Viderman, 1970), following Isakower's (1938) elaborations. The analyst's position was seen as closely related to this object, in striking contrast to the strong conflict between the ego-core of the patient and the analyst in ego-psychology. In 1967, Lacan distinguished three types of "suppositions" in unconscious knowledge. The suitability issue is strongly connected to suppositions.

- The supposition by the patient concerning the analyst's professional skills is one of the first incentives for treatment. This supposition usually includes a certain degree of distrust in neurotic patients, whereas it may include directly delusional interpretations in paranoid cases and severe inconsistencies in schizophrenic cases. This supposition is generally modified during treatment.

- In his symptoms, dreams and "psychopathology of everyday life," the patient is "subjected" to his unconscious knowledge. The analyst supposes this to be true in the analytical setting as well, but does not know what that knowledge is. This supposition is presented as one aspect of the analyst's desire.

- The analyst's knowledge is understood to be "know-how" in the processing of the unconscious knowledge to which the analyzed subject has been subjected. This "know-how" is based on ethics involving the desire of the analyst rather than his academic knowledge. It includes both specification of the chain of signifiers at the core of the symptoms, and the fostering of changes in the patient's unconscious choices.

The end of the cure was defined as the result of two "negative movements" involved in the "psychoanalytical act."

- The development of drives: determining the specificity of the "object cause of desire," its relationship to the mother's desire, and helping the patient to separate himself from it.
- The development of thoughts, leading the patient to the conclusion that sexual relationships are impossible to conceptualize, despite his unconscious craving to do so.

As a result, several types of cure termination were described:

- Cases in which temporary relief was gained from the analyst's supposition of the "meaning behind the suffering," with the patient refusing to go any further.
- Cases in which treatment provided the patient with a certain amount of knowledge about the object of desire, and his own unconscious choices, but in which the patient refused or was not able to go any further.
- Complete cases, in which the "double psychoanalytical act" was completed, with the analyzed subject asked if he himself would like to become an analyst (provided that the supervised management of his first cases is successful).

    The most common reasons for not going further during the first step of therapy include the patient having a psychotic structure, threatening to decompensate, the patient being patently immoral ("canaillerie"), or lacking curiosity, or personal interest in mental matters. Most of the reasons for not going further in the second step concern the patient finding sufficient equilibrium, becoming able to assert unconscious decisions involving a separation from misleading ideals or dangerous desires, with the patient not wishing to seek a more precise characterization of the object cause of desire, and not quite having abandoned the pathological idealizations causing symptoms.

4. *The fourth theory*, "analytical discourse" and "rehabilitation of the symptom" focused on two issues directly related to suitability: the psychosocial and political conditions determining the possibility of an analytical cure,

and the positive aspects of the symptoms (Lacan, 1975/2005). The steps described in the third theory were redeveloped as follows:

- The preliminary state of the disease is described as dominated by the "discourse of the master," in which the subject has been subjected to mental events related to the specificities of his sociopolitical and religious environment. The general idea is that his symptoms and the structure of his unconscious are the direct result of current sociopolitical dilemmas, as interpreted by the language of unconscious culpability.

- The analyst's intervention, during preliminary interviews involves mostly the "hysterization of discourse," in which the subject is made to question the situation in which he has been placed, and the way he has symbolized the conflict in his symptoms,

- The next step involves setting up the "analytic discourse," in which "object a" comes to the fore. As in previous models, the analyst incarnates some aspects of this object, and the patient's elaborations concerning the object are directly supported by the analyst.

This raises three types of suitability issues:

- Social censure and its intrapsychic equivalents: individuals belonging to social groups with strict censure practices may be unsuitable for treatment; this may also be the case for individuals with intangible characters and personality conformity.

- The capacity for hysterization: during the preliminary interviews, some individuals may find it very difficult to display minimal "hysterization" of the conflict underlying the symptom. The preliminary evaluation should propose explanations for this, making it possible to distinguish between cases of neurotic counter-cathexis amenable to amelioration within the cure, and psychotic structures with low-key symptoms. Conversely, in some individuals, what appears to be a striking readiness for "hysterization" may in the long term prove to be a reflection of schizophrenic or manic disorders.

- The issue of suitability for analytic discourse itself, is paralleled by the capacity of the subject to accept the full process of the analytical cure, and the analyst's ability to cope with being identified with the type of object particular to the patient, and to help him to develop appropriate modifications of his object-relations.

Lacan subsequently (especially in the Le Sinthome seminar, [Lacan, 1975/2005]) focused on the treatment of psychotics, developing his "real, symbolic and imaginary" model from Philippe Chaslin's (1912) concept of "discordance"—the basic relationship the schizophrenic patient has with his body. This work led to the systematic study of modes of compensation for psychotic diseases and had implications for the treatment of neurotics as well. Within this theoretical framework, the most fundamental symptom of an individual was considered to have two distinguishable aspects: (1) a clearly pathological aspect, and (2) an element of "personal style" that could be developed in an acceptable way to counterbalance distress and anxiety. This personal style element has also been invoked to prevent negative therapeutic reactions.

Subsequent Developments of the Theory

A number of issues relating to suitability have been developed since Lacan's death.

1. *The treatment of psychoses:* The issue of the suitability of psychoanalytic treatment for psychotics has been systematically explored. Particular attention has been paid to the following aspects: counterbalancing auditory hallucinations, limiting delusional intuitions and interpretations, developing limited symptoms to counterbalance delusional experiences, encouraging artistic practices involving a limitation of depersonalization and psychotic manifestations. A few cases of patients becoming stable in the long term have been reported and it is generally thought that many psychotic patients may benefit from such modified practices.

2. *Predicting negative therapeutic reactions:* Emphasis on the differences in "psychoanalytic trajectories" possible for each patient, already evident in Lacan's two last periods, has continued, leading to discussions on the extent of preliminary interviews, the management of interpretations, and the possibility of organizing discontinuous treatments.

3. *Treatment of perversions:* The French school has been divided for years between those considering that perversions are generally not suitable for analytic treatment, and those claiming the opposite. In recent years, efforts have been made to specify the situations under which a favorable outcome could be predicted. In general, the suitability of these individuals is currently considered similar to that of neurotics. The wish to change sexual orientation is no longer seen as a valid criterion. There is a consensus that the ability to discuss inner anxiety and family concepts and the acceptance of such discussions indicates suitability for treatment. Inaccuracy in the reporting of one's known conflicts, "playing a double game" without reporting it to the analyst, and criminal behavior seem to be obstacles to suitability.

Analyzability: Practical and Technical Perspectives

The Individual Dimension

Analysts evaluate the structural aspects of the personality, the strength of internal operating models, the nature of intrapsychic conflicts, awareness of these conflicts, motivations and the ability to talk about oneself. They also evaluate the duration of these problems, diseases in the parents and prior treatments. Some also insist on the absence of certain elements: psychosis, risk of acting out, etc. Others feel that it is very important to be able to tolerate frustration and anguish. Some accept to manage patients in a "heroic" manner, guided primarily by the lack of indication for other types of management and considering analytical treatments as the last resort for the patient.

Analysts generally look for the following features in a patient:

- The capacity for "psychological insight," defined as the possibility to speak of one's dreams and fantasies and to observe oneself. The treatment is considered a progressive process, making use of material from further and further back in time (dreams, fantasies, memories, reconstructions, conscious and unconscious conflicts).

- The capacity to count on one's own personal resources and not solely on what the treatment can provide.

- The ability to develop transference. A distinction is made between the *development* and the *analysis* of transference.

- The personal defense characteristics of the patient are also important in that the patient must temporarily renounce his symptoms and defenses. We can distinguish between two different types of defensive organization. The first uses defenses such as denial, disavowal, retreat, repression and displacement. Individuals using such defenses are more sensitive to the interpersonal aspect and are therefore more suitable for a more "psychotherapeutic" approach. The second uses intellectualization, reactional training, rationalization, negation and projection. Individuals with such defenses are interested in developing a concept of themselves, respond well to interpretations and are therefore more suitable for a more "purely psychoanalytic" approach.

The Inter-Individual Dimension

The therapist factor is very important. The therapist must have general competence resulting from his training, but must also have a personal capacity to identify with, and to adapt his practices to, the different transference modes in which he is involved by the patient, particularly at the start of therapy. In other words, the capacity of the therapist to assume the identity of the patient's particular type of object, and to help the patient to develop the appropriate modifications in his relationship with that object, is essential. In this context, insight is not simply an awareness of a situation fixed in the unconscious. Instead, it is participation in a process identifying associated signifiers and their development. The security base incarnated by the analyst should be associated with a capacity for hysterization and role-playing in the relationship involved in the construction of mental objects. Bowlby (1988) highlighted the importance of identifying the different memories involved in transference relationships (semantic and procedural).

Suitability and Aim of Psychoanalytical Treatment

Before leaving the subject of analyzability, we should raise one point initially brought up by Freud that continues to excite debate: the goals of psychoanalytical treatment. Consideration of these goals is important when trying to identify the end point of analysis, but is also important right from the preliminary interviews. The distinction made by Ticho (1972) is interesting in this respect. Ticho distinguished between the life goals and the goals of treatment. Life goals are the goals that the patient would like to attain if he could achieve his full potential. Treatment goals concern the removal of obstacles to the discovery by the patient of his true potential. It may therefore prove useful to identify what should be changed in the patient's psychic organization to enable certain goals to be reached, right from the preliminary interviews, based on explicit and implicit life goals. Treatment goals are continually rediscussed during the course of the analysis. Enabling the patient to become aware of and to clarify his life goals, even if not all of them can be attained, is the sign of a successful analytical process. It would not be realistic to go beyond this, because, as pointed out by Freud, in most cases we must content ourselves with transforming hysterical misery into ordinary unhappiness.

Practical Applications

Various tools are available to the clinician to help him reflect on the possibility of a patient entering into and participating in a psychoanalytic process.

Capacities of the Patient to Engage in Psychoanalytic Psychotherapy

Definition: Probability that the patient will be able to develop the psychic working methods required for the therapeutic process.

Factors
- Acceptance of the treatment
  - *Conscious*
    - Capacity of the patient to represent and to describe the treatment
    - Circumstances of the demand and attitudes of the patient

- *Unconscious*
  - Cultural acceptability
  - Support of friends and family
  - Ambivalence of the patient
- Acceptance of the therapeutic framework
  - Understanding of the framework and of its constraints—anticipation of frustrations
- Personal dispositions
  - Ability to engage in a positive transference
  - Preparation for the expected mental work
  - Observation of one's own thought processes
  - Capacity for insight
  - Associative capacities
  - Tolerance: for preconscious and unconscious psychic representations

Patients for Whom Psychoanalytical and Psychodynamic Approaches Are Appropriate

- Acceptance of the treatment
  - Knowledge of the principles underlying the treatment and of its expected therapeutic goals.
  - Circumstances of the request for treatment (short treatment or treatment of indefinite length). Previous treatment.
  - Cultural background. Interest in the psychoanalytical process.
  - Role of the environment. Pressure for or hostility towards the treatment.
  - Degree of autonomy. Role of the patient within his environment, with evaluation of difficulties or conflicts, capacities, strengths and non-conflictual factors. Relationship with work (type of work, professional success etc.)
  - Level of motivation (degree of ambivalence, masochism etc.).
  - Rational and irrational expectations of treatment (view that treatment will magically change everything, determination to change others)
- Acceptance of the setting and the psychoanalytical process
  - Knowledge of the setting and its constraints.
  - Capacity to tolerate expected frustrations and the length of the treatment.
  - Object relations likely to indicate the capacity to develop an analyzable transference (relationship with parents, experience of loss and separation,

any blocking factors during previous therapy, and the object investment of the analyst).

- Capacity to fantasize, to dream, and to be interested in the meaning of dreams.
- Capacity to establish ties between a past and a present event.
- Capacity to associate.
- Capacity to observe oneself and to ensure that conflicts are from within and not just from outside of oneself
- Control of emotional reactions and impulsiveness.
- Capacity to tolerate negative emotions.

Alarm Signals: Probable Problems of Insecurity and Attachment

- Discourse indices: content
  - Things often heard: what is conscious/analytical approach
    - Denigration
    - Fear of dependence
    - Sign of fragility or weakness
    - Danger, mental manipulation
    - Guinea pig, expects no benefit from the analysis
    - Forced to attend because does not feel has a problem
    - Other
  - Surprising attitudes in the first encounter or after a first session of high quality
    - Unbroken silence
    - Factual logorrhoea that bores us and leaves us empty
    - Clinging aggressiveness
    - Submission
  - Situational indices (security base behavior)
    - Waiting room
    - On entering the office
    - Attitude towards the professional
    - Response to possible emotional manifestations on the part of the psychoanalyst
  - Biographical indices
    - Antecedents for relevant attachment (early separation or loss, repeated affective ruptures, maltreatment, sexual abuse, negligence)

Evaluation of the Representation of Assistance

- "Epidsodic" indices. Experience of assistance
  - Previous experience of this type of help?
  - Previous experience of professional help in general?
  - What did you think when this help was suggested?
  - In general, what does it mean for you to ask for help, to not be able to manage by yourself?
  - Your own ideas?
    - Examples? What specific memories do you have of asking for help?
  - Family traditions? In general, what are the views of your family on assistance?
    - Examples?

Attitude Towards Relevant Attachment

- How important is attachment?
- How important are relationships?
- How important are negative emotions (anger, sadness, fear)?
- How important were the possible attacks on attachment experienced by the subject?

"Procedural" Indices

- What was the client's discourse like when situations concerning the attachment system were raised?
- How does the client behave with the psychoanalyst in relevant "attachment" situations?
- What subverbal changes are observed?
  - Voice, emotion
- Reactions to "dysfunctions" of the therapeutic framework:
  - Errors, lateness, absences etc.

For Parents of Young Children Who Come to Talk About or to Seek Help Concerning Parenting Difficulties

- Does not feel the need to respond to vital needs of protection, closeness and security
  - Does not hear the baby's signals
    - Why is he crying? Why does he cling to me?

- Interprets the signals of the baby in a surprising manner
    - He only does it to annoy me!
- It's all an act!
    - It's capricious!

- The parent gives the response that seems the most appropriate, based on his or her own theory on what helps babies to grow up
    - You shouldn't be weak!
    - You shouldn't get attached to people!
    - You should be able to manage on your own!
    - I never had anything and that didn't stop me from getting on!

- The lack of an "instruction manual" or how to prevent fatality when exposed to vulnerability?
    - I would like you to have more than I had!
    - Why aren't you well-behaved, docile or grateful like I was, even though I had nothing?
    - Who's looking after me, a nostalgic and wounded child?
    - I explode. I can't cope!
    - How does a child think or feel?

First Step: Evaluate What Asking For Help Represents for the Subject in the Immediate Conditions of Minimal Alliance

- Construct hypothesis concerning the principal system of motivation
    - How is the attachment system activated?
    - What strategies appear?
    - Can you immediately count on a certain security?
- If not, the priority is to render the meeting less dangerous

REFERENCES

Alexander, F., & French, T. M. (1946). *Psychoanalytic therapy: Principles and application.* New York: Ronald Press.

Bowlby, J. (1969/1982) *Attachment and loss.* New York: Basic Books.

Bowlby, J. (1988). *A secure base: Clinical applications of attachment theory.* London: Routledge.

Bretherton, I. (1990). Communication patterns: Internal working models and the intergenerational transmission of attachment relationships. *Infant Mental Health Journal, 11,* 237-252.

Brisch, K. H. (2002). *Treating attachement disorders: From theory to therapy.* New York: Guilford Press.

Cassidy, J., & Kobak, R. R. (1988). *Avoidance and its relation to other defensive processes.* In J. Belski & T. Nezworski (Eds.), *Clinical implications of attachment* (pp. 300-319). Mahwah, NJ: Lawrence Erlbaum Associates.

Chaslin, P. (1912). *Eléments de sémiologie et clinique mentales.* Paris: Asselin & Houzeau.

Crowell, J. A. (2003). Assessment of attachment security in a clinical setting: Observations of parents and children. *Developmental and Behavioral Pediatrics, 24,* 199-204.

Dornes, M. (2000). *Die emotionale Welt des Kindes.* Frankfurt: Fischer.

Dozier, M., Cue, K. L., & Barnett, L. (1994). Clinician as caregivers: Role of attachment organization in treatment. *Journal of Consulting and Clinical Psychology, 62,* 793- 800.

Etchegoyen, R. H. (1991). *The fundamentals of psychoanalytic technique.* London: Karnac.

Farber, B., Lippert, R. A., & Nevas, D.B. (1995). The therapist as attachment figure. *Psychotherapy, 32,* 204- 212.

Federn, P. (1952). *Ego psychology and the psychoses.* New York: Basic Books.

Freud, A. (1936/1967). *Writings of Anna Freud: Vol. II: The ego and the mechanisms of defense.* New York: International Universities Press.

Freud, S. (1905). On psychotherapy. *Standard Edition, 7,* 255-268.

Freud, S. (1913). On beginning the treatment (Further recommendations on the technique of psycho-analysis, I). *Standard Edition, 12,* 121-144.

Freud, S. (1937). Analysis terminable and interminable. *Standard Edition, 23,* 209-253.

Gill, M. M., Newman, R., Redlich, E. C., & Sommers, M. (1954). *The initial interview in psychiatric practice.* New York: International Universities Press.

Glover, E. (1958). *The technique of psycho-analysis.* 2nd Edition. New York: International Universities Press.

Greenson, D. P. (1992). *Assessment of analyzability.* In A. Sugarman, R. A. Nemiroff, & D. P. Greenson (Eds.), *The technique and practice of psychoanalysis: 2. A memorial volume to Ralph R. Greenson,* (pp. 43-62). Madison, CT: International Universities Press.

Greenson, R. R. (1992). *Beginnings: The preliminary contacts with the patients.* In A. Sugarman, R. A. Nemiroff, & D. P. Greenson (Eds.), *The technique and practice of psychoanalysis: 2. A memorial volume to Ralph R. Greenson,* (pp. 1-42). Madison, CT: International Universities Press.

Hartmann, H. (1958). Ego psychology and the problem of adaptation (D. Rapaport, Trans.). New York: International Universities Press. (Original work published 1939).

Isakower, O. (1938). A contribution to the patho-psychology of phenomena associated with falling asleep. *International Journal of Psychoanalysis, 19,* 331-45.

Jakobson, R., & Halle, M. (1956). *Fundamentals of language.* The Hague, Netherlands: Mouton.

Kivlighan, M.D., Patton, M. J., & Foote, D. (1998). Moderating effects of client attachment on the counselor experience-working alliance relationship. *Journal of Counseling Psychology, 45,* 274- 278.

Klein, M. (1948). *Contributions to psychoanalysis: 1921-1945.* London: Hogarth Press.

Lacan, J. (1936). *Le stade du miroir.* Paris: Seuil.

Lacan, J. (1956). *Seminar on 'The purloined letter.'* In J. P. Muller & W. J. Richardson (Eds), *The Purloined Poe* (Jeffrey Mehlman, Trans.), (pp. 28-54). Baltimore and London: Johns Hopkins University Press.

Lacan, J. (1962). *Le Séminaire l'Angoisse.* Paris: Seuil.

Lacan, J. (1966). *Ecrits: A selection.* Paris: Seuil.

Lacan, J. (2001). *Proposition of 9 October 1967 on the psychoanalyst of the school* (R. Grigg, Trans.). In *Autres Écrits,* Paris: Seuil. (Original work published in 1967.)

Lacan, J. (2005). *Le séminaire livre XXIII: Le sinthome.* Paris: Seuil. (Original work published in 1975.)

Lévi-Strauss, C. (1963). *Structural anthropology.* (C. Jacobsen & B. Schoepf, Trans.). New York: Basic Books.

Lichtenberg, J. D., Lachmann, F. M., & Fosshage, J. L. (1992). *Self and motivational systems: Toward a theory of psychoanalytic technique.* London: The Analytic Press.

Liotti, G. (2004). Trauma, dissociation and disorganized attachment: Three strands of a single braid. *Psychotherapy: Theory, Research, Practice, Training, 41,* 472-486.

Main, M., & Hesse, E. (1990). *Parents' unresolved traumatic experiences are related to infant disorganized attachment status: is frightened and/or frightening parental behavior the linking mechanism?* In M. T. Greenberg, D. Cicchetti, & E. M. Cummings (Eds.), *Attachment in preschool years: Theory, research, and intervention,* (pp. 161-184). Chicago: Chicago University Press.

Main, M., Kaplan, N., & Cassidy, J. (1985). *Security in infancy, childhood and adulthood: A move to the level of representation.* In I. Bretherton & E. Waters, *Growing points in attachment theory and research,* (pp. 66-104). *Monographs of the Society for Research in Child Development, 50* (Serial No. 209).

Mallinckrodt, B. (2000). Attachment, social competencies, social support and interpersonal process in psychotherapy. *Psychotherapy Research, 10,* 239-266.

Myers, W. A. (1990). *On beginning with an elderly patient.* In T. J. Jacobs & A. Rothstein (Eds.), *On beginning an analysis,* (pp. 261-272). Madison, CT: International Universities Press.

Rosen, J. N. (1953). *Direct analysis: Selected papers.* New York: Grune & Stratton.

Rosenfeld, H. (1965) *Psychotic states.* London: Hogarth.

Roudinesco, E. (1994). *Histoire de la psychanalyze en France.* Vol. 1, 1982, Vol. 2, 1986. Paris: Fayard.

Sauvagnat, F. (1994). Psychanalyze et neurosciences. In P*sychanalyze et recherche universitaire* (Actes du colloque). France: Université de Rennes.

Sechehaye, M. (1951). *A new psychotherapy of schizophrenia: Relief of frustrations by symbolic realization* (G. Rubin-Rabson, Trans.). New York: International Universities Press.

Slade, A. (1999). *Attachment theory and research: Implications for the theory and practice of individual psychotherapy with adults.* In J. Cassidy & P. R. Schavers (Eds.), *Handbook of attachment: Theory, research, and clinical applications,* (pp. 575-594). New York: Guilford Press.

Sugarman, A., Nemiroff, R. A., & Greenson, D.P. (1992). *The technique and practice of psychoanalysis: 2. A memorial volume to Ralph R. Greenson.* Madison, CT: International Universities Press.

Ticho, E. A. (1972). Termination of psychoanalysis: Treatment goals, life goals. *Psychoanalytic Quarterly, 41,* 315-333.

Tyrrell, C. L., Dozier, M., Teague, G. B., & Fallot, R. D. (1999). Effective treatment relationships for persons with serious psychiatric disorders: The importance of attachment states of mind. *Journal of Consulting and Clinical Psychology, 67,* 725-733.

Tyson, R., & Sandler, J. (1971). Problems in the selection of patients for psychoanalysis: Comments on the application of concepts of 'indications,' 'suitability,' and 'analyzability.' *British Journal of Medical Psychology, 44,* 211-228.

Viderman, S. (1970). *La construction de l'espace analitique.* Paris: Demaël.

West, M., & Keller, A. (1994). *Psychotherapy strategies for insecure attachment in personality disorders.* In M. B. Sperling & W. H. Berman (Eds.), *Attachment in adults: clinical and developmental perspectives,* (pp. 313–330). New York: Guildford.

Winnicott, D. (1953). Transitional objects and transitional phenomena: A study of the first not-me possession. *International Journal of Psychoanalysis, 34,* 89-97.

Zetzel, R. (1968). The so-called good hysteric. *International Journal of Psychoanalysis, 49,* 256-260.

A Developmental Framework for Depth Psychology and a Definition of Healthy Emotional Functioning

Stanley I. Greenspan, MD[1] and Stuart G. Shanker, DPhil[2]

Editor's Note: The third paper draws on both the psychoanalytic and the non-psychoanalytic developmental literature—both conceptual and empirical—to present an integrated perspective on the development and the functional nature of healthy (adaptive) and impaired (maladaptive) mental activity.

The authors accomplish this through the delineation of six progressive early organizational levels of mental and emotional functioning, providing for each level both clinical observations and empirical research findings, and indicating the understandings for organized mental (ego) functioning. The six developmental levels outlined range from the so-called homeostatic level of self-regulation and interest in the world characteristic of the first three months of post-natal life, to the (sixth) level of representational differentiation, the capacity to build logical bridges between ideas and emotions that mark the approximate period from 30 to 48 months. The effort throughout is to integrate empirical research findings with the data of close clinical observation in a manner that provides meaningful and usable understanding of the increasing complexity of mental and emotional functioning throughout the developmental process. This provides substantial empirical and conceptual underpinning for a psychoanalytic understanding of human mental life.

PREFACE

In order to classify psychopathology, it is essential to have a working definition of healthy mental or emotional functioning. With such a working definition, deviations from healthy functioning can be elucidated. Without it, it is difficult to classify disordered functioning. For example, does the presence of symptoms, such as transient anxiety or feelings of depression or preoccupations with certain thoughts, constitute a sign of disorder or a sign of healthy responses to selected experiences? Is a tendency to be interested in oneself first and interested in others only to the degree that they meet one's own needs a

---

[1] Clinical Professor of Psychiatry and Pediatrics, George Washington University Medical School
[2] Distinguished Research Professor of Philosophy and Psychology, York University

disordered pattern or simply a position on a healthy continuum of different types of relationships?

The definition of healthy emotional functioning is especially important when developing treatment approaches and assessing outcomes. For example, should the focus of a particular treatment be the amelioration of an isolated symptom or the broadening of the range of internal emotional experience, such as a deepening of empathy, of which a person is capable? In evaluating the effectiveness of a particular medication or type of focused therapy, is it necessary to look at the change in a target symptom alone, or look also at changes in what defines healthy social and emotional functioning? For example, if a particular antidepressant reduces depressive symptoms, is it helpful to have a model whereby one also looks at changes in the person's relationships and level of self-awareness?

A concrete example of the importance of this point is the clinical observation that certain types of antidepressants, MAO inhibitors, tended to increase feelings of self-involvement, narcissism, and grandiosity. These types of feelings, however, were rarely looked for in the early studies of MAO inhibitors. In general medicine, pathology and pathophysiology are a part of a broader framework of healthy physical functioning, and interventions are always viewed to whatever degree possible, in the context of a "profile" of the individual's functioning.

In the psychiatric and psychological field, by contrast, we have not sufficiently embraced a model of mental health that can be agreed to by all. As a consequence, it is difficult to achieve consensus on what constitutes pathology and what constitutes meaningful therapeutic results. Debates about different hypothetical constructs or theories have unfortunately, at times, distracted us from formulating a model of mental health that is based on direct observation. Such a model would lend itself to operational concepts that could be employed in a variety of research studies and be used as a basis for classifying mental health disorders.

In this article, we approach this challenge from the perspective of studies of human development. Observing how infants and young children develop their distinctively human characteristics offers a model for healthy emotional functioning. Together with clinical observations and empirical research on adults, observations of infants and young children may be able to contribute to a much-needed framework for healthy emotional and social functioning.

INTRODUCTION

It was not until late in the 20th century that a true developmental perspective began to emerge in psychology. Prior to this time, interest in the question "How does the mind develop?" was really concerned with some variant of the question:

"How does one produce an upright or productive member of our society?" This utilitarian perspective remained prominent until well into the 20th century, as can be seen, for example, in Watson's famous boast:

> Give me a dozen healthy infants, well-formed, and my own specified world to bring them up in and I'll guarantee to take any one at random and train him to become any type of specialist I might select—doctor, lawyer, artist, merchant, chief, and yes, even beggar man and thief, regardless of his talents, penchants, tendencies, abilities, vocations and race of his ancestors. (1930).

This behaviorist leitmotif can be traced back to the Romans, if not beyond (see Greenspan & Shanker, 2004, Ch. 13). But the psychological question of how the *mind* develops—how a child begins to regulate her affects, to act purposefully and recognize others as intentional agents with minds of their own, how she learns how to speak and reason and form abstract concepts—emerged as a *scientific* concern only in the latter part of the 20th century.

In the early days of the psychoanalytic movement, theorists explored this issue by attempting to reconstruct early development from their research on older children and adults. Margaret Mahler and Anna Freud were among the first to conduct observational studies on preverbal infants, where the focus was that of inferring from their external behaviors what the internal life of the child must be like. Independent of this line of research, the 20th century saw the enormous growth of developmental psychology as an academic discipline. It is difficult to summarize the full extent of the important findings that have been made in these studies (Bremmer & Fogel, 2001).

Depth psychology concerns itself with levels of the mind that influence mental health and illness but are often not manifest directly in surface behaviors and in non-clinical settings. For example, depth psychology considers the deepest levels of intimacy and sexuality, anger and fear, the tendencies to split our inner worlds into polar opposites, to project our own wishes and thoughts onto others, and to incorporate the wishes and thoughts of others into ourselves. It concerns itself with the formation of our sense of self and of others and the way that these tendencies are internalized at different levels of differentiation and integration. It also concerns itself with the differentiation of our affects and emotions, their transformation from discharge modes to signals of symbolized feelings, the formation of defensive and coping strategies, and the development of personality patterns and personality disorders. Depth psychology is thus preoccupied with some of the most critical and yet perplexing dimensions of human functioning.

Developmental psychology is concerned with the empirical study of the development of physical functioning (e.g., motor skills, growth, the psychological effect of hormonal changes); neurophysiological patterns (e.g., cortical organization, neural plasticity, the relationship between neural and cognitive development); perception (e.g., visual, auditory, tactile, and olfactory functioning); cognition (e.g., attention, learning, memory, problem-solving, causal reasoning); communication (e.g., gesturing, eye gaze, vocalizations); linguistic facility (e.g., comprehension, production, morphology, pragmatics, reading); social functioning (e.g. attachment, peer relationships); emotional functioning (e.g., mechanisms of development; influence of emotions on behavior, perception and cognition; influence of emotions on the growth of the mind); personality (e.g., temperament and behavior, genetic and environmental influences on temperament); and morality (e.g., prosocial attitudes, empathy, moral reasoning).

Developmental psychologists use a number of formal techniques to study these domains, such as high-amplitude sucking, habituation, and preferential looking; naturalistic, laboratory, and psychophysiological studies; and ethnographic research. But they have been constrained to look at children's behaviors in situations which, unlike clinical settings, involve relatively little affective challenge. In order to construct a developmental framework for depth psychology, therefore, we need to integrate not only these important bodies of research, which have hitherto operated in relative isolation from one another, but also, to add clinical work with children and infants. In clinical settings, children encounter situations of affective challenge, in which their minds are inevitably stretched, providing another critical source of information about both the normal and pathological ways in which the mind can grow.

There now exists an impressive literature seeking to relate the work being done in depth psychology with findings from developmental psychology. The missing piece in this literature is the formulation of a theory explaining the developmental pathways to the essential depth psychological capacities, including the capacities for self-regulation, forming relationships, engaging in co-regulated affect signaling, constructing internalized representations of self and objects, and forming differentiated and integrated self and object representational structures at successively higher levels of organization. Such a formulation also must explain the development of derivative ego functions, including reality-testing, defensive and coping capacities, and various levels of reflective or "observing ego" capacities. As part of the conceptualization of the developmental pathways leading to these critical human capacities, it is essential not only to look at the observations from each of these fields, but also to articulate the strengths and limitations of their respective findings. These must be woven together with fresh clinical observations of developing infants and children into a cohesive theory that explains the pathways to the capacities that define our humanity.

A developmental model that would prove useful to mental health practitioners and policy advisors should meet four criteria:

- It should consider adaptive or healthy as well as psychopathologic human mental functioning. Consideration of adaptive psychological functioning has always been an essential feature of in-depth psychological approaches.
- It should address the deeper levels of the mind.
- It should be based on a confluence of empirical, observable, and clinical studies.
- Perhaps most critically, it should be relevant to clinical work by providing an understanding of developmental pathways toward healthy and pathologic development, respectively.

Thus, as we construct a developmental framework for depth psychology, we need to take into account the levels of the mind that explain clinically relevant healthy and disordered functioning. At the same time, we need to attend to the enormous number of empirical studies on cognitive, perceptual, motor, social, and emotional development in the past half century. The challenge to depth psychoanalytic approaches is to make sense of these findings—to interpret their implications for our understanding of the deepest levels of the mind.

The Distinction Between Depth and Surface Approaches

Depth psychological understanding of the mind has, for the most part, emerged from clinical studies where the mind's capacities are stretched to deal with such challenges as conflict, anxiety, overwhelming affect, trauma, unusual family patterns, and biological differences. Developmental psychology has largely followed a normative model in which age-related averages are computed from measures of behavior taken on large numbers of children. Most of the latter studies focus on the capacities or behavior of infants and young children in non-clinical contexts: that is, in situations that are relatively familiar to the child and involve minimal stress. Even those experiments that do challenge infants and children do so within the expectable range of healthy experiences; for to do otherwise is unethical.

The observations of infants and young children confronting extreme challenges, such as John Bowlby's studies (e.g., 1951) of prolonged separation from caregivers, Rene Spitz's studies of institutionalized infants (e.g., 1965), Anna Freud and Dorothy Burlingham's observations of children in war situations (Burlingham & Freud, 1942), Wayne Dennis's research (e.g., 1960) on children in impoverished orphanages, as well as more recent work on children exposed to trauma or responding to various types of extreme stress (see, e.g., Hilweg & Ullman, 1999, La Greca, et al., 2002), constitute landmark studies. Yet, they are relatively few in number compared to the countless studies of emotional, social, and cognitive development in normative contexts that have contributed to the current field of developmental psychology. While many of the findings of normative studies are highly important, they have often been made on *surface* phenomena.

Such studies would be akin to observations one might make of undergraduate students in familiar situations where their behavior, emotional expressions, and cognitive operations are operating in a fairly narrow range. Even in situations in which undergraduates are exposed to a stress, such as watching a horror movie or undergoing a difficult job interview, they are still operating in a relatively safe and secure environment. But, as indicated earlier, clinical situations often reveal very different levels of functioning, precisely because they occur in much more stressful and often traumatic situations. We are certainly no longer surprised to hear of a student who functions very well in her studies and exams, but who is deeply anxious or depressed in her private life.

To amplify the significance of this fundamental distinction between *depth* and *surface* phenomena and the tendency to mix these two realms of experience together uncritically, we might consider the case of attachment research. Studies of attachment have obvious implications for depth psychology, given the importance of caregiver-infant relationships in the development of the mind (Fonagy, Gergely, Jurist, & Target, 2002). The original paradigm in attachment research involved the "strange situation," typically conducted with children between the ages of one and two years (Ainsworth, Blehar, Waters, & Wall, 1978).[3] Different infant and toddler patterns have been observed using this paradigm, including secure, avoidant, and disorganized patterns. But does this situation allow for the full range and intensity of affects or emotion that would reveal an infant's or young child's defenses and coping strategies, or their psychological make-up in depth? Does the experimental "strange situation" paradigm reveal the depth of their intimacy, the degree of pleasure they experience in their relationships, their capacity to cope with anger or fear? In other words, do the observed patterns in such studies reveal the full range of functioning that children might show in relationship to their capacity for attachment?

Perhaps all that can be said definitively about the significance of findings from the "strange situation" for depth psychology is that these studies confirm that short-term, even seemingly minor disruptions in children's primary relationships lead to some interesting feelings and consequences. Furthermore, some very interesting predictions can be made on the basis of these findings; for example, about personality characteristics (e.g., self-esteem, self-knowledge, enthusiasm, resilience); peer relationships (e.g., sociability, friendliness, cooperativeness, empathy, popularity); relationships with adults (e.g., independence, confidence with strangers, compliance); frustration tolerance and impulse control;

---

[3] A parent and baby play in a room with toys when a stranger enters, sits down, and talks to the parent; the parent leaves the room and the stranger remains, responding to the infant if she is upset; the parent returns and greets her baby, comforting her if necessary, and the stranger leaves the room; the parent leaves the room again and the stranger re-enters, again offering comfort to the baby if necessary; finally, the parent returns and, if necessary, comforts her child and endeavors to get her re-interested in the toys.

persistence in problem-solving, curiosity, and attention span; adjustment (e.g., antisocial behavior, psychopathy); and attitudes towards child-rearing.

Important research procedures and related findings inform clinical evaluations and practice, but should not become clinical practice. When we assess toddlers clinically, for example, we use a much broader construct of attachment. We look to see how children deal with challenges in a variety of contexts (including past and present) and we try to ascertain the depth and range of their affects; the subtlety of the pleasure that they experience in their relationships, their warmth, openness, assertiveness, curiosity; the way they cope with anger; and so on. We look for the richness of the nonverbal communicative behavior with which they negotiate their affects and the degree of differentiation in their co-regulated signaling about different sorts of affects. For example, some toddlers excel at negotiating their feelings of assertiveness or aggression but have trouble engaging in co-regulated affect signaling about their feelings of dependency; or one might see the exact reverse pattern.

The basic problem with attachment research, therefore, is that it is often used to say a great deal more than is warranted. In fact, it has been used to define attachment *per se*. The assumption here is that a narrow, experimental situation captures the full range of human relationships and intimacy characterized by the word "attachment," or that the few different responses observed are an adequate representation of the full range of a child's functioning vis-à-vis attachment. While in a general sense this research supports an important perspective on the vital nature of relationships, the findings are often inappropriately generalized because of the confusion between *surface approaches* and *depth approaches*. Data from surface approaches should thus be interpreted within an overall depth psychological framework.

The underlying problem here, when we contrast surface with depth approaches, is the tendency of the former to narrow the conditions in which a phenomenon is studied in such a way as to narrow one's understanding of the very phenomenon one is seeking to understand. Indeed, there could be no better example of this tendency than attachment research. Bowlby's original studies on attachment were informed by his readings in ethology, which led him to formulate his famous hypothesis that attachment behaviors (in both infants and caregivers) are naturally selected in order to protect the infant from predation.[4] Even more profound than its role in negotiating security, however, is the role that attachment plays in the co-regulated affect signaling that takes place between infants and caregivers.

---

[4] To this day, Bowlby's relatively narrow picture of the evolutionary origins of attachment behavior has continued to inform research in the area, as can be seen, for example, in the numerous attempts to reduce attachment to a psychobiological phenomenon, e.g., Polan & Hofer, 1999.

As we have described elsewhere (Greenspan & Shanker, 2004), by the time we come to test infants in the "strange situation," they have already undergone a considerable amount of development. It is through their earliest attachment behaviors that babies begin to learn to tame their catastrophic reactions and transform them into interactive signals. For example, a mother smiles and the baby smiles back. She coos and the baby coos back. The baby smiles, raises his arms as if to say, "Hey!" and vocalizes emotionally needy sounds that convey, "Look at me!" The mother looks his way. Baby then smiles and flirts and the mother flirts back. For this type of emotional signaling to occur, a baby needs to have been wooed into a warm, pleasurable relationship with one or a few caregivers. Only in that case is there another being toward whom he experiences deep emotions, and, therefore, with whom he wants to communicate.

Herein lies a critical deeper function of attachment: the baby needs opportunities to be "intentional," to express an emotion or need by making a sound, using a facial expression, or making a gesture with an arm, and to have his efforts confirmed by being responded to. Attachment thus provides continuous opportunities to learn and fine-tune the skills of emotional signaling that are used to communicate and negotiate emotional states. By no means, then, is attachment confined to the sort of intense, even catastrophic emotions that we observe in infants when they are exposed to stressful situations. But even in terms of survival, the role of attachment is more complex than is suggested by Bowlby's narrowly ethological point-of-view. For in order for humans to have survived, they not only had to protect their infants from predators; more fundamentally, they had to develop the capacity to live in groups. As we explained in *The First Idea* (Greenspan & Shanker, 2004), the very growth of this capacity, and thus human survival itself, is derived from the same formative emotional processes that underlie various levels of affective synchrony, and in turn lead to symbol formation and logical problem-solving. Thus, it is through attachment with their primary caregivers that babies come to learn their group's distinctive manner of communication.

The upshot of this argument is that the full depth of attachment cannot be gleaned from conditions that simply stress an infant's sense of security. Bowlby's attachment paradigm was based on the assumption that chronically stressful conditions must have prevailed in our evolutionary past and that attachment developed as an adaptation. To the degree that these situations prevailed, Bowlby's ideas represent an enduring contribution to our understanding one of the foundations of human relationships. However, modern studies of primates in the wild suggest that the original paradigm, as important as it was, was too narrow. Nonhuman primate dyads operate in a broad range of environmental contexts and ecologies, and under less threatening conditions we observe a broad array of relational behaviors underlying complex affective signaling and interactions similar to those described above (see Falk, 2000; Greenspan & Shanker, 2004; Small, 1998).

In other words, even nonhuman primates are able to transform emotions from the catastrophic level, which would be operative under conditions of threat, to more differentiated affective expressions in a variety of patterns of co-regulation that typically permit the complex social negotiation of subtle affects dealing with themes of dependency, independence, assertiveness, curiosity, and a variety of problem-solving capacities. What we glean from a more depth-oriented approach to the study of attachment, therefore, is that in the evolutionary sense, attachment had come to serve other purposes besides simply that of survival during catastrophic or threatening conditions. Attachment also had to serve as the foundation for co-regulated affect signaling, leading both to higher cognitive and communicative functions and to the formation and coherence of groups.

CONSTRUCTING A DEVELOPMENTAL FRAMEWORK FOR DEPTH PSYCHOLOGY

As indicated, in order for the valuable findings from normative experimental studies to contribute to depth psychology (and they should), these findings cannot be translated directly and have to be interpreted within the framework of a depth developmental psychology. For this we need a clinically relevant developmental model that subsumes the broad range of experiences in clinical and non-clinical contexts.

Constructing a developmental framework for depth psychology is important for a number of reasons. Primarily, it serves to define the development of a person (i.e., what it means to be a human being). It helps us avoid the tendency to define a person based on a few narrow capacities, such as a particular cognitive capacity (e.g., IQ). Any developmental framework of human functioning must use a model that captures the full range and depth of what it means to be human. From developmental studies of children forming their minds, we can now systematize the stages whereby children:

- Perceive, attend and regulate, and move
- Form relationships and develop the capacity for sustained intimacy
- Learn to interact, read social/emotional cues, and express a wide range of emotions
- Form a sense of self that involves many different feelings, expressions, and interaction patterns
- Construct a sense of self that integrates different emotional polarities (e.g., love and hate)
- Create internal representations of a sense of self, feelings, and wishes, as well as impersonal ideas

- Categorize internal representations in terms of reality vs. fantasy (reality testing), sense of self and others (self and object representations), wishes and feelings, defenses and coping capacities, and use these for judgment, peer relationships, and a range of higher-level self-observing and reflective capacities

The above capacities of the human mind, as well as others, have adaptive developmental sequences and are compromised to varying degrees in different types of psychopathology. Depression involves symptoms such as feeling, "I am a bad person." It also involves, at a more fundamental level, a limitation in the capacity to regulate affect or emotions. Symptoms such as irrational beliefs ("Everyone knows I'm an evil person") may be more fundamentally related to a deficit in the capacity to construct and maintain a stable sense of reality (i.e., a stable, differentiated internal self-object representation). Our definition of a human being and our framework for a depth psychology are based on core capacities that characterize the most essential aspects of human functioning. In the next section of this chapter, we construct a developmental model that addresses the deeper levels of the mind, and we review the literature supporting this model.

THE STAGES OF MENTAL (EGO) DEVELOPMENT

The psychoanalytic literature is characterized by a long history of developmental observations illustrated by the work of such pioneers as Anna Freud (1965), Bowlby (1969), Escalona (1968), Kernberg (1975), Kohut (1971), Mahler (1972), and Spitz (1945). More recent observers and theoreticians of infancy and early childhood have built on this foundation, discussing preverbal interaction patterns and their psychotherapeutic implications (e.g., Beebe 1992; Emde 1976; Fonagy 1997; Greenspan 1979, 1981; 1989b; 1992; 1997b; Lichtenberg 1983; Stern 1974a). Beebe and Lachman (2002) have particularly described the implications of dyadic interactions for the psychotherapeutic process.

Over the past 30 years, we have been able to add to this work and formulate a developmental framework for depth psychology from our clinical work with infants, young children, and their families with a variety of challenges, including severe environmental and biological risks.

In an attempt to understand early emotional development, we conducted a number of clinical, observational, and intervention studies on emotional development in infants, young children, and their families. These have included multi-risk infants and families, infants and children with biologically based developmental problems such as autism, and infants and families without significant challenges or problems (Greenspan, 1981; Greenspan, et al. 1987; 1992; 1998; 1998; Interdisciplinary Council on Developmental and Learning Disorders Clinical Practice Guidelines Workgroup, 2000). Interestingly, it was the clinical work with infants, young children, and their families with both environmental and biological risks that led to an understanding of how different aspects of development work together. This led to the formulation of the Developmental Structuralist Theory and the Developmental, Individual-Difference, Relationship-Based model (DIR™) (Greenspan, 1979; 1989b; 1992; 1997a; Greenspan & Lourie, 1981).

Based on this theory and model, we formulated the Functional Emotional Developmental Approach (Greenspan, 1992; 1997a) which describes the critical emotional capacities that characterize development. These capacities, as noted previously, are broader than the expression of specific affects, such as pleasure or anger. They also serve as the foundations for adaptive development.

According to the Functional Emotional Developmental Approach, affect and affective interaction are responsible not only for emotional development and the formation of intrapsychic capacities, but for cognitive capacities as well. As we have shown elsewhere (e.g., Greenspan, 1979; 1997b), in constructing the child's intelligence, Piaget focused on impersonal cognition and the role of motor explorations of the environment. He missed the fact that affective interactions actually lead the way. At each stage of intelligence, they construct both emotional and cognitive capacities (Greenspan, 1979; 1997b). For example, by three to four months of age, way before they can pull a string or ring a bell, infants are learning about preverbal causality ("means-end" relationships) when their smile evokes a caregiver's smile. The functional emotional developmental framework also serves as an organizing construct for the other aspects of development, including motor, sensory, language, and cognitive functioning. For example, when we describe the child's capacity for two-way interactive, emotional communication at around eight months (reciprocal affect-cueing), in addition to the specific emotional features of affect cueing, we take into account the cognitive component (cause and effect interaction), the motor component (reaching), the language component (exchanging vocalizations that convey affect), and the sensory component (using sight, touch, and perception of sound as part of a co-regulated, reciprocal emotional interaction). Therefore, the Functional Emotional Developmental Approach provides a way of characterizing emotional functioning and, at the same time, a way of looking at how all the components of development (cognition, language, and motor skills) work together (as a mental team) organized by the designated emotional goals. It enables us to observe not only emotional capacities that are present, including emotional challenges, but also emotional capacities that are missing that should be present (for example, the capacity for pleasure and intimacy). In this model, emotional expression enables the full range of expected developmental abilities to work together in a functional manner (Greenspan, 1997b).

THE DEVELOPMENTAL LEVELS OF EMOTIONAL FUNCTIONING

There are six early, basic organizational levels of emotional experience and a number of subsequent ones. For each of these developmental levels, relevant research, clinical observations, and implications for mental (ego) functioning is discussed.

Self-Regulation and Interest in the World (Homeostasis): 0-3 Months

The first level of development involves regulation and shared attention, that is, self-regulation and emerging interest in the world through sight, sound, smell, touch, and taste. Children and adults build on this early developing set of capacities when they act to maintain a calm, alert, focused state, and organize their behavior, affect, and thoughts. The infant is capable at birth, or shortly thereafter, of initial states of regulation to organize experience in an adaptive fashion. The infant's ability for regulation is suggested by a number of basic abilities involving forming cycles and establishing basic rhythms, perceiving and processing information, and exploring and responding to the world (Berlyne, 1960; Deci, 1977; Harlow, 1953; Hendrick, 1939; Hunt, 1965; Meltzoff & Moore, 1977; Sander, 1962; White, 1963).

The early regulation of arousal and physiological states is critical for successful adaptation to the environment. It is important in the modulation of physiological states including sleep-wake cycles and hunger and satiety. It is needed for mastery of sensory functions and for learning self-calming and emotional responsivity. It is also important for regulation of attentional capacities (Als, Lester, Tronick, & Brazelton, 1982; Brazelton, Koslowski, & Main, 1974; Field, 1981; Sroufe, 1979; Tronick, 1989). It is generally recognized that self-regulatory mechanisms are complex and develop as a result of physiological maturation, caregiver responsivity, and the infant's adaptation to environmental demands (Lachmann & Beebe, 1997; Lyons-Ruth & Zeanah, 1993; Rothbart & Derryberry, 1981; Tronick, 1989).

In the early stages of development, the caregiver normally provides sensory input through play and caretaking experiences, such as dressing and bathing, and soothes the young infant when distressed to facilitate state organization (Als, 1982). Infant and caregiver engage in an interactive process of mutual co-regulation whereby the infant uses the parent's physical and emotional state to organize himself (Feldman, Greenbaum, & Yirmiya, 1999; Sroufe, 1996). This synchronization of states between parent and child is the basis for affect attunement and the precursor to social referencing and preverbal communication.

During this early stage, the infant learns to tolerate the intensity of arousal and to regulate his internal states so that he can maintain the interaction while gaining pleasure from it (Sroufe, 1979). This achievement has been described as "affective tolerance"; that is, the ability to maintain an optimal level of internal arousal while remaining engaged in the stimulation (Fogel, 1982). The parent first acts to help regulate this arousal and then, once the infant can regulate himself, works to facilitate the infant's responses. If the infant does not develop affective tolerance, he may develop a pattern of withdrawal, with resulting challenges to the formation and stability of relationships. Brazelton and his colleagues (1974) observed how the caregiver attempts to synchronize her behavior with the infant's natural cycles. For example, mothers generally reduce their facial expressiveness when the infant gazes away, but maintain it when the infant looks at them (Kaye & Fogel, 1980).

Clinical Observations

As indicated, the infant's first task in the developmental structuralist approach sequence is simultaneously to take an interest in the world and to regulate himself. To compare infants who can simultaneously self-regulate and take an interest in the world with those who cannot, it has been clinically useful to examine each sensory pathway individually and also to examine the range of sensory modalities available for phase-specific challenges (Greenspan, 1992).

Each sensory pathway may be:

- Hyperarousable (e.g., the baby who overreacts to normal levels of sound, touch, or brightness)
- Hypoarousable (e.g., the baby who hears and sees but evidences no behavioral or observable affective response to routine sights and sounds—often described as the "floppy" baby with poor muscle tone who is unresponsive and seemingly looks inward)
- Neither hypo- nor hyperarousable but having a subtle type of early processing disorder (hypo- or hyperarousable babies may also have a processing difficulty)

It is important to note that the differences in sensory reactivity and processing were observed many years ago and continue to be discussed in the occupational therapy literature (Ayres, 1964). If an individual sensory pathway is not functioning optimally, the range of sensory experience available to the infant is more limited. This limitation determines, in part, the options or strategies the infant can employ and the types of sensory experience that are organized. Some babies can employ the full range of sensory capacities. At the stage of regulation and interest in the world (i.e., homeostasis), for example, one can observe that such babies look at mother's face or an interesting object and follow it with their eyes. When such a baby is upset, the opportunity to look at mother helps him become calm and happy (i.e., showing a calm smile). Similarly, a soothing voice, a gentle touch, rhythmic rocking, or a shift in position (offering vestibular and proprioceptive stimulation) can also help such a baby relax, organize, and self-regulate.

There are also babies who functionally employ only one or two sensory modalities. We have observed babies who brighten up, become alert, and become calm with visual experience, but who, with auditory stimuli, either become relatively unresponsive, become hyper-excitable, or appear to become "confused." (A 2-month-old baby may be operationally defined as confused when, instead of looking toward a normal, high-pitched maternal voice and alerting, she makes random motor movements suggesting that the stimulus has been taken in, looks past the object repeatedly, and continues the random movements). Other babies appear to use vision and hearing to self-regulate and take an interest in the world but have a more difficult time with touch and movement. They often become irritable even with gentle stroking, become hyperaroused when held upright, and are calm only when held horizontally. Still other babies calm down only when rocked to their own heart rate, respiratory rate, or mother's heart rate. Studies of the role of vestibular and proprioceptive pathways in psychopathology in infancy are important areas for continuing research.

As babies use a range of sensory pathways, they also integrate experiences across the senses (Spelke & Owsley, 1979). Yet, there are babies who are able to use each sensory pathway but who have difficulty, for example, integrating vision and hearing. They can alert to a sound or a visual cue but are not able to turn and look at a stimulus at the same time. Instead, they appear confused and may even have active gaze aversion or go into a pattern of extensor rigidity and avoidance.

The sensory pathways are usually observed in the context of sensorimotor patterns; turning toward the stimulus or brightening and alerting, for example, involve motor "outputs." There are babies who have difficulties in the way they integrate their sensory experience with motor output. The most obvious case is a baby with severe motor difficulties. At a subtle level, it is possible to observe compromises in such basic abilities as self-consoling or nuzzling in the corner of mother's neck or relaxing to rhythmic rocking. In this context, Escalona's classic descriptions (1968) of babies with multiple sensory hypersensitivities require further study as part of a broader approach to assessing subtle difficulties in each sensory pathway, as well as understanding associated master patterns.

In this first stage, there are babies who cannot organize their affective-thematic proclivities in terms of phase-specific tasks. Babies who are uncomfortable with dependency often evidence specific sensory hypersensitivities or higher-level integrating problems, as well as maladaptive infant-caregiver interactions. Babies with a tendency toward hyper- or hypoarousal may not be able to organize the affective-thematic domains of joy, pleasure, and exploration. Instead, they may show apathy and withdrawal or display a total disregard for certain sensory realms while over-focusing on others (e.g., babies who stare at an inanimate object while ignoring the human world).

Children with sensorimotor dysfunction typically have difficulty utilizing the range of sensory experiences available to them for learning, and, as a result, may be unable to organize purposeful, goal-directed movement and socially adaptive behaviors. These children often have maladaptive responses in forming affective relationships or attachments. An infant who is hypersensitive to touch and movement, for example, may avoid tactile contact, resist being held and moved in space, and avert his gaze to avoid face-to-face interactions. Both the touch-hypersensitive child and the socially limited child exemplify how sensorimotor dysfunction may affect emotional behaviors.

In addition, difficulties with muscle tone or coordination can affect the infant's ability to signal interest in the world. For example, the young baby who arches away from the mother's breast during feeding affects the level of engagement that occurs during a normal feeding experience. In turn, these problems affect the caregiver's ability to respond to her infant's signal, particularly when she does not understand what the baby's responses mean. The mother whose baby arches away every time he is held may feel that she is a defective mother, particularly if the baby's tactile hypersensitivities or increased muscle tone are not identified.

Some investigators explore sensory, motor, and affective differences in terms of temperament. Temperamental differences have been shown to influence the organization and regulation of inter- and intrapersonal processes (Campos, Campos, & Barrett, 1989). Temperamental qualities that are associated with the child's being characterized as "difficult," for example, have been linked to later psychopathology (Thomas & Chess, 1984). The difficult temperament might create challenges in self-regulatory processes and affect infant-caregiver interaction adversely. Of course, neither sensory nor temperamental characteristics alone necessarily predict pathology. The effects of particular sensory or temperamental characteristics can be modulated by the attention of a sensitive, responsive caregiver. Because temperament involves overall patterns of behavior, while the sensory processing pathways described above involve specific capacities that may underlie and even account for temperament, it is especially important to understand an individual's particular sensory processing ability. A sensorily overreactive infant, for example, is very likely to be temperamentally difficult to comfort.

Even when the infant is quite competent from a regulatory standpoint, a caregiver might fail to draw her baby into a regulating relationship. Dysregulation may occur, for example, with a caregiver who is exceedingly depressed or who is so self-absorbed that she fails to soothe or woo the new baby. A caregiver who is impatient with or threatened by the infant's manifestation of sensory or temperamental sensitivity, and who reacts with abuse, withdrawal, or other maladaptive responses, may encourage an infant's reliance on ineffective patterns of behavior, thus contributing to the infant's inability to achieve self-regulation.

Implications for Mental (Ego) Functioning

It may be postulated that there are adapted sensorimotor patterns that are part of what psychoanalytic theorists have called the "autonomous ego functions" that are present shortly after birth. It is then useful to consider how these capacities (e.g., perception and discrimination) are used to construct an emerging organization of an experiential world, including drive derivatives, early affects, and emerging organizations of self and object(s). It would be a logical error to assume that these seemingly innate capacities are themselves a product of early interactional learning or structure building, even though secondarily they are influenced by experiences.

In this early phase of development, one cannot yet postulate differentiated self-object experiential organizations. The infant's main goals appear to include a type of sensory awakening, interest and regulation, without evidence of clear intentional object seeking or self-initiated differentiated affective interactions. With both at-risk and normal infants, we have observed that they respond to the overall stimulus qualities of the environments, especially human handling. Likewise, there is little evidence for a notion that the infant is impervious to his emotional surroundings. In fact, in our studies of multi-risk families (Greenspan, et al. 1987), the quality of self-regulation, attention, and sensory-affective interest in the world in the first month to two of life was influenced to a great degree by the physical and emotional qualities of the infant-caregiver patterns (i.e., soothing and interesting care-giving patterns rather than hyper-or hypo-stimulating ones). But this does not mean that those who, like Mahler and colleagues (1975), suggest a qualitative difference in this early stage (i.e., her concept of a normal autistic phase) may not have an important insight. Even though mother's voice can be discriminated from other sounds, even in utero, this capacity does not indicate that there is a conceptual discrimination between mother and the physical environment, between the meaning of her voice and that of the sound of a car, for example. In other words, the baby cannot yet abstract and organize types of experiences according to general characteristics. One must distinguish what the infant is capable of (e.g., complex discriminations) from how the infant is functionally involved in phase-specific tasks and goals. For example, the 3-year-old who becomes severely anxious about the loss of his human, affective object may have excellent capacities for conserving his impersonal objects. A 6-year-old capable of advanced logic in math or science may lag considerably in the logic of reality testing, confusing fantasy and reality. A cognitive capacity may or may not be used for organizing in-depth emotional experience. Our clinical observations suggest that early in life, the capacities the infant uses to organize in-depth emotional experience lag behind the capacities he uses to process either relatively impersonal experience or affective experience lacking in psychological depth.

One may consider a preintentional stage of object relatedness (i.e., prewired patterns that gradually come under interactive control) and a stage in the organization of experience in which the sense of self and object are not yet organized as distinct entities. At this stage, the experiences of "self" and "other" are closely intertwined and are unlikely to be yet separate from other sensory experiences involving the physical world. It is worth repeating that differential infant responses do not necessarily mean differentiated internal experiences. Responses or behaviors can simply be constitutional, reflexive (e.g., to heat or cold), and/or conditioned (whether via classical or operant modes).

Therefore, the concept of an experiential organization of a *world object*, including what later becomes a self-other-physical world, may prove useful. This state of ego organization may be considered to be characterized by two central tendencies: to experience sensory and affective information through each sensory (motor) channel, and to form patterns of regulation. These tendencies may be further characterized by the level of sensory pathway arousal (i.e., sensory hyper- and hypoarousal) in each sensory (motor) pathway and by emerging sensory (motor) discrimination and integration capacities. Under optimal conditions, the early sensory and affective processing, discrimination, and integration capacities, the early functions of the ego, are being used for the gradual organization of experience. Under unfavorable conditions, these early ego functions evidence undifferentiated sensory hyperarousal, undifferentiated sensory hypoarousal, and lack of discrimination and integration in all or any of the sensory-affective (motor) pathways. Therefore, the early stage of global undifferentiated self-object worlds may remain or progress to higher levels of organization, depending on innate maturational patterns and early experiences, as together they influence each sensory-affective (motor) pathway in terms of arousal, discrimination, and integration.

In addition, as early drive-affect organizations are now being harnessed and integrated by the emerging ego functions of sensory-affect (motor) processing, differentiation, and integration, it is useful to consider drive-affect development from the perspective of the ego. From this perspective, the Freudian concept of the oral phase may be considered more broadly as part of a system of "sensory-affective" pleasure involving all the sensory-affective (motor) pathways, of which the mouth is certainly dominant (in terms of tactile, deep pressure, temperature, pain, and motor, especially smooth muscle, patterns). The mouth's dominance is due to the highly developed nature of its sensory-affective and motor pathways. From the perspective of the ego, however, drive-affect derivatives are elaborated throughout the "sensory surface" of the body.

Forming Relationships, Attachment, and Engagement: 2-7 Months

Another early level concerns engagement, or a sense of relatedness, a lifelong capacity. Once the infant has achieved some capacity for self regulation and interest in the world between two and four months of age, she becomes more engaged in social and emotional interactions. There is greater ability to respond to the external environment and to form a special relationship with significant primary caregivers. The infant's capacity for engagement is supported by early maturational abilities for selectively focusing on the human face and voice and for processing and organizing information from the senses (Meltzoff, 1985; Papousek, 1981; Papousek & Papousek, 1979; Stern, 1985). A sense of shared humanity, a type of synchrony of relating, is evident in the ways that both the infant and parent use their senses, motor systems, and affects to resonate with each other (Butterworth & Jarrett, 1980; Scaife & Bruner, 1975).

As we saw above, the quality of early engagement has implications for later attachment patterns and behavior (Ainsworth, Bell, & Stayton, 1974; Bates, Maslin, & Frankel, 1985; Belsky, Rovine, & Taylor, 1984; Grossmann, Grossmann, Spangler, Suess, & Unzner, 1985; Lewis & Feiring, 1987; Miyake, Chen, & Campos, 1985; Pederson, et al., 1990). Attachment or relating with the caregiver is important not only because it represents the capacity to form human relationships, but also because it has been shown that atypical attachment patterns can have a negative impact on developmental outcomes (Carew, 1980). Longitudinal studies have found that securely attached children tend to have better emotional adaptability, social skills, and cognitive functioning (Cassidy & Shaver, 1999). During the school-aged and adolescent years, children who were securely attached as infants are more likely to be accepted by their peers and were better able to form intimate relationships with them (Sroufe, Egeland, & Carlson, 1999). In addition, a secure attachment seems to provide a protective mechanism for children whose families experience a high level of stress (Egeland & Kreutzer, 1991). The key element that underlies a secure attachment is sensitive and responsive care-giving (Ainsworth, Blehar, Waters, & Wall, 1978; De Wolff & van Ijzendoorn, 1997).

Attachment has a specific research meaning in the studies cited above and in others. As we emphasized, however, in a clinical as well as normative developmental context, it is useful to consider a broader framework for relationships involving the overall pattern of relating between an infant and caregiver. This broader focus involves the depth of pleasure, range of feelings, and meanings given to relationships. The processes that define relationships go significantly beyond definitions used in various research paradigms (Greenspan, 1997a).

Clinical Observations

In this stage, which involves a growing intimacy with the primary caregiver(s), one can observe babies who are able to employ all their senses to orchestrate highly pleasurable affect in this relationship. The baby with a beautiful smile, looking at and listening to mother, experiencing her gentle touch and rhythmic movement and responding to her voice with synchronous mouth and arm and leg movements, is perhaps the most vivid example. Clinically, however, we observe babies who are not able to employ their senses to form an affective relationship with the human world. The most extreme case is a baby who actively avoids sensory and, therefore, affective contact with the human world. Human sounds, touches, and even scents are avoided with chronic gaze aversion, recoiling, flat affect, or random or nonsynchronous patterns of brightening and alerting. We also observe babies who use one or another sensory pathway to experience a pleasurable relationship with the human world but who cannot orchestrate the full range and depth of sensory experience. The baby who listens to mother's voice with a smile but averts his gaze and looks pained at the sight of her face is an example.

Forming an attachment or relationship organizes a number of discrete affective proclivities—comfort, dependency, pleasure, and joy, as well as assertiveness and curiosity in the context of a pleasurable caregiver-infant relationship. In the adaptive pattern, protest and anger are organized along with the expected positive affects as part of a baby's emotional interest in the primary caregiver. A healthy 4-month-old can, as part of his repertoire, become negative, but then can also quickly return to mother's beautiful smiles, loving glances, and offers of comfort. Relationship patterns, once formed, continue and develop further throughout the course of life.

By this phase, infants and children can already have major limitations in certain affect proclivities. Rather than evidencing joy, enthusiasm, or pleasure with their caregivers, they may seem emotionally flat. Similarly, rather than evidencing (periodic) assertive, curious, protesting, or angry behavior in relationship to their primary caregiver, they may only look very compliant and give shallow smiles. In addition to being constricted in their affective range, babies may also show a limitation in their organizational stability. An example is a baby who, after hearing a loud noise, cannot return to his earlier interests in the primary caregiver. Where environmental circumstances are unfavorable, or where for other reasons development continues to be disordered, early attachment or relationship difficulties may occur. If these difficulties are severe enough, they may form the basis for an ongoing deficit in the baby's capacity to form affective human relationships and to form the basic personality structures and functions that depend on the internal organization of human experience.

Implications for Mental (Ego) Functioning

The pleasurable preference for the human world suggests interactive object seeking. Apathy in reaction to caregiver withdrawal, preference for the physical over the interpersonal world, and chronic active aversion in clinically disturbed populations also suggest emerging organized object-related patterns, albeit mal-adaptive ones.

At this phase there is no evidence yet of the infant's ability to abstract all the features of a human object in terms of a concept of the whole object. Infants seek the voice, smiling mouth, twinkly eyes, or rhythmic movements alone or in some combinations, but not yet as a whole. In addition, the tendency toward global withdrawal, rejection, or avoidance suggests undifferentiated reaction patterns as compared to differentiated patterns in which the influence of a "me" or a "you" is felt. The 3-month-old does not show the repertoire of the 8-month-old in "wooing" a caregiver into a pleasurable interaction. The 3-month-old under optimal conditions displays synchronous interactive patterns, smiling and vocalizing in rhythm with the caregiver. When in clinical distress, he evidences global reactivity; in contrast, the 8-month-old can explore alternative ways of having an impact on his caregiver. This difference suggests that not until the next stage is there a full behavioral (prerepresentational) comprehension of cause and effect or self and object differentiation. Representation/comprehension does not occur until late in the second year of life.

During this stage the infant ordinarily progresses from the earlier stage of a self/other/world object (where both human and not-human worlds are not yet distinct, and the human self and nonself are also not distinct) to a stage of intentional undifferentiated human self-object organization. There is the sense of synchrony and connectedness to a human object, suggesting that the infant's experiential organization differentiates the human object from physical objects. But even at a behavioral level there is not yet evidence of a self-object differentiation. In this sense the concept of symbiosis (Mahler, Pine, & Bergman, 1975) is not at odds with the clinical observation of a lack of self and object differentiation.

The functioning of the ego at this stage is characterized by intentional object seeking, differentiated organizations of experience (self from human object), and global patterns of reactivity to the human object. These patterns of reactivity include pleasure-seeking, protest, withdrawal, rejection (with a preference for the physical world, based on what appears to be a clear discrimination), hyper-affectivity (diffuse discharge of affects), and active avoidance.

To the degree that later self and object organization are undifferentiated, aspects of experience may combine or organize in different ways. This process reflects a lack of full structure formation and is perhaps a precursor to condensations, displacements, and projective and incorporative-introjective mechanisms. Projection, incorporation, and introjection in a differentiated sense, where distinct images are transferred across boundaries, are not yet in evidence. We therefore see a progression from a stage of undifferentiated world self/object to an undifferentiated human self/object.

Two-Way, Purposeful Communication (Somatopsychological Differentiation): 3-10 Months

The next stage involves purposeful communication. It is characterized by the development of intentional, nonverbal communications or gestures. These gestures include affective communication, facial expressions, arm and leg movements, vocalizations, and spinal posture. From the middle of the first year of life onward, individuals rely on gestures to communicate. Initially during the stage of purposeful communication, simple reciprocal gestures, such as head nods, smiles, and movement patterns, serve a boundary-defining role. The "me" communicates a wish or intention, and the "other" or "you" communicates back some confirmation, acknowledgment, or elaboration on that wish or intention.

The stage of two-way, causal, intentional communication indicates processes occurring at the somatic (sensorimotor) and emerging psychological levels. The arrival of this phase is evidenced in the infant's growing ability to discriminate primary caregivers from others and to differentiate her own actions from their consequences—affectively, somatically, behaviorally, and interpersonally.

These capacities are first seen as the infant develops complex patterns of communication in the context of her primary human relationship. Parallel with development of the baby's relationship to the inanimate world, in which basic schemes of causality (Piaget, 1962) are being developed, the infant becomes capable of complicated human emotional communication (Brazelton, Koslowski, & Main, 1974; Charlesworth, 1969; Stern, 1974b; Tennes, Emde, Kisley, & Metcalf, 1972). There is both a historic and a newly emerging consensus among clinicians, developmental observers, and researchers that affects are used for intentional communication (Bowlby, 1973; Brazelton & Cramer, 1990; Mahler, Pine, & Bergman, 1975; Osofsky & Eberhart-Wright, 1988; Spitz, 1965; Stern, 1985; Winnicott, 1965) and that these affective patterns—for example, for happiness, distress, anger, fear, surprise, and disgust—are similar in different cultures and in both children and adults (Campos, Barrett, Lamb, Goldsmith, & Stenberg, 1983; Darwin, 1872; Ekman, Friesen, & Ellsworth, 1972; Izard, 1971). Intentional communication, which involves both intuiting and responding to the caregiver's emotional cues, gradually takes on qualities that are particular to relationships, family, and culture (Brazelton & Als, 1979; Bruner, 1982; Feinman & Lewis, 1983; Kaye, 1982; Kimmert, Campos, Sorce, Emde, & Svejda, 1983; Kleinman, 1986; Markus & Kitayama, 1990; Schweder, Mahapatra, & Miller, 1987; Stern, 1977; Trevarthen, 1979; Tronick, 1980).

Clinical Observations

When there are distortions in the emotional communication process—as occurs when a primary caregiver responds in a mechanical, remote manner or projects some of her own dependent feelings onto her infant—the infant may not learn to appreciate causal relationships between people at the level of compassionate and intimate feelings. This situation can occur despite the fact that causality seems to be developing in terms of the inanimate world and also the impersonal human world.

Some babies do not possess the capacity to orchestrate their sensory experiences in an interactive cause-and-effect pattern. For these infants, a look and a smile on mother's part do not lead to a consequential look, smile, vocalization, or gross motor movement on baby's. Such a baby may perceive the sensory experiences mother is making available, but seems unable to organize these experiences, and either looks past mother or evidences random motor patterns.

We also observe babies who can operate in a cause-and-effect manner in one sensory pathway but not another. For example, when presented with an object, they may clearly examine it in a purposeful way. When presented with an interesting auditory stimulus, however, instead of responding vocally or reaching toward it, the infant behaves chaotically, with increased motor activity and discharge behavior such as banging and flailing. Similarly, with tactile experience, some babies, instead of touching mother's hand when she is stroking their abdomen, begin emitting random-seeming or chaotic motor responses that appear unrelated to the gentle stimulus.

We observe even more profoundly the differential use of the senses as infants are now also learning to process information in each sensory mode and between modes. Infants differ in how and when they begin to see relations between elements in a pattern. Some babies learn quickly and some slowly that a sound leads to a sound or a look to a look. It is intriguing to consider the implications for later learning problems if certain sensory pathways are not fully incorporated into a cause-and-effect level of behavioral organization. Such early differences may account, for example, for the differences between children with auditory-verbal abstracting and sequencing problems and those with visual-spatial problems. Motor differences, such as high or low muscle tone or lags in motor development or in motor planning, also obviously influence the infant's ability to signal his wishes. In organizing cause-and-effect communications, therefore, a compromise in a sensory or motor pathway not only limits the strategies available for tackling this new challenge, but may also restrict the sensory and motor modalities that become organized at this new developmental level. In addition, as we elaborate further, it may restrict the associated drive and affect patterns as well.

As babies learn to orchestrate their senses in the context of cause-and-effect interactions, we observe an interesting clinical phenomenon in relationship to what was described in the early neurological literature as "proximal" and "distal" modes. At this time, we may begin seeing a shift toward distal rather than proximal modes of communication. Proximal modes of communication include direct physical contact, such as holding, rocking, and touching. Distal modes encompass communication via vision, auditory cueing, and affect signaling. The distal modes can obviously occur across space, whereas the proximal modes require, as the word implies, physical closeness. The crawling 8-month-old can remain in emotional communication with his primary caregiver through reciprocal glances, vocalizations, and affect gestures. Some babies, however, seem to rely on proximal modes for a sense of security. Early limitations in negotiating space are seen later on to affect the capacity to construct internal representations.

If one divides the emotional terrain into its parts, one can see cause-and-effect signaling with the full range of emotions. In terms of dependency, the 8-month-old can make overtures to be cuddled or held. Unless he has tactile hypersensitivity, he shows pleasure with beatific smiles and love of touching. There is curiosity and assertiveness as the 8-month-old reaches for a rattle in mom's hand. There is also anger and protest as he throws his food on the floor in a deliberate, intentional manner and looks at his caregiver as if to say, "What are you going to do now?" There is protest, even defiance, often expressed by biting, banging, and sometimes butting. At 8 months, children express anger this way because they have better motor control of their mouths, heads, and necks than of their arms and hands.

Where the caregiver does not respond to the baby's signal by, for example, returning a smile or a glance, we have observed that the baby's affective-thematic inclinations may not evidence this differentiated organization. Instead the infant may remain either synchronous, as in the attachment phase, or may shift from synchrony to a more random quality. The expected range may be present but not subordinated into a cause-and-effect interchange.

There are also many babies who, because of a lack of reciprocal responses from their caregiver, evidence affective dampening or flatness and a hint of despondency or sadness. This may occur even after the baby has shown a joyfulness and an adaptive attachment. In some cases at least, it seems as though when not offered the phase-specific "experiential nutriments" (the cause-and-effect interactions of which he is now capable), but only the earlier forms of relatedness, the baby begins a pattern of withdrawal and affective flattening. It is as though he needs to be met at his own level to maintain his affective-thematic range. Most interesting are the subtle cases in which the baby can reciprocate certain affects and themes, such as pleasure and dependency, but not others, such as assertiveness, curiosity, and protest. Depending on the baby's own maturational tendencies and the specificity of the consequences in the care-giving environment, one can imagine how this uneven development occurs. For example, caregivers who are uncomfortable with dependency and closeness may not afford opportunities for purposeful reciprocal interactions in this domain but may, on the other hand, be quite "causal" in less intimate domains of assertion and protest.

Implications for Mental (Ego) Functioning

It is useful to think of this stage of development as a first step in reality testing. At this time, pre-representational causality is established. The intentionality of the infant in both adaptive (reaching out) and maladaptive (rejecting) modes suggests at least a behavioral comprehension of a "self" influencing an "other." It also suggests self-object differentiation at the behavioral level. Behavioral level in this context means the organization of behavior patterns or tendencies rather than the later organization of symbols. Only late in the second year does a child begin to have the ability to create mental representations through higher-level abstractions. At this time, however, the "I" is likely an "I" of behavior ("If I do this it causes that") rather than the "I" of a mental representation ("If I feel or think or *am* a certain way, it has this or that impact"). The capacity to construct mental representations allows the growing child to organize and even rearrange different elements of the "self" or "other" into mental images. Because there is behavioral cause-and-effect or differentiated interaction, one can think of a behavioral or pre-representational type of reality testing.

There is no evidence yet for the child's having the ability to abstract all aspects of the "self" or "other." Experiences are still in fragments. Temporal and spatial continuity, while rapidly developing, are not yet fully established. The "I" is a physical and behavioral "I"; an "I" that can make things happen in the behavior pattern of the "other." The "I" and the "other" are not yet an "I" or "other" that represents or organizes all the aspects of the self or other. Hence, it is possible to consider this stage as characterized by somatic and behavioral part self/ part object differentiation. The ego is characterized now by a capacity to differentiate aspects of experience in both the impersonal and drive-affect domains. It is worth emphasizing again that only at this stage are differentiated internal relationships possible. But even at this stage, there are likely to be differentiated part-object schemes of behavior, not whole objects in a representational form. This view differs from interpretations of infant behavior that are based on normative samples of infants in experimental situations.

Behavioral Organization, Problem-Solving, and Internalization: A Complex Sense of Self: 9-18 Months

The next stage involves the child's capacity for engaging in a continuous flow of complex, organized problem-solving interactions and the formation of a pre-symbolic sense of self. With appropriate reading of cues and differential responses, the infant's or toddler's behavioral repertoire becomes complicated, and communications take on more organized, meaningful configurations. By 12 months of age, the infant is connecting behavioral units into larger organizations as she exhibits complex emotional responses such as affiliation, wariness, and fear (Ainsworth, Bell, & Stayton, 1974; Ainsworth, et al. 1978; Bowlby, 1969;

Sroufe & Waters, 1977). As the toddler approaches the second year of life, in the context of what Mahler (Mahler, Pine, & Bergman, 1975) called the practicing subphase of the development of individuation, there is an increased capacity for forming original behavioral schemes (Piaget, 1962), for imitative activity and intentionality, and for behavior suggesting functional understanding of objects (Werner & Kaplan, 1963).

It is recognized that at this stage the infant takes a more active role in developing and maintaining the reciprocal relationship with the caregiver (Bell, 1977; Goldberg, 1977; Reingold, 1969). In addition, much has been written about the growing complexity of the reciprocal dyadic interaction (Cicchetti & Schneider-Rosen, 1984; Greenspan & Porges, 1984; Talberg, Couto, O'Donnell, & Cuoto Rosa, 1988; Tronick & Gianino, Jr., 1986). These complex interactions enable the child to utilize and respond to social cues and eventually to achieve a sense of competence as an autonomous being in relationship with a significant other (Brazelton & Als, 1979; Lester, Hoffman, & Brazelton, 1985).

There is now in evidence, therefore, a stage of behavioral organization of a complex sense of self. Interactions become more complex, and social patterns involve many circles of intentional communication that negotiate intimacy exploration, aggression, and limit setting. For example, a baby at this age can use emotional signals to figure out whether or not a behavior is acceptable (Dunn, 1988; Emde, Johnson, & Easterbrooks, 1988; Kagan, 1981; Radke-Yarrow, Zahn-Waxler, & Chapman, 1983; Zahn-Waxler & Radke-Yarrow, 1982).

Clinical Observations

This stage involves a baby's ability to sequence many cause-and-effect units into a chain or an organized behavior pattern (e.g., the 14-month-old who can take mother's hand, walk her to the refrigerator, bang on the door, and, when the door is opened, point to the desired food). Wish and intention are organized under a complex behavior pattern. This organized behavior pattern can be viewed as an accomplishment that involves coordinated and orchestrated use of the senses. Here the toddler who is capable of using vision and hearing to perceive various vocal and facial gestures, postural cues, and complex affect signals is able to extract relevant information from his objects and organize this information at new levels of cognitive and affective integration. A toddler who is not able to incorporate certain sensory experiences as part of his early cognitive and affective abstracting abilities (Werner & Kaplan, 1963) may evidence a very early restriction in how his senses process information.

Balanced reliance on proximal and distal modes of communication becomes even more important during this phase of development. The mobile toddler enjoying his freedom in space presumably can feel secure through his distal communication modes (e.g., looking and listening across space). It is interesting in this context to examine traditional notions of separation anxiety in light of the conflicts that some toddlers have over separation and individuation(Mahler, Pine, & Bergman, 1975). With the use of the distal modes, the toddler can "have his cake and eat it too." If he can bring the care-giving object with him through the use of distal contact with her, he does not have to tolerate a great deal of insecurity. He can "refuel" distally, by looking at mother or listening to her voice, and signal her back with vocalizations or arm gestures. He can use proximal contact, such as coming over for a cuddle when necessary. The youngster who has difficulty in using his distal modes to remain in contact with the primary caregiver may need more proximal contact. While this reliance on proximal contact can occur because of feelings of insecurity generated by an ambivalent primary caregiver, the limitations of a child's own sensory organization may also be an important factor in this pattern. From a motor and sensory perspective, therefore, to master this stage, the toddler needs to be able to process sounds and sights, employ reciprocal motor gestures, and comprehend spatial relationships.

The piecing together of many smaller cause-and-effect units of experience involves integrating a range of types of experiences, such as pleasure, assertiveness, curiosity, and dependency, into an organized pattern. For instance, it is not uncommon for a healthy toddler to start with a dependent tone of cuddling and kissing his parents, to shift to a pleasurable, giggly interchange with them, and then to get off their laps and invite them to engage in an assertive chase game in which he runs to a room that is off-limits. When the parents say, "No, you can't go in there," protest and negativism may emerge. Under optimal circumstances, the interaction may come to a relative closure with the toddler back in the playroom, sitting on his parent's lap, pleasurably exploring pictures in his favorite book. Here the child has gone full circle, suggesting that he has connected the many affective-thematic areas.

Around 18 months, as children begin to abstract the meaning of objects, their understanding of the functions of the telephone or brush may have its counterpart in their experiencing the caregiver as a "functional" being invested with many affective-thematic proclivities. Although children are able to integrate many behavioral units between 12 and 18 months, they do not seem to be able to make a full integration of intense emotions. For the moment at least, they do not fully realize that the person they are mad at is the same person they love and enjoy. It is not until the end of the next stage that the sense of split-off fury seems, at least in clinical observations, to be modified at some level by an awareness of love and dependency.

Implications for Mental (Ego) Functioning

The new capacities for behavioral organization, affective integration, and behavioral sense of self and object in functional terms (a conceptual stand toward the world) characterize this stage of ego development. We can observe three levels:

- Fragmented (little islands of intentional problem-solving behavior)
- Polarized (organized patterns of behavior expressing only one or another feeling states, e.g., organized aggression and impulsivity or organized clinging, needy, dependent behavior, or organized fearful patterns)
- Integrated (different emotional patterns—dependency, assertiveness, pleasure, etc.—organized into integrated, problem-solving affective interactions such as flirting, seeking closeness, and then getting help to find a needed object)

Now, there is what may be thought of as a conceptual self-object relationship. Different self-behaviors and object behaviors are not only discriminated from each other (as in the earlier stage), but are now also viewed as part of a whole. Teasing behavior, jokes, anticipation of emotional reactions, and awareness of how to get others to respond emotionally all point to this new conceptual affective ability. But even more important is the toddler's new ability to organize in all dimensions of life. This is illustrated by his tendency, under stress, to organize his negativism, or become sophisticated in his clinging dependency, or develop intricate aggressive patterns, or exploit or manipulate peers and adults in new interpersonal patterns. In worrisome situations, one also observes the toddler regress from organized behavior patterns to highly fragmented patterns, or become withdrawn or rejecting.

The ego can now organize experience in terms of functional expectancies. This capacity of the ego also facilitates integrated functional identifications. Instead of simply copying a behavior, a child can copy or identify with a functional interpersonal pattern. These functional patterns can also be projected or incorporated. Now not simply an isolated behavior (e.g., hitting) but a "behavioral attitude" (e.g., being controlling) can be projected or incorporated. Most defenses may exist on such a hierarchy related to stages in the functioning of the ego.

During this stage ego structure formation is undergoing rapid progress. Both deficits of experience and conflicts between behavioral-affective tendencies likely undermine structure formation. One, therefore, does not need to postulate deficit models and conflict models of the mind as in opposition. Rather, the two tendencies can be seen to be working together. For example, Kohut (1971) would suggest that lack of parental empathy leads the toddler to experience a deficit in terms of his self-esteem regulation (an early affective self-object pattern). Kernberg (1975) would suggest that the unadmiring, overcontrolling, or intrusive caregiver creates a condition in which the toddler experiences rage and conflict and then resorts to primitive splitting defenses in order to cope. We have concluded, based on both clinical and observational studies of toddlers, that both tendencies are operative.

A lack of empathy, combined with intrusive overcontrol, leads to painful humiliation, rage, and fear of object loss as well as to deficits in self-object experiences and in the formation of structures regulating self-esteem. For example, the 18-month-old experiencing rage and fear, without therapy, usually resorts to passive compliance, indifferent impulsivity, and avoidance. This regressive way of dealing with conflict during this phase leads to structural deficit because the ability to abstract affective polarities is not learned. Likewise, a lack of empathic admiration and a lack of emotional availability seem to leave the toddler feeling too uncertain about his objects to experiment with his behavioral and affective polarities. In addition, a toddler who evidences overreactivity to sensory and affective experience is likely to experience loss and fear more readily than the sensory-craving, assertive, and sometimes aggressive toddler who does more readily experience rage. Reconstructive work with older children and adults must deal with both the reality of the early object relationship and the rage, humiliation, fear, conflict, and consequent primitive strategies employed at the time and subsequently repeated. At this age, conflict leads to deficits, and deficits create the increased probability of irresolvable conflicts. Appropriate structure is necessary to resolve conflict, and conflicts at an early age often lead to structural deficits. Which comes first is a chicken-or-egg question.

This stage of ego development is characterized by many new capacities and is transitional to the next stages, in which mental representations and differentiated self-object representational structures are possible.

Representational Capacity: 18-30 Months

The next level involves the creation, elaboration, and sharing of symbols and meanings. The individual's ability to represent or symbolize experience is illustrated in pretend play, the verbal labeling of feelings ("I feel happy"), and the functional use of language.

This level begins as the toddler approaches the end of the second year. Internal sensations and unstable images become organized as multisensory, affective images or representations that can be evoked and are somewhat stable (Bell, 1970; Fenson & Ramsay, 1980; Gouin-Decarie, 1965; Piaget, 1962). While this capacity is fragile between 16 and 24 months, it soon becomes a dominant mode in organizing the child's behavior.

Related to the ability to create representations is the capacity for "object permanence." This capacity, which is relative and goes through a series of stages, refers to the toddler's ability to search for hidden inanimate objects(Gouin-Decarie, 1965).

Infants progress from engaging in actions with themselves (e.g., feeding self) to using themselves as the agents to act upon others (e.g., toddler uses a doll to feed another doll). The development of language and the capacity to share meanings with others facilitates children's capacity to describe themselves and to understand the difference between themselves and others. This development of perspective coincides with the early stages of empathy and prosocial behavior (Butterworth, 1990; DesRosiers & Busch-Rossnagel, 1997; Meltzoff, 1990; Pipp-Siegel & Pressman, 1996; Stern, 1983).

The elaboration of ideas or representations gradually becomes more complex, as does the sense of self, which now involves symbols, not just behaviors (e.g., use of words for intent and descriptions, use of personal pronouns, improved recognition of self in mirror) (Fein & Apfel, 1979; Fenson, Kagan, Kearsely, & Zelazo, 1976; Inhelder, Lezine, Sinclair, & Stambak, 1972; Pipp, Fischer, & Jennings, 1987; Rubin, Fein, & Vandenberg, 1983). Pretend play and intentional interpersonal use of language illustrate these new capacities (Erikson, 1940; Fein, 1975; Kraus & Glucksberg, 1969; Lowe, 1975; Nelson, 1973; Peller, 1954; Waelder, 1933).

Over time, causal schemes are developed at a representational level (McCune-Nicholich, 1977; Sinclair, 1970), leading to thinking capacities. In addition, as ideas and behaviors are being elaborated, they reflect not only ongoing relationships, but prior negotiations as well. A large number of studies on early attachment patterns and later behavior illustrate the importance of early patterns as well as later relationships (Aber & Baker, 1990; Arend, Gove, & Sroufe, 1979; Cassidy, 1990; Cassidy & Marvin, 1988; Easterbrooks & Goldberg, 1990; Egeland & Farber, 1984; Goldberg & Easterbrooks, 1984; Main, Kaplan, & Cassidy, 1985; Marvin & Stewart, 1991; Maslin-Cole & Spieker, 1990; Matas, Arend, & Sroufe, 1978; Pastor, 1981; Sroufe, 1983; Sroufe, Fox, & Pancake, 1983; Waters, Wippman, & Sroufe, 1979). As children elaborate their ideas, they use them to make more sense of their experiences and themselves (Bretherton & Beeghly, 1982; Dore, 1989; Dunn, 1988; Dunn, Bretherton, & Munn, 1987; Nelson & Gruendel, 1981; Schank & Abelson, 1977).

Clinical Observations

A mental representation or idea is a multisensory image that involves the construction of objects from the perspective of all the objects' properties. Where the range, depth, and integration of sensory experiences are limited, the very construction of the object and representation is obviously limited in either its sensory range and depth or affective investment and meaning.

As the child learns to construct his own multisensory, affective-thematic image of his experiential world, he organizes affective-thematic patterns at a level of meanings. This new level of organization can be thought of as operating in two ways. The youngster with a representational capacity now has the tool to interpret and label feelings rather than simply act them out. A verbal 2½-year-old can evidence this interpretive process by saying "me mad" or "me happy." Because many children have language delays, pretend play may be a more reliable indicator than language of the child's ability to interpret and label. For example, a child soon provides a picture of her representational world as she plays out dramas in different thematic realms (e.g., conveying her concept of dependency by having two dolls feed or hug each other).

The representational capacity also provides a higher-level organization with which to integrate affective-thematic domains. Thus, we observe new experiences as the child develops from two to five years of age. These include empathy and more consistent love. This more mature love for self and others includes object constancy; it is stable over time and survives separations and affect storms (Mahler, et al., 1975). Later on, it embraces the ability to experience loss, sadness, and guilt.

Because of the complexities of representational elaboration, the conceptualization of this stage may be aided by subdividing the representational capacity into three levels or subcategories. The first level is the descriptive use of the representational mode (the child labels pictures and describes objects). The second level is the limited interactive use of the representational mode (the child elaborates one or two episodes of thematic-affective interactions, such as statements of "give me candy," "me hungry," or the construction of a play scene with two dolls feeding, fighting, or nuzzling). The third level is behavioral and/or symbolic elaboration of representational, affective-thematic interactions.

Implications for Mental (Ego) Functioning

This stage of ego organization is characterized by the capacity to elevate experiences to the representational level. Current experience can be organized into multisensory-affective images that are mobile in time and space (e.g., children imagine images of objects in the absence of the object). The representational system can also construct multisensory images of sensations or patterns from within the organism that may have occurred in the past. These earlier patterns of somatic sensation and simple and complex chains of behavior and interaction are now interpreted via representation. How well formed, accurate, or distorted these representations of earlier prerepresentational experience are depends on the character of the early patterns, their repetition in the present, the abstracting ability of the ego, and the emerging dynamic character of the ego; that is, its ability to represent some areas of experience better than others.

To the degree that there is a less than optimal interactive experience available (the caregiver is concrete or ignores or distorts certain representational themes), we observe a series of mental (ego) operations, which include:

- Concretization of experience (access to representation is never achieved)
- Behavioral-representational splitting (some areas gain access, but core areas remain at behavioral level)
- Representational constriction (global dynamically relevant areas remain outside the representational system)
- Representational encapsulation—limited dynamically relevant areas remain in more concrete form
- Representational exaggeration or lability—domains of experience that are ignored or distorted become exaggerated and/or labile; their opposites become exaggerated and/or labile; or other "displaced" dynamically related thoughts, affects, or behaviors become exaggerated or labile.

At this time we can postulate an undifferentiated representational self-object built on a foundation of somatic and behavioral differentiated self-objects. Often, at this stage of development, representational elaboration is associated with primary process thinking. Because behavioral and somatic differentiation is already occurring, and because representational differentiation occurs simultaneously with representational elaboration, we may need to rethink our notions of primary process thinking.

Representational Differentiation (Building Logical Bridges Between Ideas and Emotional Thinking): 30-48 Months

The next level involves creating logical bridges between ideas. Shared meanings are used both to elaborate wishes and feelings and to categorize meanings and solve problems. The child elaborates and eventually differentiates those feelings, thoughts, and events that emanate from within from those that emanate from others. The child begins to differentiate the actions of others from her own. This process gradually forms the basis for the differentiation of self-representations from representations of the external world, animate and inanimate. It also provides the basis for such crucial personality functions as the capacity to discriminate real from unreal, the capacity to regulate impulse and mood, and the capacity to focus attention and concentration in order to learn and interact.

As logical bridges between ideas are established, reasoning and appreciation of reality grow, including distinguishing what is pretend from what is believed to be real, dealing with conflicts, and finding prosocial outcomes (Dunn & Kendrick, 1982; Flavell, Green, & Flavell, 1986; Harris, Brown, Marriott, Whittall, & Harmer, 1991; Harris & Kavanaugh, 1993; Wolf, Rygh, & Altshuler, 1984; Wooley & Wellman, 1990). As children become capable of emotional thinking, they begin to understand relationships between their own and others' experiences and feelings. They illustrate these relationships in their narratives. Emotional thinking also enables children to begin to reason about right and wrong

(Buchsbaum & Emde, 1990; Emde & Buchsbaum, 1990; Harris, 1989; Nelson, 1986; Smetana, 1985; Stewart & Marvin, 1984; Wolf, 1990). As children move into subsequent stages and become more concerned with peers, they begin to appreciate emotional complexities such as mixed feelings (Donaldson & Westerman, 1986; Harter & Whitesell, 1989).

The capacity for differentiating internal representations becomes consolidated as object constancy is established (Mahler, et al. 1975). As the child moves into the oedipal stage, both reality and fantasy become more complex (Bruner, 1986; 1990; Dore, 1989; Fivush, 1991; Greenspan, 1993; Singer & Singer, 1990). In middle childhood, representational capacity becomes reinforced with the child's ability to develop derivative representational systems tied to the original representation and to transform them in accordance with adaptive and defensive goals. This achievement permits greater flexibility in dealing with perceptions, feelings, thoughts, and emerging ideals. Substages for these capacities include representational differentiation, the consolidation of representational capacity, and the capacity for forming limited and also multiple derivative representational systems (structural learning) (Greenspan, 1979). Throughout these stages, but especially in the formation of complex behavior patterns and rituals, the elaboration of ideas, and the creation of bridges between ideas, one observes cultural influences, e.g., in the way girls and boys construct aspects of their inner worlds (Reiss, 1989). The well-known finding that in Western cultures men tend to be more assertive and competitive and women more caring and relationship-oriented (Gilligan, 1982) is evident during development. Girls show more empathy and show it earlier than boys; parents talk to boys more about anger and to girls more about sadness (Zahn-Waxler, Robinson, & Emde, 1992).

At the level of building bridges between ideas, the child can make connections between different ideas and feelings ("I am mad because you took my toy") and can balance fantasy and reality. An adult using capacities begun during this stage can similarly hold logical conversations about wishes and feelings and make connections. ("I feel lonely and needy, and I get helpless when I feel that way. Sometimes I get mad because I can't stand being so vulnerable.")

Clinical Observations

For the child to meet the challenges of organizing and differentiating his internal world according to "self" and "other," "inside" and "outside," dimensions of time and space and affective valence, he is, in part, dependent on the integrity of the sensory organization that underlies his experiential world. Now, as earlier, the capacity to process sensory information is critical, including sequencing auditory-verbal and visual-spatial patterns according to physical, temporal, and spatial qualities in the context of abstracting emerging cognitive and affective meanings. The child is now challenged to understand what he hears, sees, touches, and feels, not only in terms of ideas, but in terms of what is "me" and "not-me"; what is past, present, and future; what is close and far; and so forth. These learning tasks depend on the ability to sequence and categorize information through each of the sensory systems and through their all working together. Therefore, if anywhere along the pathway of sensory processing there are difficulties, the subsequent ability to organize impersonal or affective information is likely to be compromised.

For example, if sounds are confused, words are not easily understood. Similarly, if spatial images are confused, spatial configurations are not easily negotiated. If short-term memory for either verbal or spatial symbols is vulnerable, information is lost before it can be combined with, and compared to, other information in abstracting meanings. And if higher level auditory-verbal symbolic or visual-spatial symbolic abstracting capacities are less than age-appropriate, the very capacity to categorize experience is limited. When one considers that the challenge is now to process and organize not only impersonal, cognitive experiences, but also highly emotional, interpersonal experiences (which keep moving, so to speak), this challenge to the sensory system is formidable. Furthermore, categories such as "me," "not me," "real," and "make-believe" are high-level constructs that depend on organizing sensory information.

In contrast to earlier views by Freud (1900) and Mahler and colleagues (1975), the child appears to use his new representational capacity to elaborate and differentiate experience simultaneously. There does not appear to be a period of magical representational thinking followed by one of reality thinking. The child continually differentiates affective-thematic organizations along lines that pertain to self and other, inner and outer, time, space, and so forth. This differentiation is based on the child's capacity to experience the consequences of his representational elaborations with the emotionally relevant people in his world, usually parents, family, and friends. The parent who interacts with the child, using emotionally meaningful words and gestures, and who engages in pretend play in a contingent manner (offering, in other words, logical representational feedback), provides the child with consequences that help him differentiate his representational world. In this view, reality testing—the capacity to separate magical from realistic thought—appears to be a gradual process beginning with the onset of the representational capacity proper, and reaching some degree of selective stabilization prior to the child's formal entry into school.

One observes the child's elaborate representational themes along two dimensions. In the horizontal dimension, the child broadens the range of his or her themes to include a range of emotional domains or drive-affect realms, including closeness or dependency, pleasure and excitement, assertiveness, curiosity, aggression, self-limit-setting, the beginnings of empathy, and consistent love. One frequently observes repetitive pretend play of a feeding or hugging scene, suggesting nurturance and dependency. Over time, however, the dramas the child may initiate (with interactive parental support) expand to include, among others, scenes of separation (one doll going off on a trip and leaving the other behind), competition, assertiveness, aggression, injury, birth, death, and recovery (the doctor doll trying to fix the wounded soldier). At the same time, the logical infrastructure of the child's pretend play and functional use of language becomes more complex and causally connected. The "He-Man" doll is hurt by the "bad guys" and therefore "gets them." After the tea party, the little girl doll goes to the "potty" and then decides it is time to begin cooking dinner. In discussions, the 3½ year old sounds more and more like a lawyer with "buts" and "becauses"—"I don't like that food because it looks yucky and will make me sick." Thus, one sees both thematic elaboration and differentiation. Even though the themes may be pretend and phantasmagoric, the structure of the drama becomes more and more logical. The rocket ship to the land of "He-Man" uses N.A.S.A. rocket fuel.

As indicated, representational differentiation depends not only on a child's being representationally engaged in thematic-affective areas but also on his experiencing cause-and-effect feedback at the representational level. Parents have to be able not only to engage but also to interpret experiences correctly. The parents who react to playing with a toy gun as aggression one day, as sexuality another day, and as dependency on a third day, or who keep shifting meanings within the same thematic play session, confuse the child. This child may not develop meanings with a reality orientation. Parents who confuse their own feelings with the child's feelings, or who cannot set limits, may also compromise the formation of a reality orientation.

Implications for Mental (Ego) Functioning

During this stage one may postulate a self-object relationship characterized by a differentiated, integrated representational self-object. Ego organization, differentiation, and integration are characterized by an abstraction of self-object representations and drive-affect dispositions into a higher-level representational organization, differentiated along dimensions of self-other, time, and space.

Mental (ego) functioning during this stage and the prior stage can be divided into a number of patterns, including the following:

- Words and actions may be used together (ideas are acted out in action, but words are also used to signify the action)
- Somatic or physical words may be used to convey feeling state ("My muscles are exploding," "Head is aching")
- Action words may be used instead of actions to convey intent ("Hit you!")
- Feelings may be conveyed as real rather than as signals ("I'm mad" or "Hungry" or "Need a hug," as compared with "I feel mad" or "I feel

hungry" or "I feel like I need a hug"). In the first instance, the feeling state demands action and is very close to action, whereas in the second, it is more a signal for something going on inside that leads to a consideration of many possible thoughts and/or actions.

- Feeling states may be global ("I feel awful," "I feel OK," etc.)

- Feeling states may be polarized (characterized as all good or all bad)

- Feelings may be differentiated (gradually there are more and more subtle descriptions of feeling states—loneliness, sadness, annoyance, anger, delight, happiness, etc.)

- Connections may be created between differentiated feeling states ("I feel angry when you are mad at me")

What operations are now available to deal with anxiety and conflict? In addition to the primitive mechanisms described earlier, the ego now has new approaches. Observations of both normal and disturbed young children suggest that these include:

- Global lack of differentiation (reality and the object ties that provide reality feedback are too disruptive or "scary.")

- Selective dedifferentiation (blurring of boundaries and changing meanings, as with "my anger won't make mother leave because we are the same person.")

- Thought-drive-affect de-differentiations ("I can think anything, but I won't have feelings so I won't be scared.")

- Thought-behavior (impulse) dedifferentiation ("If I do it without thinking, it's not me. Only when I think and plan it is it me.")

- Selective constrictions of drive-affect-thematic realms (areas such as anger or sexual curiosity are avoided and may remain relatively undifferentiated, often because they are associated with disorganizing interactive experience such as withdrawal or overstimulation)

- Affect, behavioral, or thought intensification ("If I exaggerate it or its opposite, it can't scare me.")

- Differentiated representational distortions (changing meanings along lines of drive-affect dispositions—"I am supergirl, the strongest." But basic reality testing is maintained—e.g., "It is only pretend.")

- Encapsulated distortions (dynamically based, conflict-driven, highly selective shifts of meanings; e.g., "I am the cause of mother's anger.")

- Transforming differentiational linkages (an early form of rationalization: As the child's capacity to connect representational units is forming, she can elaborate, as in "I like mommy because she is home all the time and am mad at daddy because he travels a lot." These logical links can undergo subtle shifts to change meanings for defensive purposes, as in "I like daddy to travel a lot because he brings me presents. I am mad at mommy.")

- Compromises in representational integration and representational identity (the integration of somatic, behavioral, and associated drive-affect proclivities is not fully maintained, as evidenced by the irritable-looking three-year-old who "feels fine" or the hitting three-year-old who "loves everyone")

Higher Levels Of Mental (Ego) Functioning

These six basic foundations create the opportunity to master higher levels of mental (ego) functioning. Later levels of capacity build on the basic ones. They include *multi-cause and triangular reasoning about emotions* (e.g., a child can figure out several reasons why he has a feeling and can comprehend emotional relationships between three people); *gray-area, differentiated, reflective thinking about his own and others' feelings* (a child can weigh the relative ways in which different feelings contribute to his or others' behavior or the relative impacts of different reasons for the way he feels); and *reflective thinking from a growing internal sense of self and internal standard* (the child is developing an affectively-integrated sense of self that she can use to make judgments and form opinions about experiences, such as "I usually don't get this angry in this situation"). Once these advanced stages are in place, they enable an individual to increase the range and depth of affective experience and negotiate a series of additional stages during adolescence and adulthood (Greenspan, 1997b; Greenspan & Shanker, 2004).

From Affects to Symbols: The Developmental Pathway to the Formation of Internal Representations

How symbols and internal representations emerge from earlier infant behavior is one of the most important unsolved mysteries in modern psychology. This empirically derived developmental framework for depth psychology suggests some answers.

We have observed that two conditions must be present for children to progress to creating meaningful internal representations and symbols. The first is that relevant affective or emotional experiences invest symbols as they form (Greenspan, 1997b). Affectively meaningful symbols of self and others become the basis for internal representations. Images without affect can lead to memories without meaning. We see this phenomenon in some children with autism. They may repeat words rather than conveying what the words mean.

The second condition for creating meaningful internal representations and symbols was a dramatic new insight for us. Yet, it is so basic in its simplicity that it also surprised us. This second condition is that *a representation or symbol emerges when perception is separated from its action*. The developmental process that enables a child to separate perception from action provides the missing link in understanding symbol formation, the construction of internal representations, and higher levels of consciousness, thinking, and self-reflection (Greenspan & Shanker, 2004).

Why does perception have to be separated from action to create symbols or internal representations? In animals, very young infants, and impulsive humans, perception is tied closely to action. They perceive something (e.g., an animal perceives a food source or an enemy) and they react (with approach, attack, flight or other response). The perception triggers an action. There is a closely linked perceptual/motor pattern, with little pause or delay in carrying out the action.

To understand what perception is like when it is not tied to one or a few predetermined actions, first consider that a perception usually involves a multisensory picture of the world. Next, imagine forming such a multisensory picture and not taking an immediate action. Such a multisensory picture is a perception or image in its own right, a freestanding image.

A person who can form a freestanding image can accumulate more affective experience with this perception. For example, over time, an image of mother can be imbued with many experiences with her, such as emotional interactions in playing, eating, and comforting. In this way, the image of mother gradually acquires more and more emotional meanings.

As images or perceptions become seasoned with more and more emotional experiences, they gradually form into an affectively meaningful symbol or internal representation. A symbol for something as complex and important as "mother" eventually involves many complex meanings, such as love, devotion, control, annoyance, and sacrifice. Over time, meaningful symbols can coalesce into integrated internal representations of "self" and "other" with greater and greater degrees of integration and differentiation (Greenspan, 1988; 1989b; 1989a).

Individuals who remain tied to global perceptual motor patterns (e.g., "catastrophic" affects or emotions tied to global, fixed perceptual motor actions such as the fight/flight reaction or massive avoidance) often do not progress to a stage where they can use internal representations to deal with affective experience. They tend to remain in an action mode.

To separate perception from action, one has to go beyond catastrophic emotions that are part of a primitive perceptual motor/action level. To tame catastrophic emotions involves a developmental process through which emotions become transformed into regulated affect signals. In the prior section, we described a number of different levels of affect signaling. Of particular importance for the formation of symbols is the transition from the stage in which

affects are used intentionally to the stage in which they can be used in co-regulated problem-solving affective interactions. During these two stages (3 and 4),
there is a dramatic transformation from catastrophic affect to co-regulated affect
signaling. Affects change from pressing for action to being used for communication, negotiation, and regulation. This transformation frees perceptions from
their fixed actions and enables them to operate as freestanding images that can
then acquire a variety of affective meanings.

As affect signals are used to communicate and negotiate, they come to
govern cognitive, social, emotional, motor and sensory functioning. In addition,
and most consequentially, as affects become transformed into regulated signals,
they integrate prerepresentational (subsymbolic) and representational (symbolic)
systems. They remain separate only in pathologic development (Greenspan &
Shanker, 2004).

This transformation of affects from catastrophic states to co-regulated affect
signals occurs over a long period of time. Human beings are unique among mammals in having a long period during which an infant or toddler is dependent on
caregivers. During this time, she can learn to use nonverbal, gestural, emotional
signals, an ability she shares with many other mammals, but she can also
develop a distinctively human capacity to meet basic needs, to interact, to communicate, and to negotiate.

IMPLICATIONS OF A FRAMEWORK FOR DEPTH PSYCHOLOGY FOR UNDERSTANDING MENTAL HEALTH AND MENTAL DISORDERS

The model presented in this chapter provides a framework for understanding
mental health, mental disorders, and psychotherapeutic approaches. (See Greenspan & Shanker, 2004 and Greenspan, 1997a; 1997b for further discussion.)
Each level in early development identifies a realm of experience that includes
basic capacities which define mental health and are relatively impaired in mental
disorders. These include the capacity to attend and regulate; to participate in relationships; to express, comprehend, and signal with a broad range of emotions; to
construct internal representations and progress to differentiating them as a basis
for reality testing; and to develop higher levels of reflective thinking and social
interaction. For each of these realms of experience and capacities we can observe
deficits or varying degrees of constriction (limitations).

In addition, we can observe affects and associated defenses and character patterns. For example, at early levels of catastrophic affect expression, we can
observe global defensive patterns, such as massive avoidance, passivity, or aggression. At levels of prerepresentational affect signaling, we can observe more differentiated defensive patterns such as negativism, selective aggression, and
compulsive rituals. At representational levels, we can observe affects being used

as internal signals to mobilize defenses that alter internal experience. These range from condensations and displacements to reaction formations, rationalizations, and sublimations.

This developmental model of mental health suggests that in terms of the relative mastery of the core functional emotional developmental capacities, mental health disturbances or problems can be defined, as indicated, in terms of varying degrees of limitations in these same core capacities. For example, the capacity for healthy relationships characterized by warmth, intimacy, stability, and flexibility can be limited with challenges involving constrictions (e.g., the individual who is aloof) or deficits (the individual who is completely withdrawn). Similarly, the healthy capacity for experiencing, comprehending, and expressing a range of age-appropriate affects can be contrasted with the maladaptive patterns of only experiencing a few selective affects, such as anger and suspiciousness.

As indicated earlier, we have conceptualized mental health and mental disorders in terms of a Developmental, Individual-Difference, Relationship-Based (DIR) model (Greenspan & Wieder, 1999). This model enables us to simultaneously consider the individual's relative mastery of his or her functional emotional developmental capacities ("D"), as described earlier; the contributions of the individual sensory-affective processing differences ("I"); and formative and ongoing relationships ("R"). For example, consider some elements in the developmental pathways leading to depression.

While there is a general consensus that depression has genetic and biological origins, it also involves environmental or experiential factors as well. The challenge has been to understand how all these factors interact. We observed that children at risk for depression express aspects of their biological patterns with increased sensitivity to sensations such as sound and touch and, as a consequence, evidence a great deal of emotional reactivity.

We have also observed a specific pattern of co-regulated, reciprocal, emotional interactions that tend to lead to a vulnerability towards depression. When the toddler or preschooler evidences emotional reactivity due to his sensory differences, and expresses strong affects, the adaptive reciprocal partner pattern is to modulate up or down to help keep the child regulated and in an even mood. As the toddler speeds up and intensifies his affective interactions, the adaptive partner soothes, engages, and attempts to calm and slow down the rhythm of affective energy. As the toddler begins to be overly subdued or self-absorbed, the adaptive caregiver might increase the saliency of his emotional cues, energize up, and increase the rhythm of affective interactions. This process of co-regulating is often a subtle one where both partners are "up" and "down" regulating each other, even before there are obvious extremes. The result is a relatively well-modulated mood. If, instead of "up" or "down" regulating, however, the reciprocal partner tends to either withdraw (even temporarily), or slow down significantly in her own responses, it may be experienced by the child as a withdrawal. The reciprocal partner may also overreact and intrude, disrupting a calm sense of relating. In these instances, instead of a pattern of modulation where the caregiver up- or down-regulates to help the child's mood stay regulated, there is a temporary rupture in the co-regulated pattern of emotional interaction. This results in dysphoric or unpleasant affects, often a sense of loss, and sometimes humiliation or anger. For example, a caregiver may personalize a toddler's intense affective responses. Instead of providing extra soothing, she may feel "He doesn't want to play with me" and, therefore, withdraw for a moment. In this situation, rather than modulated emotional interactions, the child experiences a sense of loss or catastrophic affects. The child can come to experience these dysphoric or catastrophic affects anytime feelings become intense. Dysphoric affects often then lead to expectations that go along with them (e.g., loss, humiliation, or other depressive ideation). In contrast, the child who has experienced soothing regulating affects when feelings become intense may come to have expectations that go along with adaptive interactions (e.g., optimism that one can feel better).

As the child moves into the representational and symbolic realm (assuming co-regulated interactions have not been severely disrupted), dysregulated patterns make it difficult for the child to construct a nurturing image of a caregiver that can be represented and felt in times of loss, stress, or anger. An internal representation characterized by nurturing images and affects can serve as a type of internal security blanket that a person can call on when needed. When this type of internal security blanket is not constructed, however, the child may also come to expect that intense feelings of any type lead to loss of soothing and nurturing. In this context, object constancy (Mahler, Pine, & Bergman, 1975) can be viewed in terms of the internal representations of the regulating affective qualities of pre-representational experiences with primary caregivers.

We have seen these patterns frequently in adults with depression. Often an event in their lives may involve loss, which routinely would precipitate some feelings of sadness. However, they cannot call on a nurturing internal image (or internal representation) to help them feel better. Therefore, they feel either "empty," "alone," "despondent," or self-critical. In addition, they do not have enough mastery of co-regulated emotional interactions to engage with their current relationships in a soothing and modulating manner.

More analytic types of depressive feelings tend to be associated with expectations of loss. Self-critical feelings are often associated with anger at the affectively dysregulating caregiver.

Individuals vulnerable to depression may tend to express their biological differences in being sensory and affectively hypersensitive. They need modulating, soothing, co-regulating emotional interactions even more than would otherwise be the case. When the care-giving environment has a hard time providing it and/

or the caregiver engages in withdrawal, slowing down or rigidity, we see a tendency toward associating needs and strong feelings with loss and other depressive affects and ideation, which, in turn, influences subsequent stages of development.

A developmental framework for depth psychology can also inform our understanding of the psychotherapeutic process (Greenspan, 1997). It suggests that in addition to clarifying and interpreting internal experience, the therapeutic process must focus on constructing experiences with the patient that foster mastery of the basic capacities associated with each developmental level (i.e., relationships, affect signaling, range of affective expression, and representation, differentiation, and integration of affective experience). It also suggests that the therapeutic process must concern itself with both the prerepresentational and representational levels of experience. The therapeutic process must deal with the patient's unique way of processing experience (i.e., her unique sensory-affective processing profile) and enable the patient to cope with the full range of experiences, from dependency and sexuality to assertiveness and aggression. For example, consider the following highlights from a case illustration of a woman who was very bright and a talented professional. She talked about being in a meeting and experiencing some competition from a peer. She felt that she was being put down and had a feeling of loss. She got depressed and could not function for the rest of the meeting. This sequence occurred routinely when she experienced competition. As she described a profound sense of "being all alone" during these moments, I asked her if she could bring to mind an image of her husband, who tended to nurture her, and picture him nurturing her at these times. She said, "You know what's interesting? I can't picture him at all in that way, even though he's a very caring person." She could not create a nurturing internal image. I later learned that she had a mother who could not nurture her through strong affects. Whenever she had strong feelings, her mother would "shut down" and "become stone-faced."

A clue to this pattern was this patient's reaction to her therapist's periodic temporary loss of empathy and relatedness. If, for example, the therapist moved in his seat or looked out the window for a second, she would immediately look quite sad. Instead of trying to pull the therapist back in, she would look down and her voice would go into more of a monotone, as though she were giving up.

It was not sufficient, however, just to verbally point out this pattern. It was necessary to create a different type of affective interaction and rhythm as well. The therapist needed to pull her back in with animated affective gestures and literally challenge her with his affective gestures to take the initiative. He did this with very distinct "expectant" looks, which communicated, "Can you keep the affective rhythm going or are you going to intensify my momentary lapse with an even bigger one?" Eventually, they were able to verbally explore this pattern as well.

Initially, this patient did not have the basis for recreating a multisensory, affective experience of nurturing in her own imagination. She did not have the internal affective image or feelings to get her through a tough time. Instead, she would get depressed because there would be no internal, representational "security blanket" for her to fall back on. The missing security blanket was absent at two levels—at the presymbolic affective interactive level and the symbolic level. As she learned to initiate affective interactions at times of loss, she also gradually became able to imagine and symbolize an internal representational security blanket (of images). She could feel and picture her husband or children in nurturing interactions.

This patient was also much stronger in her verbal processing capacities than her visual-spatial processing—a pattern we have observed in many individuals prone to depression. She was much better with details than big-picture thinking. Because of these processing patterns, she took a long time to progress to the level of feeling and "picturing" nurturing interactions, first describing them, and then gradually feeling and picturing them. This emerging capacity evolved in the context of transference explorations, and related considerations of past and present experiences.

As her explorations broadened, she was able to deal with many additional conflicts. For example, she was very competitive with her "stone-faced" mother and had sought out her father as an "ally" in the family triangles. Only after she was able to construct internal, nurturing images, however, was she able to explore her own competitiveness, triangular relationship, and other conflicts.

One goal, then, for working with the child or adult with depressive tendencies is for the therapist to work on the flow of interaction, up-regulating with the person when necessary and, at the same time, helping the person understand what might have happened in his or her own background to bring on these tendencies. As this capacity becomes established, the patient is often able to experience, express, and verbally explore a broad range of affects, including feelings of anger, entitlement, and fear of loss. The patient is often also able to organize pre-oedipal and oedipal fantasies into a more integrated narrative, which is then able to serve as a basis for further self-exploration.

CONCLUSION

A developmental framework for depth psychology explores the formation of our most distinctly human capacities, such as relating, feeling, and reflecting. It informs a distinctly psychoanalytic way of defining mental health and mental health disorders and the therapeutic process. In addition to overcoming symptoms and specific behaviors or maladaptive patterns, mental health must be defined by the realms of experience and capacities that arise and define human development during the course of life. Therefore, in addition to addressing discrete symptoms and modifying specific behaviors, a depth psychological, developmental framework enables us to understand mental health and mental illness as defined by capacities and limitations in the realms of experience that characterize the deepest levels of human development and functioning.

REFERENCES

Aber, J., & Baker, A. J. (1990). Security of attachment in toddlerhood: Modifying assessment procedures for joint clinical and research purposes. In M. T.Greenberg, D. Cicchetti, & E. M. Cummings (Eds.), *Attachment in the Preschool Years* (pp. 427-463). Chicago: University of Chicago Press.

Ainsworth, M., Bell, S. M., & Stayton, D. (1974). Infant-mother attachment and social development: Socialization as a product of reciprocal responsiveness to signals. In M. Richards (Ed.), *The integration of the child into a social world* (pp. 99-135). Cambridge, England: Cambridge University Press.

Ainsworth, M., Blehar, M., Waters, E., & Wall, S. (1978). *Patterns of attachment: A psychological study of the strange situation.* New York: Lawrence Erlbaum Associates.

Als, H. (1982). Patterns of infant behavior: Analogs of later organizational difficulties? In F. H. Duffy & N. Geschwind (Eds.), *Dyslexia: A neuroscientific approach to clinical evaluation* (pp. 67-92). Boston: Little, Brown, & Co.

Als, H., Lester, B. M., Tronick, E., & Brazelton, T. B. (1982). Towards a research instrument for the assessment of preterm infants' behavior (APIB). In H. Fitzgerald & M. W. Yogman (Eds.), *Theory and research in behavioral pediatrics* (pp. 35-132). New York: Plenum Press.

Arend, R., Gove, F. L., & Sroufe, L. A. (1979). Continuity of individual adaptation from infancy to kindergarten: a predictive study of ego-resiliency and curiosity in preschoolers. *Child Development, 50,* 950–959.

Ayres, J. (1964). Tactile functions: Their relation to hyperactive and perceptual motor behavior. *American Journal of Occupational Therapy, 18,* 6-11.

Bates, J. E., Maslin, L. A., & Frankel, K. A. (1985). Attachment, security, mother-child interaction, and temperament as predictors of problem behavior ratings at age three years. Monographs of the Society for Research in Child Development, 50(1-2, Serial No. 209).

Beebe, B., Jaffe, J., & Lachmann, F. (1992). A dyadic systems view of communication. In N. Skolnik & E. Waters (Eds.), *Relational perspectives in psychoanalysis* (pp. 61-81). Hillsdale, NJ: Analytic Press.

Beebe, B., & Lachmann, F. (2002). *Infant research and adult treatment: Co-constructing interactions.* Hillsdale, NJ: Analytic Press.

Bell, R. (1977). Socialization findings re-examined. In R. Bell & L. Harper (Eds.), *Child effects on adults.* New York: John Wiley .

Bell, S. M. (1970). The development of the concept of the object as related to infant-mother attachment. *Child Development, 41,* 219-311.

Belsky, J., Rovine, M., & Taylor, D. G. (1984). The Pennsylvania Infant and Family Development Project, III: The origins of individual differences in infant-mother attachment: Maternal and infant contributions. *Child Development, 55,* 718-728.

Berlyne, D. E. (1960). *Conflict, arousal, and curiosity.* New York: McGraw Hill.

Bowlby, J. (1951). Maternal care and mental health. *Monographs of the World Health Organization, 51.* Geneva: World Health Organization.

Bowlby, J. (1969). *Attachment and loss.* (Vol. 1) London: Hogarth Press.

Bowlby, J. (1973). *Attachment and loss*. (Vol. 2) New York: Basic Books.

Brazelton, T. B., & Als, H. (1979). Four early stages in the development of mother-infant inter-action. *The Psychoanalytic Study of the Child, 34*, 349-369.

Brazelton, T. B., & Cramer, B. (1990). *The earliest relationship: Parents, infants, and the drama of early attachment*. Reading, MA: Addison-Wesley Publishing Co.

Brazelton, T. B., Koslowski, B., & Main, M. (1974). The origins of reciprocity; the early mother-infant interaction. In M. Lewis & L. Rosenblum (Eds.), *The Effect of the Infant on Its Caregiver*. New York: John Wiley .

Bremmer, R., & Fogel, A. (2001). *Handbook of infant development*. London: Blackwell.

Bretherton, I., & Beeghly, M. (1982). Talking about inner states: The acquisition of an explicit theory of mind. *Developmental Psychology, 18*, 906-921.

Bruner, J. S. (1982). *Child's talk: Learning to use language*. New York: Norton.

Bruner, J. S. (1986). *Actual minds, possible worlds*. Cambridge, MA: Harvard University Press.

Bruner, J. S. (1990). *Acts of meaning*. Cambridge, MA: Harvard University Press.

Buchsbaum, H. K., & Emde, R. N. (1990). Play narratives at 36 months: Moral development and family relationships. *Psychoanalytic Studies Child, 45*, 129-155.

Burlingham, D., & Freud, A. (1942). *Young children in wartime: A year's work in a residential war nursery*. London: Allen & Unwin.

Butterworth, G. (1990). Self perception in infancy. In D. Cicchetti & M. Beeghly (Eds.), *The self in transition: Infancy to childhood*. Chicago: Chicago University Press.

Butterworth, G., & Jarrett, N. (1980). *The geometry of preverbal communication*. Edinburgh.

Campos, J., Barrett, K., Lamb, M. E., Goldsmith, H. H., & Stenberg, C. (1983). Socioemotional development. In M. M. Haith & J. Campos (Eds.), *Handbook of Child Psychology, Vol. II*. New York: John Wiley .

Campos, J., Campos, R., & Barrett, K. (1989). Emergent themes in the study of emotional development and emotion regulation. *Developmental Psychology, 25*, 394-402.

Carew, J. V. (1980). Experience and the development of intelligence in young children at home and in day care. Monographs of the Society for Research in Child Development, 45(6-7).

Cassidy, J. (1990). Theoretical and methodological considerations in the study of attachment and self in young children. In M. T. Greenberg & D. Cicchetti (Eds.), *Attachment in the Pre-school Years* (pp. 87-120). Chicago: Chicago University Press.

Cassidy, J.,& Marvin, R, with the Attachment Working Group of the John D. and Catherine T. MacArthur Network on the Transition from Infancy to Early Childhood (1988). *A system for coding the organization of attachment behavior in 3 or 4 year old children*. Washington, DC.

Cassidy, J., & Shaver, P. R. (1999). *Handbook of attachment*. New York: Guilford Press.

Charlesworth, W. R. (1969). The role of surprise in cognitive development. In D. Elkind & J. H. Flavell (Eds.), *Studies in Cognitive Development: Essays* (pp. 257-314). London: Oxford University Press.

Cicchetti, D., & Schneider-Rosen, K. (1984). Toward a transactional model of childhood depression. *New Directions for Child Development, 26*, 5-27.

Darwin, C. (1872). *The expression of emotions in man and animals*. London: Murray (Republished by University of Chicago Press, 1965).

De Wolff, M. S., & van Ijzendoorn, M. H. (1997). Sensitivity and attachment: A meta-analysis on parental antecedents of infant attachment. *Child Development, 68*, 571-591.

Deci, E. (1977). *Intrinsic motivation*. New York: Plenum.

Dennis, W. (1960). Causes of retardation among institutional children: Iran. *Journal of Genetic Psychology, 96*, 47-59.

DesRosiers, F. S., & Busch-Rossnagel, N. A. (1997). Self-concept in toddlers. *Infants and Young Children, 10,* 15-26.

Donaldson, S., & Westerman, M. (1986). Development of children's understanding of ambivalence and causal theories of emotions. *Developmental Psychology, 22,* 655-662.

Dore, J. (1989). Monologue as reenvoicemnt of dialogue. In K.Nelson (Ed.), *Narratives from the crib* (pp. 27-73). Cambridge, MA: Harvard University Press.

Dunn, J. (1988). *The beginnings of social understanding.* Cambridge, MA: Harvard University Press.

Dunn, J., Bretherton, I., & Munn, P. (1987). Conversations about feeling states between mothers and their young children. In I.Bretherton (Ed.), *Symbolic play: The development of social understanding.* New York: Academic Press.

Dunn, J., & Kendrick, C. (1982). *Siblings.* Cambridge, MA: Harvard University Press.

Easterbrooks, M. A., & Goldberg, W. A. (1990). Security of toddler-parent attachment: Relation to children's sociopersonality functioning during kindergarten. In M. T. Greenberg, D. Cicchetti, & E. M. Cummings (Eds.), *Attachment in the Preschool Years* (pp. 221-245). Chicago: University of Chicago Press.

Egeland, B., & Farber, E. A. (1984). Infant-mother attachment: Factors related to its development and changes over time. *Child Development, 55,* 753-771.

Egeland, B., & Kreutzer, T. (1991). A longitudinal study of the effects of maternal stress and protective factors on the development of high risk children. In A. L. Green, E. M. Cummings, & K. H. Karraker (Eds.), *Life-span developmental psychology: Perspectives on stress and coping* (pp. 61-84). Hillsdale, NJ: Lawrence Erlbaum Associates.

Ekman, P., Friesen, W., & Ellsworth, P. (1972). *Emotions in the human face.* Elmsford, NY: Pergamon.

Emde, R. N., & Buchsbaum, H. K. (1990). "Didn't you hear my mommy?" Autonomy with connectedness in moral self-emergence. In D. Cicchetti & M. Beeghly (Eds.), *The self in transition: Infancy to childhood* (pp. 35-60). Chicago: University of Chicago Press.

Emde, R. N., Gaensbauer, T. J., & Harmon, R. J. (1976). *Emotional expression in infancy: A biobehavioral study.* Psychological Issues Monograph No. 37. New York, International Universities Press.

Emde, R. N., Johnson, W. F., & Easterbrooks, M. A. (1988). The dos and don'ts of early moral development: Psychoanalytic tradition and current research. In J. Kagan & S. Lamb (Eds.), *The emergence of morality* (pp. 245–277). Chicago: University of Chicago Press.

Erikson, E. H. (1940). Studies in interpretation of play: I. Clinical observation of child disruption in young children. *Genetic Psychology Monographs, 22.*

Escalona, S. (1968). *The roots of individuality.* Chicago: Aldine.

Falk, D. (2000). *Primate Diversity.* New York: W. W. Norton.

Fein, G. G. (1975). A transformational analysis of pretending. *Developmental Psychology, 11,* 291-296.

Fein, G. G., & Apfel, N. (1979). Some preliminary observations on knowing and pretending. In N. Smith & M. Franklin (Eds.), *Symbolic Functioning in Childhood.* Hillsdale, NJ: Lawrence Erlbaum Associates.

Feinman, S., & Lewis, M. (1983). Social referencing and second order effects in ten-month-old infants. *Child Development, 54,* 878-887.

Feldman, R., Greenbaum, C. W., & Yirmiya, N. (1999). Mother-infant affect synchrony as an antecedent of the emergence of self-control. *Developmental Psychology, 35,* 223-231.

Fenson, L., Kagan, J., Kearsely, R. B., & Zelazo, P. R. (1976). The developmental progression of manipulative play in the first two years. *Child Development, 47,* 232-235.

Fenson, L., & Ramsay, D. (1980). Decentration and integration of play in the second year of life. *Child Development, 51,* 171-178.

Field, T. (1981). Gaze behavior of normal and high-risk infants during early interactions. *Journal of the American Academy of Child and Adolescent Psychiatry, 20,* 308-317.

Fivush, R. (1991). Gender and emotion in mother-child conversations about the past. *Journal of Narrative and Life History, 1,* 325-341.

Flavell, J. H., Green, F. L., & Flavell, E. R. (1986). Development of knowledge about the appearance-reality distinction. With commentaries by M. W. Watson and J. C. Campione. *Monographs of the Society for Research in Child Development, 51*(1, Serial No. 212).

Fogel, A. (1982). Affect dynamics in early infancy: Affective tolerance. In T. Field & A. Fogel (Eds.), *Emotion and early interaction.* Hillsdale, NJ: Lawrence Erlbaum Associates.

Fonagy, P., Gergely, G., Jurist, E., & Target, M. (2002). *Affect regulation, mentalization, and the development of the self.* New York: Other Press LLC.

Fonagy, P., & Target, M. (1997). Attachment and reflective function: their role in self-organization. *Development and Psychopathology, 9,* 679-700.

Freud, A. (1965). *Normality and pathology in childhood; assessments of development.* New York: International Universities Press.

Freud, S. (1900/1958). The interpretation of dreams. Parts I and II. *Standard Edition, 4,* 1-625.

Gilligan, C. (1982). *In a different voice: Psychological theory and women's development.* Cambridge, MA: Harvard University Press.

Goldberg, S. (1977). Social competence in infancy: A model of parent-infant interaction. *Merrill-Palmer Quarterly, 23,* 163-177.

Goldberg, W. A., & Easterbrooks, M. A. (1984). Toddler development in the family: Impact of the father involvement and parenting characteristics. *Developmental Psychology, 55,* 740-752.

Gouin-Decarie, T. (1965). *Intelligence and affectivity in early childhood: An experimental study of Jean Piaget's object concept and object relations.* New York: International Universities Press.

Greenspan, S. I. (1979). Intelligence and adaptation: An integration of psychoanalytic and Piagetian developmental psychology. *Psychological Issues Monographs No. 47-48.* New York: International Universities Press.

Greenspan, S. I. (1981). *Psychopathology and adaptation in infancy and early childhood: Principles of clinical diagnosis and preventive intervention.* Clinical Infant Reports, No. 1. New York, International Universities Press.

Greenspan, S. I. (1988). The development of the ego: Insights from clinical work with infants and young children. *Journal of the American Psychoanalytic Association, 36,* 3-55.

Greenspan, S. I. (1989a). The development of the ego: Biological and environmental specificity and the psychopathological developmental process. *Journal of the American Psychoanalytic Association, 37,* 605-638.

Greenspan, S. I. (1989b). *The development of the ego: Implications for personality theory, psychopathology, and the psychotherapeutic process.* New York: International Universities Press.

Greenspan, S. I. (1992). *Infancy and early childhood: The practice of clinical assessment and intervention with emotional and developmental challenges.* Madison, CT: International Universities Press.

Greenspan, S. I. (1993). *Playground politics: Understanding the emotional life of your school-age child.* Reading, MA: Addison Wesley.

Greenspan, S. I. (1997a). *Developmentally-based psychotherapy.* Madison, CT: International Universities Press.

Greenspan, S. I. (1997b). *The growth of the mind and the endangered origins of intelligence.* Reading, MA: Addison Wesley Longman.

Greenspan, S. I. (1998). Commentary: Guidance for constructing clinical practice guidelines for developmental and learning disorders: Knowledge vs. evidence-based approaches. *Journal of Developmental and Learning Disorders, 2,* 171-192.

Greenspan, S. I., & Lourie, R. S. (1981). Developmental structuralist approach to the classification of adaptive and pathologic personality organizations: Infancy and early childhood. *American Journal of Psychiatry, 138,* 725–735.

Greenspan, S. I., & Porges, S. W. (1984). Psychopathology in infancy and early childhood: clinical perspectives on the organization of sensory and affective-thematic experience. *Child Development, 55,* 49-70.

Greenspan, S. I., & Shanker, S. (2004). *The first idea: How symbols, language, and intelligence evolve, from primates to humans.* Reading, MA: Perseus Books.

Greenspan, S. I., & Wieder, S. (1998). *The child with special needs: Encouraging intellectual and emotional growth.* Reading, MA: Perseus Books.

Greenspan, S. I., Wieder, S., Lieberman, A., Nover, R., Lourie, R., & Robinson, M. (1987). *Infants in multirisk families: Case studies in preventive intervention.* Clinical Infant Reports. (3). New York, International Universities Press.

Grossmann, K., Grossmann, K. E., Spangler, G., Suess, G., & Unzner, L. (1985). Maternal sensitivity and newborns' orientation responses as related to quality of attachment in Northern Germany. *Monographs of the Society for Research in Child Development, 50*(1-2, Serial No. 209).

Harlow, H. F. (1953). Motivation as a factor in the acquisition of new responses. In *Current theory and research in motivation: A symposium* (pp. 24-29). Lincoln: University of Nebraska Press.

Harris, P. L. (1989). *Children and emotion.* Oxford: Basil Blackwell.

Harris, P. L., Brown, E., Marriott, C., Whittall, S., & Harmer, S. (1991). Monsters, ghosts, and witches: Testing the limits of the fantasy-reality distinction in young children. *British Journal of Developmental Psychology, 9,* 105-123.

Harris, P. L., & Kavanaugh, R. (1993). Young children's understanding of pretense. *Monographs of the Society for Research in Child Development, 58*(1, Serial No. 231).

Harter, S., & Whitesell, N. (1989). Developmental changes in children's emotion concepts. In C. Saarni & P. L. Harris (Eds.), *Children's understanding of emotion.* New York: Cambridge University Press.

Hendrick, I. (1939). *Facts and theories of psychoanalysis.* New York: Knopf.

Hilweg, W., & Ullman, E. (Eds.) (1999). *Childhood and trauma, separation, abuse, war.* Bath, UK: Ashgrove Press

Hunt, J. M. (1965). *Intrinsic motivation and its role in psychological development.* Lincoln, NE: University of Nebraska Press.

Inhelder, B., Lezine, I., Sinclair, H., & Stambak, M. (1972). Le debut de la function symbolique. In E. M. Hetherington & P. H. Mussen (Eds.), *Handbook of child psychology,* Vol. 4 (pp. 187-243). New York: John Wiley .

Interdisciplinary Council on Developmental and Learning Disorders Clinical Practice Guidelines Workgroup, S. I. G. C. (2000). *Interdisciplinary Council on Developmental and Learning Disorders' Clinical practice guidelines: Redefining the standards of care for infants, children, and families with special needs.* Bethesda, MD: Interdisciplinary Council on Developmental and Learning Disorders.

Izard, C. E. (1971). *The face of emotion.* New York: Meredith & Appleton-Century-Crofts.

Kagan, J. (1981). *The second year: The emergence of self-awareness.* Cambridge, MA: Harvard University Press.

Kaye, K., & Fogel, A. (1980). The temporal structure of face-to-face communication between mothers and infants. *Developmental Psychology, 16,* 454-464.

Kaye, K. (1982). *The mental and social life of babies: How parents create persons.* Chicago: University of Chicago Press.

Kernberg, O. F. (1975). *Borderline conditions and pathological narcissism.* New York: Jason Aronson.

Kimmert, M. D., Campos, J., Sorce, F. J., Emde, R. N., & Svejda, M. J. (1983). Social referencing: Emotional expressions as behavior regulators. In R. Plutchik & H. Kellerman (Eds.), *Emotion: Theory, research and experience: Vol. 2. Emotions in early development* (pp. 57-86). Orlando: Academic Press.

Kleinman, A. (1986). *Social origins of distress and disease.* New Haven: Yale University Press.

Kohut, H. (1971). *The analysis of self: A systematic approach to the psychoanalytic treatment of narcissistic personality disorders.* New York: International Universities Press.

Kraus, R., & Glucksberg, S. (1969). The development of communication: Competence as a function of age. *Child Development, 40,* 255-266.

Lachmann, F. M., & Beebe, B. (1997). The contribution of self and mutual regulation to therapeutic action: A case illustration. In M. Moskowitz, C. Monk, C. Kaye, & S. Ellman (Eds.), *The neurobiological and developmental basis for psychotherapeutic intervention* (pp. 94-121). Northvale, NJ: Jason Aronson.

La Greca, A. M., Silverman, W. K., Vernberg, E. M., & Roberts, M. C. (Eds.) (2002). *Helping children cope with disasters and terrorism.* Washington, DC: American Psychological Association.

Lester, B. M., Hoffman, J., & Brazelton, T. B. (1985). The rhythmic structure of mother-infant interaction in term and preterm infants. *Child Development, 56,* 15-27.

Lewis, M., & Feiring, M. (1987). Infant, maternal and mother-infant interaction behavior and subsequent attachment. *Child Development, 60,* 831-837.

Lowe, M. (1975). Trends in the development of representational play in infants from one to three years-an observational study. *Journal of Child Psychology and Psychiatry and Allied Disciplines, 16,* 33-47.

Lyons-Ruth, K., & Zeanah, C. (1993). The family context of infant mental health: I. Affective development in the primary caregiving relationship. In C. Zeanah (Ed.), *Handbook of infant mental health* (pp. 14-37). New York: Guilford Press.

Mahler, M. S., Pine, F., & Bergman, A. (1975). *The psychological birth of the human infant: Symbiosis and individuation.* New York: Basic Books.

Main, M., Kaplan, N., & Cassidy, J. (1985). Security in infancy, childhood and adulthood: A move to the level of representation. *Monographs of the Society for Research in Child Development, 50*(1-2, Serial No. 209).

Markus, H., & Kitayama, S. (1990). Culture and the self: Implications for cognition, emotion, and motivation. *Psychological Review, 98,* 224-253.

Marvin, R., & Stewart, R. B. (1991). A family systems framework for the study of attachment. In M. T. Greenberg, D. Cicchetti, & E. M. Cummings (Eds.), *Attachment in the preschool years* (pp. 51-87). Chicago: University of Chicago Press.

Maslin-Cole, C., & Spieker, S. J. (1990). Attachment as a basis of independent motivation: A view from risk and nonrisk samples. In M. T. Greenberg, D. Cicchetti, & E. M. Cummings (Eds.), *Attachment in the preschool years* (pp. 245-272). Chicago: University of Chicago Press.

Matas, L., Arend, R., & Sroufe, L. (1978). Continuity of adaptation in the second year: The relationship between quality of attachment and later competence. *Child Development, 49,* 547-556.

McCune-Nicholich, L. (1977). Beyond sensorimotor intelligence: Measurement of symbolic sensitivity through analysis of pretend play. *Merrill-Palmer Quarterly, 23,* 89-99.

Meltzoff, A. (1985). The roots of social and cognitive development: Models of man's original nature. In T. M. Field & N. A. Fox (Eds.), *Social perception in infants.* Norwood, NJ: Ablex Publishing Co.

Meltzoff, A. (1990). Foundations for developing a concept of self: The role of imitation in relating self to other and the value of social mirroring, social modeling, and self practice in infancy. In D. Cicchetti & M. Beeghly (Eds.), *The self in transition: Infancy to childhood.* Chicago: Chicago University Press.

Meltzoff, A., & Moore, K. (1977). Imitation of facial and manual gestures by human neo-nates. *Science, 198,* 75–78.

Miyake, K., Chen, S., & Campos, J. (1985). Infant temperament, mother's mode of interaction, and attachment in Japan: An interim report. *Monographs of the Society for Research in Child Development, 50*(1-2, Serial No. 209).

Nelson, K. (1973). Structure and strategy in learning to talk. *Monographs of the Society for Research in Child Development, 38*(1-2, Serial No. 149).

Nelson, K. (1986). *Even knowledge: Structure and function in development.* Hillsdale, NJ: Lawrence Erlbaum.

Nelson, K., & Gruendel, J. M. (1981). Generalized even representations: Basic building blocks of cognitive development. In A. L. Brown & M. E. Lamb (Eds.), *Advances in developmental psychology, Vol. 1.* Hillsdale, NJ: Lawrence Erlbaum.

Osofsky, J. D., & Eberhart-Wright, A. (1988). Affective exchanges between high risk mothers and infants. *International Journal of Psychoanalysis, 69 (Pt 2),* 221-231.

Papousek, H. (1981). The common in the uncommon child. In M. Lewis & L. Rosenblum (Eds.), *The uncommon child* (pp. 317-328). New York: Plenum Press.

Papousek, H., & Papousek, M. (1979). Early ontogeny of human social interaction: Its biologi-cal roots and social dimensions. In K. Foppa, W. Lepenies, & D. Ploog (Eds.), *Human ethol-ogy: Claims and limits of a new discipline* (pp. 456-489). New York: Cambridge University Press.

Pastor, D. (1981). The quality of mother-infant attachment and its relationship to toddlers' initial sociability with peers. *Developmental Psychology, 23,* 326-335.

Pederson, D. R., Moran, G., Sitko, C., Campbell, K., Ghesquire, K., & Acton, H. (1990). Mater-nal sensitivity and the security of infant-mother attachment: a Q-sort study. *Child Develop-ment, 61,* 1974-1983.

Peller, L. (1954). Libidinal phases, ego development, and play. *The Psychoanalytic Study of the Child, 9,* 178–198.

Piaget, J. (1962). The stages of intellectual development of the child. In S. Harrison & J. McDermott (Eds.), *Childhood psychopathology* (pp. 157-166). New York: International Univers-ities Press.

Pipp-Siegel, S., & Pressman, L. (1996). Developing a sense of self and others. *ZERO TO THREE, 17,* 17-24.

Pipp, S., Fischer, K. W., & Jennings, S. (1987). Acquisition of self-and-mother knowledge in infancy. *Developmental Psychology, 47,* 86-96.

Polan, H. J., & Hofer, M. A. (1999). Psychobiological origins of infant attachment and separa-tion responses. In J. Cassidy & P. R. Shaver (Eds.), *Handbook of attachment: Theory, research, and clinical application* (pp. 162-180). New York: Guildford Press.

Radke-Yarrow, M., Zahn-Waxler, C., & Chapman, M. (1983). Children's prosocial dispositions and behavior. In E. M. Hetherington & P. H. Mussen (Eds.), *Handbook of child psychology, Vol. 4* (pp. 469-545). New York: John Wiley.

Reingold, H. (1969). The social and socializing infant. In D. Goslin (Ed.), *Handbook of socializa-tion theory and research.* Chicago: Rand McNally.

Reiss, D. (1989). The represented and practicing family: Contrasting visions of family continu-ity. In A. J. Sameroff & R. N. Emde (Eds.), *Relationship disturbances in early childhood* (pp. 191-220). New York: Basic Books.

Rothbart, M. K., & Derryberry, D. (1981). Development of individual differences in tempera-ment. In M. E. Lamb & A. L. Brown (Eds.), *Advances in Developmental Psychology, Vol. 1.* Hills-dale, NJ: Lawrence Erlbaum.

Rubin, K. H., Fein, G. G., & Vandenberg, B. (1983). Play. In E. M. Hetherington & P. H. Mussen (Eds.), *Handbook of Child Psychology, Vol. 4* (pp. 136-148). New York: John Wiley.

Sander, L. (1962). Issues in early mother-child interaction. *Journal of the American Academy of Child & Adolescent Psychiatry, 1,* 141-166.

Scaife, M., & Bruner, J. S. (1975). The capacity for joint visual attention in the infant. *Nature, 253,* 265–266.

Schank, R. C., & Abelson, R. P. (1977). *Scripts, plans, goals and understanding.* Hillsdale, NJ: Lawrence Erlbaum.

Schweder, R., Mahapatra, M., & Miller, J. (1987). Cultural and moral development. In J. Kagan & S. Lamb (Eds.), *The emergence of morality in young children* (pp. 1-90). Chicago: University of Chicago Press.

Sinclair, H. (1970). The transition from sensorimotor to symbolic activity. *Interchange, 1,* 119-126.

Singer, D. G., & Singer, J. L. (1990). *The house of make-believe: Children's play and developing imagination.* Cambridge, MA: Harvard University Press.

Small, M. (1998). *Our babies, ourselves: How biology and culture shape the way we parent.* New York: Anchor Books.

Smetana, J. (1985). Preschool children's conceptions of transgressions: Effects of varying moral and conventional domain-related attributes. *Developmental Psychology, 21,* 18-29.

Spelke, E. S., & Owsley, C. (1979). Intermodal exploration and knowledge in infancy. *Infant Behavior and Development, 2,* 13-27.

Spitz, R. A. (1945). Hospitalism: An inquiry into the genesis of psychiatric conditions in early childhood. *The Psychoanalytic Study of the Child, 1,* 53-74.

Spitz, R. A. (1965). *The first year of life: A psychoanalytic study of normal and deviant development of object relations.* New York: International Universities Press.

Sroufe, L. A. (1979). Socioemotional development. In J. Osofsky (Ed.), *Handbook of infant development.* New York: John Wiley.

Sroufe, L. A. (1983). Infant-caregiver attachment and patterns of adaptation in preschool: The roots of maladaptation and competence. In M. Perlmutter (Ed.), *Minnesota Symposium in Child Psychology, Vol. 16* (pp. 41–91). Hillsdale, NJ: Lawrence Erlbaum.

Sroufe, L. A. (1996). *Emotional development: The organization of emotional life in the early years.* New York: Cambridge University Press.

Sroufe, L. A., Egeland, B., & Carlson, E. (1999). One social world: The integrated development of parent-child and peer relationships. In W. A. Collins & B. Laursen (Eds.), *Relationships as developmental context: The 29th Minnesota Symposium on Child Psychology.* Hillsdale, NJ: Lawrence Erlbaum.

Sroufe, L. A., Fox, N. A., & Pancake, V. (1983). Attachment and dependency in developmental perspective. *Child Development, 54,* 1615-1627.

Sroufe, L. A., & Waters, E. (1977). Attachment as an organizational construct. *Child Development, 48,* 1184–1199.

Stern, D. (1974a). Mother and infant at play: The dyadic interaction involving facial, vocal, and gaze behaviors. In M. Lewis & L. Rosenblum (Eds.), *The effect of the infant on its caregiver.* New York: John Wiley.

Stern, D. (1974b). The goal and structure of mother-infant play. *Journal of the American Academy of Child and Adolescent Psychiatry, 13,* 402-421.

Stern, D. (1977). *The first relationship: Mother and infant.* Cambridge, MA: Harvard University Press.

Stern, D. (1983*). The early development of schemas of self, of other, and of various experiences of 'self with other.' In J. Lichtenberg & S. Kaplan (Eds.), *Reflections on self psychology.* Hillsdale, NJ: Analytic Press.

Stern, D. (1985). *The interpersonal world of the infant: A view from psychoanalysis and developmental psychology.* New York: Basic Books.

Stewart, R. B., & Marvin, R. (1984). Sibling relations: The role of conceptual perspective-taking in the ontogeny of sibling caregiving. *Child Development, 55,* 1322-1332.

Talberg, G., Couto, R. J., O'Donnell, M. L., & Cuoto Rosa, J. A. (1988). Early affect development: empirical research. *International Journal of Psychoanalysis, 69,* 239-259.

Tennes, K., Emde, R. N., Kisley, A., & Metcalf, D. (1972). The stimulus barrier in early infancy: An exploration of some formulations of John Benjamin. In R. Hold & E. Peterfreund (Eds.), *Psychoanalysis and contemporary science, Vol. 1* (pp. 206-234). New York: MacMillan.

Thomas, A., & Chess, S. (1984). Genesis and evolution of behavioral disorders: from infancy to early adult life. *American Journal of Psychiatry, 141,* 1-9.

Trevarthen, C. (1979). Communication and cooperation in early infancy: A description of primary intersubjectivity. In M. Bullowa (Ed.), *Before speech: The beginning of interpersonal communication* (pp. 321–347). Cambridge, England: Cambridge University Press.

Tronick, E. (1980). The primacy of social skills in infancy. In D. B. Sawin, R. C. Hawkins, L. O. Walker, & J. Penticuff (Eds.), *Exceptional infant, Vol. 4* (pp. 144-158). New York: Brunner/Mazel.

Tronick, E. Z. (1989). Emotions and emotional communication in infants. *American Psychologist, 44,* 112-119.

Tronick, E. Z., & Gianino, A. F., Jr. (1986). The transmission of maternal disturbance to the infant. *New Directions in Child Development,* 5-11.

Waelder, R. (1933). The psychoanalytic theory of play. *Psychoanalytic Quarterly, 2,* 208-224.

Waters, E., Wippman, J., & Sroufe, L. A. (1979). Attachment, positive affect, and competence in the peer group: two studies in construct validation. *Child Development, 50,* 821-829.

Watson, J. B. (1930). *Behaviorism.* Revised edition. Chicago: University of Chicago Press.

Werner, H., & Kaplan, B. (1963). *Symbol formation. An organismic-developmental approach to language and the expression of thought.* New York: John Wiley.

White, R. W. (1963). *Ego and reality in psychoanalytic theory. Psychological Issues. 11.* New York, International Universities Press.

Winnicott, D. W. (1965). Ego distortion in terms of true and false self. In *The maturational processes and the facilitating environment* (pp. 140-152). New York: International Universities Press.

Wolf, D. (1990). Being of several minds. In D. Cicchetti & M. Beeghly (Eds.), *The self in transition* (pp. 183–213). Chicago: University of Chicago Press.

Wolf, D., Rygh, J., & Altshuler, J. (1984). Agency and experience: Actions and states in play narratives. In I. Bretherton (Ed.), *Symbolic play* (pp. 195-217). Orlando, FL: Academic Press.

Wooley, J. D., & Wellman, H. M. (1990). Young children's understanding of realities, nonrealities, and appearances. *Child Development, 61,* 946-964.

Zahn-Waxler, C., & Radke-Yarrow, M. (1982). The development of altruism: Alternative research strategies. In M. Eisenberg (Ed.), *The development of prosocial behavior.* New York: Academic Press.

Zahn-Waxler, C., Robinson, J. D., & Emde, R. N. (1992). The development of empathy in twins. *Developmental Psychology, 28,* 1038-1047.

The Contribution of Cognitive Behavioral and Neurophysiological Frames of Reference to a Psychodynamic Nosology of Mental Illness

Editor's Note: This fourth paper, parallel to the preceding paper's combined clinical and research contributions to a developmental formulation of a complex depth psychological understanding of human mental functioning, describes the same combining of clinical and research contributions to the understanding of unconscious mental processes, and their neurophysiological substrates, in elucidating the full complexity of human mental functioning.

Shevrin, an empirical psychoanalytic researcher, draws upon the range of studies in cognitive psychology and in neurophysiology, his own and that of others, to show how they complexly interdigitate with (correlate with) psychoanalytic conceptualizations to build a multisided explanatory framework of the phenomena of mental and emotional illness, in his words, to explain comprehensively their 'irrational,' 'peremptory,' and 'unbidden' aspects. Like the previous chapter on the developmental perspective, this one, on the cognitive behavioral and the neurophysiological perspectives, provides conceptual underpinning to a full psychoanalytic understanding of human mental life.

The effort to develop an atheoretical, purely descriptive nosology for mental health disorders has in recent years come under increasing criticism (Blatt & Levy, 1998; Shedler, 2002; Westen, 1997; Westin & Morrison, 2001). Several revisions have been undertaken to correct the serious difficulties identified by users of the system as well as critics. Another revision is now in progress. Many have pointed out that aspiring to create a diagnostic system qualifying as atheoretical is a scientific non-starter (Blatt & Levy, 1998). Mental health disorders confront the diagnostician with highly complex and ambiguous phenomena, ranging from fragmentary and often tendentious self-reports and flawed history to a multiplicity of behaviors occurring in the consulting room such as silence, tics, eye

---

[1] Professor of Psychology, Director University of Michigan Program of Research in Neuro-Psychoanalysis, University of Michigan

aversion, tears, angry explosions, demands, accusations, pleading, resignation, expressions of hopelessness, submission, and much more that human suffering elicits. From all of these the clinician must select, weigh, and determine the factors presumably constituting or causing the patient's disorder. It is highly unlikely that the clinician presented daily with this kind of complexity would not draw upon some frame of reference or conceptualization to assist in selecting, weighing, and ultimately separating what is important from what is unimportant as determined by guiding principles, often not explicitly identified.

Currently there are at least three major frames of reference that inform, to one extent or another, in one combination or another, the way clinicians evaluate their patients: (1) cognitive behavioral, (2) biological, and (3) psychodynamic. Each of these approaches is based on assumptions that are usually implicit and are to a greater or lesser extent supported by independent evidence. As a result it is not difficult to note blatant conceptual inconsistencies among these three reference frames. For example, the cognitive behavioral approach assumes that depressive beliefs cause depressed mood from which it follows that if beliefs are changed, moods will change. On the other hand, the biological approach assumes that abnormal amounts of certain neurotransmitters cause depressed moods from which it follows that if the amounts of these neurotransmitters are normalized, depressed moods will lift. For the former it is of little interest what is happening to neurotransmitters; they play no role in the theory nor are they accessible to the cognitive method. For the latter, it makes no difference what the beliefs are; they play no role in the theory nor are they accessible to the biochemical method. Yet findings from quite a few studies point to the augmentation in treatment benefit if both depressive beliefs and neurotransmitter levels are simultaneously addressed (Ressler, Rothbaum, & Tannenbaum, 2000). There are also recent neuroimaging studies appearing to show that each treatment modality affects different parts of the brain (Etkin, Pittenger, Polan, & Kandel, 2005). These findings would seem to require some metatheory that would explain the relationship between beliefs and neurotransmitters, how they interact, or if they work as independent factors. The other possibility is that practitioners subscribe to no theory, implicit or explicit, but rely on what one could call the "kitchen sink" approach to diagnosis and treatment: You throw in whatever seems to work either by some measure of clinical usefulness or reputation. Often this is the mark of clinicians at the end of their rope.

The psychodynamic frame of reference, although far from being an agreed upon set of interrelated concepts, is in agreement with the cognitive behavioral view in accepting that psychological factors such as beliefs can play a role, and in agreement with the biological view that significant brain processes are involved, but adds the important proviso that both beliefs and neurotransmitter levels are either secondary effects or concomitants of other causes, psychological in nature that are unconscious and thus unreportable by the patient. These considerations do not enter into cognitive behavioral or biochemical description. Yet in the respect that patients are unaware of neurotransmitter levels, there is a similarity to the neurotransmitter approach but for radically different reasons. Moreover, it is further assumed that the influence of unconscious factors is seldom direct and, in common sense terms, rational or reasonable. Interestingly, something similar can be said about neurotransmitter levels, whose effect is of a different order (psychological) from its cause (biochemical), posing intriguing questions about how mind and brain relate to one another. On the other hand, the relationship between depressive beliefs and depressive mood seems to be fairly direct and rational, once granting the validity of the beliefs.

Although it would be generally agreed that beliefs can influence behavior, it is not so clear about the means through which this is accomplished. Ordinarily we think that a changed belief would work through changing a person's motivation or attitude. If I learn that someone I believed was trustworthy turns out to be a scoundrel, my belief would change as a function of my disappointment, self-criticism for having been duped, and wariness in my further dealings with that person. There would not seem to be an automatic, unmediated impact of a changed belief, anymore than we continue to believe that the relationship between conditioned and unconditioned stimuli is automatic in the sense that the early behaviorists assumed. Rescorla, (1988) and others going back to Pavlov himself introduced such cognitive considerations as expectation and awareness of the relationship to account for some forms of conditioned learning.

The same can be said about changing neurotransmitter levels. It is highly unlikely that a meaningful change in a neurotransmitter in one important part of the brain does not affect other parts of the brain that instantiate such processes as thought and motivation, strongly implying that these local effects are mediated by many other functions related to other parts of the brain (Friston, 2000). In short, whether we are talking about beliefs or neurotransmitters, an explanation of their presumed effects must entail a much more complex picture of mediating factors that includes considerations of memory, affect, and motivation, in particular as these concern the significant people and important events in patients' lives. If we are to move from a descriptive to an explanatory basis for mental health nosology, then we must be prepared for a multi-factorial approach: What psychological factors mediate between specific beliefs and mood? What neurophysiological factors mediate between specific neurotransmitter levels and mood? What unconscious factors mediate between conscious experience and behavior?

Once one views the psychodynamic approach in this context it is entirely possible for both the cognitive behavioral and biological approaches to be drawn upon in a psychodynamic approach to nosology insofar as the psychodynamic clinician must give beliefs their due, and keep in mind that powerful genetic factors may strongly predispose to one mental health disorder or another. Freud early on described the complementary series in which at one end neurosis was mainly determined by heredity and on the other end mainly by environment. Most disorders, falling on the continuum in between, result from an interaction of both factors. The major outcome of depression research conforms to this series, starting with Bowlby's observations (Bowlby, 1986). Two main factors have been identified: (1) frequency of familial depression assumed to be gene related and (2) an experience of loss or failure, an adventitious environmental cause. The psychodynamic clinician, however, is forced to view these factors as contributory to the formation of unconscious desires, needs and interpersonal expectations that are causes not accounted for by the content of beliefs or the existence of hereditary factors alone. From a theoretical standpoint the psychodynamic approach stands or falls on the existence of such unconscious factors and the way they affect the nature of mental health disorders. At the same time, the psychodynamic approach can lay claim to being more comprehensive than either of the other approaches insofar as it incorporates the full panoply of psychological factors as well as brain processes. This comprehensiveness has been explicitly acknowledged by Kandel, a Nobel Laureate in physiology, who noted that psychoanalysis was the only comprehensive theory available to psychiatry (Kandel, 1999).

THE IRRATIONAL, THE PEREMPTORY, AND THE UNBIDDEN

Relevant to the psychodynamic approach are several characteristics of the behavior of all psychiatric patients that have seldom been noted outside the psychoanalytic literature and yet decisively distinguish these disorders from what we would consider to be normal or healthy behavior. A consideration of these characteristics leads into a more thorough examination of the psychodynamic approach and what it specifically has to offer other approaches, both diagnostically and as a mode of treatment. Thereafter, we are in a position to address the psychological and neuroscience evidence supporting the existence of the assumed unconscious factors and the way in which they operate to cause mental disorder. Let us start with a spider phobia as an instance of a mental health disorder. The description to be offered can be applied to any symptom or for that matter to any personality disorder. First, the symptom is irrational by common sense standards. The extent of the fear and the resultant avoidant behavior is inconsistent with the actual danger posed by spiders. Phobic patients are usually painfully embarrassed by this realization. Second, despite this realization the fear is obligatory, not under conscious control, and peremptory in the important sense that its dictates must be obeyed—the spider must be avoided, or great anxiety is experienced. Third, the appearance of the symptom is not the result of a conscious, voluntary decision to avoid spiders, but appears unbidden and unwanted.

To generalize from phobias to any mental health disorder, it can be said that such disorders are distinguishable from more or less normal behavior because they are irrational, peremptory, and unbidden. This applies to personality disorders as well as Axis I-type symptoms like phobias, if we view personality disorders as the outcome of gradual changes occurring over relatively long stretches of time in which what is irrational, peremptory, and unbidden become "second nature," or the customary way the person deals with the world that psychodynamic clinicians refer to as "ego syntonic." The borderline patient alternates between outrageous demands and suicidal threats; both are irrational and peremptory, as the patient attempts to either ignore their origin or to rationalize them, when in fact these actions are intrinsically unbidden and not under conscious control.

There is, however, one important and instructive exception—dreams. We know that everyone dreams nightly whether the dreams are remembered or not. They are considered to be a normal phenomenon despite their notorious irrationality, their peremptory appearance several times a night, and are entirely unbidden insofar as we cannot ordinarily control the when and how of their appearance. It is also instructive to note that dreaming can result in extremely pathological behavior when the normal inhibition of motor expression is absent. Individuals have attacked bedmates and others as they irrationally, peremptorily, and beyond waking control have enacted their dreams (Schenck & Mahowald, 2002). One can say that what saves dreams from being considered a mental disorder is the normal presence of motor inhibition, a factor of central importance that is an instance of a much larger category of inhibitory behaviors to be described later.

But insofar as dreams share the three features with mental health symptoms (being irrational, peremptory, and unbidden), and furthermore, are a normal occurrence, we see that there is a level of mental organization undoubtedly instantiated in the brain that is present in all of us all of the time, and can eventuate in overt behavioral disturbance when this level of psychophysiological organization is released from inhibition. One can also strike a comparison with physical diseases. Harmful bacteria and viruses are continuously present in our bodies, but are kept from producing overt symptoms by the strength of our immunological system and its capacity to generate antibodies that serve the same purpose as motor inhibition in dreams, to keep otherwise harmful processes in check.

In short, this brief excursion into dreaming serves to illustrate the two important presuppositions of psychodynamic theory: (1) the critical role of unconscious psychological factors and (2) the irrational, peremptory, and unbidden manner in which they can affect consciousness and action. The first factor is more specifically referred to as the dynamic unconscious, to differentiate it from the cognitive unconscious, which deals with relatively rational ideas generally under conscious control and retrieved voluntarily. In psychodynamic theory, the cognitive unconscious is referred to as the preconscious. The second factor Freud called the primary process. It operates on the basis of different hypothesized principles of thought, feeling, and action. To those who practice on the basis of these two presuppositions, they appear to be both necessary and useful. However, they are not in and of themselves coercive to those who believe otherwise, as many do who adhere to cognitive behavioral or biological frames of references. To be coercive each presupposition must be supported by evidence independent of its use in the clinical situation.

Once psychopathology is viewed in the manner just described, another implication emerges. Psychopathology is best conceived not in terms of hard and fast categories (e.g., depression, anxiety, etc), but as a continuum in which the diagnosis would incorporate degrees of the irrational, peremptory, and unbidden. On one extreme we would identify psychotic symptoms of hallucination and delusion; on the other, mental health diagnoses would merge into transient and reversible experiences of depression, anxiety, or obsessions that never become fully irrational, peremptory, or unbidden. It is well established, for example, that anxiety states can be remarkably acute, but quickly pass. It is well known clinically that symptoms wax and wane for no apparent reason. The particular content of the disorder, whether it was comprised of depressive moods, anxiety states, obsessions or compulsive preoccupations, hallucinations and delusions, would be ascertained mainly from the content of self-report and observable behavior and would continue to comprise the descriptive dimension of a mental health disorder. But the extent of the pathological nature of the condition described would depend on the extent to which it is irrational, peremptory, and unbidden. These qualities would point to the causative presence of powerful unconscious dynamic forces that have to some significant extent escaped inhibitory control and are affecting thought, feeling, and action in grossly irrational ways. Such patterns can be acute and appear as symptoms, or can settle into life-long character patterns that are then identified as personality disorders. The position taken here is that it is not necessarily the content of the disorder that renders it pathological, but its behavioral and experiential form. In delusions and hallucinations, for example, the very same content may meet the three criteria or not with significantly different outcomes. An instructive illustration occurs in the biographical film, *A Beautiful Mind* (Howard, 2001), in which the paranoid hero after drug treatment still experiences his delusions and hallucinations but no longer feels impelled to act on them. They have lost their peremptory character and thus they can be contained and ignored. A qualitative improvement in inhibition has occurred, almost as if a dream, previously pathologically enacted, is now safely inhibited from motor expression. How this change occurs and what role the drug, at that time Thorazine, played in this change could well be a focus of research, rather than largely being ignored once the psychotic symptoms are no longer worrisome.

However, the requirements of treatment in these respects are quite different from the requirements of diagnosis. In treatment we are concerned not only with the degree to which the content is irrational, peremptory, and unbidden, but with the highly specific life experiences that have contributed to making it so. From a psychodynamic standpoint, to modify the formal properties of the disorder identified in the diagnosis, the specific sources in the dynamic unconscious must be identified and reenacted in the transference relationship with the clinician. It is mainly through the transference enactment that the irrational, peremptory, and unbidden nature of the psychopathology can be fully experienced, and the step taken to make it less so. As with the hero in *A Beautiful Mind*, the patient may continue to feel tendencies to act as before, and be aware of these proclivities, but now the need to act is under control and much unhappiness can be avoided. At the same time, the illustration from *A Beautiful Mind* suggests that similar effects can be achieved through medication, thus opening up a useful avenue of clinical and basic research, only possible if one conceives of mental disorder in the manner described.

Finally, this brings us to a closer consideration of the role of inhibition, taken in its most generic sense, as some process or act keeping something from happening that would otherwise happen. Perhaps the most basic and primitive instance of a successful inhibition is what ordinarily happens in rapid eye movement sleep when dreaming is in progress. We do not act out our dreams because of a built in motor inhibition. Psychodynamic theory posits that degrees and types of inhibition are central to our understanding of how the mind works. It should also be mentioned that a fundamental principle of neural functioning is the presence of inhibition as the necessary counterpart of excitation. The nervous system could not function without inhibitory as well as excitatory processes. What makes mental health symptoms so troublesome is the failure of inhibition at some level that accounts for the peremptory nature of the disorder. The compulsive cannot not wash his hands. And since it doesn't matter if the hands are absolutely clean, since very likely they have just been washed, the act is irrational. And finally the act is forced upon the compulsive who would prefer not to do it, thus unbidden.

The role of inhibition, amply evidenced throughout the nervous system, is a major and essential factor in psychodynamic theory, where it is referred to as a defense. Defenses serve to moderate the influences of those psychological processes that would result in irrational, peremptory, and unbidden actions, that is, the appearance of mental and emotional symptoms, or the slower influence of the same factors that would result in gradual and persistent character changes. The point that needs emphasis is that psychological defenses are essentially in the same category as neural inhibitions and the motor block (another instance of neural inhibition) active in rapid eye movement sleep. Defenses are thus biologically as well as psychologically based. A relevant instance might be drawn from a recently published study by Shevrin, Ghannam, and Libet (2002) dealing with repression based on Libet's discovery that it takes an average of 500 msec of neural recruitment before a stimulus enters consciousness (Libet, Alberts, Wright & Feinstein, 1967). The actual range among the individuals tested was 200 to 750 msec. It was hypothesized that this spread would be positively correlated with the tendency to repress as determined by a battery of psychological tests, including a reasonably objective paper and pencil test (Caine & Hawkins, 1963). The hypothesis was supported. The result was interpreted to mean that the neurophysiological tendency to take longer to become conscious of a stimulus was a necessary condition for developing repression as a defense. Moreover, during that time interval between stimulus registration and awareness, much could happen to the still unconscious processing of the stimulus. This effect is related in turn to the growing literature based on subliminal stimulus exposures, in which the stimulus remains unconscious yet has determinable effects on consciousness and action unbeknownst to the person (Bernat, Shevrin, & Snodgrass, 2001; Shevrin, 1973, 1990, 2000, 2001; Shevrin & Fritzler, 1968; Shevrin, Smith, & Fritzler, 1971; Snodgrass, Bernat, & Shevrin, 2004; Snodgrass & Shevrin, 2005).

The picture that emerges can best be summarized as follows. In order to develop the foundation for a comprehensive conceptual frame of reference for mental health nosology, it is essential to integrate the cognitive behavioral emphasis on beliefs and other cognitive factors, the biological emphasis on neurophysiological factors such as neurotransmitters as well as recent evidence of interactive neuronal systems, within a psychodynamic frame of reference, emphasizing the importance of unconscious processes that can produce the hallmark indicators of mental and emotional disturbance—the irrational, peremptory, and unbidden—unless defended against or inhibited. Although this integration is certainly conceptually possible, it is clearly essential that evidence needs to be adduced to support the two key assumptions: (1) the existence of unconscious processes, and in particular dynamic unconscious processes and (2) the irrational, peremptory, and unbidden way that these processes work unless successfully defended against. It is relevant in this regard, that two cognitive behaviorists, Power and Brewer (1991), have attempted a comparable conceptual integration from a cognitive behaviorist perspective, arguing mainly on clinical grounds that the notions of an unconscious and defenses must be incorporated into cognitive behavioral treatment. Power and Brewer, however, lean toward a cognitive preconscious, non-dynamic view of unconscious factors, and do not appear to include the different way in which dynamic unconscious processes affect consciousness and behavior. But they have taken an important step in accommodating into their cognitive behavioral approach concepts also amenable to a psychodynamic view. The time may be ripe for the kind of integration here advocated if a sound theoretical framework for mental health diagnosis is to be devised. But what is the current evidential base for the two assumptions stressed as central in the account thus far developed?

THE CURRENT STATUS OF COGNITIVE AND NEUROSCIENCE EVIDENCE FOR UNCONSCIOUS MENTAL PROCESSES AND THE NATURE OF THEIR INFLUENCE ON CONSCIOUSNESS AND BEHAVIOR

A good place to start in our consideration of the cognitive and neuroscience evidence is with dreaming, which we have offered as a paradoxically normal condition that appears to have the characteristics of overt mental disorder, kept from becoming so by successful inhibition. The reader is referred to a recent publication in which the rich psychological, neurophysiological, and neuroanatomical literature on dreams is presented by its key contributors (Pace-Schott, Solms, & Blagrove, 2003). For my present purposes, I only draw upon the well established neurophysiological differences between rapid eye movement (REM) and non-rapid eye movement (NREM) sleep. Awakenings from these two quite different psychophysiological states result in a significantly greater incidence of dream reports in REM than NREM sleep, and generally speaking with more bizarre dream reports in REM than in NREM sleep. In studies of these differences no attention has been given to the role that unconscious processes might be playing in accounting for the differences. It occurred to Shevrin and Fisher, both pioneering investigators of subliminal perception and memory to be dealt with more extensively later, that it would be instructive to combine subliminal stimuli presented in the pre-sleep waking state with the effects that these stimuli might have on REM and NREM sleep (Shevrin & Fisher, 1967). The subliminal stimulus could serve as a tracer or tag revealing the nature of the unconscious processes involved in the two different states of sleep. In this way something might be learned about the differential bizarreness obtained in the REM state, a consideration with theoretical implications beyond dreaming itself.

A special subliminal stimulus had previously been devised that made it possible to track different levels of linguistic processing that were related to what Freud as early as his monograph *On Aphasia* had identified as critical to our understanding of how unconscious processes operate on language (Freud, 1891). I refer to the semantic and phonemic levels. The special stimulus was a picture of a pen pointed at knee making up the rebus representation of the word "penny." Quite easily and reliably three levels could be traced in various responses after the "penny" rebus had been flashed subliminally: The usual semantic level related to the words "pen" and "knee," the clang level in which the "pen" and "knee" sounds could be traced in words like "pennant" or "neither," and finally the rebus word itself "penny" and its associates like "nickel," "dime," etc. Shevrin and Fisher (1967) hypothesized that the clang and rebus levels would be more prominent following REM awakenings, and the semantic level more prominent after NREM awakenings. Associations based on concrete phonemic connections should produce seemingly irrational consequences. For example, if one associated to the picture of the knee a memory in which one had had two equally bad choices, one would be hard pressed to see a rational, semantic connection to the knee unless one knew that an intermediate associate was "neither," a clang associate of knee. Similarly Shevrin and Fisher (1967) predicted that if more bizarre, irrational levels of unconscious processing were involved in REM sleep, the clang and rebus levels would emerge following REM awakenings. The results supported both hypotheses: More clang and rebus associates after REM and more semantic, rational associates after NREM. The same subliminal stimulus had qualitatively different effects depending on responses obtained in two different psychophysiological states. The results also implied that two different levels of unconscious processing were operative, one rational and the other seemingly irrational. The former might be considered closer to the cognitive preconscious and the latter to the dynamic unconscious. From a psychiatric standpoint, it should be noted that the non-semantic, phonemic use of language is overtly present in manic states and in schizophrenic thought disorder. We would add that it is also found in normally occurring REM states where this use of language enters into the unconscious contribution to the bizarre and irrational nature of the dream experience. The evidence from this study strongly supports the view that unconscious processes, once inhibitions (defenses) weaken, cause conscious experience and actions to become irrational. The bizarre content of REM dreams is saved from becoming gross overt psychopathology by being inhibited at a motor level.

In this regard it is intriguing to cite observations reported by Schenck and Mahowald (2002) of patients suffering from RBD (Rapid Eye Movement Behavior Disorder) a condition in which neurodegenerative disease has damaged the neurological basis for muscle atonia. Often these patients are older men described by their spouses as mild-mannered and seldom given to overt expressions of anger. But with the onset of REM sleep they begin to pummel their wives violently. Remarkably, their dream reports are of protecting their wives from an assault. It is as if the loss of inhibition provided by the muscle atonia allows the inhibited (defended against) anger to erupt, while the dream simultaneously turns the enacted anger into its opposite, quite irrationally given the actual circumstances, yet in keeping with the patients' waking personality. Parenthetically, it might also be observed that this evidence supports Freud's position that disguise and defense are operative in the construction of the dreams themselves, an important instance of the role of inhibitions and defenses in dream formation.

The evidence from the Shevrin and Fisher study supports the two assumptions described previously—that unconscious processes exist and that they are characterized by qualitatively different forms of thought, taken in the broadest sense.

The Shevrin and Fisher study was published in 1967, some ten years after the first subliminal dream studies were published by Fisher (1956, 1957; Shevrin, 2003a). These first publications began what has since become a veritable avalanche of subliminal investigations in such diverse fields as perception, memory, social attitudes, prejudice and neuroscience investigations of unconscious fear and implicit memory (see Greenwald & Banaji, 1995; Snodgrass, Bernat, & Shevrin, 2004; Snodgrass & Shevrin, 2005). This widespread interest in investigating unconscious processes is perhaps one of the most remarkable developments in psychology currently under way. It is tantamount to a paradigm shift away from the previous behaviorist view according to which mental processes as such, whether conscious or unconscious, had no scientific standing. The behaviorist position has almost completely been replaced with a cognitive science view that is fully concerned with mental processes and their unconscious as well conscious character, at least as concerns perception and memory.

Of more than historic interest is the fact that the empirical investigation of unconscious processes was introduced to contemporary psychology by a number of psychoanalytic investigators beginning in the fifties of the last century at a time when academic psychology had not yet freed itself from its behaviorist manacles. Over the subsequent half century the basic findings of these psychodynamic researchers, that perception as well as memory formation could occur without consciousness, have been amply replicated and validated by countless cognitive experiments. Although important debates continue concerning the nature of unconscious processes, there is now widespread acceptance within psychology, and in neuroscience, that unconscious processes exist and play an important role in the workings of the mind and brain. This significant development is of great importance to any theory of mental health nosology. It means that the beliefs studied by cognitive behaviorists and the neurotransmitter levels studied by biological psychiatrists, insofar as they must rely on perceptions and memories reported by their patients (e.g., in the form of accounts of moods and their changes), must now take into consideration that these perceptions and memories are influenced by unconscious processes, meaning that irrational connections and defensive requirements may modify the content and the reliability of these accounts. At the same time, these effects might provide significant signposts to the diagnostician as to what is happening unconsciously.

Any theory that would be a useful basis for a mental and emotional diagnostic system must at the very least draw upon the latest developments in the sciences contributing to the understanding of the basic processes involved in mental and emotional disorders. This is plainly the case for the biological frame of reference. Psychiatrists draw upon not only the most recent clinical trials, but also upon bench research on neurotransmitters and the nature of their chemical and neurophysiological properties. Only in this way can a secure theoretical foundation be assured while also opening the door to further advances based on new findings. Yet it is notable that advances in cognitive psychology and cognitive neuroscience have not as readily been drawn upon in a similar manner. There is no call for incorporating findings on unconscious perception and implicit memory into mental health nosology. These advances, however, relate closely to the psychodynamic frame of reference and begin to provide the evidential basis for its relevance to this nosology.

Aside from unconscious aspects of perception and memory, the net has been cast much wider in the search for the effects of unconscious processes. There is, for example, evidence for unconscious affect that directly impinges on the understanding of depressive and manic moods, their origin and persistence (Bernat, Bunce, & Shevrin, 2001; Berridge & Winkeilman, 2003). Unconscious influences have also been identified by social psychologists in the study of attitudes and prejudice (Greenwald & Banaji, 1995). All of these investigations, however, do not directly deal with the dynamic unconscious, or those unconscious processes that exist in some state of inhibition that we have identified as critical to our understanding of mental and emotional disorders.

Evidence for the Dynamic Unconscious

As I turn to reviewing the psychological and neuroscientific evidence for the dynamic unconscious, it is important to keep clearly in mind the purpose for this review. It is to demonstrate that, (1) there is such evidence and (2) the evidence cannot be ignored if we are to have a sound theoretical basis for mental health diagnosis. Perhaps the best way to approach the difficult methodological issues involved in the investigation of the dynamic unconscious is to draw upon the model proposed by Fisher, important parts of which have independently been incorporated into contemporary cognitive views of the unconscious (Fisher, 1956, 1957). Fisher's model starts with the assumption, based largely on subliminal research, that every stimulus initially registers preconsciously, a position that is also taken by most cognitive psychologists. Once registered, the subliminal stimulus can go in three different directions: (1) immediately become conscious, the path for most but not all supraliminal stimuli, (2) remain in the preconscious until attention is directed to it, or (3) be drawn into the dynamic unconscious where it is subject to repression (inhibition) and becomes part of, or influences, conscious processes or actions in not necessarily rational ways. Fisher referred to these influences as "indirect" to distinguish them from the "direct" path followed by most supraliminal stimuli. In point of fact, these "indirect" influences would be considered by cognitive psychologists to be forms of "implicit" memory by which they would mean that these influences are not identified by the person as "explicitly" deriving from the memory left by the subliminal stimulus.

How and why a memory left by the unconscious perception of a subliminal stimulus is not consciously identified as such poses some interesting questions that do not concern us, except for one consideration. The "indirect" or "implicit" character of the influence on consciousness may reflect the irrational associations by which these influences act upon consciousness and are thus more difficult to relate to its source. Fisher's research on using conscious images as ways to detect the effects of subliminal stimuli has shown that the kind of irrational associations found in the Shevrin and Fisher dream study also are evident in these images, suggesting that dream-like thinking can take place in the awake state. These findings were further supported by a number of studies by Shevrin and colleagues showing that clang and rebus effects appear in free associations collected after the penny and other rebuses had been presented subliminally in the fully awake state (Shevrin, 1973). Again it must be noted that, as in dreams, the images and free associations while revealing irrational associations do not rise to the level of mental symptoms because they are successfully defended against enactment or persistence. Yet it should be noted further that the psychodynamic clinician may learn a good deal of what might be going on unconsciously from these markers. In place of the experimental subliminal stimulus the clinician would take note, for example, of how the patient responds to the clinician's queries and challenges.

The Fisher (1956,1957), Shevrin and Fisher (1967), and Shevrin (1973) studies tell us something about the way subliminal stimuli are processed unconsciously and how they influence consciousness, but in and of themselves they do not distinguish independently between the preconscious and the dynamic unconscious. Shevrin and colleagues (1992, 1996) have conducted a study in which for the first time an effort was made to integrate three different methods essential to investigating the dynamic unconscious in a clinically relevant and objective way: (1) psychodynamically based, unstructured, diagnostic interviews and projective tests, (2) subliminal and supraliminal stimulus presentations, and (3) brain responses in the form of event-related potentials. From a methodological standpoint, it was intended that each method would provide its own particular strength, while countering the limitations of the other two methods. Thus the highly subjective, inferential, clinical method would be moderated by the more objective, subliminal and brain response methods, while contributing the full richness of psychological content that only the psychodynamic clinical method can provide. At the same time the psychological subliminal method would be counterbalanced by the totally non-psychological event-related potential method, as well as providing markers for the underlying brain processes. Results would emerge from a convergence of these methods. For a complete description of the methodology the reader is referred to two publications (Shevrin, et al. 1992;

Shevrin, Bond, Brakel, Hertel, & Williams, 1996). For present purposes, only the results are presented and enough of the method to make the results understandable.

Subjects were eleven patients meeting DSM-IV criteria for social phobia. The main dependent variable in the study was words selected from interview and test transcripts by the clinicians on the basis of a consensually arrived at psychodynamic formulation, mainly stressing the nature of the presumed unconscious conflict, and its relationship to the social phobia. The primary findings were that the words selected to capture the unconscious conflict were better classified as belonging together by the brain waves when presented subliminally than when presented supraliminally. Words related to the conscious symptom experience did not show this relationship. Moreover, the same paper and pencil test of repression (Caine & Hawkins, 1963) that had been used in the previously mentioned study on delay to consciousness (Shevrin, Ghannam, & Libet, 2002) correlated significantly with the difference in correct brain wave classification of the unconscious conflict words, subliminally and supraliminally. Subjects more repressive on the test showed a greater difference in favor of better classification subliminally than supraliminally. This was further supported by the finding that when subjects were asked at the end of the study to place all the words in the experiment in as many different categories as they wished, the unconscious conflict words were placed in significantly more categories than the symptom-related words, even though their brain responses had correctly classified the unconscious conflict words as belonging together subliminally.

The main value of the study is to demonstrate that the complex judgments and inferences of psychodynamically-oriented clinicians performing their diagnostic task, based on unstructured interviews and projective tests, can be convergently validated by experimental psychological methods and brain responses. This complements the work of Westen and Shedler (1999), who have shown that such clinical judgments can also be made reliably, as well as correlating with predictable behavioral differences. Beyond that, our results provide independent evidence for the existence of a dynamic, as well as cognitive, unconscious instantiated in the brain that must be taken into account if we are to understand the nature of mental and emotional disorders.

In another study dealing with spider phobics, we have been able to demonstrate operationally the existence of defense-based inhibition operating entirely unconsciously (Shevrin, Brakel, Abelson, & Snodgrass, 2004). In that study we employed a standard method of threshold determination referred to as signal detection. Pictures of spiders were flashed at 1 msec, our standard subliminal speed, to ten spider phobics and six snake phobics. In addition to the spiders, an equal number of blank cards were interspersed. Subjects were asked simply to say whether they saw something or nothing and to give an approximately equal number of each response. From these responses a measure of stimulus detectability is derived (d') that indicates the degree to which the stimulus, in this case the spider, is detected. Overall for both groups d' was not significantly different from zero, indicating that the stimulus was unconscious or at the objective detection threshold. When, however, detectability was correlated with the same measure of repression used in the other studies mentioned, we found a highly negative correlation but only for the spider phobics. In fact, for those spider phobics high in repression their spider detectability was below zero, or chance, indicating that they were responding to the spider stimulus subliminally, but reacted by inhibiting this response. The evidence favors the interpretation, consistent with Fisher's model, that the spider, flashed subliminally at 1 msec, registered preconsciously, but because of its phobic status interacted with the dynamic unconscious and, for those subjects who favored repression as a defense, resulted in an inhibition of detection. The same results were obtained for another personality measure also related to repression, the Marlowe-Crowne inventory (Crowne & Marlowe, 1964).

In this same study, electrophysiological evidence for inhibition was obtained in event-related potentials. At the P200 amplitude component (occurring 200 msec post-stimulus) the greater the difference in favor of the control stimulus over the spider stimulus, the more repressive the spider-phobic subject, strongly suggesting that the spider stimulus was subject to inhibition. Two more recent studies demonstrate that anxiety influences subliminal but not supraliminal processing of the same stimuli (Etkin, et al. 2004; Villa, Bazan, Shevrin, Snodgrass, & Brakel, in press). The Etkin study is of further interest because fearful stimuli were used in an fMRI design.

Related to these studies of phobics is research by Bradley and colleagues (1996) on depression. These investigators found an interesting dissociation between conscious and unconscious sensitivity to depression-related words depending on whether or not overt symptoms of depression were present. People who gave evidence on a self-report questionnaire that they might be subject to depression showed sensitivity to depression-related words only when they were presented subliminally. Overtly depressed people, however, showed both supraliminal and subliminal sensitivity to depression-related words. One might surmise that at some point the overtly depressed people were like the first group marked by only unconscious reactivity to depressive stimuli that remained non-symptomatic until some environmental trigger such as a loss or failure undermined defenses and sent them into an overt depression. Our study on social phobics strongly suggests that what produced inhibition in spider phobics given to repression was related to some defended against conflict that remained unconscious until inhibitory defenses were weakened. A major depressive reaction bears all the hallmarks of a mental disorder previously identified—the depth of despair often bordering on suicide is irrational in the context of the individual's actual life circumstances, it cannot be controlled or contained and is thus peremptory, and it often appears to occur seemingly out of nowhere ("I woke up one morning and everything had turned black.").

Before proceeding to consider evidence for qualitatively different processing going on unconsciously, I briefly summarize the key results favoring the existence of unconscious processes and strongly arguing for the inclusion of the notion of an unconscious in any theory of mental disorder nosology:

- Since the 1950's and with accelerating tempo, many experiments have established the existence of unconscious processes in perception, memory, and affect.

- Other studies have demonstrated that unconscious processes play an important role in dream formation, and in social and simple phobias.

- There is also evidence that defenses are active in the processing of subliminal stimuli of unconscious conflictual significance.

- Brain processes have been found to provide markers for the presence of unconscious processes and more specifically for unconscious conflict.

Overall the evidence argues for the presence and importance of unconscious processes in general and for their relevance to psychopathology. Any diagnostic system to be useful and valid would need to take into account the existence of unconscious processes and the existence of defensive, inhibitory processes. What is not as yet clear is the way in which these influences operate to produce the irrational, peremptory, and unbidden nature of mental and emotional disorders.

A Psychodynamic View of What Causes the Irrational, Peremptory, and Unbidden Nature of Mental Symptoms

Although it is relatively easy to identify behavior as irrational, peremptory and unbidden, it becomes a matter for psychodynamic theory supported by collateral evidence to account convincingly for these characteristics as caused by underlying unconscious processes and failures in inhibition or defense. It should be noted that neither the cognitive/behavioral nor biological frames of reference offer any explanation of these three omnipresent characteristics, although recent neuroimaging studies have begun tentatively to identify certain regions of the frontal cortex as the locus of inhibition, a finding consistent with the psychodynamic frame of reference (Blair, 2001, Damasio, Tranel, & Damasio, 1990, Malloy, Bihrle, & Duffy, 1993, Soloff, et al., 2003). With these considerations in mind, I examine each of the three characteristics in turn.

The Irrational

Ordinarily the irrational is defined by reference to the rational; it is simply the absence of the rational. In the currently prevalent philosophical view the irrational is defined as what is not rational by reason of error or inadequate knowledge. Yet this view does not take into consideration the possibility that there could be some substantive reason why the person might be behaving irrationally. In the case of a spider phobia, we might wonder if the person at one time, usually in childhood, had been very frightened by a spider, and that this fright had persisted. Or a more sophisticated explanation might draw on evolutionary theory and posit that, at one time in the prehistory of homo sapiens, fear of spiders was adaptive and that this has persisted as an atavistic instinctive response like a psychological appendix that can become inflamed but serves no useful function.

Another approach consistent with psychoanalytic theory and in keeping with some recent cognitive views, is to posit that the irrational is not simply the consequence of error or inadequate knowledge, but follows its own rules. In fact, a number of cognitive theorists have argued in favor of a dual process theory of cognition according to which irrational thought has its own underlying principles (Stanovich & West, 2000). An outstanding advocate of this position and a recent Nobel Prize winner in economics, Kahneman (2003), has shown that people do not behave simply as rational decision makers in pursuing their economic well being, nor is their behavior fully accounted for by errors and inadequate knowledge.

Brakel and Shevrin (2003) have pointed out that the first dual process theorist was Freud. As early as his monograph *On Aphasia* (Freud, 1891), he sought to explain aphasic and other language disorders as based on two different aspects of language—words used as referents for objects or concepts (word meaning) and words used as concrete entities based on their sound, appearance, or vocalization (word presentation). Over time, and with increasing clinical experience with neurotic and psychotic patients, he broadened the application of this dual process theory of language so that it entered into his explanation of hysterical conversions, obsessional preoccupations, slips of the tongue, manic and schizophrenic thought disorder, and dreams. What began as a purely linguistic distinction, he eventually broadened into two general principles of mental functioning: the primary and secondary process—in contemporary cognitive terms, a true dual process theory. The dual nature of language use constituted a special but important instance of the more general phenomenon. The Shevrin and Fisher (1967) dream study, as already described, exploited the linguistic dimension of this dual process theory, demonstrating that word presentations, in this instance the sound of the word (i.e., 'ny'), were mainly active in rapid eye movement sleep and contributed to the bizarre (irrational) character of dreaming in that state, while word meanings (i.e., "knee") were mainly active in non-rapid eye movement sleep and contributed to the relative rational character of dreaming in that state. Furthermore, these effects were entirely unconscious. These transformations of language were part of what Freud called the dream work, or the unconscious processes giving rise to the dream, rather than the dream content itself. This point merits further careful consideration because it bears on an important aspect of psychiatric diagnosis—the reliability of self-reports. It is entirely possible for the word "penny" to appear in a dream by way of a secondary process (i.e., related to considerations of money), or in a primary process way (i.e., related to "pen" and "knee" when combined to form the rebus word "penny"). The manifest content alone does not betray its origins. Similarly the belief that "someone is following me" may in fact be true (secondary process), or a delusion (primary process). The differential diagnosis is based on just those characteristics I have been emphasizing—the irrational, peremptory, and unbidden. The delusion does not yield to reason. The main point to underscore with respect to the irrational is that the content is produced by a different and unconscious mental process in which the rational has already been compromised. In the dream study, word meanings have been supplanted by word presentations in producing rapid eye movement dreams. It is this difference in the underlying process that produces the overt irrationality and why the irrational is an indicator of psychopathology. It is not the content in and of itself. At the same time it should be kept in mind that the dream itself is not a form of psychopathology, although it could become so when inhibition fails. By the same token, dreams tell us that the potential for psychopathology is present in all of us.

But there is still another consideration of prime importance. What role does the unconscious play in primary and secondary process mentation? It has been our contention that the unconscious plays a key role. It is in what the patient cannot report that the pathological causes reside. Another question also requires a response. If the primary and secondary process are general principles of mental life as Freud contended, then their operation should not be restricted to language. Parenthetically, this is also the position of most cognitive dual process theorists. Yet language pathology is not the only form mental symptoms assume, although they are clearly prominent in obsessive, manic, and schizophrenic disorders.

Brakel (2004) and Brakel and colleagues (2000, 2002, 2005) have addressed the role of the unconscious, and the generality of the primary and secondary process in a series of studies using geometric figures, rather than relying on the mediation of language as in the rebus studies. The theoretical basis for generalizing beyond language can, however, be illustrated from the rebus studies. One can look at the word presentation as a feature unrelated to word meaning; it is of a different order. The phoneme "ny" has no bearing on the meaning of "knee." A very different word presentation can carry the same meaning as, for example, "genou" in French. Word meaning depends on a relationship of reference that can arbitrarily be assigned to any combination of sounds. On the other hand, features are concrete and perceptual in nature and do not depend on a relationship of reference. This is at the core of the qualitative difference between the primary and secondary process.

In three studies dealing with different implications drawn from Freud's theory of primary and secondary process, Brakel and colleagues (2000, 2002, 2005) asked subjects to make a similarity judgment between a master figure and two choices. One choice is based on seeing a similarity of relationships among the features even though the individual features are different from the master figure. The other choice is based on seeing a similarity of individual features even though the relationship among the features is entirely different from the master figure. In effect, the relational judgment is comparable to word meaning insofar as relationships are involved that are not dependent on particular features. The feature-based judgment is comparable to the word presentation insofar as it is entirely based on individual features and not the relationships among them. This distinction between feature and relationship has also been investigated in the cognitive literature on similarity judgments where they are referred to as attributional (based on features or attributes) and relational (based on relationships) similarity judgments (Medin & Heit, 1999).

We derived three hypotheses from Freud's dual process theory that attributional similarity judgments should be more frequent, (1) in very young children (Brakel, Kleinsorge, Snodgrass, & Shevrin, 2000), (2) when performed subliminally (Brakel, Shevrin, & Villa, 2002), and (3) when people are under stress or anxious (Brakel & Shevrin, 2005). All three hypotheses were supported. Taken together the verbal rebus studies and the non-verbal attributional/ relational studies demonstrate that the primary process is a general principle of mental organization. The alternative to the rational is not the irrational resulting from error and inadequate information, but another form of thought that Brakel has suggested should be called arational (Brakel, 2002). It follows from this conclusion that the irrational character of mental and emotional disorder is intrinsic to the disorder and has underlying unconscious mental causes. In a mental or emotional disorder something happens to the way in which the world and the self are perceived, remembered, thought about, felt, and acted upon that have their origins in arational unconscious processes.

The Peremptory

There is nothing in this account of the irrational that would explain the peremptory character of mental disorders, why the pathological act cannot be controlled but must be performed. We can begin our inquiry with some recent neuroscience findings that resonate with other aspects of the psychodynamic frame of reference than those we have thus far identified. These findings have their origin in the discovery that there is a place in the brain which, when activated by electrical stimulation or certain drugs, causes the affected animal, usually a rat, to keep on wanting that activation to continue. When the animal is in control of delivering the activation, it does so without pause until it can no longer perform the act. The apparent need to perform the act is peremptory. The rat could not not do it. At first it was thought that this was a pleasure center associated with some need state—hunger, thirst, or sex. But when the rat was made hungry, it not only responded to food in this state of activation, but it would respond to water or a mate indiscriminately. Parenthetically, one could observe that it was not behaving rationally because it was not thirsty or sexually aroused, but hungry. It was also observed that when this part of the brain was activated, the rat would immediately engage in exploratory behavior. Furthermore, when this region of the brain was ablated the result was an inert, inactive animal which would not seek food when hungry, or water when thirsty, or a mate when sexually aroused. But if the means of satisfaction were placed right before it so that it needn't engage in any activity, it would avidly satisfy its needs.

Clearly, this particular part of the brain had more to do with motivation and action than it did with pleasure or specific need gratification. A leading affective neuroscientist, Panksepp, has identified this part of the brain as what he called a SEEKING system (Panksepp, 1998). Another neuroscientist, Berridge, has called it an unconscious "wanting" system that is behaviorally and neuroanatomically separate from "liking" (Berridge, 1996). Intriguingly "wanting" need not result in obtaining what one "likes.' Pleasure and desire are anatomically and functionally distinguishable.

This brain system is activated by dopamine (DA), a neurotransmitter found in various parts of the brain. Of particular relevance to our subject is its presence in the ventral tegmental area (VTA) that innervates the nucleus accumbens septi (NAS), usually referred to as the meso-accumbens DA system. It is this NAS DA system that is involved in SEEKING and in "wanting." Perhaps the most impressive demonstrations of how this system works has been reported by Berridge (1996) with rats. Rats were conditioned beforehand to press a lever to obtain a sugar pellet; the conditioned stimulus was either a light or a buzzer. In the next phase of the experiment, only the conditioned cue, the light or sound, is presented for 30 seconds to see how hard the rat now works to receive its reward. The rat in this phase of the experiment does not receive any reward. The normal expectation is that the rat gradually reduces its lever pressing once it learns that the light or buzzer is no longer followed by a reward. But if the NAS DA circuits are directly activated by injected amphetamine, the rat's behavior changes dramatically. It shows very little tendency to diminish its lever pressing in the absence of reward, but every time the conditioned stimulus appears, the animal goes into a frenzy of lever pushing that ceases immediately once the conditioned stimulus disappears. As Berridge points out, this is irrational behavior. No reward is forthcoming, yet the rat treats the conditioned stimulus each time it appears as if it is. In Panksepp's view this is delusional (Panksepp, 1999).

Berridge demonstrates that the NAS DA activated rat has not lost its liking for sugar. Sugar placed in its mouth elicits the appropriate facial and behavioral response. When the DA circuits are not activated, it acts normally, diminishing its lever pressing in the absence of reward. Berridge calls this irrational behavior, 'wanting' in single quotes to distinguish it from rational wanting. He also allows for the possibility that 'wanting' can be activated unconsciously and cites subliminal research in this regard (Berridge & Winkielman, 2003). According to Berridge what happens as a result of the NAS DA activation is a *sensitization* of these NAS DA circuits so that the conditioned cue acquires intense *incentive salience*. An incentive is a call to action, and is thus similar to Panksepp's emphasis on "energized expectation" or anticipatory action as a key element in the SEEKING system. Note that the NAS DA activated rat doesn't simply sit by and wait for the sugar reward to appear. It energetically goes after the light on the lever as if it were the sugar pellet.

The amphetamine activated animal's behavior had become peremptory, uncontrollable, and one could add as indeed Berridge observed, irrational. Berridge and Robinson (1995) have also developed a theory to explain addiction by positing that addiction is a pathology of 'wanting' and not of pleasure seeking as often maintained. In fact, they adduce evidence that drug 'wanting' can occur in addictive people in the absence of any experienced 'liking.' Panksepp takes the relationship between activated DA circuits and irrational behavior much further, suggesting that schizophrenic thought disorder may be the outcome of pathologically intense NAS DA circuit activation. As evidence, he points out that most anti-psychotic medication reduces NAS DA activity. He also cites evidence that the usual expected REM dream rebound effect after REM dream deprivation can be moderated by NAS DA circuit activation between sleep periods, suggesting the build up of an unexpended intense anticipatory impetus. For him the key defining aspect of the SEEKING system is to an extent dissipated by intervening activation of the SEEKING system.

We thus have an animal model for peremptory and irrational behavior as well as human models for addiction and schizophrenia that are also instantiated in the brain. The relationship of these neuroscience models to a psychodynamic frame of reference are not difficult to identify. Berridge's 'wanting' and Panksepp's intense anticipatory state parallel the psychodynamic concepts of drives and wishes (see Shevrin, 2003b). Furthermore these drives or wishes under certain circumstances can become peremptory and result in arational influences on action. Just as rats keep on pressing the lever in the absence of actual reward, compulsives keeps on washing their hands despite the absence of any payoff. We do know that if compulsives or phobics are kept from responding with their pathological actions that they become intensely uncomfortable. It might be interesting to see what would happen to the NAS DA activated rat if it were kept from performing its peremptory lever pressing. We might predict that it would become extremely stressed.

What we learn from Berridge and Panksepp is that a motivational pressure of some kind is involved in activation of the NAS DA. Panksepp reported that when this system is ablated the animal becomes inert, still having needs but with no urgency to act to gratify them. Underlying the peremptory aspect of psychopathological behavior are powerful motivations that cannot be directly discerned because they influence these behaviors in arational ways, working unconsciously, much as Berridge's unconscious 'wanting.' If we now take a closer look at the NAS DA activated rat, we can see that it continues to respond to a feature (one isolated part) of the conditioning relationship rather to the relationship between the conditioned and unconditioned stimulus. It continues to act almost as if the light or buzzer is the reward because it is unable any longer to keep the conditioning relationship in mind. Its behavior is dominated by features rather than by relationships and is thus primary process and arational. Our psychodynamic model generalizes what Berridge has applied to drug addicts and Panksepp to schizophrenics to all forms of psychopathology. The differences reside in the particular content of the disorder, not in the underlying principles, much as the germ theory of disease is based on the principle that microorganisms cause disease, while any specific disease is caused by a particular microorganism.

The Unbidden

The arational has to do with the unconscious causal nexus involved in creating a mental disorder. The peremptory has to do with the absolute necessity to enact or express the disorder because of a powerful motivational impetus. The unbidden, on the other hand, has to do with the involuntary nature of the disorder as seen from the vantage point of the patient's conscious wishes or desires. There is thus a conflict between what the patient consciously wishes to do and what these powerful arationally expressed motivations insist the patient do. The conflict is between two sets of motivations, one conscious, the other unconscious, the one rational, the other arational. However, it is the unconscious impetus that is considerably less controllable and more powerful than the conscious motivation. More accurately from a psychodynamic standpoint, some compromise eventuates between drive strength and defenses such that complete enactment is avoided along with its consequences. From this standpoint the symptom itself may be such a compromise keeping the person from committing less desirable actions. On the basis of the revealing research of Panksepp and Berridge it would seem that unconscious 'wanting' has an insistence and persistence that cannot readily yield to conscious, rational control. Hyperactivation of the NAS DA system, that we might suppose is involved in all mental disorders and in particular in schizophrenia, renders unconscious 'wanting' both unbidden and undeniable.

Within the psychodynamic frame of reference the counterpart of hyperactivation of the NAS DA system is an intensification of drive strength and a comparable weakening of defenses. As I have spelled out elsewhere there is a striking parallel between both Panksepp's SEEKING system and Berridge's unconscious 'wanting' and Freud's concept of drives (Shevrin, 2003b). Panksepp identifies four dimensions of the SEEKING system: (1) regulatory imbalances, (2) the object through which regulatory balance is restored, (3) consummatory behavior, and (4) actual seeking activity accompanied by indications of energizing expectation. Although the terms of Freud's definition of drive differ, their referents are similar: (1) somatic source *(regulatory imbalance)*, (2) object *(same)*, (3) aim *(consummatory behavior)*, and (4) motor action *(seeking activity)*. It is the fourth dimension that defines the uniqueness of the SEEKING system for Panksepp and the unique nature of the drive for Freud. It is the impetus toward action, the motor factor or galvanizing expectancy, that makes the demand on the mind for work, as Freud put it in "Instincts and Their Vicissitudes" (1915), and motivates seeking as the means through which to meet the organism's vital needs. In health these four dimensions of drive, or SEEKING, or 'wanting,' work harmoniously together; in mental disturbance they become irrational (arational), peremptory, and unbidden causing actions that defeat the person's efforts to achieve satisfaction.

SUMMARY AND CONCLUSIONS

It is clear that efforts over the last 50 years to develop a purely descriptive nosology of mental illness have encountered increasing difficulty that has necessitated several unsuccessful revisions with yet another revision currently in progress. Lurking behind this descriptive effort are three conceptual frames of reference: cognitive behavioral, biological, and psychodynamic. In some respects these frames of reference are incompatible; in other ways they are complementary. There is a need for a comprehensive conceptual frame of reference. The psychodynamic frame of reference is offered as the only approach capable of the comprehensiveness needed to incorporate the cognitive/behavioral and biological frames of reference. This approach would require that the nosology of mental illness shift from a category and content base, resulting in non-explanatory descriptions, to a process and formal property base, making possible an explanatory account.

Three formal properties are offered as together defining a mental disorder and providing the springboard for an explanatory account: the irrational, peremptory, and unbidden. It is further argued that the mental processes characterized by these properties are always present, but are kept in some state of inhibition so that they do not give rise to symptomatic enactments. Dreams are offered as a normal instance that, but for motor inhibition, would result in overt disturbed enactments. This explanation is likened to the microorganism theory of disease in which disease is explained as the result of microorganisms, usually present in the body, at some point overcoming the body's natural defenses and causing illness.

It is shown how each of these properties is related to underlying causative unconscious processes characterized by a fundamentally different form of mentation. Cognitive experimental and neuroscience evidence is cited supporting this theoretical account of mental disorders.

REFERENCES

Bernat, E., Bunce, S., & Shevrin, H. (2001). Event-related brain potentials differentiate positive and negative mood adjectives during both supraliminal and subliminal visual processing. *International Journal of Psychophysiology, 42,* 11-34.

Bernat, E., Shevrin H., & Snodgrass, M. (2001). Subliminal visual oddball stimuli evoke a P300 component. *Journal of Clinical Neurophysiology, 112,* 159-171.

Berridge, K. C. (1996). Food reward: Brain substrates of wanting and liking. *Neuroscience and Biobehavioral Review, 20,* 1-25.

Berridge, K. C., & Robinson, T. (1995). The mind of the addictive brain: Neural sensitization of wanting versus liking. *Current Directions in Psychological Science, 4,* 71-76.

Berridge, K. C., & Winkeilman, P. (2003). What is an unconscious emotion? The case for unconscious "liking." *Cognition and Emotion, 17,* 181-211.

Blair, R. J. (2001). Neurocognitive models of aggression, the antisocial personality disorders and psychopathy. *Journal of Neurology, Neurosurgery, and Psychiatry, 71,* 727-731.

Blatt, S. J., & Levy, K. N. (1998). A psychodynamic approach to the diagnosis of psychopathology. In J. W. Barron (Ed.), *Making diagnosis meaningful* (pp. 73-109). Washington DC: American Psychological Association Press.

Bowlby, J. (1986). *Loss: Sadness and depression.* New York: Basic Books.

Bradley, B. P., Mogg, I., & Millar, N. (1996). Implicit memory bias in clinical and non-clinical depression. *Behavior Research and Therapy, 34,* 865-879.

Brakel L. A. W. (2002). Phantasy and wish: A proper function account for human arational primary process mediated mentation. *The Australasian Journal of Philosophy, 80,* 1-16.

Brakel, L. A. W. (2004). The psychoanalytic assumption of the primary process: Extra-psychoanalytic evidence and findings. *Journal of the American Psychoanalytic Association, 52,* 1131-1161.

Brakel, L. A. W., Kleinsorge, S., Snodgrass, M., & Shevrin, H. (2000). The primary process and the unconscious: Experimental evidence supporting two psychoanalytic presuppositions. *International Journal of Psychoanalysis, 81,* 553-569.

Brakel, L. A. W., & Shevrin, H. (2003). Freud's dual process theory and the place of the arational. *Behavioral and Brain Science, 26,* 527-534.

Brakel, L. A. W., & Shevrin, H. (2005). Anxiety, attributional thinking, and the primary process. *International Journal of Psychoanalysis, 86,* 1679-1693.

Brakel, L. A. W., Shevrin, H., & Villa, K. (2002). The priority of primary process categorizing: Experimental evidence supporting a psychoanalytic developmental hypothesis. *Journal of the American Psychoanalytic Association, 50,* 483-505.

Caine, T. M., & Hawkins, L. G. (1963). Questionnaire measures of the hysteroid/obsessoid component of personality: The HOQ. *Journal of Consulting Psychology, 27,* 206:209.

Crowne, D., & Marlowe, D. (1964). *The approval motive.* New York: John Wiley.

Damasio, A. R., Tranel, D., & Damasio, H. (1990). Individuals with psychopathic behavior caused by frontal damage fail to respond autonomically to social stimuli. *Behavior and Brain Research, 41,* 81-94.

Etkin, A., Klernenhage, K. C., Dudman, J. T., Rogan, M. T., Hen, R., & Kandel, E. R. (2004). Individual differences in trait anxiety predict the responses of the basolateral amygdale in unconsciously processed fearful faces. *Neuron, 44,* 1043-1055.

Etkin, A., Pittenger, C., Polan, J., & Kandel, E. R. (2005). Toward a neurobiology of psychotherapy: Basic science and clinical applications. *Journal of Neuropsychiatry and Clinical Neuroscience, 17,* 145-158.

Fisher, C. (1956). Dreams, images, and perception: A study of unconscious-preconscious relationships. *Journal of the American Psychoanalytic Association, 4,* 5-48.

Fisher, C. (1957). A study of the preliminary stages of the construction of dreams and images. *Journal of the American Psychoanalytic Association, 5,* 5-60.

Freud, S. (1891/1953). *On aphasia,* New York: International Universities Press.

Freud, S. (1915/1957). Instincts and their vicissitudes. *Standard Edition, 14,* 105-140.

Friston, K. J. (2000). Imaging neuroscience: 1. Neuronal transients and nonlinear coupling. *Philosophical Transactions of the Royal Society of London, B, 355,* 215-236.

Greenwald, A. G., & Banaji, M. R. (1995). Implicit social cognition: Attitudes, self-esteem, and stereotypes. *Psychological Review, 102,* 4-27.

Howard, R. Grazer, B. (Producers), & Howard, R. (Director). (2001). *A beautiful mind.* [Motion picture]. United States: Universal Pictures.

Kahneman, D. (2003). A perspective on judgment and choice: Mapping bounded rationality. *American Psychologist, 58,* 697-720.

Kandel, E. R. (1999). Biology and the future of psychoanalysis: A new intellectual framework for psychiatry revisited. *American Journal of Psychiatry, 156,* 505-524.

Libet, B., Alberts, W. W., Wright, E. W., & Feinstein, B. (1967). Response of human somatosensory cortex to stimuli below threshold for conscious sensation. *Science, 158,* 1597-1600.

Malloy, P., Bihrle, A., & Duffy, J. (1993). The orbitomedial frontal syndrome. *Archives of Clinical Neuropsychology, 8,* 185-201.

Medin, D. C., & Heit, E. J. (1999). Categorization. In D. Rumelhart & B. Martin (Eds.), *Handbook of cognition and perception* (pp. 99-143). San Diego: Academic Press.

Pace-Schott, E. F., Solms, M., & Blagrove, M., (Eds.) (2003). *Sleep and dreaming: Scientific advances and reconsiderations.* Cambridge: Cambridge University Press.

Panksepp, J. (1998). *Affective neuroscience: The foundations of human and animal emotions.* New York: Oxford University Press.

Panksepp, J. (1999). The role of nucleus accumbens dopamine in motivated behavior: A unifying interpretation with special reference to reward-seeking. *Brain Research Reviews, 31,* 6-41.

Power, M. J., & Brewer, C. R. (1991). From Freud to cognitive science: A contemporary account of the unconscious. *British Journal of Clinical Psychology, 30,* 289-310.

Rescorla, R. A. (1988). Pavlovian conditioning: It's not what you think it is. *American Psychologist, 43,* 151–160.

Ressler, K. J., Rothbaum, B. O., & Tannenbaum, L. (2000). Cognitive enhancers as adjuncts to psychotherapy: Use of d-cycloserine in phobic individuals to facilitate extinction of fear. *Archives of General Psychiatry, 61,* 1136-1144.

Schenck, C. H., & Mahowald, M. W. (2002). REM sleep behavior disorder: Clinical, developmental, and neuroscience perspectives 16 years after its formal identification in SLEEP. *Sleep, 25,* 293-308.

Shedler, J. (2002). A new language for psychoanalytic diagnosis. *Journal of the American Psychoanalytic Association, 50,* 429-456.

Shevrin, H. (1973). Brain wave correlates of subliminal stimulation, unconscious attention, primary-and secondary-process thinking and repressiveness. *Psychological Issues, 30*(8), 56-87.

Shevrin, H. (1990). Subliminal perception and repression. In J. Singer (Ed.), *Repression and dissociation: Implications for personality, psychopathology and health.* Chicago: University of Chicago Press.

Shevrin, H. (2000). The experimental investigation of unconscious conflict, unconscious affect, and unconscious signal anxiety. In M. Velmans (Ed.), *Investigating phenomenal consciousness: New Methodologies and maps* (pp. 33-65). Amsterdam/Philadelphia: John Benjamins Publishing.

Shevrin, H. (2001). Event-related markers of unconscious processes. *International Journal of Psychophysiology, 42,* 209-218.

Shevrin, H. (2003a). *Subliminal explorations of perceptions, dreams, and fantasies: The pioneering contributions of Charles Fisher* (Monograph). Madison, CT: International Universities Press.

Shevrin, H. (2003b, September 15). The psychoanalytic theory of drive in the light of recent neuroscience theories and findings. 1st Annual C. Philip Wilson, MD Memorial Lecture. New York: Lenox Hill Hospital.

Shevrin, H., Bond, J. A., Brakel, L. A. W., Hertel, R., & Williams W. (1996). *Conscious and unconscious processes: Psychodynamic, cognitive, and neurophysiologic convergences.* New York: Guilford Press.

Shevrin, H., Brakel, L. A. W., Abelson, J., & Snodgrass, M. (2004, August). Evidence of unconscious inhibition in spider phobics. Presented at International Neuro-Psychoanalysis Society, Rome.

Shevrin, H., & Fisher C. (1967). Changes in the effects of a waking subliminal stimulus as a function of dreaming and non-dreaming sleep. *Journal of Abnormal Psychology, 72,* 362-368.

Shevrin, H., & Fritzler, D. (1968). Visual evoked response correlates of unconscious mental processes. *Science, 161,* 295-298.

Shevrin, H., Ghannam, J. H., & Libet, B. (2002). A neural correlate of consciousness related to repression. *Consciousness and Cognition, 11,* 334-341.

Shevrin, H., Smith, W. H., & Fritzler, D. (1971). Average evoked response and verbal correlates of unconscious mental processes. *Psychophysiology, 6,* 149-162.

Shevrin, H., Williams, W. J., Marshall, R. E., Hertel, R. K., Bond, J. A., & Brakel, L. A. W. (1992). Event-related potential indicators of the dynamic unconscious. *Consciousness and Cognition, 1,* 340-366.

Snodgrass, M., Bernat, E., & Shevrin, H. (2004). Unconscious perception: A model based approach to method and evidence. *Perception and Psychophysics, 66,* 846-867.

Snodgrass, M., & Shevrin, H. (2005). Unconscious inhibition and facilitation at the objective detection threshold: Replicable and qualitatively different unconscious perceptual effects. *Cognition. Epublication in advance of publication in journal.*

Soloff, P. H., Meltzer, C. C., Becker, C., Greer, P. J., Kelly, T. M., & Constantine, D. (2003). Impulsivity and prefrontal hypometabolism in borderline personality disorder. *Psychiatry Research, 123,* 153-163.

Stanovich, K., & West, R. (2000). Individual differences in reasoning: Implications for the rationality debate. *Behavioral and Brain Science, 23,* 645-726.

Villa, K. K., Bazan, A., Shevrin, H., Snodgrass, M., & Brakel, L.A.W. (in press). Lexical modularity in unconscious primary process cognition. *Neuropsychoanalysis.*

Westen, D. (1997). Divergences between clinical and research methods for assessing personality disorders: Implications for research and the evolution of Axis II. *American Journal of Psychiatry, 154,* 895-903.

Westen, D., & Morrison, K. (2001). A multidimensional meta-analysis of treatments for depression, panic, and generalized anxiety disorder: An examination of the status of empirically supported therapies. *Journal of Consulting and Clinical Psychology, 69,* 875-899.

Westen, D., & Shedler, J. (1999). Revising and assessing Axis II: Part 1. Developing a clinically and empirically valid assessment method. *American Journal of Psychiatry, 156,* 258-272.

Psychoanalytic Therapy Research: Its History, Its Present Status, and Its Projected Future

Robert S. Wallerstein, MD[1]

Editor's Note: This essay is a historical survey of psychoanalytic therapy research, back to its beginnings with a first contribution in Boston close to a century ago, in 1917, through a slow and quite simplistic early unfolding over its first half-century, and into a recently burgeoning and increasingly sophisticated methodological and substantive development, into two differentiated, outcome and process, streams, related, but also distinctive, that characterizes its present status.

This historical accounting is parsed conceptually, first into four distinct generations of outcome research starting, in the first generation, with the simple descriptions by the treating clinicians of their assessments of the therapeutic outcomes they feel they had achieved, through to the sophistication and complexity of present-day fourth generation conceptions that bring together current process research studies—which have lagged behind the development of outcome research studies by several decades—with a whole new generation of therapy outcome measures created in the past two decades, and in conceptual sophistication (being reflections of underlying change in personality structure and functioning) beyond anything that existed in earlier research generations.

The same development is described for process research, parsed also into four generations, but not really starting until a half-century later, with the development and deployment of suitable technology—namely audio and video recording, and computerization with high-speed word or situation searches. It is now possible to bring the array of current process measures into conjunction with the current array of advanced outcome measures of underlying personality (or structural) change most relevant to the therapeutic claims of psychoanalytic therapies, and all in relation to a centralized shared data base, permitting comparison and contrast between the findings that each of these separate instruments is designed to, and does, elicit. It is now a quantum leap beyond where this research field started almost a century ago.

ABSTRACT

Systematic research into the processes and outcomes of psychoanalytic therapy has had a chequered history within psychoanalysis. Though Freud conceived

[1] Emeritus Professor and Former Chair, Department of Psychiatry, University of California San Francisco, School of Medicine

of psychoanalysis as a *science* of the mind, he was indifferent to the usefulness of, and the need for, the formal research by which science, any science, incrementally grows and enlarges its knowledge base. And this attitude exerted a seriously chilling effect upon the possibilities for formal psychoanalytic research during Freud's lifetime. Nonetheless, formal research into psychoanalytic therapy did start as far back as 1917, and has truly burgeoned since the middle of the twentieth century. I describe the history of psychoanalytic outcome research from its beginnings, through four generations of increasing conceptual sophistication and methodological comprehensiveness; and then the counterpart history of psychoanalytic process research, starting several decades later when the technology necessary for it—recording of therapeutic sessions and computerization of transcribed hours—became both available and increasingly clinically acceptable. The process history is also divided into four (telescoped) generations. I end with a statement of current integrated possibilities for quantum advance in this research arena.

INTRODUCTION

As an organized enterprise, formal psychoanalytic research has had a checkered history in psychoanalysis, a discipline developed through the *clinical* data of the therapeutic consulting room. The whole corpus of psychoanalysis, comprehending the phenomena of both normal and abnormal personality functioning, attests brilliantly to the explanatory power of the theory derived from the data generated in the consulting room. It flourished in the hands of its founding genius, and all of us who have come after, and it has provided a truly extraordinary range of insights into the structure of the mind, the organization of mental illness, and the forces at work in the treatment situation.

Although Freud was deeply committed to his conception of the psychoanalysis that he had single-handedly brought into being as a *science*, a natural science embedded in an evolutionary biological framework, he himself was indifferent, and even antipathetic, to the systematic research by which science, any science, grows incrementally and accrues a deepening knowledge base. Though he respected the experimental support of his dream theory offered by Otto Pötzl (1917/1960), in general he felt that the thousands of hours that he and his adherents spent with their analysands provided proof enough of his theories. And, when in 1934 the American psychologist Saul Rosenzweig wrote to Freud about his experimental observations that offered a method for studying repression, Freud responded politely but curtly:

> My dear Sir: I have examined your experimental studies for the verification of the psychoanalytic assertions with interest. I cannot put much value on these informations because the wealth of reliable observations on which

these assertions rest make them independent of experimental verification. Still, it can do no harm. Sincerely yours, Freud. (cited in Shakow & Rapaport, 1964, p. 129).

It was the chilling effect of this bias upon the discipline that Freud so dominated until his death that played its very significant role in the painfully slow development of psychoanalytic research over the first half-century history of the discipline and that led to the sober appraisal in 1960 by Hans Strupp, a dedicated psychotherapy researcher, that whatever considerable growth formal research into psychotherapy had undergone to that point, it had exerted but slight influence on the theory and practice of therapy. He stated bluntly:

> Clinical perception and scientific rigor have varied inversely . . . . If the advances of psychoanalysis as a therapeutic technique are compared with experimental research contributions, there can be little argument as to which has more profoundly enriched the theory and practice of psychotherapy. To make the point more boldly, I believe that up to the present, research contributions have had exceedingly little influence on the practical procedures of psychotherapy. (Strupp, 1960).

Such was the parlous state of the psychoanalytic therapy research enterprise when I entered into it in 1954, six years prior to Strupp's published lament. I have described in detail elsewhere (Wallerstein, in press) my own career trajectory through medical school, psychiatry and psychoanalysis, and into a position, offered to me in 1954 by Gardner Murphy, Director of Research, as Assistant Director of Research at The Menninger Foundation in Topeka, Kansas.

My charge was to develop research that could link the Research Department directly to the central clinical activity—the practice of psychoanalytic therapy—to which the entire clinical staff devoted its time. The topic which I and a group of colleagues decided to address was, not surprisingly, the effort to learn more about two simple, but not simple-minded, questions: (1) *What* changes take place in psychoanalysis and psychoanalytic psychotherapies—what are the reach and the limitations of these therapeutic modalities when appropriately deployed, i.e., the outcome question, and (2) *How* do these changes come about, through the interaction of what factors in the patient, in the therapist and the therapy, and in the concomitant life situation of the patient, i.e., the process question.

In creating this research program, which became the 30-year-long Psychotherapy Research Project (PRP) of The Menninger Foundation, we did find a small reservoir of prior work in this arena to draw upon. In an overview of the entire field of psychoanalytic therapy research that I recently published (Wallerstein, 2001), I divided this history, which actually went back to a first article by Coriat (1917) until its current state, into four generations, meaning generations not only in terms of temporal onset and duration, but also in terms of increasing conceptual sophistication and methodological comprehensiveness.

First Generation Outcome Studies: Statistical Counts

The first generation of early statistical studies of therapeutic outcomes began as early as 1917, when Coriat, in Boston, reported on the results achieved in 93 cases, of whom 73% were declared either recovered or much improved, these rates being nearly equal across all diagnostic categories (Coriat, 1917). As with all these statistical studies in this first generation, the judgments of improvement were made by the treating clinician, according to unspecified criteria, and without individual clinical detail or supporting evidence.

In the decade of the 1930s, several comparable but larger scale simple statistical reports emerged from the experiences of some of the pioneering psychoanalytic training institutes. In 1930, Fenichel reported results with 721 patients from the initial decade of the Berlin Institute (Fenichel, 1930), and this was followed by a similar report by Jones in 1936 on 738 applicants to the London Psychoanalytic Clinic (Jones, 1936), and by Alexander in 1937 on 157 cases from the Chicago Psychoanalytic Clinic (Alexander, 1937). They all reported substantial benefits with the great majority of the neurotic patients, and in the Chicago Psychoanalytic Clinic cases an even higher percentage of positive results with those in the separated-off category of the psychosomatic; however, contrary to Coriat's earlier results, they found much lower improvement percentages in those labeled psychotic.

In a review article evaluating the overall results of psychoanalysis, Knight (1941) combined the findings of all these prior studies, and added 100 patients treated at the Menninger Clinic. Again the results were judged to be completely comparable with those of the other studies in the outcomes with so-called neurotic and psychotic patients. Knight made reference to the pitfalls of these simple statistical accounts; the absence of consensually agreed definitions and criteria, the crudeness of nomenclature and diagnostic classification, and the failure to address issues of therapeutic skill with cases of varying severity.

The most ambitious study of this first generation genre was the report of the Central Fact-Gathering Committee of the American Psychoanalytic Association (Hamburg, et al., 1967)—as late as 1967. Data were collected over a 5-year period; altogether there were 10,000 initial responses to questionnaires submitted by 800 analysts, with some 3,000 termination questionnaires on treatment completion. As with the other studies cited thus far, criteria for diagnosis and improvement were not specified, and these and other flaws resulted ultimately in a report that was declared to be simply an "experience survey" consisting of (1) facts about the demographics of analysts' practices, (2) analysts' opinions on their patients' diagnoses, and (3) analysts' opinions on the therapeutic results. Not unexpectedly, the great majority of the patients were declared to be substantially improved. And a year later, in 1968, there appeared the last of these first generation surveys of psychoanalytic clinic experiences, a report from the Southern California

Institute (Feldman, 1968), with again, very comparable findings, and a similar statement of inherent limitations.

Altogether, this sequence of so-called first-generation outcome studies, spanning a half-century, from 1917 to 1968, was scientifically simplistic and failed to command much interest in the psychoanalytic clinical world. Most practitioners agreed with Glover's (1954) dour assessment: "Like most psycho-therapists, the psycho-analyst is a reluctant and inexpert statistician" (p. 393)—and, it could be added, researcher. It was such conclusions that spurred what I call second-generation studies, the efforts at more systematic outcome research geared towards overcoming the glaring methodological simplicity that marked each of the studies described to this point.

In addition to the lack of consensually agreed criteria at every step of these first-generation studies—from initial diagnostic assessments to outcome judgments of therapeutic results—and the use of these judgments (derived from unspecified criteria) by the (necessarily biased) therapist, as the sole evidential primary database, there was also the methodological difficulty that these studies were all retrospective, with all the potential therein for bias, for confounding of judgments, for *post hoc ergo propter hoc* reasoning, and the like. Efforts to address these issues, including the introduction of prospective inquiry, and even the fashioning of predictions to be confirmed or refuted by subsequent assessment, began in earnest in the 1950s and 1960s in America, and have since spread worldwide.

SECOND GENERATION OUTCOME STUDIES: FORMAL RESEARCH

I will briefly indicate six major American projects from this second-generation research, three based on group-aggregated studies of clinic cases from the Boston, Columbia, and New York Psychoanalytic Institutes, and three based on individually focused studies in New York, San Francisco, and Chicago. I also mention here, out of the many current programs elsewhere in the world, four major European projects of this kind: (1) the Anna Freud Centre review of 765 cases treated over four decades with psychoanalysis or psychotherapy (Fonagy & Target, 1994, 1996; Target & Fonagy, 1994a, 1994b), (2) the German Psychoanalytical Association (DPV) study of the long-term results of psychoanalytic therapies involving the study by the researchers of 190 patients drawn from cooperating DPV members (Leuzinger-Bohleber, 1997), (3) the European multicenter collaborative study of intensive psychoanalytic treatment involving analysts from Sweden, Finland, Norway, Holland, and Italy (Szecsody, et al., 1997), and (4) the Swedish outcome study of patients in state-subsidized psychoanalysis and long-term therapy (Sandell, et al., 2000).

Boston Psychoanalytic Institute

Now to the earlier American second-generation studies: In 1960, Knapp and his colleagues reported on 100 supervised psychoanalytic patients from the Boston Institute Clinic (Knapp, 1960), rated initially for suitability for analysis, of whom 27 were followed up a year later to ascertain just how suitable the patients had indeed turned out to be. The evaluation procedures were blind. There turned out to be very limited success in this assessment of suitability for analysis from the initial evaluation. However, two significant limitations of this study should be mentioned: First, the testing of the predictions took place at the one-year mark rather than more suitably at termination; clearly much can change in this regard—in both directions—later in analysis. Second, the patients selected by psychoanalytic clinic committees are already carefully screened, with clearly unsuitable cases already rejected. The range of variability in the accepted cases is thus considerably narrowed, making differential predictions within that group inherently less reliable.

Inspired by this work, Sashin, Eldred, and van Amerongen (1975) subsequently studied 183 patients treated at the same clinic from 1959 to 1966—but in this case data were collected after an average of 675 hours, at a point averaging 6 years *after* termination. Predictor variables were assessed with a 103-item questionnaire, via six major outcome criteria: (1) restriction of functioning by symptoms, (2) subjective discomfort, (3) work productivity, (4) sexual adjustment, (5) interpersonal relations, and (6) availability of insight. Only ten of the predictor items demonstrated some predictive value in relation to outcomes, and these only with modest correlations. And as a group, these ten variables "made little clinical sense." Overall, the Boston Institute studies yielded only fair prediction to judgments of analyzability as assessed at the one-year mark, and no effective prediction at all to final treatment outcomes from the patients' characteristics as judged initially.

Columbia Psychoanalytic Center

The Columbia Psychoanalytic Center project, contemporaneous with the Boston studies, was written up in a sequence of published reports in 1985 (Bachrach, Weber, & Solomon, 1985; Weber, Bachrach, & Solomon, 1985a, 1985b; Weber, Solomon, & Bachrach, 1985). This project consisted of prospective studies of a large number of patients (1,348 in Sample 1 and 237 in Sample 2), all treated by the same body of therapists. Data were collected from multiple perspectives, with opportunities to compare findings in psychoanalysis (40% of the total) with those in analytic psychotherapy (the other 60%). The authors stated that all previous studies had been limited in at least one of the following ways: small sample size, inadequate information about outcomes, not based on terminated cases, or restricted to retrospective data. Further, no other studies had permitted comparison between large numbers of terminated analyses and psycho-therapies conducted by the same therapists. In addition, criteria for therapeutic benefit were established distinct from criteria for the evolution of a psychoanalytic process.

The most striking finding from this project was that across every category of patient, therapeutic benefit measures always substantially exceeded measures of an evolved analytic process. For example, only 40% of those who completed analyses with good therapeutic benefits were characterized as having been "analyzed." An equally striking finding was that the outcomes of these treatments, in terms of both therapeutic benefit and analyzability, were only marginally predictable from the initial evaluation. This finding was, of course, in keeping with the Boston studies just cited—and for the same reasons. As noted by the authors (Weber, Bachrach, & Solomon, 1985a), "The . . . conclusion . . . is *not* that therapeutic benefit or analyzability are *per se* unpredictable, but that once a case has been carefully selected as suitable . . . its eventual fate remains relatively indeterminate" (p. 135).

In overall conclusion, the authors stated that Sample 1 was three times larger than in any previous study, and that the project was the first to have a psychotherapy comparison group, and one of the first to make the conceptual distinction between analyzability and therapeutic benefit. Sample 2 was smaller, assembled a decade later, with some refinements in data collection and some differences in observational vantage points, but in almost every particular, the findings of Sample 1 were replicated. In the final article in this series (Bachrach, Weber, & Solomon, 1985), the authors stressed the advantages of their project over other studies: (1) the N was very large; (2) it was a prospective study with predictive evaluations made before outcomes were known; (3) they used clinically meaningful scales; (4) aside from evaluations by patients and therapists, they used independent judges; and (5) psychoanalysis and psychotherapy were assessed comparatively.

New York Psychoanalytic Institute

The third of these group-aggregated studies, from the New York Institute (Erle, 1979; Erle & Goldberg, 1979, 1984), was similarly constituted, although with a significant focus on the study of treatments carried out by more experienced analysts. There were two samples. The first (Erle, 1979) consisted of 40 supervised cases in the Treatment Center of the New York Institute. The results were completely comparable with those at the Boston and Columbia centers. The majority of the patients were judged to have benefited substantially, but only half of those were judged to have been involved in a proper psychoanalytic process. The authors compared this with another sample of 42 private patients, treated by seven analytic colleagues, who had begun their treatments in the same time period and were assessed in the same manner as the Treatment Center patients. The results were substantially the same. The second sample (Erle & Goldberg, 1984) extended the work to a group of 160 private patients gathered over a subsequent five-year span from sixteen experienced analysts. The outcomes with these experienced analysts were completely comparable with the results of all the earlier studies of clinic patients treated by candidates.

Two decades subsequently, the same authors published still another study comprising two samples (Erle & Goldberg, 2003). Since 63 of the patients in the earlier second report were still in treatment at the time of the study, the authors decided on a new Sample 1 consisting of a further report on this same group now carried through to their treatment terminations, plus a Sample 2 consisting of 92 cases treated subsequently by 20 analysts (including 12 of the 16 who had participated in the earlier study). What was new here was that this last sample was not a retrospective study as the earlier ones had been, but was prospective, starting with initial diagnostic evaluations, and predictions about anticipated course in regard to expected analyzability and therapeutic benefit. The outcomes were again completely comparable with the results of all the earlier studies reported here. However, the authors did find a significantly higher predictive accuracy in regard to issues of analyzability and therapeutic benefit than anyone had previously reported.

Individually Focused Studies: New York, San Francisco, Chicago

I turn now to the individually focused American studies. Over a time span parallel to that of these relatively large-scale outcome studies of psychoanalytic clinic patients (and some comparison private patients), assessed by pre- and post-treatment rating scales and grouped statistically, Pfeffer at the New York Psychoanalytic Treatment Center initiated a wholly other kind of study of terminated psychoanalyses, by intensive individual study of a small research-procured population (Pfeffer, 1959, 1961, 1963). He reported on nine patients who had completed analyses under Treatment Center auspices, and agreed to a series of interviews by a "follow-up analyst" who had not conducted the treatment. The interviews were open-ended, weekly, "analytic" in character, and ranged from two to seven in number before the participants agreed on a natural close. The chief finding, in all instances, consisted of the rapid reactivation of characteristic analytic transferences, including even transitory symptom flare-ups, as if in relation to the original treating analyst, with subsequent rapid subsidence, at times aided by pertinent interpretations, and in a manner that reflected the new ways of neurotic conflict management achieved in the analysis.

In the last of these three reports, Pfeffer (1963) attempted a metapsychological explanation of these "follow-up study transference phenomena" (p. 230). His conclusion was:

The recurrence in the follow-up study of the major preanalytic symptom-atology in the context of a [momentarily] revived transference neurosis as well as the quick subsidence of symptoms appear to support the idea that conflicts underlying symptoms are not actually shattered or obliterated by analysis but rather are only better mastered with new and more adequate solutions. (p. 234)

The neurotic conflicts thus "lose their poignancy."

Two other research groups, one in San Francisco (Norman, Blacker, Orem-land, & Barrett, 1976; Oremland, Blacker, & Norman, 1975), and one in Chicago (Schlessinger & Robbins, 1974, 1975, 1983), replicated Pfeffer's studies, with some slight alterations in method, and in both instances confirmed what has come to be called "the Pfeffer phenomenon." This overall finding from all three groups—that even in analyses considered highly successful, neurotic conflicts are not obliterated, as was once felt, but rather are muted, or lose their poig-nancy—is echoed in the well-known analytic quip that we still recognize our good friends after their analyses.

I note one final consideration: A shared characteristic of these second-genera-tion studies—whether the group-aggregated broad statistical outcome account-ings (Boston, Columbia, Erle & Goldberg in New York), or the individually more process focused in-depth studies (Pfeffer in New York, San Francisco, Chicago)—was the failure to segregate results at termination from the issue of the stability (or not) of these results as revealed at some established follow-up point subse-quent to termination, with all the different possibilities—for consolidation and enhancement of treatment gains, for the simple maintenance of treatment achievements, or for actual regression back toward the pretreatment state.

Conceptually, this was a failure to accord specific theoretical status to what Rangell (1966/1990) called the "postanalytic phase." Rangell described a variety of possible courses that can characterize this phase and concluded that "the desired goal should be a transition to a normal interchange in which the analyst can be seen and reacted to as a normal figure and no longer as an object for con-tinued transference displacement" (p. 722). In the third-generation studies, next to be described, the distinction between results at termination and those at a sub-sequent follow-up study point (anywhere from 2 to 5 years later) becomes a clearly demarcated research focus—among the advances over the second-genera-tion studies.

THIRD GENERATION OUTCOME STUDIES: COMBINED PROCESS AND OUTCOME

What I call the third-generation studies of the outcomes of psychoanalysis have actually been contemporaneous in time with the second-generation studies

just described. These third-generation studies are systematic psychoanalytic therapy research projects that have attempted both to assess outcomes across a significant array of different kinds of cases, and to also examine the processes through
which these outcomes have been achieved via intensive longitudinal study of
each individual case. In this, these projects have combined the methodological
approaches of the group-aggregated with those of the individually focused second-generation studies. Like the best second-generation studies, they have carefully defined their terms, constructed rating scales, and tried to operationalize
their criteria at each assessment point. These third-generation studies have been
constructed prospectively, starting with pretreatment assessment. Unlike the second-generation studies, they have separated outcomes at termination from functioning at a specified follow-up point and have attempted to account for further
changes, in either direction, that took place during this "postanalytic phase."
Bachrach and colleagues (1991), in their comprehensive survey of research on the
efficacy of psychoanalysis, singled out the newer Boston Institute studies (Kantrowitz, 1986; Kantrowitz, Paolitto, Sashin, Solomon, & Katz, 1986; Kantrowitz,
Katz, Paolitto, Sashin, & Solomon, 1987a, 1987b; Kantrowitz, et al., 1989; Kantrowitz, Katz, & Paolitto, 1990a, 1990b, 1990c) and the Psychotherapy Research
Project of The Menninger Foundation (Wallerstein, 1986, 1988a) that our group
created in Topeka in the 1950s, as the only ones to fully meet their state-of-the-
art specifications for outcomes studies—state-of-the-art as of their time of publication, over a dozen years ago. These two I review here as exemplars of this third
generation research approach.

Boston Psychoanalytic Institute

The Boston studies of Kantrowitz and her group were undertaken in the
1970s and were published in the following decade. Twenty-two supervised cases
at the Boston Institute Clinic were selected for prospective study, with the initial
assessment based upon a projective psychological test battery used to yield measures of (1) affect availability and modulation, (2) quality of object relations, (3)
adequacy of reality testing, and (4) motivation for change. Approximately a year
after termination, the initial test battery was repeated, and both the patient and
analyst were interviewed.

A series of three articles (Kantrowitz, et al., 1986, 1987a, 1987b) described the
results. Of the 22 patients, 9 were felt to have had a successful analytic outcome,
5 a more limited outcome, and 8 to be unanalyzed. Nonetheless, the greater number achieved therapeutic benefits along each of the change dimensions, and
along each dimension the therapeutic benefit surpassed the analytic result, as
measured by the degree of successfully completed analytic work. That is, a consistent and important finding—fully in accord with the second-generation studies
of Weber and colleagues at the Columbia Institute (Weber, Solomon, &

Bachrach, 1985; Web, Bachrach, & Solomon, 1985a, 1985b) and Erle and Goldberg at the New York Institute (Erle & Goldberg, 1979, 1984, 2003)—was that therapeutic benefit was achieved by a substantial majority, and was regularly in excess of what could be accounted for by the evocation and interpretive resolution (as best as possible) of the transference neurosis. However, although most patients derived significant benefit from their analytic experience, successful outcome could not be predicted from any of the predictor variables—again, in accord with the second-generation studies.

This finding led these investigators to speculate that "a particularly important omission [from the predictor variables] might have been consideration of the effect of the [therapist-patient] match in shaping the two-person psychoanalytic interaction" (Kantrowitz, et al. 1989, p. 899). By "match" they meant, "an interactional concept; it refers to a spectrum of compatibility and incompatibility of the patient and analyst which is relevant to the analytic work" (p. 894). They further noted that although "this mesh of the analyst's personal qualities with those of the patient has rarely been a special focus of [research] attention . . . most analysts when making referrals do consider it; few assume that equally well-trained analysts are completely interchangeable" (Kantrowitz, 1986, p.273).

This same team returned for follow-up interviews with the same cohort in1987, 5 to 10 years after the terminations, this time including the retrospective assessment of the goodness of the analyst-patient match as one of the variables contributing to the outcomes (Kantrowitz, Katz, & Paollitto, 1990a, 1990b, 1990c). Nineteen of the original 22 patients could be located, and 18 agreed to be interviewed. Again, a variety of change measures were used; global improvement ratings, affect management, quality of object relations, adequacy of reality testing, work accomplishment, and overall self-esteem. Overall results at the follow-up point comprised 3 of the 18 further improved, 4 stable, 6 deteriorated but restored with additional treatment, 4 deteriorated despite additional treatment, and 1 returned to the original analyst and still in treatment, and therefore not counted.

The most striking finding was that, again, the stability of the achieved gains in the follow-up period could not be predicted from the assessments at termination—that is, according to Kantrowitz and colleagues (1990a), "the psychological changes were no more stable over time for the group of patients assessed as having achieved a successful [analysis] concomitant with considerable therapeutic benefit than for the other group of patients assessed as having achieved therapeutic benefit alone" (p. 493). In focusing on the assessment of analyst-patient match (Kantrowitz, Katz, & Paolitto, 1990c), the authors concluded that with 12 of the 17 patients, the kind of match did play a role in the achieved outcome. They gave examples of facilitating matches with good outcomes, impeding matches with poor outcomes, and more complex situations in which the match was at first facilitating to the analytic process, but later seemed to have an influence in preventing the completion of the analytic work.

The Menninger Foundation

The other third-generation analytic therapy research study to be described here is The Psychotherapy Research Project (PRP) of The Menninger Foundation that our group brought into being in 1954. Of this project Bachrach and colleagues said in their comprehensive review: "Systematic, methodologically informed research about psychoanalytic outcomes began with The Menninger Foundation Psychotherapy Research Project . . . [It] is by far the most comprehensive formal study of psychoanalysis yet undertaken and remains the only study of outcomes that spans almost the entire life cycle of many of its patients" (1991, p. 878).

Certainly, PRP was the most ambitious such research program ever carried out (Wallerstein, 1986, 1988a; Wallerstein, Robbins, Sargent, & Luborsky, 1956). Its intent was to follow the treatment careers and subsequent life careers of a cohort of patients (42 in number), half in psychoanalysis, and half in psychoanalytic psychotherapies—and each in the treatment clinically indicated—to follow them from the initial pretreatment comprehensive evaluation, through the entire natural span of their treatments (for however many years that entailed), and then into formal follow-up inquiries several years after termination, and with as much of an open-ended follow-up thereafter as circumstance might make possible and the span of interested observation might last. The patients entered their treatments over the span of the mid-1950s; their period of treatment ranged from 6 months to a full 12 years; all were reached—100%—for follow-up study at the 2- to 3-year mark; and more than one third could be followed for periods ranging from 12 to 24 years beyond their treatment terminations, with four still in treatment when my book *Forty-Two Lives in Treatment* (Wallerstein, 1986), the overall clinical accounting of this project, was published at the 30-year mark, in 1986.

The aim of PRP was to learn as much as possible about (1) *what* changes take place in psychoanalysis and the psychoanalytic psychotherapies (the outcome question), and (2) *how* those changes come about—through the interactions of what factors in the patient, in the therapy and the therapist, and in the patient's concomitantly evolving life situation, as they, in interaction, codetermine those changes (the process question). Three overall treatment groups were set up—psychoanalysis, expressive analytic psychotherapy, and supportive analytic psychotherapy—in accord with the then-consensus (in the 1950s) in the literature regarding the defining characteristics of these three therapeutic modes, together with differential indications for their deployment, derived from the dynamic formulations of the patients' lives, characters, and illness structures.

The project goals within this framework were to specify the particular reach and limitation of the therapeutic outcome for each kind of patient, treated appropriately, within each of the proffered approaches. There was a special interest in the empirical elaboration of the psychological change mechanisms operative within both the interpretive uncovering (i.e., expressive) and the "ego strengthening" (i.e., supportive) therapeutic modes. *Forty-Two Lives in Treatment* represents the full statement of the project's organization, its method and design, its instruments and operations, and its findings and conclusions (Wallerstein, 1986). For a capsule summarization of its overall results, I can best report by paraphrasing a several-page segment from the conclusions of a summarizing paper about the project (Wallerstein, 1988a, pp. 144-149).

The overall conclusions, as of 1986, can be brought together as a series of sequential propositions regarding the appropriateness, efficacy, reach, and limitations, of psychoanalysis and of psychoanalytic therapies (variously expressive and supportive)—always with the caveat that this segment of the patient population (i.e. those sicker individuals who seek their intensive analytic treatment within a psychoanalytic sanatorium setting) is not necessarily representative of the usual outpatient therapy population.

1. The first proposition concerns the distinction between "structural change" in personality, presumably based on the interpretive resolution, within the transference-countertransference matrix, of unconscious intrapsychic conflicts, and "behavioral change," or just "altered techniques of adjustment," presumably all that can come out of the other, non-interpretive, non-insight-aiming, change mechanisms. The PRP experience clearly questioned the continued usefulness of this effort to tightly link the kinds of changes achieved to the intervention mode—expressive or supportive—by which they are brought about. The changes reached in the supportive therapies seemed often enough to represent just as much structural change, with its greater stability, durability, and capacity to weather environmental vicissitudes, as the changes reached in the most expressive-analytic cases.

2. The second proposition concerns the proportionality argument—that therapeutic change will be at least proportional to the degree of conflict resolution. This proposition is almost unexceptionable, as it is clear that there can be significantly more change than on the basis of conflict resolution, in all the supportive ways through which change can be brought about. But inversely, it would be hard to image real conflict resolution without at least proportional changes in behaviors, dispositions, and symptoms.

3. The third proposition, often linked to the proportionality argument, but clearly separate, concerns the necessity argument—that effective conflict resolution is a necessary condition for at least certain kinds of change, i.e. true "structural change." An overall PRP finding—almost an overriding one—has been the repeated demonstration that a substantial range of

changes—in personality functioning and in life-style—have been brought about via the more supportive therapeutic modes, cutting across the gamut of declared supportive and expressive (even fully psychoanalytic) therapies.

4. Counterpart to the proposition based on the tendency to overestimate the necessity of the expressive treatment mode's operation via conflict resolution in order to effect structural change has been the other proposition, that supportive therapeutic approaches so often achieved far more than expected—and often enough reached the kinds of changes expected to depend upon insightful conflict resolutions—and did so in ways that represented indistinguishably "structural changes." Within both the psychotherapy and the psychoanalysis groups, the changes predicted, although more often predicated on more expressive techniques, were achieved to a greater-than-expected degree on the bases of more supportive techniques.

5. Considering these treatments from the perspective of psychoanalysis, just as more was accomplished than expected with psychotherapy, especially in its supportive modes, so psychoanalysis, as the quintessentially expressive therapeutic mode, often achieved less—at least with these sicker patients—than had been predicted. This more limited success reflected the ethos of the psychoanalytic sanatorium, dedicated to the ongoing life management of that segment of more disorganized patients who cannot be helped sufficiently with any other approach than psychoanalysis, but cannot tolerate the rigors of the treatment within the usual outpatient setting. This is the concept of so-called "heroic indications" for psychoanalysis, and in the PRP experience this group of patients did poorly with psychoanalysis, however modified, or buttressed by concomitant hospitalization, while they tended to have good outcomes in appropriately modulated supportive-expressive psychotherapy. On this basis, we can speak of the relative failure of so-called heroic indications for psychoanalysis, and invite a repositioning of the pendulum, more in the direction of narrowing indications for (proper) psychoanalysis.

6. Finally, the predictions made for prospective courses and outcomes tended to be for more substantial and enduring change where the treatment was to be more expressive-analytic, and *pari passu*, the predicted results were for more limited and less stable changes the more supportive the treatment was intended to be—and all these presumptions were consistently tempered in the actual implementation in the treatment courses. Psychoanalysis and expressive psychotherapies were systematically modified to introduce more supportive components, and they often achieved less than predicted, and with a varying but often substantial amount of those outcomes reached by supportive means. The supportive therapies, on the other hand, often accomplished a good deal more than expected, and

again, with more of the change on the bases of more supportive techniques than originally specified.

In conclusion, these overall results can be summarized as follows: (1) The treatment results in psychoanalysis and in varying mixes of expressive-supportive psychotherapies tend to converge, rather than diverge, in outcome; (2) across the whole spectrum, the treatments carried more supportive elements than originally projected, and these elements accounted for substantially more of the changes achieved than had been originally anticipated; (3) the supportive aspects of psychoanalytic therapy deserve far more respectful consideration than they have been accorded in the analytic literature; and (4) the kinds of changes achieved by this patient cohort—divorced from how they were brought about—often seemed quite indistinguishable from each other, in terms of reflecting "structural changes" in personality functioning.

FOURTH GENERATION STUDIES: NEW POSSIBILITIES

In a summarizing address that I gave a number of years ago on the field of psychoanalytic therapy research (Wallerstein, 2001), I sketched the outlines of what I felt to be the nascent fourth generation of this research, which I and others were trying to prod into being through the Collaborative Analytic Multi-Site Program (CAMP), which I organized under the auspices of the American Psychoanalytic Association (Wallerstein, 2001). CAMP has been an effort to coordinate the activities of the whole known array of psychoanalytic therapy research groups, both process and outcome study groups, in the United States—and with participants from abroad, the UK, Germany, Sweden and Holland—in contrasting and comparing their findings on a shared database of audiotaped psychoanalytic therapy hours.

In tribute to what is now a rapidly expanding field, those then hopeful but preliminary formulations can now be expanded in a major way, bringing together at this time the whole development of the field of psychotherapy research *process* studies—lagging behind the development of outcome studies by several decades—together with the possibilities inhering in a whole new generation of therapy *outcome* measures created in the past two decades, and in conceptual sophistication beyond anything indicated to this point.

PROCESS RESEARCH: INTRODUCTION

First, to the outlines of the process research domain. Because of its inherently greater conceptual and methodological complexity, research into the processes by which change is brought about in psychoanalytic therapies—the answers to the "how" question—has been far more recent in origin, and only now can be segmented into its counterpart generations. Since it necessarily entails a detailed focus on moment-to-moment therapeutic interactions, process research has indeed only become feasible on a significant scale through the more recent development and deployment of suitable technology—namely, the possibilities for audio and video recording, and computerization with high-speed word or situation searches.

Audio recording had been actually introduced into psychoanalytic research as early as 1933, when Earl Zinn made Dictaphone recordings of psychoanalytic treatments at Worcester State Hospital (Carmichael, 1956). Early on, it made very slow headway, basically because of the strong conviction within psychoanalytic circles that any such intrusion into the privacy of the treatment situation would seriously compromise, if not altogether vitiate, the therapeutic endeavor. In a major overview in 1971, a colleague and I (Wallerstein & Sampson, 1971) reviewed the literature to that date on audio recording in therapy sessions, and discussed the arguments for and against such use. Briefly, the major pro arguments were the greater completeness, verbatim accuracy, permanence and public character of the database, as well as the facilitation of the separation of the therapeutic from the research responsibility, with the ability then to bypass the subjectivities of the analyst as a contaminant of the data filter. The major con arguments were the indeterminate impact of this (research) intrusion on the 'naturalness' of the therapeutic process (including the compromise of full confidentiality and the insertion into the treatment of goals other than therapeutic) and the sheer enormity, complexity, and cost of the database thus made available, cost being not just for recording, but also for faithful transcription.

Since then, however, a fair number of analytic psychotherapies and even full analyses have been carried out while being recorded, with ample research gain, and without evident hurtful impact on the clinical outcome, and a growing segment of the psychoanalytic world has come to accept this as a benign as well as a potentially valuable procedure. One marker was the experience of Merton Gill in the late 1960s (personal communication), when he was a member of the then Downstate Institute in New York and was conducting a research-recorded psychoanalysis at the Downstate Medical Center. Gill undertook to present his work with this patient to a monthly seminar of the institute's training analysts, and after a year of presentations the group expressed its conviction that a properly psychoanalytic process was indeed transpiring, and that the impact of the recording—like any other condition surrounding a psychoanalytic treatment—could be brought under analytic scrutiny for its many meanings, as indeed it needed to be, and in this case could be clearly demonstrated.

FIRST GENERATION PROCESS STUDIES: DEVELOPMENT OF MEASURES

It is within the framework of this gradually increasing acceptance of recorded treatments as bona fide within an ever growing segment of the psychoanalytic community that Wilma Bucci in a current manuscript (Bucci, in press) creates a complementary perspective, spelling out what she calls four generations—conceptually, not temporally—of psychoanalytic process research. The first generation consisted of the development of a range of objective process measures, and the establishment of their reliability and usefulness, mostly accomplished in the seventies. At the risk of slighting equally worthwhile others that may not be known to me, let me list (alphabetically) eight of the best known and widely cited of these micro-analytic measures of therapy process: (1) Bucci's Multiple Code Theory (MCT) and Referential Cycle, based on the fluctuations of referential connections between nonverbal systems and the communicative verbal code; (2) Dahl's studies of Fundamental Repetitive and Maladaptive Emotion Structures (FRAMES), built upon a classification of emotional expression; (3) M. Horowitz's Configurational Analysis and Role Relationship Model (CARR), based on the interaction of mental schemas as they affect thought and action concerning the self and others; (4) L. Horwitz's Menninger Treatment Intervention Project (TRIP), exploring the evolving relationship between the therapeutic alliance and the interpretation of the transference; (5) Jones's Psychotherapy Process Q-Set (PPQS), a Q-sort providing for the description and classification of treatment processes in a form suitable for quantitative analysis; (6) Luborsky's Core Conflictual Relationship Theme (CCRT), a categorization of transference expressions and of responses to them; (7) Perry's Defense Mechanism Rating Scales (DMRS), a hierarchy of the maturity of defense development; and (8) Waldron's Analytic Process Scales (APS), assessing the contributions of the analyst, of the patient, and of the interactional characteristics of their relationship, to the evolving analytic process. A formidable array indeed of process measures, centrally based on the assessment of audiotaped and transcribed therapeutic sessions.

SECOND GENERATION PROCESS STUDIES: SHARED DATA SETS

What Bucci designates as second-generation process studies consists of the application of these instruments to shared data sets. A major example is represented in the contents of a 1988 book, edited by Dahl and colleagues, *Psychoanalytic Process Research Strategies* (Dahl, Kächele, & Thomä, 1988), the proceedings of a workshop of American and German therapy process researchers held in Ulm, Germany, just prior to the 1985 International Psycho-Analytical Association Congress in Hamburg.

The Ulm workshop brought together some of the most productive research groups in America and Germany engaged in the study of moment-to-moment interaction processes, in single hours, or in segments of hours, using audiotaped and transcribed treatment sessions. Each of the participating groups (including several of those just listed) had developed its own concepts of the basic units of the psychoanalytic process, and its own instruments to measure them, and had used its measures in relation to its own available data set. The book described efforts to compare findings from these disparate groups—as much as possible when there had been sharing of the database—in a search for elements of convergence.

In the introduction to that book, Dahl expressed the hope that this convergence could be found in the principle enunciated by Strupp and colleagues (1988) in the initial chapter: "that the description and representation, theoretically *and* operationally, of a *patient's conflicts,* of the *patient's treatment,* and of the *assessment of the outcome* must be congruent, which is to say, must be represented in comparable, if not identical, terms" (Dahl, Kächele, & Thomä, 1988, p. ix). This fundamental integrative principle—proposed to subsume conceptually the entire array of process and outcome measures—is put this way by Strupp and colleagues:

> The principle of the [Problem-Treatment-Outcome] P-T-O Congruence proposes that the intelligibility of psychotherapy research is a function of the similarity, isomorphism, or congruence among how we conceptualize and measure the clinical problem (P), the process of therapeutic (T) change, and the clinical outcome (O)," (1988, p. 7).

Another major and currently ongoing effort in this direction is the Collaborative Analytic Multi-Site Program (CAMP), which, as already indicated, I organized under the auspices of the American Psychoanalytic Association now more than a dozen years ago (Wallerstein, 2001). This has been an effort at the ingathering of all the known active psychoanalytic therapy research groups, process and outcome, including all those mentioned to this point and a good many others, to meet, originally for a whole day twice yearly, and now only once yearly in New York, in connection with the mid-winter meeting of the American Association.

The CAMP program is designed to accommodate all the participating groups' own concepts and instruments in relation to a shared agreed-upon database of available audiotaped and transcribed sessions from already completed psychoanalytic treatments, as well as from new cases—this last has not yet been undertaken—so that before-and-after outcome studies can be prospectively built in. The comparing and contrasting of findings in relation to the same database by all these process and outcome groups would finally make it possible to determine the degrees of convergence of the concepts and instruments elaborated by the different research groups, and also to determine the degree of imbrication of process and outcome studies—that is, the degree to which the Principle of PTO Congruence can be realized. Unhappily, the inability to date to secure the necessary funding for this ambitious program has limited the CAMP endeavor to only partial fulfillments, the collaboration of subgroups from the involved process research programs in comparative work on shared data.

THIRD GENERATION PROCESS STUDIES: CLINICAL-RESEARCH INTEGRATION

And further, in Bucci's schema, there is now emerging a third generation of therapy process research, a further integration of these various process studies with concomitant, equally intensive, *clinical* studies of the same patient population—clinical studies at least as intensive as those described in *Forty-Two Lives in Treatment* (Wallerstein, 1986)—in order to create a more direct bridge between research findings and the clinical activities of the psychoanalytic practitioner community. Two studies now underway at International Psychoanalytical Association institutes—one at the Institute for Psychoanalytic Training and Research (IPTAR) in New York (Freedman, Lasky, & Hurvich, 2003), and the other at two collaborating groups, the Argentine Psychoanalytic Association and Belgrano University, both in Buenos Aires (Lopez-Moreno, et al., 1999)—provide models for this third-generation work. Bucci in her article (in press) gives a detailed description of both projects: the IPTAR project providing a unique and innovative approach to incorporating multiple perspectives on the therapeutic process by what they call a method of "sequential specification," through phases of clinical scan, and then clinical confirmation, followed by specification of changes of psychological functioning, with finally the application of objective research methods including Bucci's Referential Activity, Luborsky's Core Conflictual Relationship Theme, and Perry's Defense Mechanism Rating Scale to the researchers' indicated descriptors—in all, a complexly imbricated clinician and researcher partnership; and the Buenos Aires project, again the collaborative integration of the clinical observations of the analyst with an array of empirical research methods, including, along with some of the process measures already mentioned, a measure newly devised by the Argentine research group, the DEPD or Differential Elements for Psychodynamic Diagnosis. Constraints of space preclude my describing either of these programs more fully.

FOURTH GENERATION PROCESS STUDIES: PROCESS-OUTCOME INTEGRATION

Which brings me to Bucci's conception of a projected fourth generation process research, the inclusion, alongside all these already presented elements, of new psychoanalytically conceived *outcome* measures that assess structural changes in the ego (changes in personality functioning), which in turn makes possible my portrayal here, via a better elaborated version of the possibilities for fourth generation outcome research than could be made when I first tried to sketch out a platform for this effort a full decade ago, all together making possible a bringing together of a fourth generation therapy research enterprise embracing both domains, the current state-of-the-art outcome instruments with the current state-of-the-art process instruments. This I state as my proposal of where this psycho-analytic therapy research arena is (can be) at this point in time.

New Outcome Measures for Structural Personality Change

But first a statement of the new outcome study possibilities. Throughout the several generations of therapy outcome research described to this point, the assessments of outcome were based on the judgments of experienced clinicians and/or a variety of standardized measures of symptom change or changes in manifest behavior patterns. These outcome measures were not designed to tap underlying changes in personality organization usually described as structural change, which are putatively the specific kinds of change that psychoanalytic therapies are designed to achieve, beyond just changes in symptoms or altered techniques of adjustment that are presumably all that non-psychoanalytic psycho-therapies can bring about.

It was to fill this glaring gap in our outcome research armamentarium that a group in San Francisco created a successor to the Menninger Psychotherapy Research Project (PRP), PRP-II, during the second half of the decade of the '80s (Wallerstein, 1988b; DeWitt, Hartley, Rosenberg, Zilberg, & Wallerstein, 1991; Zilberg, Wallerstein, DeWitt, Hartley, & Rosenberg, 1991). This involved the creation of a set of scales, designated Scales of Psychological Capacities (SPC), 17 in number, designed to create a profile of personality functioning, which, if altered in configuration over the course of therapy, would reflect changes in underlying personality organization, i.e. structural changes in the ego, in a way that would be agreed by the adherents of the varying theoretical perspectives within our currently pluralistic psychoanalytic world.

At the time that our San Francisco research group created the SPC, we felt we were the first to venture in this direction; and our scales did take root and are now deployed quite widely in therapy research, both in the United States and in a range of countries in Europe, with extant translations into five European languages. However, similar efforts (unknown to us at the time) were going on, to fill the same need, in other analytic research centers, both here and abroad, some simultaneous with our own, and some in the years since—and as far as I can tell, each independent of every other. By my count—and once more, I may be slighting some equally accomplished programs that have not yet come to my attention—there are at least eight other sets of scales designed to the same end, developed in other centers, tested to good psychometric qualities, and in use in various research programs around the world.

The others I have in mind—again, just to list them—are: (1) the Karolinska Psychodynamic Profile (KAPP), created in Sweden, simultaneously with our SPC, but totally independently, with also, coincidentally, 17 scales of *personality attributes,* conceptually very comparable to our *capacities,* and in a significant number, quite identical; (2) the Operationalized Psychodynamic Diagnosis (OPD), again, a conceptually very comparable instrument, this one created by German researchers; (3) the Structured Interview of Personality Organization (STIPO), created by the Kernberg-Clarkin group at Cornell, covering 94 areas of inquiry, divided into six overall domains of personality functioning; (4) the McGlashan Semistructured Interview (MSI), similar to the STIPO, covering 32 areas of personality functioning; (5) the Analytic Process Scales (APS), created by Waldron and his group in New York, designed as a *process* measure to assess the contributions of the analyst, of the patient, and of the interactional characteristics of their relationship, to the evolving analytic process, and already listed under process measures, but usable (and used) in before-and-after application, to assess personality *outcome* as well; (6) the Psychotherapy Process Q-Set (PPQS), a Q-sort providing for the description and classification of treatment *processes* in a form suitable for quantitative analysis, and also already listed under process measures, but also usable, in similar before-and-after application, as an *outcome* measure of personality; (7) the Shedler-Westen Assessment Procedure (SWAP), also a Q-sort, but differently constructed, and geared to assessment of overall personality functioning; and (8) the Object Relations Inventory (ORI), created by Blatt and his colleagues at Yale, organized, as a measure of personality structure, into two separate scales of personality organization, a Differentiation-Relatedness Scale of Self and Object Representations, and a trait sequence, Qualitative and Structural Dimensions of Parental Description. Again, like the array of the major process research instruments, previously listed, an impressive ensemble indeed.

FULFILLMENT OF A RESEARCH VISION

Which brings me to the present and the projected future for analytic therapy research, the possibility for the realization of the original vision of CAMP, when the necessary material resources can be generated. It is to bring the array of process measures into conjunction with the now assembled array of outcome measures that are most relevant to the claims of the psychoanalytic therapies, i.e., the outcome measures of structural change just listed, all in relation to a centralized shared database, not only of currently available audiotaped and transcribed hours, but ultimately and ideally, to new analytic therapies, starting prospectively from their initial diagnostic process, and carrying through to the natural terminations of the treatments, and beyond that, to predetermined points of follow-up study some years later. The structure for this fully elaborated program has been laid out in the original prospectus of CAMP (Wallerstein, 1991).

It is a breathtakingly grand vision, for which we collectively do have the conceptual and technical resources at this point in time, and a far cry indeed from where we were at the beginnings of this work, back in 1917, with the first report of a simple estimation by the treating clinician of how successful he felt he had been with a significant cohort of patients treated in the first decade of psychoanalysis in America. This vision represents my research convictions as to where we currently stand, and my research credo as well. It contains the promise of filling out the substantive knowledge base for each kind of patient along the psychopathological spectrum, of what psychoanalytic therapy can achieve, and how, through what means, it is achieved—the affirmative response to the two simple questions, with which our own research program, along with so many other research programs, was begun; and in this sense giving needed added meaning to psychoanalysis as a science of the mind, and needed added help to those who come to psychoanalytic therapy. It is up to our current and its successor generations of psychoanalytic therapy researchers to fulfill that dream.

REFERENCES

Alexander, F. (1937). *Five-year report of the Chicago Institute for Psychoanalysis: 1932-1937.* Chicago: Chicago Institute for Psychoanalysis.

Bachrach, H. M., Galatzer-Levy, R., Skolnikoff, A. Z., & Waldron, S., Jr. (1991). On the efficacy of psychoanalysis. *Journal of the American Psychoanalytic Association, 39,* 871-916.

Bachrach, H. M., Weber, J. J., & Solomon, M. (1985). Factors associated with the outcome of psychoanalysis (clinical and methodological considerations). Report of the Columbia Psychoanalytic Center Research Project (IV). *International Review of Psychoanalysis, 12,* 379-388.

Bucci, W. (in press). Building the interface of research and practice: Achievements and unresolved questions. In W. Bucci & N. Freedman (Eds.), The integration of clinical and research perspectives in psychoanalysis: A tribute to the work of Robert Wallerstein. *Psychological Issues Monograph.* Madison, CT: International Universities Press.

Carmichael, H. T. (1956). Sound film recording of psychoanalytic therapy: A therapist's experiences and reactions. In L. A. Gottschalk & A. H. Auerbach (Eds.) *Methods of Research in Psychotherapy* (pp. 50-59). New York: Appleton-Century-Crofts.

Coriat, I. (1917). Some statistical results in the psychoanalytical treatment of the psychoneuroses. *Psychoanalytic Review, 4,* 209-216.

Dahl, H., Kächele, H., & Thomä, H. (1988). *Psychoanalytic Process Research Strategies.* Berlin: Springer-Verlag.

DeWitt, K. N., Hartley, D. E., Rosenberg, S. E., Zilberg, N. J., & Wallerstein, R. S. (1991). Scales of psychological capacities: Development of an assessment approach. *Psychoanalysis and Contemporary Thought, 14,* 343-361.

Erle, J. B. (1979). An approach to the study of analyzability and analysis: The course of forty consecutive cases selected for supervised analysis. *Psychoanalytic Quarterly, 48,* 198-228.

Erle, J. B., & Goldberg, D. A. (1979). Problems in the assessment of analyzability. *Psychoanalytic Quarterly, 48,* 48-84.

Erle, J. B., & Goldberg, D. A. (1984). Observations on assessment of analyzability by experienced analysts. *Journal of the American Psychoanalytic Association, 32,* 715-737.

Erle, J. B., & Goldberg, D. A. (2003). The course of 253 analyses from selection to outcome. *Journal of the American Psychoanalytic Association, 51,* 257-293.

Feldman, F. (1968). Results of psychoanalysis in clinic case assignments. *Journal of the American Psychoanalytic Association, 16,* 274-300.

Fenichel, O. (1930). Statistischer bericht über die therapeutische tätigkeit, 1920-1930. *Intern. Psychoanal. Verlag,* 13-19.

Fonagy, P., & Target, M. (1994). The efficacy of psychoanalysis for children with disruptive disorders. *Journal of the American Academy of Child and Adolescent Psychiatry, 33,* 45-55.

Fonagy, P., & Target, M. (1996). Predictors of outcome in child psychoanalysis: A retrospective study of 763 cases at the Anna Freud Centre. *Journal of the American Psychoanalytic Association, 44,* 27-77.

Freedman, N., Lasky, R., & Hurvich, M. (2003). Two pathways towards knowing psychoanalytic process. In M. Leuzinger-Bohleber, A. Dreher, & J. Canestri (Eds.), *Pluralism and unity? Methods of research in psychoanalysis* (pp. 207-221). London, International Psychoanalytical Association.

Glover, E. (1954). The indications for psycho-analysis. *Journal of Mental Science, 100,* 393-401.

Hamburg, D. A., Bibring, G. L., Fisher, C., Stanton, A. H., Wallerstein, R. S., Weinstock, H. I., et al. (1967). Report of ad hoc committee on Central Fact-Gathering Data of the American Psychoanalytic Association. *Journal of the American Psychoanalytic Association, 15,* 841-861.

Jones, E. (1936). *Decannual report of the London Clinic of Psychoanalysis, 1926-1937.* London: London Clinic of Psychoanalysis.

Kantrowitz, J. L. (1986). The role of the patient-analyst "match" in the outcome of psychoanalysis. *Annual of Psychoanalysis, 14,* 273-297.

Kantrowitz, J. L., Katz, A. L., Greenman, D. K., Morris, H., Paolitto, F., Sashin, J., et al. (1989). The patient-analyst match and the outcome of psychoanalysis: A pilot study. *Journal of the American Psychoanalytic Association, 37,* 893-919.

Kantrowitz, J. L., Katz, A. L., & Paolitto, F. (1990a). Follow-up of psychoanalysis five to ten years after termination: I. Stability of change. *Journal of the American Psychoanalytic Association, 38,* 471-496.

Kantrowitz, J. L., Katz, A. L., & Paolitto, F. (1990b). Follow-up of psychoanalysis five to ten years after termination: II. Development of the self-analytic function. *Journal of the American Psychoanalytic Association, 38,* 637-654.

Kantrowitz, J. L., Katz, A. L., & Paolitto, F. (1990c). Follow-up of psychoanalysis five to ten years after termination: III. The relation between the resolution of the transference and the patient-analyst match. *Journal of the American Psychoanalytic Association, 38,* 655-678.

Kantrowitz, J. L., Katz, A. L., Paolitto, F., Sashin, J., & Solomon, L. (1987a). Changes in the level and quality of object relationships in psychoanalysis: Follow-up of a longitudinal prospective study. *Journal of the American Psychoanalytic Association, 35,* 23-46.

Kantrowitz, J. L., Katz, A. L., Paolitto, F., Sashin, J., & Solomon, L. (1987b). The role of reality testing in psychoanalysis: Follow-up of 22 cases. *Journal of the American Psychoanalytic Association, 35,* 367-385.

Kantrowitz, J. L., Paolitto, F., Sashin, J., Solomon, L., & Katz, A. L. (1986). Affect availability, tolerance, complexity, and modulation in psychoanalysis: Follow-up of a longitudinal prospective study. *Journal of the American Psychoanalytic Association, 34,* 529-559.

Knapp, P. H., Levin, S., McCarter, R. H., Wermer, H., & Zetzel, E. (1960). Suitability for psychoanalysis: A review of one hundred supervised analytic cases. *Psychoanalytic Quarterly, 29,* 459-477.

Knight, R. P. (1941). Evaluation of the results of psychoanalytic therapy. *American Journal of Psychiatry, 98,* 434-446.

Leuzinger-Bohleber, M. (1997). " . . . die Fähigkeit zu lieben, zuarbeiten und des Leben zu geniessen." *Zu den vielen Facetten psychoanalytischer Katamneseforschung.* Giessen, Germany: Psychosozial Verlag.

López-Moreno, C., Dorfman-Lerner, B., Roussos, A., & Schalayeff, C., (1999). Investigación empírica en Psicoanálisis. *Revista de Psicoanálisis,* APA. Tomo LVI, 677-693.

Norman, H. F., Blacker, K. H., Oremland, J. D., & Barrett, W. G. (1976). The fate of the transference neurosis after termination of a satisfactory analysis. *Journal of the American Psychoanalytic Association, 24,* 471–498.

Oremland, J. D., Blacker, K. H., & Norman, H. F. (1975). Incompleteness in "successful" psychoanalysis: A follow-up study. *Journal of the American Psychoanalytic Association, 23,* 819-844.

Pfeffer, A. Z. (1959). A procedure for evaluating the results of psychoanalysis: A preliminary report. *Journal of the American Psychoanalytic Association, 7,* 418-444.

Pfeffer, A. Z. (1961). Follow-up study of a satisfactory analysis. *Journal of the American Psychoanalytic Association, 9,* 698-718.

Pfeffer, A. Z. (1963). The meaning of the analyst after analysis: A contribution to the theory of therapeutic results. *Journal of the American Psychoanalytic Association, 11,* 229-244.

Pötzl, O. (1960). The relationship between experimentally induced dream images and indirect vision. *Psychological Issues, 2,* 41-120. (Original work published in 1917.)

Rangell, L. (1990). An overview of the ending of an analysis. In *The human Core: The intrapsychic base of behavior* (Vol. 2, pp. 703-725). Madison, CT: International Universities Press. (Original work published in 1966.)

Sandell, R., Blomberg, J., Lazar, A., Carlsson, J., Broberg, J., & Schubert, J. (2000). Varieties of long-term outcome among patients in psychoanalysis and long-term psychotherapy: A review of findings in the Stockholm Outcome of Psychoanalysis and Psychotherapy Project (STOPP). *International Journal of Psychoanalysis, 81,* 921–942.

Sashin, J. I., Eldred, S. H., & van Amerongen, S. T. (1975). A search for predictive factors in institute supervised cases: A retrospective study of 183 cases from 1959 to 1966 at the Boston Psychoanalytic Society and Institute. *International Journal of Psychoanalysis, 56,* 343-359.

Schlessinger, N., & Robbins, F. P. (1974). Assessment and follow-up in psychoanalysis. *Journal of the American Psychoanalytic Association, 22,* 542-567.

Schlessinger, N., & Robbins, F. P. (1975). The psychoanalytic process: Recurrent patterns of conflict and changes in ego functions. *Journal of the American Psychoanalytic Association, 23,* 761-782.

Schlessinger, N., & Robbins, F. P. (1983). *A developmental view of the psychoanalytic process: Follow-up studies and their consequences.* New York: International Universities Press.

Shakow, D., & Rapaport, D. (1964). *The influence of Freud in American psychology. Psychological Issues Monograph*(13). New York: International Universities Press.

Strupp, H. H. (1960). Some comments on the future of research in psychotherapy. *Behavioral Science, 5,* 60–70.

Strupp, H. H., Schacht, T. E., & Henry, W. P. (1988). *Problem-treatment-outcome congruence: A principle whose time has come.* In H. Dahl, H. Kächele, & H. Thomä (Eds.), *Psychoanalytic process research strategies* (pp. 1-14). Berlin: Springer-Verlag.

Szecsody, I., Varvin, S., Amadei, G., Stoker, J., Beenen, F., Klockars, L., et al. (1997 August). *The European Multi-Site Collaborative Study of Psychoanalysis (Sweden, Finland, Norway, Holland & Italy).* Paper presented at the Symposium on Outcome Research, International Psychoanalytical Association Congress, Barcelona, Spain.

Target, M., & Fonagy, P. (1994a). The efficacy of psychoanalysis for children with emotional disorders. *Journal of the American Academy of Child and Adolescent Psychiatry, 33,* 361-371.

Target, M., & Fonagy, P. (1994b). The efficacy of psychoanalysis for children: Prediction of outcome in a developmental context. *Journal of the American Academy of Child and Adolescent Psychiatry, 33,* 1134-1144.

Wallerstein, R. S. (1986). *Forty-two lives in treatment: A study of psychoanalysis and psychotherapy.* New York: Guilford Press.

Wallerstein, R. S. (1988a). Psychoanalysis and psychotherapy: Relative roles reconsidered. *Annual of Psychoanalysis, 16,* 129-151.

Wallerstein, R. S. (1988b). Assessment of structural change in psychoanalytic therapy and research. *Journal of the American Psychoanalytic Association, 36 (Supplement),* 241-261.

Wallerstein, R. S. (1991). *Proposal to the Ludwig Foundation for a collaborative multi-site program of psychoanalytic therapy research.* Unpublished manuscript.

Wallerstein, R. S. (2001). The generations of psychotherapy research: An overview. *Psychoanalytic Psychology, 18,* 243-267.

Wallerstein, R. S. (in press). My life as a psychoanalytic therapy researcher and in CAMP. In, W. Bucci & N. Freedman (Eds.), *The integration of clinical and research perspectives in psychoanalysis: A tribute to the work of Robert Wallerstein.* Psychological Issues Monograph. Madison, CT: International Universities Press.

Wallerstein, R. S., Robbins, L. L., Sargent, H. D., & Luborsky, L. (1956). The Psychotherapy Research Project of The Menninger Foundation. *Bulletin of the Menninger Clinic, 20,* 221-278.

Wallerstein, R. S., & Sampson, H. (1971). Issues in research in the psychoanalytic process. *International Journal of Psychoanalysis, 52,* 11-50.

Weber, J. J., Bachrach, H. M., & Solomon, M. (1985a). Factors associated with the outcome of psychoanalysis: Report of the Columbia Psychoanalytic Center Research Project (II). *International Review of Psychoanalysis, 12,* 127-141.

Weber, J. J., Bachrach, H. M., & Solomon, M. (1985b). Factors associated with the outcome of psychoanalysis: Report of the Columbia Psychoanalytic Center Research Project (III). *International Review of Psychoanalysis, 12,* 251-262.

Weber, J. J., Solomon, M., & Bachrach, H. M. (1985). Characteristics of psychoanalytic clinic patients: Report of the Columbia Psychoanalytic Center Research Project (I). *International Review of Psychoanalysis, 12,* 13-26.

Zilberg, N. J., Wallerstein, R. S., DeWitt, K. N., Hartley, D., & Rosenberg, S. E. (1991). A conceptual analysis and strategy for assessing structural change. *Psychoanalytical and Contemporary Thought 14,* 317-342.

Evaluating Efficacy, Effectiveness, and Mutative Factors in Psychodynamic Psychotherapies

Sidney J. Blatt, PhD,[1] John S. Auerbach, PhD,[2] David C. Zuroff, PhD,[3] Golan Shahar, PhD[4]

Editor's Note: This paper demonstrates that therapeutic process variables contribute to outcome more significantly than the type of treatment per se. The authors also show that a psychodynamic framework defines and informs clinical work with these formative therapeutic processes, further documenting the importance of the therapeutic relationship and patient personality factors. The authors present the development by Blatt and his collaborators of the conceptions of two distinctive major character configurations, the anaclitic, or relational, based centrally on the wish and need for relatedness with others, and the introjective, or self-definitional, based centrally on the wish and need for a differentiated and integrated identity and self-agency. They describe—and support with empirical demonstration—the differences in life experience, in drive focus, and in defensive organization, of these predominant character styles, and then in the distinctive configurations of psychopathology that characteristically can eventuate within each, as well as finally, in their differential amenability to more supportive (ego-strengthening) or more expressive (insight-aiming) therapeutic approaches.

Alongside their conceptual development, the authors present the development and deployment of their instruments, centrally the Object Relations Inventory (ORI), to operationalize and to empirically test their premises in both non-clinical (psychologically healthy) and clinical (mentally and emotionally ill) populations. In this they demonstrate in detail how their measure (one of those indicated in the review by Wallerstein in the immediately preceding chapter) can be used to test efficacy, effectiveness, and mutative factors in psychoanalytically-based psychotherapies.

[1] Professor of Psychiatry and Psychology, Departments of Psychiatry and Psychology, Yale University
[2] Professor, East Tennessee State University; Coordinator of the Post-Traumatic Stress Program, J. H. Quillen Veterans Affairs Medical Center
[3] Professor, Department of Psychology, McGill University
[4] Assistant Professor of Psychiatry and Psychology, Departments of Psychiatry and Psychology, Yale University

ABSTRACT

Analyses of data from several studies of the therapeutic process in intensive psychodynamic treatment of outpatients and of seriously disturbed, treatment-resistant inpatients, as well as from brief outpatient treatment of patients with major depression, led to several conclusions that are consistent with psychodynamic formulations. First, evaluation of therapeutic progress must go beyond assessment of symptom reduction as the primary outcome measure and include assessments of decreased vulnerability to stress and the development of enhanced adaptive capacities as well as more mature and adaptive representations (i.e., cognitive-affective schemas) of self and of others. These changes in personality organization and structure are essential in most forms of psychopathology if symptomatic improvement is to be sustained without extensive relapse. Second, therapeutic outcome is primarily determined not by the type of treatment provided, as guided by treatment manuals (e.g., cognitive behavioral therapy [CBT] and interpersonal therapy [IPT]), but by the therapist's ability to appreciate the nature of the patient's disturbances and personality organization, an understanding that is essential for establishing a therapeutic relationship that enables the patient to feel trust and confidence in the therapist and to participate actively in the treatment process. These findings indicate that psychodynamic formulations provide a basis for understanding important differences in patients' personality organization and their psychological disturbance, and that this understanding is central to treatment efficacy and effectiveness.

INTRODUCTION

Responsibility to our patients and to our disciplines demands that we systematically evaluate our interventions in mental health services. Considerable effort has recently been devoted to developing guidelines for the identification of evidence-based treatments (EBTs) in mental health. Most of these attempts have been based on two fundamental assumptions: that the type of treatment is the primary factor determining therapeutic outcome, and the therapeutic outcome is most effectively assessed by a reduction of manifest symptoms. Meta-analyses of a wide range of studies (e.g., Lambert & Barley, 2002), extensive literature reviews (e.g., Westen, Novotny, & Thompson-Brenner, 2004), and analyses of data from probably the most comprehensive data set ever established in psychotherapy research (Blatt & Zuroff, 2005), the Treatment for Depression Collaborative Research Program (TDCRP), sponsored and implemented by the National Institute of Mental Health (NIMH) (Elkin, Parloff, Hadley, & Autry, 1985), however, indicate a number of limitations of these assumptions in the attempts to identify empirically supported treatments. In particular, our findings (Blatt & Zuroff, 2005; Zuroff & Blatt, in press) indicate that the quality of the therapeutic relationship, established very early in the treatment process, and not the type of treatment provided, is critical to treatment outcome. These limitations suggest that a necessary first step in identifying effective treatments is a fuller understanding of the processes that facilitate therapeutic change (Blatt, Shahar & Zuroff, 2002).

Much treatment research has compared various forms of treatment with either waiting list controls or treatment as usual (TAU), as defined by contemporary clinical practice in the community. Both of these designs, however, frequently involve weak control groups. Comparison with waiting list controls indicates only that doing something is better than doing nothing, but this design provides little information about the nature of the treatment process and the mechanisms of therapeutic change (Blatt, Shahar, & Zuroff, 2002). Also, TAU is usually a weak control because most studies using a TAU control group provide relatively little information about the treatment offered by individual clinicians in the community. Additionally, several important collateral differences, beyond the type of the treatment provided, often exist within a research context by members of a research team and the treatment provided by a clinician in solo practice in the community. Participation in a research team usually involves a degree of commitment and enthusiasm, a social support structure, and an organization that facilitates communication among the participating clinicians. A similar context is usually lacking for the community clinician in solo practice. These differences in treatment context could contribute to important differences in therapeutic outcome (Blatt & Zuroff, 2005).

Given these limitations of waiting lists and of TAU as control conditions in psychotherapy research, a more effective and possibly more powerful research design is the comparison of active treatments, but findings from comparative treatment trials are usually equivocal about the superiority of particular forms of treatment. Extensive meta-analyses of comparative treatment trials usually indicate relatively few differences in therapeutic efficacy and effectiveness among various forms of active treatment (e.g., American Psychiatric Association, 1982; Frank, 1979, 1982; Luborsky, 1962; Shapiro & Shapiro, 1982; Smith, Glass, & Miller, 1980). This lack of significant differences among active treatments is so frequent that it has been labeled, from Alice in Wonderland, the Dodo bird effect (Frank 1973; Luborsky, Diguer, McLellan, & Woody, 1995; Luborsky, et al., 2002; Luborsky, Singer, & Luborsky, 1975) in which the declaration is made that "everyone has won and all must have prizes."

This functional equivalence suggests that either our research methods are insensitive to differences among various forms of treatment (e.g., Kazdin, 1986; VandenBos & Pino, 1980; Wortman, 1983) or that these various forms of treatment share common processes (e.g., Frank, 1979; Strupp & Binder, 1984) that make them functionally equivalent (Lambert, Shapiro, & Bergin, 1986; Stiles, Shapiro, & Elliott, 1986). These shared processes, including the therapeutic alliance, are often referred to as nonspecific effects. Additionally, the recent identification of the impact of allegiance effects in influencing therapeutic outcome (Luborsky, et al., 1999), again possibly through the effects of enthusiasm and commitment, raises further complications about many of the findings from the comparison of active treatments. Thus, although a few types of treatment have been identified as effective in reducing some specific symptoms, most studies report a functional equivalence among various forms of treatment.

A possible factor underlying the dodo bird effect is the use of manifest symptoms as the primary criterion of therapeutic outcome, mainly because some symptom reduction can be realized not only through psychotherapy but also through support from family and friends (e.g., Brown & Harris, 1978; Cohen & Wills, 1985) or through activities like writing about stressful experiences (e.g., Pennebaker, 1997). Symptom-focused approaches to psychotherapy usually reveal few, if any, differences in treatment outcome among many psychotherapeutic approaches (Blatt & Zuroff, 2005). In addition, symptom reduction without a reduction in vulnerability can result in relapse.

The limitations of symptom reduction as the primary measure of therapeutic change have recently been demonstrated in further analyses of data collected as part of the NIMH-sponsored TDCRP (Blatt & Zuroff, 2005). Although medication resulted in a more rapid decline in symptoms than psychotherapy (Gibbons, et al., 1993), analyses of data from this comprehensive research program found no differences in the degree of symptom reduction among the three active treatments evaluated in this extensive and comprehensive study (cognitive-behavioral therapy [CBT], interpersonal therapy [IPT] and Imipramine with clinical management [IMI-CM]) at termination, after 16 weeks of treatment (e.g., Elkin, 1994), and at a follow-up assessment 18 months after termination (Blatt, Zuroff, Bondi & Sanislow, 2000). Further analyses of the TDCRP data (e.g., Blatt, et al., 2000; Zuroff, Blatt, Krupnick & Sotsky, 2003), however, revealed significant treatment differences in patients' ratings of the impact of the treatment on their life adjustment at three follow-up assessments conducted 6, 12, and 18 months after termination. Specifically, patients in both CBT and IPT reported significantly greater increase in their capacity to establish and maintain interpersonal relationships and to recognize, understand, and cope with their symptoms of depression than did patients receiving medication (IMI-CM). Additional analyses (Zuroff, et al., 2003) highlight the importance of this impact of treatment on patients' reports of their adaptive capacities. Patients who reported that treatment contributed substantially to their adaptive capacities at the 6-month follow-up assessment had significantly fewer depressive symptoms in response to stressful life events during the remaining 12 months of the follow-up period. Thus, reports by the patients early in the follow-up period, of an enhanced adaptive capacity (EAC), predicted a significantly reduced vulnerability to stressful life events later in the follow-up period.

In addition to indicating the long-term advantage of psychotherapy over medication, these findings suggest that treatment effects are more likely to be found in measures that assess change in adaptive capacities, or a reduction in vulnerability, than in symptom reduction. Thus, evaluations of therapeutic gain, in addition to symptom reduction, should include assessments of the reduction of the vulnerability to depression and the development of resilience as expressed in increased adaptive capacities and in the ability to manage stressful life events (Blatt & Zuroff, 2005).

Extensive further analyses of data from the TDCRP (see summary in Blatt & Zuroff, 2005; Zuroff & Blatt, in press) also indicate that primary among the determinants of therapeutic outcome in the brief outpatient treatment for serious depression are the quality of the therapeutic relationship that patient and therapist establish very early in the treatment process (by the second treatment session) and the pretreatment personality characteristics of the patients, especially their level of pretreatment perfectionism. Specifically, a good therapeutic alliance and a low level of pretreatment perfectionism both independently predicted significantly greater reductions of symptoms and of vulnerability to depression, as well as a significantly greater increase in adaptive capacities and stress resilience.

These findings, consistent with the recent emphasis on the importance of the therapeutic relationship in the treatment process (e.g., Norcross, 2002; Wampold, 2001), suggest that efforts to identify empirically based treatments (EBT's) require a much more complex view of the treatment process than just evaluating the effects of particular treatments in reducing focal symptoms. Rather, these findings indicate that it is important to include dimensions of the treatment process, especially the quality of the therapeutic relationship and patients' pretreatment characteristics, and to consider their impact on the therapeutic process across a range of outcome measures beyond symptom reduction. Psychotherapy research must go beyond the simple comparisons of the efficacy and effectiveness of particular forms of treatment in the reduction of focal symptoms. Rather, treatment research needs to address more complex questions like what kinds of treatments are effective, for what kinds of patients, in what kinds of ways, and through what kinds of mechanisms (Blatt, Shahar, & Zuroff, 2002; Blatt & Shahar, 2004a; Zuroff, Blatt, Krupnick, & Sotsky, 2003; Paul, 1969).

This paper addresses three issues that must be considered in any attempt to identify empirically-based treatments, especially long-term, intensive, psychodynamically oriented treatment:

1. The role of patient pretreatment characteristics in determining therapeutic outcome,
2. The development of appropriate measures of therapeutic change beyond symptom reduction, particularly the development of reliable methods for systematically assessing change in aspects of personality organization, and
3. A consideration of the possible mechanisms of therapeutic change.

The sections to follow are devoted to these fundamental issues:

- The importance of pretreatment personality characteristics and the quality of the therapeutic relationship, as experienced by the patient, in determining differential responses to treatment,

- The importance of assessing aspects of personality organization (psychic structure) in evaluating both long-term, intensive psychodynamic as well as brief, manual-directed treatments, and

- The identification of mutative factors in the treatment process.

PATIENT PRETREATMENT CHARACTERISTICS AND THERAPEUTIC OUTCOME

Lee Cronbach (1953), the distinguished research methodologist, noted the importance of evaluating patient-treatment and patient-outcome interactions in psychotherapy research because different types of patients may be responsive to different aspects of the treatment process and may respond to treatment in different, but in equally desirable, ways. Cronbach and others since (e.g., Beutler, 1991) have argued that differences in therapeutic outcome may be a function of the congruence of patient characteristics with aspects of the treatment process. Different types of patients may respond more effectively to different types of treatment or respond to the same type of treatment in divergent, but in equally desirable, ways (Blatt & Felsen, 1993). Kiesler (1966, p. 110) noted that among the most salient obstacles to the development of methodologically sophisticated psychotherapy research are assumptions of "patient and therapist uniformity"— that "patients at the start of treatment are more alike than they are different." Kiesler (1966, p. 113) therefore stressed the need to abandon these uniformity myths in favor of "designs that can incorporate relevant patient variables and crucial therapist dimensions so that one can assess which therapist behaviors are more effective with which type of patients." The inclusion of patient-treatment and patient-outcome interactions in psychotherapy research, however, requires a conceptual model that identifies meaningful personality variables that could mediate the relationships among patient characteristics, type of treatment, and type of therapeutic outcome (Beutler, 1991), a theoretical framework that links patients' characteristics with central aspects of the therapeutic process. Research not guided by theoretically derived considerations and supported by previous empirical investigations can lead researchers into a "hall of mirrors" (Cronbach, 1975) because of the complexity of the potential interactions. According to Beutler (1991, p. 222), "one can avoid entering (this) hall of mirrors by exploring the interactions between theoretically meaningful ... variables" that are relevant to the processes assumed to underlie psychological change (see also Smith & Sechrest, 1991; Snow, 1991).

One model for introducing patient variables into psychotherapy research has been a psychodynamic theory of personality development and psychopathology developed by Blatt and colleagues (e.g., Blatt, 1974, 1991, 1995, in press; Blatt & Blass, 1990, 1996; Blatt & Shichman, 1983) that focuses on two fundamental developmental lines in personality development: (1) a relational or anaclitic line that involves the development of the capacity to establish increasingly mature and mutually satisfying interpersonal relationships, and (2) a self-definitional or introjective line that involves the development of a consolidated, realistic, essentially positive, differentiated, and integrated identity. These two developmental lines normally evolve throughout life in a reciprocal or dialectic transaction. An increasingly differentiated, integrated, and mature sense of self is contingent on establishing satisfying interpersonal relationships, and, conversely, the continued development of increasingly mature and satisfying interpersonal relationships is contingent on the development of a more mature self-concept and identity. In normal personality development, these two developmental processes evolve in an interactive, reciprocally balanced, mutually facilitating fashion (Blatt, in press; Blatt & Blass, 1990, 1992, 1996; Blatt & Shichman, 1983).

The identification of the centrality of the two dimensions of relatedness and self-definition in personality development is consistent with formulations from a wide range of personality theories, both psychoanalytic and nonpsychoanalytic. Freud (1930), for example, differentiated between egotistic and altruistic urges, between erotic individuals who focus on emotional relationships and narcissistic individuals who are inclined to be self-sufficient, between object and ego libido, and between libidinal drives in the service of attachment and aggressive drives necessary for autonomy, mastery, and self-definition (Freud 1914, 1926). Loewald (1962, p. 490) noted that Freud's explorations of

> ... these various modes of separation and union ... [identify a] polarity inherent in individual existence of individuation and 'primary narcissistic union'—a polarity that Freud attempted to conceptualize by various approaches and that he recognized and insisted upon from beginning to end by his dualistic conception of instincts, of human nature, and of life itself.

Shor and Sanville (1978) discussed psychological development as involving a fundamental oscillation between "necessary connectedness" and "inevitable separations" or between "intimacy and autonomy." A wide range of nonpsychoanalytic personality theorists (e.g., Angyal, 1951; Bakan, 1966; Benjamin, 1974; McAdams, 1985; McClelland, 1986; Wiggins, 1991) has also discussed relatedness and self-definition as two primary dimensions of personality organization.

The delineation of relatedness and self-definition as two fundamental psychological dimensions has enabled investigators from different theoretical orientations (e.g., Arieti & Bemporad, 1978, 1980; Beck, 1983; Blatt, 1974, 1998, 2004;

Blatt, D'Afflitti, & Quinlan, 1976; Blatt, Quinlan, Chevron, McDonald & Zuroff, 1982; Bowlby, 1988a, 1988b) to identify two types of depression (Blatt & Maroudas, 1992)—an anaclitic depression centered on feelings of loneliness, abandonment, and neglect and an introjective depression focused on issues of self-worth and feelings of failure and guilt (see, e.g., Blatt, 1974, 1998; Blatt, D'Afflitti, et al., 1976; Blatt, et al., 1982). Extensive empirical investigation (see Blatt, 2004; Blatt & Zuroff, 1992; Luyten, 2002) indicates consistent differences in the life experiences (both current and early) of these two types of depressed individuals (Blatt & Homann, 1992), as well as major differences in their basic character styles and in the clinical expression of their depression (Blatt, et al., 1982).

The differentiation between individuals preoccupied with issues of relatedness and those with issues of self-definition has also enabled investigators to identify an empirically derived structure for integrating the diversity of personality disorders described in Axis II of DSM-IV (American Psychiatric Association, 1994). Systematic empirical investigation of outpatients (Morse, Robins, & Gittes-Fox, 2002; Ouimette, Klein, Anderson, Liso, & Lizardi, 1994) and of inpatients (Levy, et al., 1995) found that the various personality disorders can be organized into two primary configurations—one organized around issues of relatedness and the other around issues of self-definition. Ouimette, et al. and Morse, et al. with outpatients, and Levy, et al. with inpatients, found that dependent, histrionic, and borderline personality disorders (anaclitic patients) had significantly greater preoccupation with issues of relatedness than with issues of self-definition. Conversely, individuals with paranoid, schizoid, schizotypal, antisocial, narcissistic, avoidant, obsessive-compulsive, and self-defeating personality disorders (introjective patients) had significantly greater preoccupation with issues of self-definition than with issues of relatedness (Blatt & Levy, 1998).

Various forms of psychopathology can be conceptualized as involving an overemphasis and exaggeration of one of these developmental lines and the defensive avoidance of the other. This distorted overemphasis defines two distinct configurations of psychopathology, each containing several types of disordered behavior that range from relatively severe to relatively mild forms of disturbance.

Developmental and clinical considerations suggest that anaclitic psychopathologies are those disorders in which patients are preoccupied primarily with issues of relatedness and use mainly avoidant defenses (e.g., withdrawal, denial, repression) to cope with psychological conflict and stress. Anaclitic disorders involve a preoccupation with interpersonal relations and issues of trust, caring, intimacy, and sexuality; they range from more to less disturbed and include undifferentiated schizophrenia, borderline personality disorder, infantile (or dependent) character disorder, anaclitic depression, and hysterical disorders.

In contrast, introjective psychopathology includes disorders in which the patients are concerned with establishing and maintaining a viable sense of self.

Underlying issues range from a basic sense of separateness, through concerns about autonomy and control, to more complex internalized issues of guilt and self-worth. These patients use counteractive defenses (e.g., projection, rationalization, intellectualization, doing and undoing, reaction formation, overcompensation) to cope with conflict and stress. Introjective patients are more ideational and concerned with establishing, protecting, and maintaining a viable self-concept than they are with the quality of interpersonal relations and with achieving feelings of trust, warmth, and affection. Issues of anger and aggression, directed toward both self and others, are usually central to their difficulties. Introjective disorders, ranging from more to less severely disturbed, include paranoid schizophrenia; the over-ideational (or guilt-ridden) borderline, paranoid, and obsessive-compulsive personality disorders; introjective (guilt-ridden) depression; and phallic narcissism (Blatt, 1974, 1991, 1995; Blatt & Auerbach, 1988; Blatt & Shichman, 1983).

The differentiation between these two broad configurations of psychopathology can be made reliably from clinical case records (see, e.g., Blatt, 1992; Blatt & Ford, 1994). In contrast to the atheoretical DSM diagnostic scheme, based primarily on differences in manifest symptoms, the anaclitic-introjective (or relational-self-definitional) distinction derives from dynamic considerations, including differences in drive focus (libidinal vs. aggressive), types of defensive organization (avoidant vs. counteractive), and predominant character style (e.g., emphasis on an object vs. a self-orientation and on affects vs. cognition). Thus, various forms of psychopathology are no longer considered as discrete diseases but rather as interrelated disturbances that are the consequence of disruptions of normal psychological development. Continuity is therefore maintained in these theoretical formulations among normal psychological development, variations in normal character or personality organization, and different forms of psychological disturbance. Furthermore, continuity is maintained within clusters of various disorders so that pathways of potential regression and progression, as well as the processes of therapeutic change, can be understood more fully. Subsequent sections of this paper illustrate how this theoretically derived and empirically supported model of personality development and psychopathology can facilitate the introduction of patient variables into psychotherapy research.

MEASURES OF THERAPEUTIC CHANGE

All psychodynamic orientations to treatment agree that sustained symptom remission, although essential to any successful treatment outcome, is secondary to and dependent upon more basic changes in the personality structure. Yet, much of current psychotherapy research focuses primarily on the reduction of symptoms, often only at the termination of treatment, as the primary measure of therapeutic progress, partly because manifest symptoms, in contrast to dimensions of personality organization, are easier to observe and measure, and partly because patients often seek treatment primarily to obtain relief from those symptoms. But this primary focus on symptom reduction reveals little about the nature of therapeutic change.

The assessment of therapeutic change in long-term, intense psychodynamic treatment usually goes beyond evaluating the reduction of manifest symptoms and includes measures of change in personality organization. Thus, research guided by psychoanalytic conceptualizations has the potential to facilitate the examination of aspects of the processes of therapeutic change that are often ignored in symptom-focused approaches to treatment and to treatment research. The measurement of psychodynamic variables of change in personality organization is complex, however, because of the difficulty arriving at working definitions of many of these constructs and in developing reliable measures for evaluating them. One fruitful approach to this problem has involved the development of measures to assess dimensions of mental representation, specifically the developmental organization and thematic content of concepts of the self and of significant others.

Mental representation is a central theoretical construct in multiple areas within psychology (e.g., psychoanalytic object relations theory, attachment theory and research, developmental psychology, and social cognition). This emphasis on mental representation has recently had a major impact on personality assessment (Blatt, 1990, 1999; Leichtman, 1996a, 1996b). The recognition of the centrality of mental representation in personality organization, for example, has led to the development of new approaches for evaluating responses to the Rorschach, not only their content but also their structural organization. Rorschach protocols, if evaluated with scoring systems derived from fundamental psychoanalytic and developmental concepts, can provide a methodology for the independent evaluation of patients' psychological development in the treatment process. Several relatively new methods have reliably evaluated aspects of object representation in Rorschach protocols in cross-sectional studies of patients with different diagnoses (e.g., Blatt, Brenneis, Schimek, & Glick, 1976a, 1976b; Urist, 1977) as well as in the study of therapeutic change in long-term, intensive psychodynamic treatment (Blatt, 1992; Blatt & Ford, 1994; Blatt & Shahar, 2004b).[5]

Concept of the Object on the Rorschach (COR) Scale

Using concepts derived from developmental psychology (see, e.g., Werner 1948), Blatt, Brenneis, Schimek, and Glick (1976a, 1976b) developed a system for

---

[5] Blatt and Auerbach (2003) recently discussed the Object Relations Inventory (ORI; Blatt, Chevron, et al., 1988; Blatt, et al., 1979), which involves the collection of spontaneous descriptions of self and significant figures, as another method for evaluating changes in the content and structural organization of mental representations in long-term, intensive, psychodynamic treatment.

assessing the structural (cognitive) organization of the concept of the human figure on the Rorschach. The system evaluates responses with humanoid features
according to developmental principles of *differentiation* (i.e., types of human figures perceived: quasi-human part properties, human part properties, quasi-
human full figures, and full human figures), *articulation* (i.e., number and type of
perceptual and functional features attributed to figures), and *integration*, including the degree of internality in the motivation of action attributed to the figures
(unmotivated, reactive, and intentional action), the degree of integration of the
object and its action (fused, incongruent, nonspecific, and congruent action), the
content of the action (malevolent, benevolent), and the nature of any interaction
(active-passive, active-reactive, and active-active interactions). In each of these six
categories (differentiation, articulation, motivation of action, integration of the
object and its action, content of the action, and nature of interaction), responses
are scored along a developmental continuum.

This developmental analysis of responses that have human or humanoid features is made separately for responses that are accurately perceived (F +) and
inaccurately perceived (F-). Scores in each of the six categories are standardized,
and a weighted sum (developmental index, DI) and an average developmental
score (developmental mean, DM) is obtained for F + and for F-responses separately. The DI and the DM of the differentiation, articulation, and integration of
accurately perceived (F +) human forms (OR +) assess the capacity for investing
in appropriate interpersonal relationships; the DI and the DM of differentiated,
articulated, and integrated inaccurately perceived (F-) human forms (OR-) assess
the degree of investment in inappropriate, unrealistic, possibly autistic fantasies
rather than in realistic relationships. These variables can be scored reliably (see,
e.g., Blatt, et al., 1988; Blatt & Ford, 1994; Ritzler, Zambianco, Harder & Kaskey,
1980), and research indicates that the OR + variables develop longitudinally with
age from early adolescence to adulthood (Blatt, Brenneis, Schimek, & Glick,
1976b) and that the OR + and OR- variables are significantly related to independent estimates of psychopathology (see, e.g., Blatt, Brenneis, et al., 1976b; Blatt,
Schimek, & Brenneis, 1980; Lerner & St. Peter, 1984a, 1984b; Ritzler, et al.,
1980). Levy, Meehan, Auerbach and Blatt (2005) recently reviewed a wide-range
of research with this assessment method.

Mutuality of Autonomy (MOA) Scale

Another measure for assessing aspects of object representation on the Rorschach is the Mutuality of Autonomy (MOA) Scale (Urist, 1977; Urist & Shill,
1982). The MOA Scale assesses the thematic content of stated or implied interactions by rating all human, animal, and inanimate relationships in a Rorschach
protocol along a 7-point continuum ranging from mutually empathic, benevolent relatedness (scale score = 1) to themes of malevolent engulfment and

destruction (scale score = 7). Scale points 1 and 2, the most adaptive scores in the scale, refer respectively to themes of reciprocal acknowledgment and constructive parallel interactions. A score of 1, for example, is given to a response to Card II of "two people having a heated political argument." An example of a score of 2 is "two animals climbing a mountain" on Card VIII. Scale points 3 and 4 indicate an emerging loss of autonomy in interaction in which the "other" exists solely either to be leaned on (a score of 3) or to mirror oneself (a score of 4). An example of a score of 3 is a response to Card I of "two men leaning on a manikin." A score of 4 is given to the response "a tiger looking at its reflection in the water" to Card VIII. Scale points 5, 6, and 7 reflect an increasing malevolence and loss of control over one's separateness. A score of 5 is given to responses characterized by themes of coercion, hurtful influence, or threat, such as "a witch casting a spell on someone" given to the top large detail of Card IX. A score of 6 indicates violent assault and destruction of one figure by another—for example, "a bat impaled on a tree" to Card I. Finally, a score of 7 represents a larger than life destructiveness imposed usually by inanimate, calamitous force as depicted, for example, in the response to Card X, "a tornado hurtling its debris everywhere." Judges can make these distinctions at a high level of reliability.

The average (mean) MOA score expresses the individual's usual quality of interpersonal relatedness. Each subject's single most pathological and single most adaptive MOA scores reflect his or her range or repertoire of interpersonal interaction. MOA scores have been shown to correlate significantly with measures of interpersonal and social functioning in clinical and nonclinical groups (see, e.g., Blatt, et al., 1988; Harder, Greenwald, Wechsler, & Ritzler, 1984; Ryan, Avery, & Grolnick 1985; Spear & Sugarman, 1984; Tuber, 1983; Urist, 1977). Urist reported significant positive correlations of the MOA Scale with independent ratings by ward staff of interpersonal relationships, as well as with aspects of the content of autobiographical descriptions of interpersonal experiences in adult inpatients. Urist also found that the tendency for individuals to give at least one response at the more integrated end of the MOA Scale correlated significantly with ratings of constructive interpersonal behavior on the ward, whereas the tendency to give at least one response at the more disrupted end of the scale correlated significantly with ratings of disrupted relationships in autobiographical narratives. Using comprehensive case records that included developmental and family history reports, notes on clinical progress, and nursing staff notes, to assess the quality of interpersonal relationships of sixty adolescent patients, Urist and Shill (1982) found that ratings of these clinical case records correlated significantly with the mean MOA score. More disrupted MOA scores were consistently associated with reports of poorer interpersonal functioning on the clinical units and in the past history. Harder at al. (1984) found that the MOA Scale correlated significantly with ratings of the severity of psychopathology derived from both complex symptom checklists and independent diagnostic assessment according to DSM-III (American Psychiatric Association, 1980). The mean MOA score differentiated among schizophrenic, affective, and nonpsychotic conditions. More severe disorders were associated with a more disrupted mean MOA score. Spear and Sugarman (1984), using a modified version of the MOA Scale, found significant differences among infantile borderline patients, overideational borderline patients, and schizophrenic patients.

In summary, MOA ratings correlate significantly with independent assessments of interpersonal behavior from clinical case records (Harder, Greenwald, Wechsler, & Ritzler, 1984; Spear & Sugarman, 1984; Urist & Shill, 1982), ward staff ratings of social interactions (Urist, 1977), psychiatric symptoms in adults and children (Harder, et al., 1984; Tuber, 1983; Tuber & Coates, 1989), and ratings of interpersonal behavior in a nonclinical context (Ryan, et al., 1985). In addition, more disrupted interactions on the Rorschach (higher MOA scores) were significantly associated with more severe clinical symptoms and psychological test indicators of severe psychopathology, including measures of thought disorder (Blatt, Tuber, & Auerbach, 1990). The correlation between the MOA scores and the COR Scale indicate a moderate degree of convergence between the ratings of the content of interaction responses on the MOA Scale and the more structurally determined ratings with the COR (Blatt, et al., 1990). The Mean MOA score (a reverse scale) correlated significantly with the investment in inaccurately perceived human forms (OR-). The more malevolent the average MOA thematic content attributed to interactions portrayed on the Rorschach, the greater the degree of elaboration of inaccurately perceived human responses (OR-). The mean MOA score, however, does not correlate significantly with the investment in accurately perceived human forms (OR+).

Two studies of the long-term, intensive psychodynamically-oriented treatment of outpatients and of seriously disturbed inpatients used measures of the content and structural organization of mental representations, as assessed by the MOA and COR scales on the Rorschach, to evaluate therapeutic change in anaclitic and introjective patients. The distinction between anaclitic and introjective patients was made by experienced clinical judges from intake clinical case reports in these two studies of long-term, intensive, psychodynamic treatment (Blatt, 1992; Blatt & Ford, 1994; Blatt, Ford, Berman, Cook, & Meyer, 1988). Clinical judges reliably classified patients as either anaclitic or introjective on the basis of descriptions of the patients in clinical case reports prepared at admission to the treatment programs. The distinction between these two groups of patients (anaclitic and introjective) was made with a high degree of inter-rater reliability (94% and 80% agreement) by judges in these two different studies. The results of these two studies (Blatt, 1992; Blatt & Ford, 1994; Blatt, et al., 1988) indicate that anaclitic and introjective patients have different needs, respond differentially to different types of therapeutic interventions, and demonstrate different treatment outcomes. Analyses based on more conventional diagnostic differentiations (e.g., psychotic, severe borderline, and neurotic psychopathology) in these studies were less effective in understanding differences over the course of treatment.

As regards the methodology for assessing object relations, the two conceptual schemes, the COR Scale and the MOA Scale, were scored reliably in both of these studies by two judges who previously had established acceptable levels of inter-rater reliability (Intraclass Correlation [ICC] > 0.70) in scoring the various dimensions of these two schemes. The judges scoring these two measures of inter-personal relatedness were uninformed to patient demographics, including age, sex, diagnosis, and the treatment group to which the patient was assigned. Judges were also uninformed about which two Rorschach protocols were from the same patient and about whether a particular Rorschach protocol was obtained before the start of treatment or later in treatment. Additionally, the COR and MOA scales were scored by different judges.

The Riggs-Yale Project (R-YP)

Therapeutic change was studied in a sample of 90 seriously disturbed, treatment-resistant patients who, after a number of years of unsuccessful outpatient and brief inpatient treatments, sought assistance in long-term, intensive, psychoanalytically oriented, inpatient treatment in an open therapeutic facility that, in addition to an extensive therapeutic community, involved at least four-times weekly psychodynamic psychotherapy (Blatt & Ford, 1994; Blatt, et al., 1988). Extensive clinical case reports were prepared at intake and, on average, after 15 months of treatment, about a year prior to termination of treatment. Thus the second evaluation was independent of any considerations about termination and discharge from the inpatient treatment program. At the same two times, at intake and again on average 15 months later, patients were administered a series of psychological assessment procedures, including the Rorschach, Thematic Apperception Test (TAT), and a form of the Wechsler intelligence test. One research team reliably rated aspects of the patients as they were described in the clinical case reports, and a second research team independently rated various aspects of the psychological assessment procedures.

Systematic differences were found between anaclitic and introjective patients on independent measures of psychological change after, on average, 15 months of intensive, psychodynamically oriented, inpatient treatment. Introjective patients appeared to change more readily and to express their change primarily in a reduction in the intensity of clinical symptoms, as reliably rated from case reports, and in changes in cognitive functioning (measures of intelligence), as reliably assessed on psychological tests administered at the beginning and toward the end of treatment. Therapeutic change seemed to occur more slowly and in more subtle form in anaclitic patients, primarily in changes in the quality of interpersonal relationships, as reliably rated from case reports, and in representations of the human figure on the Rorschach. Thus, anaclitic and intro-jective patients changed primarily in ways congruent with their basic concerns and preoccupations.

Therapeutic change in the representation of interpersonal relationships on the Rorschach, as measured by the COR Scale, was expressed primarily in the reduction of maladaptive, inappropriate representations, and this significant reduction occurred primarily in anaclitic, but not in introjective, patients. Reduc-tion in maladaptive representations on the Rorschach, as measured by the COR Scale (OR-), was significantly correlated with increases in ratings of the quality of interpersonal behavior in the narrative reports in the independently established clinical case records only for anaclitic patients. It is noteworthy that no signifi-cant changes in representations of these seriously disturbed inpatients were observed in measures of adaptive representations (OR+).

In addition to these improvements in the structure of maladaptive representa-tions in the COR, some reduction ($p < 0.10$) in the representation of malevol-ence in interpersonal interactions on the Rorschach, as measured by the MOA Scale, occurred in introjective patients. This reduction in the representation of malevolence in interpersonal relations, as measured by the MOA Scale, was signif-icantly correlated with increases in the quality of interpersonal relationships in the narrative reports in the clinical case records.

Both anaclitic and introjective patients had significant reductions in thought disorder on the Rorschach, but this reduction occurred on different types of thought disorder (Blatt & Besser, in review).

Anaclitic patients had significant reductions in thought disorder that expressed disruptions of boundaries—in contamination and confabulation responses. In Contamination responses, two independent percepts or concepts merge or fuse into a highly idiosyncratic response (e.g., an accurately perceived "hand" and "rabbit's head," to a bottom detail on card X of the Rorschach, merge into an idiosyncratic "rabbit's hand"). In the contamination responses,

> . . . objects or concepts cannot maintain their separateness or independence and become fused in a single distorted unit . . . . The basic issue is the insta-bility of boundaries between objects and ideas . . . (expressing) a tendency not to differentiate oneself from others and to blur and confuse conven-tional boundaries. (Blatt & Ford, 1994, p.245).

Confabulation responses express an inability to maintain a boundary or sepa-ration between inside and outside, between what is perceived and how one thinks or feels about the perception. Thus, confabulation responses are character-ized by "extensive and arbitrary ideational or affective elaboration" that seriously distort a sometimes accurately perceived response (e.g., "two fetuses, representing good and evil, heaven and hell" on Card II of the Rorschach). These associative elaborations "overwhelm the perception with often grandiose and highly unrealistic personal elaborations and associations" (Blatt & Ford, 1994, p. 246). Distance is lost between perceptions and reactions and associations to the perception; reality is distorted by intense, exaggerated associations. Thus, significant reduction in thought disorder in anaclitic patients occurred in responses that express tendencies to merge and fuse with others or to lose the boundary between what is perceived and how it is experienced (Blatt & Besser, in review).

Introjective patients, in contrast, had a significant reduction in thought disorder on Fabulized Combination responses that reflect a tendency toward the attribution of an arbitrary or inappropriate relationship between separate and independent events or objects because of their spatial or temporal contiguity (e.g., two separate and independent responses, a tiger and a flower, are placed in an arbitrary relationship because of their spatial contiguity "tigers standing on a flower" on card VIII). Fabulized Combination responses are considered the less serious of these three major types of thought disorder on the Rorschach (Blatt & Ritzler, 1974; Rapaport, Gill & Schafer, 1945), and they occur primarily in more organized borderline and depressed outpatients (Wilson, 1985) who often have more paranoid features.

Also consistent with the fundamental distinctions between anaclitic and introjective psychopathology, reduction in overall thought disorder on the Rorschach in anaclitic patients correlated significantly with improvement in the ratings of affect regulation (labile and flattened affect) in the clinical case records, while reduction in overall thought disorder in introjective patients correlated significantly with reductions in clinical symptoms (psychotic and neurotic) in the clinical case records (Blatt & Ford, 1994).

In summary, therapeutic progress in the seriously disturbed, treatment-resistant inpatients in the long-term, intensive, psychodynamically oriented, patient treatment at the Austen Riggs Center was reflected in changes in the representation of interpersonal relations on the Rorschach, but the nature of these changes was contingent on the patient's type of psychopathology. Therapeutic progress, as reflected primarily by reduced investment in maladaptive representations on the COR Scale, occurred primarily in anaclitic patients. In introjective patients, therapeutic progress was reflected primarily in a reduction in the degree of malevolence attributed to human figures on the Rorschach, as measured by the MOA Scale. The COR Scale evaluates primarily structural (cognitive) organizational qualities of representations of human figures on the Rorschach while the MOA Scale evaluates primarily the thematic content of these representations. Further analyses of these data indicated that the degree of malevolence on the MOA Scale was related to therapeutic change primarily in the overideational introjective patients because the MOA Scale is closely related to the degree of thought disorder on the Rorschach (Blatt, et al., 1990), while changes in the structural organization of the representation of the human figure on the Rorschach (COR Scale) occurred in the more interpersonally oriented anaclitic patients because the COR Scale primarily assesses aspects of interpersonal relatedness (Blatt, et al., 1990).

The divergent expressions of therapeutic outcome for these two types of patients suggested that anaclitic and introjective patients change in different ways during the treatment process. These findings suggested that these two types of patients might also have divergent responses to different forms of therapy or to different aspects of the therapeutic process.

The Menninger Psychotherapy Research Project (MPRP)

The second study compared the effects of two types of treatments, psychoanalysis (PSA) and long-term supportive-expressive psychotherapy (SEP), with anaclitic and introjective outpatients (Blatt, 1992; Blatt & Shahar, 2004b).[6] Despite many prior analyses of data from the clinical evaluations and psychological assessments conducted before and after treatment in the MPRP, results failed to reveal any statistically significant differences in outcome between the two types of therapeutic intervention (Wallerstein, 1986). The anaclitic-introjective distinction was introduced into further analyses of the data from the MPRP (Blatt, 1992; Blatt & Shahar, 2004a), from ratings by two independent judges who reliably differentiated anaclitic and introjective patients on their evaluation of the clinical case records prepared at the beginning of treatment. These two senior clinicians agreed on the differentiation of 26 of the 33 patients as either anaclitic or introjective. The anaclitic-introjective differentiation of the remaining seven was made by a third senior clinician. Fifteen of the 33 outpatients (two female and seven male anaclitic; three female and three male introjective) had been seen in psychoanalysis. At intake, seven of these patients were diagnosed as neurotic and eight as having a personality disorder. Their mean age was 30 years. Eighteen of the 33 patients (six female and six male anaclitic; three female and three male introjective) had been seen in SEP. At intake, seven of these patients were diagnosed as neurotic, nine as having a personality disorder, and two as latent psychotic. Their mean age was 32.67 years.

Analyses of the data from the MPRP, using the distinction between the two types of psychopathology, indicated that anaclitic and introjective patients are differentially responsive to psychotherapy and psychoanalysis. The evaluation of psychological test data, gathered at the beginning and again at the end of treat-

---

[6] By design, the weekly frequency of treatment sessions was significantly different in the two treatment conditions (on average, SEP = 2.72 and PSA = 4.67 sessions per week; $F (1,32) = 41.26, p < .001$), but the total number of treatment sessions was not significantly different in the two treatment groups (on average, SEP = 453.16 and PSA = 733.73 sessions; $F (1, 32) = 2.17$, n.s.). Thus, SEP and PSA were both long-term intensive treatments (Blatt 1992).

ment, specifically the scales for evaluating the qualities of object representation on the Rorschach (i.e., the COR and MOA scales), revealed that anaclitic patients had significantly greater positive change in psychotherapy than in psychoanalysis. Introjective patients, in contrast, had significantly greater positive change in psychoanalysis than in psychotherapy. Thus, the relative therapeutic efficacy of psychoanalysis versus psychotherapy seems contingent to a significant degree upon the patient's pretreatment pathology and character structure. More dependent, interpersonally-oriented, anaclitic patients responded more effectively to SEP, in which there is more direct interaction with the therapist. The more ideational introjective patients, who stress separation, autonomy, and independence, responded more effectively in PSA. Thus, statistically significant ($p < 0.001$) patient-by-treatment interactions on the Rorschach measures of object representation indicated that congruence between patients' character style and important aspects of the therapeutic process contribute to the efficacy of treatment outcome. Patients come to treatment with varying problems, character styles, and needs, and appear to be responsive in divergent ways to different types of therapeutic intervention.

PSA was significantly more effective than SEP in facilitating the development of adaptive and benevolent interpersonal schemas in both anaclitic and introjective patients.[7] SEP, in contrast, actually resulted in a decline of these more adaptive representations among introjective patients. Introjective patients in the MPRP also tended ($p < 0.10$) to have greater therapeutic gains than anaclitic patients as assessed with ratings of general clinical functioning by clinicians using the Health-Sickness Rating Scale (Luborsky, 1962), especially when these patients were in PSA (Blatt, 1992; Blatt & Shahar, 2004a). In addition, both PSA and SEP were effective in reducing the intensity of maladaptive malevolent interpersonal schemas, but with different types of patients. PSA was significantly more effective than SEP in reducing the intensity of malevolent, destructive representations in introjective patients, while SEP was significantly more effective than PSA in reducing the intensity of these malevolent representations in anaclitic patients (Blatt, 1992; Blatt & Shahar, 2004a). Elements of this statistically significant patient-by-treatment interaction were found even in those few patients for whom the two primary clinical judges disagreed in classifying the patients as either anaclitic or introjective, such that the decision had to be made by a third judge (Blatt & Shahar, 2004b). Findings (Blatt & Shahar, 2004a) suggest that SEP was more effective in reducing maladaptive interpersonal schemas with the more affectively labile, emotionally overwhelmed anaclitic patients by providing a supportive–containing context. PSA, in contrast, was more effective in decreasing maladaptive interpersonal tendencies primarily with the more distant, isolated,

---

[7] It is noteworthy that therapeutic progress in the more integrated outpatients in the MPRP was expressed in increases in adaptive representations (OR+), whereas therapeutic progress in the more disturbed inpatients in the Riggs-Yale study was expressed primarily in the reduction of maladaptive representations (OR-).

over ideational and well defended introjective patients by more fully engaging these patients in the explorations and interpretations of the psychoanalytic process. These findings are discussed more fully in the section on the mechanisms of therapeutic change.

These findings suggest that PSA is particularly effective with introjective patients, whereas SEP is relatively ineffective, or even detrimental, with this type of patient. This greater therapeutic response of introjective patients in PSA in the MPRP is consistent with findings reported above that introjective patients had more extensive therapeutic gains in long-term, psychodynamically oriented, intensive, treatment of seriously disturbed, treatment-resistant, inpatients at the Austen Riggs Center. These findings of positive outcome of introjective patients in long-term psychodynamic treatment with inpatients in the R-YP and with outpatients in the MPRP are consistent with the findings of Fonagy, et al. (1996) and the conclusions by Gabbard, et al. (1994) about the constructive response of introjective patients to long-term insight-oriented psychodynamic treatment. This constructive response of introjective patients to long-term psychodynamic treatment is in marked contrast to the relatively poor response of these patients to brief manual-directed treatment for depression, to be discussed shortly.

Additional analyses of data from the MPRP also indicated that patients who had more constructive interpersonal schemas prior to treatment made significantly greater therapeutic gains in both PSA and SEP, but especially in PSA (Shahar & Blatt, in press). These findings are consistent with a series of studies by Piper and colleagues (e.g., Piper & Duncan, 1999, Piper, Joyce, McCallum, & Azim, 1998; Piper, Ogrodniczuk, McCallum, Joyce, & Roise, 2003) who demonstrated that outpatients with good object relations, as assessed in an unstructured interview, benefited more from brief, psychoanalytically oriented expressive psychotherapy than from brief supportive treatment. These findings from the MPRP are also consistent with the conclusions of Gabbard, et al. (1994) that interpretive therapeutic approaches are most effective with patients who have greater ego strength.

Taken together, these findings from the R-YP and the MPRP provide strong confirmation of Cronbach's formulations (1953) that pretreatment characteristics of patients are important dimensions that influence therapeutic response (Blatt and Felsen, 1993). These findings also indicate the importance of assessing dimensions of the representation of interpersonal relationships as measures of therapeutic change. This mounting evidence of the crucial role of patients' pretreatment characteristics reflects a major shift in psychotherapy research, in which data analyses are going beyond the comparison of two forms of treatment for the reduction of a particular focal symptom (e.g., depression or anxiety) and are beginning to address more complex questions, such as what types of treatment are more effective, in what kinds of ways, with which types of patients

(Blatt, et al., 2002; Blatt & Shahar, 2004a; Paul, 1969). The findings in both the Riggs-Yale study and in the further analyses of data from the Menninger Psychotherapy Research Project also indicate the importance of assessing both the content and structure of the representation of interpersonal interactions. The results indicate that the Rorschach, especially scored with the Concept of the Object and the Mutuality of Autonomy scales, can be an effective way of assessing therapeutic change.

Brief Treatment of Depression in the NIMH-Sponsored Treatment of Depression Collaborative Research Program (TDCRP)

The differential response of anaclitic and introjective patients in the long-term, intensive, psychodynamically-oriented treatment in the Riggs-Yale and Menninger studies suggested that the anaclitic-introjective distinction might be useful when evaluating the effectiveness of various forms of brief psychotherapy in treating depression. The NIMH-sponsored TDCRP (e.g., Elkin, et al., 1989), as noted previously, compared three forms of treatment for depression (cognitive-behavioral therapy (CBT), interpersonal therapy (IPT), and medication (Imipramine [IMI-CM]). In the primary analyses of their data, the TDCRP investigators found "no evidence of greater effectiveness of one of the psychotherapies as compared with the other and no evidence that either of the psychotherapies was significantly less effective than . . . Imipramine plus clinical management" (Elkin, 1994, p. 971).

The distinction between anaclitic and introjective forms of psychopathology, as noted earlier, has been useful in defining subtypes of depression (e.g., Beck, 1983; Blatt, 1974, 1998; Blatt, D'Afflitti, et al., 1976; Blatt, et al., 1982). Dissatisfaction with symptomatic classifications of depression had led several independent clinical investigators (i.e., Arieti & Bemporad, 1978, 1980; Beck, 1983; Blatt, 1974, 1998, 2004; Blatt, Brenneis, et al., 1976b, 1982; Bowlby, 1988a, 1988b) to differentiate types of depression on the basis of the fundamental concerns that lead individuals to become depressed. These various perspectives differentiated between relational and self-definitional forms of depression. The convergence of these conceptualizations, derived from diverse theoretical perspectives (i.e., attachment theory, cognitive-behavioral theory, psychoanalysis), clinical experiences, and research findings, suggests impressive agreement about the nature of depression, at least on a descriptive level (Blatt & Maroudas, 1992).

The anaclitic-introjective distinction was introduced into the analyses of data from the TDCRP through the Dysfunction Attitudes Scale (DAS; Weissman and Beck, 1978), a 40-item questionnaire assessing attitudes presumed to predispose an individual to depression that had been administered to the patients prior to the start of treatment. Factor analysis conducted on the DAS data obtained at intake in the TDCRP (Imber, Pilkonis, Sotsky, Elkin, Watkins, Collins, Shea,

Leber & Glass, 1990), consistent with previous analyses of the DAS (e.g., Cane, Olinger, Gotlib, & Kuiper, 1986), identified two principal factors—Need for Approval and Perfectionism. The first factor taps patients' need for approval by others and corresponds to the anaclitic or dependent form of depression; the second factor, which taps patients' tendency to set extremely high and unrealistic self-standards and to adopt a punitive attitude toward the self, corresponds to the introjective or self-critical form of depression (Blatt, 1974). Previous studies have shown links between these two DAS factors and the anaclitic (dependent) and introjective (self-critical) personality configurations, respectively (Blaney & Kutcher, 1991; Rude & Burnham, 1995; Segal, Shaw, & Vella, 1989; Segal, Shaw, Vella & Katz, 1992).

Blatt and colleagues (Blatt, Quinlan, Pilkonis, & Shea, 1995; Blatt, Sanislow, Zuroff & Pilkonis, 1996; Blatt, Zuroff, Bondi, Sanislow, & Pilkonis, 1998; Zuroff, Blatt, Sotsky, Krupnick, Martin, Sanislow, & Simmens, 2000) examined the contributions of patients' pretreatment DAS levels of Need of Approval and Perfectionism to therapeutic outcome in the TDCRP.[8] Although Need for Approval seemed to facilitate treatment outcome, these results failed to reach statistical significance. Significant effects were found in analyses involving Perfectionism, however. Specifically, patients' pretreatment level of perfectionism predicted poorer outcome at termination (i.e., after 16 weeks of treatment), as well as at the follow-up assessment conducted 18 months after the termination of treatment, on all five primary measures of therapeutic progress used in the TDCRP (Blatt, et al., 1995; Blatt, et al., 2000). Further analyses revealed that patients' pretreatment perfectionism significantly impeded therapeutic progress in two thirds of the sample, primarily in the latter half of treatment, beginning between the 9th and the 12th treatment session (Blatt, Berman, Cook, & Ford, 1998), independent of the type of treatment the patients had received.

Additional analyses indicated that pretreatment level of perfectionism affected therapeutic outcome primarily by disrupting the patients' quality of interpersonal relations both in the treatment process and in social relationships outside of treatment. Zuroff, et al. (2000), using ratings of the therapeutic alliance in the TDCRP that were developed by Krupnick and colleagues (1996) from a modified version of the Vanderbilt Therapeutic Alliance Scale (VTAS; Hartley & Strupp, 1983), found that patients' (but not the therapists') contributions to the therapeutic alliance mediated the effect of pretreatment perfectionism on treatment outcome at termination. Furthermore, the participation of more perfectionistic patients in the development of the therapeutic alliance reached a plateau at the 9th treatment session and failed to improve further in the latter half of the treatment process, thereby leading to poorer therapeutic response (Zuroff, et al.,

---

[8] In these analyses, the anaclitic and introjective distinctions are used as continuous dimensions rather than as a binary (categorical) differentiation.

2000). Shahar, Blatt, Zuroff, Krupnick, and Sotsky (2004) found that pretreatment perfectionism was also significantly related to poorer social support outside of treatment, and this impaired social support also significantly mediated the relationship of perfectionism to treatment outcome. Using the ratings by clinical evaluators on the Social Network Form (Elkin, Parloff, Hadley, & Autry, 1985) to assess patients' social network, Shahar, et al. (2004) found that patients with high levels of pretreatment perfectionism reported less satisfying social relationships over the course of treatment and that this disruption in social relationships in turn predicted poorer therapeutic outcome at termination. Thus, perfectionistic (introjective) patients appear to have greater interpersonal difficulty both in and outside of the treatment process; they have poorer therapeutic alliances (Zuroff, et al., 2000) and more limited social networks (Shahar, et al., 2004) during treatment. In addition, patients with higher pretreatment levels of perfectionism were also more vulnerable to stressful life events during the follow-up period, and this vulnerability led to increased depression (Zuroff & Blatt, 2002).

The introduction of the distinction between anaclitic and introjective dimensions into the analyses of data from the TDCRP facilitated the identification of a large segment of the patients in the TDCRP (about two thirds of the sample) who failed to make progress in the second half of the treatment process and, as we shall discuss shortly, it also enabled us to understand some of the mechanisms that disrupted the therapeutic response of these introjective patients. Thus, introjective patients appear to have limited benefit from the brief treatments in the TDCRP or from the long-term supportive-expressive psychotherapy in the MPRP, but appear to be particularly responsive to psychoanalysis and other long-term, psychodynamically oriented, intensive treatments. The constructive response of introjective patients to long-term psychodynamic treatment in the Riggs-Yale and Menninger studies stands in stark contrast to the relative ineffectiveness of several forms of brief treatment for these introjective patients, including medication (Blatt, et al., 1995, 1996, 1998) in the treatment for depression in the TDCRP. It would have been very interesting to have had some estimate of the change in the quality of mental representations in the TDCRP, either through the Rorschach or through spontaneous descriptions of self and significant others, including descriptions of the therapist (Blatt & Auerbach, 2001, 2003). These more open-ended assessments might have provided further understanding of some of the mechanisms and processes of therapeutic change in brief treatment for depression.

Findings from our further analyses of data from the TDCRP indicate the importance of including measures of therapeutic gain in addition to symptom reduction that assess changes in vulnerability to stress and the development of resilience and increased adaptive capacities (Blatt & Zuroff, 2005). These findings raise serious questions about the validity of current efforts to identify empirically supported treatments by comparing different types of treatment in their relative efficacy and effectiveness in reducing symptoms (Blatt & Zuroff, 2005). These findings suggest that efforts to identify EST's require a much more complex view of the treatment process, one that needs to include other dimensions of the treatment process, especially the quality of the therapeutic relationship and patients' pretreatment characteristics, and that investigates the impact of these factors of the therapeutic process across a range of outcome measures beyond symptom reduction. Consistent with formulations of Cronbach (1953) about the importance of possible patient-treatment and patient outcome interactions in psychotherapy research, the findings from the R-YP, MPRP, and TDCRP clearly indicate that different types of patients may be responsive to different aspects of the treatment process, and that different types of patients may respond to treatment in different, but equally desirable ways (Blatt, et al., 2002). As Blatt and Zuroff (2005) have recently demonstrated, these findings from the analysis of data from the TDCRP indicate that patients' pretreatment personality characteristics and the quality of the therapeutic relationship, rather than the type of treatment provided, are the primary factors influencing therapeutic outcome in the brief treatment of depression. These findings highlight the importance of future research being devoted to understanding more fully the processes that contribute to therapeutic gain.

MECHANISMS OF THERAPEUTIC CHANGE

The results of further analyses of data from the MPRP (Blatt, 1992; Blatt & Shahar, 2004a) suggested that PSA and SEP may involve different therapeutic mechanisms. For both anaclitic and introjective patients, SEP led to a significant reduction of the total number of responses given to the Rorschach, whereas PSA led to their increase. Thus, SEP may have been more effective with anaclitic patients possibly because it provides a supportive therapeutic context that contains the associative activities and maladaptive interpersonal schemas of these more affectively labile, emotionally overwhelmed, and vulnerable patients. PSA, by contrast, led to a significant increase in the total number of responses given to the Rorschach, suggesting that PSA facilitates the development of adaptive interpersonal schemas and the decrease of maladaptive schemas in introjective patients because the explorations and interpretations in PSA more effectively engage these more distant, well-defended, and interpersonally isolated individuals (Blatt & Shahar, 2004a).

The increased associational activity in PSA, and its decrease in SEP, and their possible role in the treatment processes evaluated in the MPRP, are consistent with clinical observations and expectations, as well as with recent findings by Fertuck, Bucci, Blatt & Ford (2004) that therapeutic progress in seriously disturbed treatment-resistant anaclitic inpatients in the Riggs-Yale Project was significantly associated with a reduction in referential activity, while progress in introjective patients was significantly associated with its increase. Fertuck, et al. assessed changes in patients' capacity for referential activity (Bucci 1984)—the degree to which connections are established between nonverbal systems and a communicative verbal code so that emotional experiences are translated into language capable of provoking corresponding experiences in a listener—using computer analyses of linguistic dimensions (e.g., Bucci, 1984) in narratives given to a standard set of TAT cards at intake and much later in the treatment process. These findings by Fertuck, et al. of therapeutic progress being associated with an increase in referential activity in introjective patients, but with its decrease in anaclitic patients in the R-YP, consistent with the results of our analyses of data from the MPRP, suggest that anaclitic patients do better in a treatment process that inhibits associational activity, whereas introjective patients do better in a treatment that facilitates it. The findings of a significant difference between PSA and SEP in changes in associational activity in the MPRP, as measured by the number of responses to the Rorschach, suggest that each modality has a unique effect on associative activity that may be part of the mechanism through which each results in constructive therapeutic change with a different type of patient.

Recent research by Fonagy, et al. (2002) indicates that reflective functioning (RF), or mentalization, is an important dimension of therapeutic progress. RF assesses the degree to which an individual has developed a theory of mind—an understanding of mental states, both one's own and those of others. Using the Adult Attachment Interview (AAI), Fonagy and colleagues (2002) evaluated individuals' capacity for RF and demonstrated how the development of this capacity is significantly related to therapeutic progress. Levy (2002) recently reported that RF increases significantly during outpatient psychotherapy. According to Fonagy, et al. the two primary dimensions of the therapeutic process, interpersonal and interpretive (see also Blatt & Behrends, 1987), both contribute to the regeneration of mentalized connections for fundamental affective experiences. Meanings are connected to affective experiences in the treatment process though the development of "second-order representations" derived from "interpersonal interpretive mechanisms" (Fonagy, et al., 2002, p. 16). Fonagy and colleagues view the establishment of linkages between affect and cognition in therapy as essential for the development of an agentic sense of self and the capacity to establish close relationships. They assume that the development of mentalization, or RF, is critical to therapeutic progress with all patients. But, as Fonagy, et al. note, therapeutic progress stems from both interpersonal and interpretive mechanisms (Blatt & Behrends, 1987), and our findings in the MPRP and the R-YP suggest that some patients may be more responsive to the former and others to the latter. The results of our analyses of data from the MPRP, the R-YP, and the TDCRP, suggest that patients may be differentially responsive to different aspects of the treatment process.

Referential thinking (see Fertuck, et al., 2004), associative activity (Rorschach responses), and mentalization, or reflective functioning, appear to have a more important role in the treatment of introjective patients with a primarily ideational orientation, who seem to be more responsive to interpretive dimensions, than in the treatment of affectively labile anaclitic patients, who appear more responsive to the interpersonal, supportive, and containing dimensions of the therapeutic process. Though a number of studies have found that changes in cognitive activity are an important aspect of therapeutic change, research groups have different conceptions of this cognitive activity and its assessment. Blatt, Shahar, and Fertuck (2003), for instance, found no significant relationship between changes in referential activity in narratives told to the TAT and changes in the number of Rorschach responses during the treatment of seriously disturbed treatment-resistant inpatients in the R-YP. Thus, future research needs to examine the conceptual assumptions and measurement procedures in these various approaches to the study of the cognitive processes considered important in the process of therapeutic change, especially with avoidant introjective patients. Research is also needed to examine further the effects of different aspects of the treatment process on cognitive activity and how different measures of this cognitive activity—reflective functioning (RF) (Fonagy, et al., 2002), referential activity (Bucci, 1984), and associative activity on the Rorschach (e.g., Blatt & Shahar, 2004a)—are interrelated and how they contribute to therapeutic change in different types of treatments with different types of patients.

The findings in the MPRP that SEP serves to contain and limit associative activity is consistent with a report by Eames and Roth (2000) that patients with a preoccupied attachment style (anaclitic patients) respond to the support and structure of psychotherapy, strive to establish a close therapeutic relationship, and appear to benefit most from a therapeutic strategy that helps them contain and modulate their overwhelming feelings. Patients with an avoidant attachment style (introjective patients), by contrast, appear to benefit most from a therapeutic strategy that facilitates their emotional engagement (see Hardy, et al., 1999).

THE ROLE OF THE THERAPEUTIC RELATIONSHIP IN THE TREATMENT PROCESS

The TDCRP provided data that enabled Blatt and Zuroff (2005) to evaluate the differential impact of three factors of the treatment process (type of treatment, patients' pretreatment personality characteristics, and the quality of therapeutic relationship) on outcome at termination (after 16 weeks of once-weekly treatment) and at an extensive follow-up assessment conducted 18 months after the termination of treatment. A detailed evaluation of data from the TDCRP (Blatt & Zuroff, 2005; Zuroff & Blatt, in press), consistent with recent extensive literature reviews (e.g., Lambert & Barley, 2002; Westen, et. al., 2004), indicated that primary among the factors that contribute to therapeutic gain in the brief outpatient treatment for serious depression were the quality of the therapeutic relationship the patient and therapist were able to establish very early, by the end of the second treatment session in the treatment process, and by the level of the patients' pretreatment introjective personality characteristics, as assessed by the level of perfectionism on the Dysfunctional Attitudes Scale (DAS) (Weissman & Beck, 1978). The quality of the therapeutic relationship assessed at the end of the second treatment session, as measured by the Barrett-Lennard Relationship Inventory (Barrett-Lennard, 1962, 1986; Gurman, 1977a, 1977b), consistent with the recent emphasis on the therapeutic relationship in the treatment process (e.g., Norcross, 2002; Wampold, 2001), was significantly related to all three outcome measures that Blatt and Zuroff (2005) constructed from data in the TDCRP: symptom reduction, reduction of vulnerability, and the development of resilience. In addition to contributing significantly to symptom reduction and the development of enhanced adaptive capacities, the quality of the therapeutic relationship, assessed early in the treatment process, significantly moderated the highly significant negative impact of pretreatment introjective personality characteristics (DAS perfectionism) on therapeutic outcome. This moderating effect occurred equally in psychotherapy (CBT, IPT) and in the medication (IMI-CM) and placebo (PLA-CM) treatment conditions (Blatt, Zuroff, et al., 1996).

To evaluate further how aspects of the therapeutic relationship facilitated therapeutic outcome, Blatt and colleagues (Blatt, Sanislow, Zuroff & Pilkonis, 1996) differentiated more effective from less effective therapists in the TDCRP by aggregating the therapeutic outcome of the 28 therapists who participated in this study in accordance with the degree of symptom reduction at termination of the patients each therapist had seen in active treatment. (Patients seen in the placebo condition were omitted from these analyses.) According to the responses of the 28 therapists to two brief questionnaires assessing aspects of the therapists' clinical practice outside their participation in the TDCRP and their values and attitudes about psychopathology and its treatment, more effective therapists (those whose patients in the TDCRP had a greater reduction in symptoms at termination) reported that they usually devoted significantly more of their clinical practice to psychotherapy alone, without the use of medication, than did the less effective therapists in the TDCRP. More effective TDCRP therapists also placed a significantly greater emphasis on a psychological rather than a biological approach to the understanding and treatment of depression. More effective therapists, for example, thought that the treatment of depression required significantly more time and eschewed biological interventions (medication and ECT) in the treatment of depression to a significantly greater extent than did less effective therapists (Blatt, Sanislow, et al., 1996). Thus, the quality of the therapeutic relationship that patient and therapist are able to establish early in the treatment process, even in manual-directed brief treatments, appears to be a significant factor determining therapeutic outcome.

SUMMARY

This paper demonstrates how psychoanalytic formulations have enabled investigators to introduce differences among patients into the study of psychotherapy process and outcome, examining how different types of patients are differentially responsive to different types of treatment, leading to different, but equally desirable, types of therapeutic outcome. This paper also demonstrates how psychoanalytic concepts have facilitated the assessment of dimensions of therapeutic change beyond symptom reduction including aspects of personality organization (e.g., the content and structural organization of representations of self and others). And this paper demonstrates how psychoanalytic formulations have facilitated the identification of some of the factors in the treatment process that possibly contribute to therapeutic gain, especially the quality of the therapeutic relationship.

Psychodynamic constructs frequently are not clearly defined, and judges often have difficulty establishing adequate levels of inter-rater reliability. As Blatt and Auerbach (2003) have noted, systematic independent assessment of patients at the beginning and the end of the therapeutic process has considerable potential for enabling investigators to introduce psychodynamic concepts into evaluations of treatment outcome and of the therapeutic process. Systematic assessment of the structure and content of mental representations on the Rorschach, or with other procedures like the Object Relations Inventory (ORI), appears to provide a way of assessing clinically relevant psychodynamic dimensions that can be assessed at acceptable levels of reliability and that appear to have substantial internal and external validity in understanding the extent and nature of therapeutic change.

In addition to developing methods for systematically assessing representations of interpersonal relationships, a psychodynamic conceptualization of personality development and psychopathology has enabled us to distinguish two broad configurations of psychopathology that appear to respond differentially to psychotherapeutic interventions. Anaclitic patients, focused on issues of interpersonal relatedness and the use of primarily avoidant defenses, and introjective patients, focused on issues of self-definition, self-control, and self-worth and the use of primarily counteractive defenses, come to treatment with differing problems, character styles, and needs, and respond in divergent ways to psychotherapy.

For many years, research methodologists (e.g., Cronbach, 1953) have urged psychotherapy investigators to include patient dimensions in their research designs, but this has been difficult to do because of a lack of a theoretically coherent and empirically supported differentiation among patients. Our findings demonstrate that psychoanalytic formulations can be used to differentiate two primary groups of patients, anaclitic (or dependent) and introjective (or self-critical), and that this model of personality development and psychopathology is an effective way of introducing patient variables into psychotherapy research designs that facilitate the exploration of the nature of therapeutic change and differential response to therapeutic interventions.

In contrast to the frequently observed dodo-bird effect, in which no significant differences are usually found among various forms of treatment, the introduction of the anaclitic-introjective distinction, as well as the assessment of the content and structure of the representation of interpersonal relationships, has enabled us to gain further insight into the mechanisms of therapeutic change, both the role of interpretations and the therapeutic relationship, in both in short-term, manual-directed treatments and in long-term, intensive, psychodynamic therapy.

In long-term, intensive psychodynamic treatment, research findings suggest that anaclitic patients are constructively responsive primarily to the more supportive interpersonal dimensions of the treatment process, while introjective patients appear to be more responsive to the interpretive aspects. Overall, introjective patients do better than anaclitic patients in long-term intensive psychodynamic treatment, but do relatively poorly in brief, manual-directed treatment, primarily because they disengage from the therapeutic relationship as they approach the predefined termination date. Introjective patients are more responsive to long-term, intensive insight oriented treatment because it more effectively engages them in the treatment process.

Overall, our findings indicate that the evaluation of the efficacy and effectiveness of treatment for psychological disturbances requires addressing complex questions about the nature of the treatment process and identifying what kinds of treatments are most effective for different kinds of patients, resulting in different types of therapeutic gain.

REFERENCES

American Psychiatric Association. (1980). *Diagnostic and statistical manual of mental disorders (3rd ed.).* Washington, DC: American Psychiatric Association.

American Psychiatric Association. (1994). *Diagnostic and statistical manual of mental disorders (4th ed.).* Washington, DC: American Psychiatric Association.

American Psychiatric Association Commission on Psychotherapies. (1982). *Psychotherapy research: Methodological and efficacy issues.* Washington, DC: American Psychiatric Association.

Angyal, A. (1951). *Neurosis and treatment: A holistic theory.* New York: John Wiley.

Arieti, S., & Bemporad, J. R. (1978). *Severe and mild depression: The therapeutic approach.* New York: Basic Books.

Arieti, S., & Bemporad, J. R. (1980). The psychological organization of depression. *American Journal of Psychiatry, 137,* 1360-1365.

Bakan, D. (1966). *The duality of human existence: An essay on psychology and religion.* Chicago: Rand McNally.

Barrett-Lennard, G. T. (1962). Dimensions of therapist responses as causal factors in thera-peutic change. *Psychological Monographs, 76*(43, Whole No. 562).

Barrett-Lennard, G. T. (1986). The relationship inventory now: Issues and advances in theory, method, and use. In L. S. Greenberg & W. M. Pinsof (Eds.), *The psychotherapeutic process: A research handbook. Guilford clinical psychology and psychotherapy series* (pp. 439-476). New York: Guilford Press.

Beck, A. T. (1983). Cognitive therapy of depression: New perspectives. In P. J. Clayton & J. E. Barrett (Eds.), *Treatment of depression: Old controversies and new approaches* (pp. 265-290). New York: Raven.

Benjamin, L. S. (1974). Structural analysis of social behavior. *Psychological Review, 81,* 392-425.

Beutler, L. E. (1991). Have all won and must all have prizes? Revisiting Luborsky, et al.'s ver-dict. *Journal of Consulting and Clinical Psychology, 59,* 226-232.

Blaney, P. H., & Kutcher, G. (1991). Measures of depressive dimensions: Are they interchange-able? *Journal of Personality Assessment, 56,* 502-512.

Blatt, S. J. (1974). Levels of object representation in anaclitic and introjective depression. *Psy-choanalytic Study of the Child, 29,* 107-157.

Blatt, S. J. (1990). Interpersonal relatedness and self-definition: Two personality configura-tions and their implications for psychopathology and psychotherapy. In J. L. Singer (Ed.) *Repression and dissociation: Implications for personality theory, psychopathology & health* (pp. 299-335). Chicago: University of Chicago Press.

Blatt, S. J. (1991). A cognitive morphology of psychopathology. *Journal of Nervous and Mental Disease, 179,* 449-458.

Blatt, S. J. (1992). The differential effect of psychotherapy and psychoanalysis on anaclitic and introjective patients: The Menninger Psychotherapy Research revisited. *Journal of the American Psychoanalytic Association, 40,* 691-724.

Blatt, S. J. (1995). Representational structures in psychopathology. In D. Cicchetti & S. Toth (Eds.), *Rochester Symposium on Developmental Psychopathology: Vol. 6. Emotion, Cognition, and Representation* (pp. 1-33). Rochester, NY: University of Rochester Press.

Blatt, S. J. (1998). Contributions of psychoanalysis to the understanding and treatment of depression. *Journal of the American Psychoanalytic Association, 46,* 723-752.

Blatt, S. J. (1999 July). *The Rorschach in the 21st century: The assessment of mental representation.* Paper presented at The International Rorschach Congress, Amsterdam.

Blatt, S. J. (2004). *Experiences of depression: Theoretical, clinical and research perspectives.* Washing-ton, DC: American Psychological Association.

Blatt, S. J. (in press). A fundamental polarity in psychoanalysis: Implications for personality development, psychopathology, and the therapeutic process. *Psychoanalytic Inquiry.*

Blatt, S. J., & Auerbach, J. S. (1988). Differential cognitive disturbances in three types of "bor-derline" patients. *Journal of Personality Disorders, 2,* 198-211.

Blatt, S. J., & Auerbach, J. S. (2001). Mental representation, severe psychopathology, and the therapeutic process. *Journal of the American Psychoanalytic Association, 49,* 113-159.

Blatt, S. J., & Auerbach, J. S. (2003). Psychodynamic measures of therapeutic change. *Psycho-analytic Inquiry, 23,* 268-307.

Blatt, S. J., & Behrends, R. S. (1987). Internalization, separation-individuation, and the nature of therapeutic action. *International Journal of Psychoanalysis, 68,* 279-297.

Blatt, S. J., Berman, W. H., Cook, B. P., & Ford, R. Q. (1998). Effectiveness of long-term, inten-sive, inpatient treatment for seriously disturbed young adults: A reply to Bein. *Psychother-apy Research, 8,* 42-53.

Blatt, S. J., Besser, A., & Ford, R. Q. (in review). Two primary configurations of psychopathol-ogy and the evaluation of change in thought disorder in long-term, intensive, inpatient treatment of seriously disturbed young adults.

Blatt, S. J., & Blass, R. B. (1990). Attachment and separateness: A dialectic model of the products and processes of psychological development. *Psychoanalytic Study of the Child, 45,* 107-127.

Blatt, S. J., & Blass, R. B. (1992). Relatedness and self-definition: Two primary dimensions in personality development, psychopathology, and psychotherapy. In J. Barron, M. Eagle, & D. Wolitsky (Eds.), *The interface of psychoanalysis and psychology* (pp. 399-428). Washington, DC: American Psychological Association.

Blatt, S. J., & Blass, R. (1996). Relatedness and self definition: A dialectic model of personality development. In G. G. Noam & K. W. Fischer (Eds.), *Development and vulnerabilities in close relationships* (pp. 309-338). Hillsdale, NJ: Lawrence Erlbaum Associates.

Blatt, S. J., Brenneis, C. B., Schimek, J. G., & Glick, M. (1976a). The normal development and psychopathological impairment of the concept of the object on Rorschach. *Journal of Abnormal Psychology, 85,* 364-373.

Blatt, S. J., Brenneis, C. B., Schimek, J., & Glick, M. (1976b). *A developmental analysis of the concept of the object on the Rorschach.* Unpublished research manual, Yale University.

Blatt, S. J., Chevron, E. S., Quinlan, D. M., Schaffer, C. E., & Wein, S. (1988). *The assessment of qualitative and structural dimensions of object representations. (Revised Edition).* Unpublished research manual, Yale University.

Blatt, S. J., D'Afflitti, J. P., & Quinlan, D. M. (1976). Experiences of depression in normal young adults. *Journal of Abnormal Psychology, 85,* 383-389.

Blatt, S. J., & Felsen, I. (1993). Different kinds of folks may need different kinds of strokes: The effect of patients' characteristics on therapeutic process and outcome. *Psychotherapy Research 3,* 245-259.

Blatt, S. J., & Ford, R. Q. (1994). *Therapeutic change: An object relations perspective.* New York: Plenum.

Blatt, S. J., Ford, R. Q., Berman, W., Cook, B., & Meyer, R. (1988). The assessment of change during the intensive treatment of borderline and schizophrenic young adults. *Psychoanalytic Psychology, 5,* 127-158.

Blatt, S. J., & Homann, E. (1992). Parent-child interaction in the etiology of dependent and self-critical depression. *Clinical Psychology Review, 12,* 47-91.

Blatt, S. J., & Levy, K. N. (1998). A psychodynamic approach to the diagnosis of psychopathology. In J. W. Barron (Ed.), *Making diagnosis meaningful* (pp. 73-109). Washington, DC: American Psychological Association.

Blatt, S. J., & Maroudas, C. (1992). Convergence of psychoanalytic and cognitive behavioral theories of depression. *Psychoanalytic Psychology 9,* 157-190.

Blatt, S. J., Quinlan, D. M., Chevron, E. S., McDonald, C., & Zuroff, D. (1982). Dependency and self-criticism: Psychological dimensions of depression. *Journal of Consulting and Clinical Psychology, 50,* 113-124.

Blatt, S. J., Quinlan, D. M., Pilkonis, P. A., & Shea, T. (1995). Impact of perfectionism and need for approval on the brief treatment of depression: The National Institute of Mental Health Treatment of Depression Collaborative Research Program revisited. *Journal of Consulting and Clinical Psychology, 63,* 125-132.

Blatt. S. J., & Ritzler, B. A. (1974). Thought disorder and boundary disturbances in psychosis. *Journal of Consulting and Clinical Psychology, 42,* 370-381.

Blatt, S. J., Sanislow, C. A., Zuroff, D. C., & Pilkonis, P. A. (1996). Characteristics of effective therapists: Further analyses of data from the National Institute of Mental Health Treatment of Depression Collaborative Research Program. *Journal of Consulting and Clinical Psychology, 64,* 1276-1284.

Blatt, S. J., & Shahar, G. (2004a). Psychoanalysis: For what, with whom, and how. A comparison with psychotherapy. *Journal of the American Psychoanalytic Association, 52,* 393-447.

Blatt, S. J., & Shahar, G. (2004b). Stability of the patient-by-treatment interaction in the Menninger Psychotherapy Research Project. *The Bulletin of the Menninger Clinic, 68,* 23-36.

Blatt, S., Shahar, G., & Fertuck, E. (2003). Unpublished data. Yale University.

Blatt, S. J., Shahar, G., & Zuroff, D. C. (2002). Anaclitic (sociotropic) and introjective (autonomous) dimensions. In J. C. Norcross (Ed.), *Psychotherapy relationships that work: Therapist contributions and responsiveness to patients* (pp. 306-324). New York: Oxford University Press.

Blatt, S. J., & Shichman, S. (1983). Two primary configurations of psychopathology. *Psychoanalysis and Contemporary Thought, 6,* 187-254.

Blatt, S. J., Schimek, J., & Brenneis, C. B. (1980). The nature of the psychotic experience and its implications for the therapeutic process. In J. Strauss, M. Bowers, T. W. Downey, S. Fleck, S. Jackson & I. Levine (Eds.), *The Psychotherapy of Schizophrenia* (pp. 101-114). New York: Plenum.

Blatt, S. J., Tuber, S. B., & Auerbach, J. S. (1990). Representation of interpersonal interactions on the Rorschach and level of psychopathology. *Journal of Personality Assessment, 54,* 711-728.

Blatt, S. J., Wein, S. J., Chevron, E. S., & Quinlan, D. M. (1979). Parental representations and depression in normal young adults. *Journal of Abnormal Psychology, 88,* 388-397.

Blatt, S. J., & Zuroff, D. C. (1992). Interpersonal relatedness and self-definition: Two prototypes for depression. *Clinical Psychology Review, 12,* 527-562.

Blatt, S. J., & Zuroff, D. C. (2005). Empirical evaluation of the assumptions in identifying evidence based treatments in mental health. *Clinical Psychology Review, 25,* 459-486.

Blatt, S. J., Zuroff, D. C., Bondi, C. M., & Sanislow, C. A. (2000). Short and long-term effects of medication and psychotherapy in the brief treatment of depression: Further analyses of data from the National Institute of Mental Health Treatment of Depression Collaborative Research Program. *Psychotherapy Research, 10,* 215-234.

Blatt, S. J., Zuroff, D. C., Bondi, C. M., Sanislow, C., & Pilkonis, P. A. (1998). When and how perfectionism impedes the brief treatment of depression: Further analyses of the National Institute of Mental Health Treatment of Depression Collaborative Research Program. *Journal of Consulting and Clinical Psychology, 66,* 423-428.

Blatt, S. J., Zuroff, D. C., Quinlan, D. M., & Pilkonis, P. A. (1996). Interpersonal factors in brief treatment of depression: Further analyses of the National Institute of Mental Health Treatment of Depression Collaborative Research Program. *Journal of Consulting and Clinical Psychology, 64,* 162-171.

Bowlby, J. (1988a). Developmental psychology comes of age. *American Journal of Psychiatry, 145,* 1-10.

Bowlby, J. (1988b) *Secure base: Clinical applications of attachment theory.* London: Routledge & Kegan Paul.

Brown, G. W., & Harris, T. (1978). *Social origins of depression: A study of psychiatric disorders in women.* London: Tavistock.

Bucci, W. (1984). Linking words and things: Basic processes and individual variation. *Cognition, 17,* 137–153.

Cane, D. B., Olinger, L. J., Gotlib, I. H., & Kuiper, N. A. (1986). Factor structure of the Dysfunctional Attitude Scale in a student population. *Journal of Clinical Psychology, 42.*

Cohen, S., & Wills, T. A. (1985). Stress, social support, and the buffering hypothesis. *Psychological Bulletin, 98,* 310-357.

Cronbach, L. J. (1953). Correlation between persons as a research tool. In O. H. Mowrer (Ed.), *Psychotherapy: theory and research* (pp. 376-389). New York: Ronald.

Cronbach, L. J. (1975). Beyond the two disciplines of scientific psychology, *American Psychologist, 30,* 116–127.

Eames, V., & Roth, A. (2000). Patient attachment orientation and the early working alliance: A study of patient and therapist reports of alliance quality and ruptures. *Psychotherapy Research, 10,* 421-434.

Elkin, I. (1994). The NIMH treatment of depression collaborative research program: Where we began and where we are. In A. E. Bergin & S. L. Garfield (Eds.), *Handbook of psychotherapy and behavior change* (pp. 114-139). Oxford, England: John Wiley.

Elkin, I., Parloff, M. B., Hadley, S. W., & Autry, J. H. (1985). NIMH Treatment of Depression Collaborative Research Program: Background and research plan. *Archives of General Psychiatry, 42,* 305-316.

Elkin, I., Shea, M. T., Watkins, J. T., Imber, S. D., Sotsky, S. M., Collins, J. F., et al. (1989). NIMH Treatment of Depression Collaborative Research Program: General effectiveness of treatments. *Archives of General Psychiatry, 46,* 971-983.

Fertuck, E., Bucci, W., Blatt, S. J., & Ford, R. Q. (2004). Verbal representation and therapeutic change in anaclitic and introjective patients. *Psychotherapy: Theory, Research, Practice, Training, 41,* 13-25.

Fonagy, P., Gergely, G., Jurist, E. L., & Target, M. (2002). *Affect regulation, mentalization, and the development of the self.* New York: Other Press.

Fonagy, P., Leigh, T., Steele, M., Steele, H., Kennedy, R., Mattoon, G., et al. (1996). The relation of attachment status, psychiatric classification, and response to psychotherapy. *Journal of Consulting and Clinical Psychology, 64,* 22-31.

Frank, J. D. (1973). *Persuasion and healing; a comparative study of psychotherapy.* Baltimore, MD: Johns Hopkins University Press.

Frank, J. D. (1979). The present status of outcome studies. *Journal of Consulting and Clinical Psychology, 47,* 310-316.

Frank, J. D. (1982). Therapeutic components shared by all psychotherapies. In J. H. Harvey & M. M. Parks (Eds.), *Psychotherapy research and behavior change* (Vol. 1, pp. 5-37). Washington, DC: American Psychological Association.

Freud, S. (1914/1957). On narcissism: An introduction. *Standard Edition, 14,* 73-102.

Freud, S. (1926/1959). Inhibitions, symptoms and anxiety. *Standard Edition, 20,* 77-174.

Freud, S. (1930/1961). Civilization and its discontents. *Standard Edition, 21,* 59-145.

Gabbard, G. O., Horowitz, L., Allen, J. G., Frieswyk, S., Newson, G., Colson, D. B., et al. (1994). Transference interpretation in the psychotherapy of borderline patients: A high-risk, high-gain phenomenon. *Harvard Review of Psychiatry, 2,* 59-69.

Gibbons, R. D., Hedeker, D., Elkin, I., Waternaux, C., Kraemer, H. C., Greenhouse, J. B., et al. (1993). Some conceptual and statistical issues in analysis of longitudinal psychiatric data: Application to the NIMH Treatment of Depression Collaborative Research Program dataset. *Archives of General Psychiatry, 50,* 739-750.

Gurman, A. S. (1977a). The patient's perception of the therapeutic relationship. In A. S. Gurman & A. M. Razin (Eds.), *Psychotherapy: A handbook of research* (pp. 503-543). New York: Pergamon.

Gurman, A.S. (1977b). Therapist and patient factors influencing the patient's perception of facilitative therapeutic conditions. *Psychiatry, 40,* 218-231.

Harder, D., Greenwald, D., Wechsler, S., & Ritzler, B. (1984). The Urist Rorschach mutuality of autonomy scale as an indicator of psychopathology. *Journal of Clinical Psychology, 40,* 1078-1082.

Hardy, G. E., Aldridge, J., Davidson, C., Rowe, C., Reilly, S., & Shapiro, D. (1999). Therapist responsiveness to patient attachment styles and issues observed inpatient-identified significant events in psychodynamic-interpersonal psychotherapy. *Psychotherapy Research, 9,* 36-53

Hartley, D., & Strupp, H. (1983). The therapeutic alliance: Its relationship to outcome in brief psychotherapy. In J. Masling (Ed.), *Empirical studies of psychoanalytic theories* (pp. 1-27). Hillsdale, NJ: Erlbaum.

Imber, S. D., Pilkonis, P. A., Sotsky, S. M., Elkin, I., Watkins, J. T., Collins, J. F., et al. (1990). Mode-specific effects among three treatments for depression. *Journal of Consulting and Clinical Psychology, 58,* 352–359.

Kazdin, A. E. (1986). Comparative outcome studies of psychotherapy: Methodological issues and strategies. *Journal of Consulting and Clinical Psychology, 54,* 95-105.

Kiesler, D.J. (1966). Some myths of psychotherapy research and the search for a paradigm. *Psychological Bulletin, 65,* 110-136.

Krupnick, J. L., Sotsky, S. M., Simmens, S., Moyer, J., Elkin, I., Watkins, J., et al. (1996). The role of the therapeutic alliance in psychotherapy and pharmacotherapy outcome: Findings in the National Institute of Mental Health Treatment of Depression Collaborative Research Program. *Journal of Consulting and Clinical Psychology, 64,* 532-539.

Lambert, M. J., & Barley, D. E. (2002). Research summary on the therapeutic relationship and psychotherapy outcome. In: J. C. Norcross (Ed.), *Psychotherapy relationships that work: Therapist contributions and responsiveness to patients* (pp. 17 -32). London: Oxford University Press.

Lambert, M. J., Shapiro, D. A., & Bergin A. E. (1986). The effectiveness of psychotherapy. In S. L. Garfield & A. E. Bergin (Eds.), *Handbook of psychotherapy and behavior change* (3rd ed.). New York: John Wiley.

Leichtman, M. (1996a). *The Rorschach: A developmental perspective.* Hillsdale, NJ: Analytic Press.

Leichtman, M. (1996b). The nature of the Rorschach task. *Journal of Personality Assessment, 67,* 478-493.

Lerner, H. D., & St. Peter, S. (1984a). Patterns of object relations in neurotic, borderline and schizophrenic patients. *Psychiatry, 47,* 77-92.

Lerner, H. D., & St. Peter, S. (1984b). The Rorschach H response and object relations. *Journal of Personality Assessment, 48,* 345-350.

Levy, K. N. (2002). *Change in attachment organization during the long-term treatment of patients with borderline personality.* Invited paper presented to S. McMain (Chair), Integrative treatments for borderline personality disorder. XVII Annual Conference of the Society for the Exploration of Psychotherapy Integration, San Francisco, CA.

Levy, K. N., Edell, W. S., Blatt, S. J., Becker, D. F., Quinlan, D. M., Kolligan, J., et al. (1995). *Two configurations of psychopathology: The relationship of dependency, anaclitic neediness, and self-criticism to personality pathology.* Unpublished manuscript.

Levy, K. N., Meehan, K. B., Auerbach, J. S., & Blatt, S. J. (2005). Concept of the object on the Rorschach Scale. In R. B. Bornstein and J. M. Masling (Eds.). *Scoring the Rorschach: Seven validated systems* (pp. 97-134). Mahwah, NJ: Lawrence Erlbaum.

Loewald, H. W. (1962). Internalization, separation, mourning, and the superego. *Psychoanalytic Quarterly, 31,* 483-504.

Luborsky, L. (1962). The patient's personality and psychotherapy change. In H. H. Strupp & L. Luborsky (eds.), *Research in psychotherapy* (Vol. 2, pp. 115-133). Washington, DC: American Psychological Association.

Luborsky, L., Diguer, L.A., McLellan, A.T., Woody, G. (1995 July). *The psychotherapist as a neglected variable: New studies of each therapist's benefits to their patients.* Paper presented at 1995 meetings of the Society for Psychotherapy Research, Vancouver, British Columbia.

Luborsky, L., Diguer, L. A., Seligman, D. A., Rosenthal, R., Kruse, E. D., Johnson, S., et al. (1999). The researcher's own therapy allegiances: A "wildcard" in comparisons of treatment efficacy. *Clinical Psychology: Science and Practice, 6,* 95-106.

Luborsky, L., Rosenthal, R., Diguer, L., Andrusyna, T. P., Berman, J. S., Levitt, J. T., et al. (2002). The dodo bird verdict is alive and well—mostly. *Clinical Psychology, 9,* 2-12.

Luborsky, L., Singer, B., & Luborsky, E. (1975). Comparation studies of psychotherapies: Is it true that "Everyone has won and all must have prizes?" *Archives of General Psychiatry, 32,* 995-1008.

Luyten, P. (2002). *Normbesef en depressie: Aanzet tot een integratief theoretisch kader en een empirisch onderzoek aan de hand van de depressietheorie van S. J. Blatt.* (*Personal standards and depression: An integrative psychodynamic framework, and an empirical investigation of S. J. Blatt's theory of depression*). Doctoral dissertation, University of Leuven, Leuven, Belgium.

McAdams, D. P. (1985). *Power, intimacy, and the life story: Personological inquiries into identity.* Homewood, IL: Dorsey.

McClelland, D. C. (1986). Some reflections on the two psychologies of love. *Journal of Personality, 54,* 334–353.

Morse, J. A., Robins, C. J., & Gittes-Fox, M. (2002). Sociotropy, autonomy, and personality disorder criteria in psychiatric patients. *Journal of Personality Disorders, 16,* 549-560.

Norcross, J. (2002). *Psychotherapy relationships that work.* New York: Oxford University Press.

Ouimette, P. C., Klein, D. N., Anderson, R., Liso, L. P., & Lizardi, H. (1994). Relationship of sociotropy/autonomy and dependency/self-criticism to DSM-III-R personality disorders. *Journal of Abnormal Psychology, 103,* 743-749.

Paul, G. L. (1969). Behavior modification research: Design and tactics. In C.M. Franks (Ed.), *Behavior therapy: Appraisal and status.* NY: McGraw Hill.

Pennebaker, J. W. (1997). *Opening up: The healing power of expressing emotions.* New York: Guilford.

Piper, W. E., & Duncan, S. C. (1999). Object relations theory and short-term dynamic psychotherapy: Findings from the Quality of Object Relations Scale. *Clinical Psychology Review, 19,* 669-685.

Piper, W. E., Joyce, A. S., McCallum, M., & Azim, H. F. (1998). Interpretive and supportive forms of psychotherapy and patient personality variables. *Journal of Consulting and Clinical Psychology, 66,* 558-567.

Piper, W. E., Ogrodniczuk, J. S., McCallum, M. J., Joyce, A. S., & Rosie, J. S. (2003). Expression of affect as a mediator of the relationship between quality of object relations and group therapy outcome for patients with complicated grief. *Journal of Consulting and Clinical Psychology, 71,* 664-671.

Rapaport, D., Gill, M. M., & Schafer, R. (1945). *Diagnostic psychological testing: Vol. 1.* Chicago: Year Book.

Ritzler, B., Zambianco, D., Harder, D., & Kaskey, M. (1980). Psychotic patterns of the concept of the object on the Rorschach test. *Journal of Abnormal Psychology, 89,* 46-55.

Rude, S. S., & Burnham, B. L. (1995). Connectedness and neediness: Factors of the DEQ and SAS dependency scales. *Cognitive Therapy and Research. 19,* 323-340.

Ryan, R., Avery, R., & Grolnick, W. (1985). A Rorschach assessment of children's mutuality of autonomy. *Journal of Personality Assessment, 49,* 6-11.

Segal, Z. V., Shaw, B. F., & Vella, D. D. (1989). Life stress and depression: A test of the congruence hypothesis for life event, content, and depressive subtypes. *Canadian Journal of Behavioural Science, 21,* 389–400.

Segal, Z. V., Shaw, B. F., Vella, D. D., & Katz, R. (1992). Cognitive and life stress predictors of relapse in remitted unipolar depressed patients: Test of congruency hypothesis. *Journal of Abnormal Psychology, 101,* 26–36.

Shahar, G., & Blatt, S. J. (in press). Benevolent interpersonal schemas facilitate therapeutic change: Further analysis of the Menninger Psychotherapy Research Project. *Journal of Psychotherapy Research.*

Shahar, G., Blatt, S. J., Zuroff, D. C., Krupnick, J., & Sotsky, S. M. (2004). Perfectionism impedes social relations and response to brief treatment of depression. *Journal of Social and Clinical Psychology, 23,* 140–154.

Shapiro, D. A., & Shapiro, D. (1982). Meta-analysis of comparative therapy outcome studies: A replication and refinement. *Psychological Bulletin, 92,* 581-604.

Shor, J., & Sanville, J. (1978). *Illusions in loving: A psychoanalytic approach to intimacy and autonomy*. Los Angeles: Double Helix.

Smith, M. L., Glass, G. V., & Miller, T. I. (1980). *The benefits of psychotherapy*. Baltimore, MD: John Hopkins University Press.

Smith, B., & Sechrest, L. (1991). The treatment of Aptitude X treatment interactions. *Journal of Consulting and Clinical Psychology, 59*, 233-244.

Snow, R. E. (1991). Aptitude treatment interactions as a framework for research on individual differences in psychotherapy. *Journal of Consulting and Clinical Psychology, 59*, 205-216.

Spear, W., & Sugarman, A. (1984). Dimensions of internalized object relations in borderline schizophrenic patients. *Psychoanalytic Psychology, 1*, 113-129.

Stiles, W. B., Shapiro, D. A., & Elliott, R. (1986). Are all psychotherapies equivalent? *American Psychologist, 41*, 161-180.

Strupp, H. H., & Binder, J. L. (1984). *Psychotherapy in a new key: A guide to time limited dynamic psychotherapy*. New York: Basic.

Tuber, S. B. (1983). Children's Rorschach scores as predictors of later adjustment. *Journal of Consulting and Clinical Psychology, 51*, 379-385.

Tuber, S., & Coates, S. (1989). Indices of psychopathology in the Rorschachs of boys with severe gender identity disorder. *Journal of Personality Assessment, 57*, 100-112.

Urist, J. (1977). The Rorschach test and the assessment of object relations. *Journal of Personality Assessment, 41*, 3-9.

Urist, J., & Shill, M. (1982). Validity of the Rorschach Mutuality of Autonomy scale: A replication using excerpted responses. *Journal of Personality Assessment, 46*, 451-454.

VandenBos, G. R., & Pino, C. D. (1980). Research on the outcome of psychotherapy. In G. R. VandenBos (Ed.), *Psychotherapy: Practice, research, policy* (pp. 23-69). Beverly Hills, CA: Sage.

Wallerstein, R. S. (1986). *Forty-two lives in treatment: A study of psychoanalysis and psychotherapy*. New York: Guilford.

Wampold, B. E. (2001). *The great psychotherapy debate: Models, methods, and findings*. Mahwah, NJ: Erlbaum.

Westen, D., Novotny, C. M., & Thompson-Brenner, H. (2004). The empirical status of empirically supported psychotherapies: Assumptions, findings, and reporting in controlled clinical trials. *Psychological Bulletin, 130*, 631-663.

Weissman, A. N., & Beck, A. T. (1978, August-September). *Development and validation of the Dysfunctional Attitudes Scale: A preliminary investigation*. Paper presented at the 86th Annual Convention of the American Psychological Association, Toronto.

Werner, H. (1948). *Comparative psychology of mental development*. New York: International Universities Press.

Wiggins, J. S. (1991). Agency and communion as conceptual coordinates for the understanding and measurement of interpersonal behavior. In W. W. Grove, & D. Cicchetti (Eds.), *Thinking clearly about psychology, Vol. 2: Personality and psychotherapy* (pp. 89-113). Minneapolis: University of Minnesota Press.

Wilson, A. (1985). Boundary disturbances in borderline and psychotic states. *Journal of Personality Assessment, 49*, 346-355.

Wortman, P. M. (1983). Meta-analysis: A validity perspective. *Annual Review of Psychology, 34*, 223-260.

Zuroff, D. C., & Blatt, S. J. (2002). Vicissitudes of life after the short-term treatment of depression: Roles of stress, social support, and personality. *Journal of Social and Clinical Psychology, 21*, 473-496.

Zuroff, D. C., & Blatt, S. J. (in press). The therapeutic relationship in the brief treatment of depression: Contributions to clinical improvement and enhanced adaptive capacities. *Journal of Consulting and Clinical Psychology*.

Zuroff, D. C., Blatt, S. J., Krupnick, J. L., & Sotsky, S. M. (2003). When brief treatment is over: Enhanced adaptive capacities and stress reactivity after termination. *Psychotherapy Research, 13*, 99-115.

Zuroff, D. C., Blatt, S. J., Sotsky, S. M., Krupnick, J. L., Martin, D. J., Sanislow, C. A., et al. (2000). Relation of therapeutic alliance and perfectionism to outcome in brief outpatient treatment of depression. *Journal of Consulting and Clinical Psychology, 68*, 114-124.

Personality Diagnosis with the Shedler-Westen Assessment Procedure (SWAP): Bridging the Gulf Between Science and Practice

Jonathan Shedler, PhD,[1] Drew Westen, PhD[2]

Editor's Note: Like the immediately preceding chapter by Blatt and his collaborators, this paper presents another of the major measures (also indicated in the review by Wallerstein in his chapter on psychoanalytic therapy research, p. 511) created to empirically delineate personality attributes and character types. The predominant focus is on the use of the SWAP for character diagnosis, with direct application as an outcome measure for underlying personality (or structural) change in psychotherapy.

The authors begin with a sophisticated discussion of the limitations of the DSM system for diagnosing personality disorders (Axis II) with respect to both diagnosis and treatment planning, before describing the development of their own diagnostic approach, the SWAP. Rather than trying to exclude clinical judgment from psychological assessment, the SWAP harnesses and systematizes clinical judgment in a manner that enhances, rather than diminishes, reliability and validity. It is an empirical approach that can bridge the longstanding schism between the experience of clinical practice and the findings of incrementally accruing science. Like Blatt et al.'s Object Relations Inventory (ORI), the SWAP can be used to test the efficacy and the effectiveness of psychoanalytically-based (as well as other) psychotherapies.

It is often easier to hear criticism when it is directed at others rather than ourselves. In this spirit, we offer an account of an unfortunate experience. During a routine medical exam, a friend had an abnormal finding on a lab test. His physician ordered more tests, then referred him to an oncologist. The oncologist ordered more tests, then referred him to a team of oncology specialists, researchers at the cutting edge of their discipline. My friend underwent a liver biopsy. The oncologists diagnosed advanced liver cancer and told him he had only months to live.

---

[1] Associate Professor of Psychology, University of Denver; Clinical Professor of Psychiatry, University of Colorado Health Sciences
[2] Professor, Department of Psychology and Department of Psychiatry and Behavioral Sciences, Emory University

In the ensuing panic there were few voices of reason. One happened to be that of a psychoanalyst, my friend's senior colleague. She asked a simple question: Had he been *feeling* sick? He had not. In fact, he had been feeling energetic and strong. The psychoanalyst raised an eyebrow. Her wordless gesture spoke volumes: Something did not add up. The pieces did not fit. If my friend had advanced liver cancer, he would likely be deathly ill.

Indeed, he did not have cancer. After additional biopsies (and ineffable emotional turmoil), the oncologists eventually concluded that his liver had an area of dense blood vessel growth (hemangioma) that had probably been present from birth and was of no medical consequence. One might reasonably ask how these research-oriented oncologists had gotten it so wrong and why an elderly psychiatrist who had not practiced medicine in decades had shown greater diagnostic acumen. No doubt many factors were at work, but we believe one factor is that the oncologists focused on laboratory findings to the exclusion of other meaningful data, including the data afforded by their own eyes and ears. Additionally, they failed to consider how the data *fit together*. Had the laboratory findings been contextualized by what else the doctors knew or could have know about their patient, they may have regarded them differently—as pieces of a diagnostic puzzle, not the diagnostic picture in its entirety. To the extent that they relied on laboratory technology to the exclusion of clinical observation, judgment, and inference, the oncologists functioned more as *technicians* than as *clinicians*.

In recent decades, the mental health professions have also emphasized data from the research laboratory over data from the clinical consulting room. Personality diagnosis once depended upon expert clinical judgment and inference about subtle, textured, and nuanced personality processes. Clinicians considered a range of data, relying not just on what patients said, but also on how they said it, drawing complexly determined inferences from patients' accounts of their lives and important relationships, from their manner of interacting with the clinician, and from their own emotional reactions to the patient. For example, expert clinicians tend not to assess lack of empathy, a diagnostic criterion for narcissistic personality disorder, by administering self-report questionnaires or asking direct questions. Often, an initial sign of lack of empathy on the part of the patient is a subtle sense on the part of the clinician of being interchangeable or replaceable, of being treated as a sounding board rather than as a fellow human being. The clinician might go on to consider whether she consistently feels this way with this particular patient, and whether such feelings are characteristic for her in her role as therapist. She might then become aware that the patient's descriptions of important others come across as somewhat two-dimensional, or that he tends to describe others more in terms of the functions they serve or the needs they meet than in terms of who they are as people. The clinician might further consider whether and how these issues dovetail with the facts the patient has provided about his life, with the problems that brought him to treatment, with information gleaned from family members or other collateral contacts, and so on. When clinicians function as clinicians and not as technicians, it is this kind of thinking, reasoning, and inference that they engage in. Such clinical inference lies at the heart of psychodynamic approaches to understanding personality.

It is just such clinical judgment and inference that psychiatry and psychology have turned away from. As successive editions of the DSM have minimized the role of clinical judgment and inference, personality diagnosis has evolved into a largely technical task of tabulating behavioral signs and symptoms with relatively little consideration for how they fit together, the psychological functions they serve, their meanings, the developmental trajectory that gave rise to them, or the present-day factors that serve to maintain them. Indeed, the diagnostic "gold standard" in personality disorder research is the structured research interview. Such assessment methods are designed to achieve interrater reliability by minimizing the role of clinical judgment or reducing it to the lowest common denominator. Instead of relying on clinical knowledge, complexly determined inferences, and consistent impressions made on the harnessed subjectivities of seasoned therapists (McWilliams, 1999), such assessment procedures substitute standardized questions and decision rules. Indeed, they are typically not administered by expert clinicians at all, but by research assistants or trainees. Like the oncologists in the story, practitioners who rely on such diagnostic methods are functioning more as technicians than as clinicians.

We must keep in mind, however, that the DSM, and the structured assessment instruments it spawned, developed in the directions they have for good reason. Prior to DSM-III, psychiatric diagnosis was unsystematic, overly subjective, and of questionable scientific merit. It often revealed more about the clinician's background and theoretical commitments than it did about the patient. The DSM and structured personality assessment methods evolved in the service of science, and in reaction against the unsystematic and overly subjective diagnostic methods of the past. In the evolution of diagnosis from a largely subjective, clinical enterprise to a largely technical, research-driven enterprise, much has been gained just as much has been lost. The solution cannot be to turn back the clock and abandon the technical developments of the past decades, any more than it would make sense for oncologists to disregard the most technically advanced laboratory tests available. The solution, rather, may be a marriage of the best aspects of clinical wisdom and empirical rigor. We need not choose between empiricism devoid of clinical realism versus a return to a pre-empirical past. To borrow the paradoxical title of a popular movie, progress may lie in going back to the future

This chapter describes the Shedler-Westen Assessment Procedure (SWAP), an approach to personality assessment designed to *harness* clinical judgment and inference rather than eliminate it, and combine the best features of the clinical and empirical traditions in personality assessment. It renders clinical constructs accessible to empirical investigation and provides a means of assessing personality that is both dynamically relevant and empirically grounded.

This chapter will (1) review problems inherent in the current DSM diagnostic system, (2) discuss difficulties associated with the use of clinical observation and inference in research, (3) describe the development of the SWAP and its use in systematizing clinical observation, (4) present a clinical case illustrating how the SWAP provides a bridge between descriptive psychiatry and psychodynamic case formulation, and (5) discuss recommendations for revising and refining DSM Axis II based on empirical findings from a national sample of patients.

WHY REVISE AXIS II?

The approach to the diagnosis of personality disorders codified by DSM finds little favor with either clinicians or researchers. There is consensus among researchers into personality disorders that the DSM classifications system for personality disorders requires major reconfiguration. Some of the problems with DSM-Axis II include the following (see Westen & Shedler, 1999a, 2000):

1. The diagnostic categories do not rest on a solid empirical foundation and often disagree with empirical findings from cluster and factor analyses (Blais & Norman, 1997; Clark, 1992; Harkness, 1992; Livesley & Jackson, 1992; Morey, 1988).

2. DSM-Axis II artificially dichotomizes continuous variables (diagnostic criteria) into present/absent, which is neither theoretically nor statistically sensible (e.g., how little empathy constitutes lack of empathy?).

3. DSM-Axis II commits arbitrarily to a categorical diagnostic system. It may be more useful to conceptualize borderline personality pathology, for example, on a continuum from none through moderate to severe, rather than classifying borderline personality disorder as present/absent (Widiger, 1993).

4. DSM-Axis II lacks the capacity to weight criteria that differ in their diagnostic importance (Davis, Blashfield & McElroy, 1993).

5. Comorbidity between diagnoses of different personality disorders is unacceptably high. Patients who receive any personality disorder diagnosis often receive four to six out of a possible ten (Blais & Norman, 1997, Grilo, Sanislow & McGlashan, 2002, Oldham, Skodol, Kellman, Hyler, et al., 1992, Pilkonis, Heape, Proietti, et al., 1995, Watson & Sinha, 1998), indicating lack of discriminant validity of the diagnostic constructs, the assessment methods, or both.

6. In trying to reduce comorbidity, DSM work groups have had to gerrymander diagnostic categories and criteria, sometimes in ways faithful

neither to clinical observation nor empirical data. For example, they excluded lack of empathy and grandiosity from the diagnostic criteria for antisocial personality disorder to minimize comorbidity with narcissistic personality disorder, despite evidence that these traits are associated with both disorders (Widiger & Corbitt, 1995).

7. Efforts to define personality disorders more precisely have led to narrower criterion sets over time, progressively eroding the distinction between personality *disorders* (multifaceted syndromes encompassing cognition, affectivity, motivation, interpersonal functioning, and so on) and simple personality *traits*. The diagnostic criteria for paranoid personality disorder, for example, are essentially redundant indicators of a single trait, chronic suspiciousness. The diagnostic criteria no longer describe the multifaceted personality syndrome recognized by most clinical theorists (Millon, 1990; Millon & Davis, 1997).

8. DSM-Axis II fails to consider personality strengths that might rule out personality disorder diagnoses for some patients. For example, differentiating between a patient with narcissistic personality disorder and a much healthier person with narcissistic dynamics may not be a matter of counting symptoms, but rather of noting whether the patient has such positive qualities as the capacity to love and to sustain meaningful relationships characterized by mutual caring and sharing.

9. DSM-Axis II does not encompass the spectrum of personality pathology that clinicians see in practice. Among patients receiving treatment for personality pathology (defined as enduring, maladaptive patterns of emotion, thought, motivation, or behavior that lead to distress or dysfunction), fewer than 40% can be diagnosed on axis II (Westen & Arkowitz-Westen, 1998).

10. The categories and criteria are not as clinically useful or relevant as they might be. For example, knowing whether a person meets DSM-IV diagnostic criteria for avoidant personality disorder or dependent personality disorder tells us little about the meaning of the person's symptoms, which personality processes to target for treatment, or how to treat them.

11. The algorithm used for diagnostic decisions (counting symptoms) diverges from the methods clinicians use, or could plausibly be expected to use, in real-world practice. Research in cognitive science indicates that clinicians are unlikely to make diagnoses by additively tabulating symptoms. Rather, they gauge the overall "match" between a patient and a mental template or prototype of the disorder (i.e., they consider the features of a disorder as a configuration or gestalt), or they use causal theories to make sense of the functional relations between the symptoms

(Blashfield, 1985; Cantor & Genero, 1986; Kim & Ahn, 2002; Westen, Heim, Morrison, Patterson, & Campbell, 2002).

12. The instruments used to assess personality disorders do not meet the standards for validity normally expected in psychological research (Perry, 1992; Skodol, Oldham, Rosnick, Kellman, & Hyler, 1991; Westen, 1997) and they show poor test-retest reliability at intervals greater than 6 weeks (First, Spitzer, Gibbon, Williams, et al., 1995; Zimmerman, 1994). The lack of test-retest reliability is especially problematic, given that personality disorders are, by definition, enduring and stable over time.[3]

Most of the proposed solutions to these problems share the assumption that progress lies in further minimizing the role of the clinician, either by developing increasingly behavioral and less inferential diagnostic criteria, or by bypassing clinical judgment entirely through self-report questionnaires. Such attempted solutions may, however, be part of the problem. By eliminating clinical observation and inference, we may unintentionally be eliminating from study the psychological phenomena that are of greatest relevance and importance. The empathically attuned clinician may still be the only "measurement instrument" sensitive enough to register crucial psychological phenomena (Shedler, Mayman, & Manis, 1993). An alternative to trying to eliminate clinical observation and inference is to *harness* it for scientific use.

THE PROBLEM WITH CLINICAL DATA

The problem with clinical observation and inference is *not* that it is inherently unreliable, as some researchers seem to assume. The problem is that it tends to come in a form that does not lend itself readily to systematic study (Shedler, 2002). Rulers measure in inches and scales measure in pounds, but what metric do psychotherapists share? Imagine three clinicians reviewing the same case material. One might speak of schemas and belief systems, another of conditioning history, and the third of transference and resistance. Even among psychoanalytic practitioners, there is little consensus about constructs and terminology. One psychoanalyst might speak of conflict and compromise formation, a second of object relations, and the third, perhaps, of self defects.

It is not readily apparent whether the hypothetical clinicians can or cannot make similar observations and inferences. There are three possibilities: (1) They may be observing and describing the same thing but using different language and metaphor systems to express it. (2) They may simply be attending to differ-

---

[3] Poor test-retest reliability has led some researchers to suggest that personality disorders may be less stable than previously believed. Another hypothesis is that the assessment instruments overemphasize transitory behavioral symptoms (e.g., self-cutting in borderline patients) and underemphasize underlying personality processes that are, in fact, more stable over time (e.g., emotional dysregulation and self-hatred in borderline patients).

ent aspects of the clinical material, as in the parable of the elephant and the blind men. (3) They may not be able to make the same clinical observations at all. *If we want to know whether clinicians can make the same observations and inferences, we must ensure that they speak the same language and pay attention to the same range of clinical phenomena.*

A STANDARD VOCABULARY FOR CASE DESCRIPTION

The *Shedler-Westen Assessment Procedure* (SWAP) is an assessment instrument designed to provide clinicians of all theoretical orientations with a standard vocabulary with which to express their observations and inferences about personality functioning (Shedler & Westen, 1998; 2004a, 2004b; Westen & Shedler, 1999a, 1999b). The vocabulary consists of 200 statements, each printed on a separate index card. Each statement may describe a given patient very well, somewhat, or not at all. A clinician who knows a patient well can describe the patient by ranking or ordering the statements into 8 categories, from those that are most descriptive of the patient (assigned a value of 7) to those that are not descriptive (assigned a value of 0). Thus, the SWAP yields a score from 0 to 7 for each of 200 personality-descriptive variables. An interactive, web-based version of the SWAP can be previewed at www.SWAPassessment.com.

The standard vocabulary of the SWAP allows clinicians to provide in-depth psychological descriptions of patients in a systematic and quantifiable form. It also ensures that all clinicians attend to the same spectrum of clinical phenomena. SWAP statements are written in a manner close to the data (e.g., "Tends to be passive and unassertive," or "Emotions tend to spiral out of control, leading to extremes of anxiety, sadness, rage, etc."), and statements that require inference about internal processes are written in clear and unambiguous language (e.g., "Tends to blame own failures or shortcomings on other people or circumstances; attributes his/her difficulties to external factors rather than accepting responsibility for own conduct or choices"). Writing items in this jargon-free manner minimizes idiosyncratic and unreliable interpretive leaps. It also makes the item set useful for all clinicians regardless of their theoretical commitments.

The SWAP is based on the Q-Sort method, which requires clinicians to place a predetermined number of statements in each category (i.e., it uses a "fixed distribution"). The SWAP distribution resembles the right half of a normal distribution or "bell-shaped curve." One-hundred items are placed in the "0" or not descriptive category and progressively fewer items are placed in the higher categories. Only 8 items are placed in the "7" or most descriptive category. The use of a fixed distribution has important psychometric advantages and eliminates much of the measurement error or "noise" inherent in standard rating procedures (see Block, 1978, for the psychometric rationale underlying the Q-sort method).[4]

---

[4] One way it does so is by ensuring that raters are "calibrated" with one another. Consider the situation with standard rating scales, where raters can use any value as often as they wish. Inevitably, certain raters will tend toward

The SWAP item set was drawn from a wide range of sources including the clinical and psychodynamic literature on personality disorders written over the past 50 years (e.g., Kernberg, 1975, 1984; Kohut, 1971, Linehan, 1993); Axis II diagnostic criteria included in DSM-III through DSM-IV; selected DSM Axis I items that could reflect aspects of personality (e.g., depression and anxiety); research on coping and defense mechanisms (Perry & Cooper, 1987; Shedler, Mayman, & Manis, 1993; Vaillant, 1992; Westen, Muderrisoglu, Fowler, Shedler, & Koren, 1997); research on interpersonal pathology in patients with personality disorders (Westen, 1991, Westen, Lohr, Silk, Gold, & Kerber, 1990); research on personality traits in non-clinical populations (e.g., Block, 1971; John, 1990; McCrae & Costa, 1990); research on personality disorders conducted since the development of Axis II (see Livesley, 1995); extensive pilot interviews in which observers watched videotaped interviews of patients with personality disorders and described them using earlier versions of the item set; and the clinical experience of the authors.

Most importantly, the SWAP-200 (the first major edition of the SWAP) is the product of a 7-year iterative revision process that incorporated the feedback of hundreds of clinician-consultants who used earlier versions of the instrument (Shedler & Westen, 1998) to describe their patients. We asked each clinician-consultant one crucial question: "Were you able to describe the things you consider psychologically important about your patient?" We added, rewrote, and revised items based on this feedback, then asked new clinician-consultants to describe new patients. We repeated this process over many iterations until most clinicians could answer "yes" most of the time. A newer, revised version of the SWAP item set, the SWAP-II incorporates the additional feedback of over 2000 clinicians of all theoretical orientations. The iterative item revision process was designed to ensure both the comprehensiveness and the clinical relevance of the SWAP item sets.

Because the SWAP is jargon-free and clinically comprehensive, it has the potential to serve as a universal language for describing personality pathology. Our studies demonstrate that experienced clinicians of diverse theoretical orientations understand the items and can apply them reliably to their patients. In one study, a nationwide sample of 797 experienced psychologists and psychiatrists of diverse theoretical orientations, who had an average of 18 years practice experience post training, used the SWAP-200 to describe patients with personality pathology (Westen and Shedler, 1999a). These experienced therapists provided similar SWAP-200 descriptions of personality disorders regardless of their theoretical commitments, and fully 72.7% agreed with the statement, "I was able to

---

extreme values (e.g., values of 0 and 7 on a 0-7 scale) whereas others will tend toward middle values (e.g., values of 4 and 5). Thus, the ratings reflect not only the characteristics of the patients but also the calibration of the raters. The Q-Sort method, with its fixed distribution, eliminates this kind of measurement error, because all clinicians must use each value the same number of times. If use of a standard item set gives clinicians a common vocabulary, use of a fixed distribution can be said to give them a common "grammar" (Block, 1978).

express most of the things I consider important about this patient" (the highest rating category). In a subsequent sample of 1201 psychologists and psychiatrists who used the SWAP-II, over 80% "agreed" or "strongly agreed" with the statement, "The SWAP-II allowed me to express the things I consider important about my patient's personality" (less than 5% disagreed). These ratings were unrelated to clinicians' theoretical orientation. Virtually identical agreement rates were obtained in a national sample of clinicians who used the adolescent version of the instrument, the SWAP-II-A.

PSYCHODYNAMICS WITHOUT JARGON

Some investigators have assumed that clinical concepts, especially psychodynamic constructs, are too vague, theoretical, or hypothetical to study empirically. The following SWAP-II items illustrate how the instrument operationalizes some psychodynamic concepts (focusing, for purposes of illustration, on defensive processes). Note that the constructs—rinsed of theoretical jargon—are relevant to a wide range of clinicians, irrespective of theoretical commitments. The traditional psychoanalytic terms for the concepts (which are not included in the SWAP) are in brackets:

SWAP item #	SWAP Item Text
116	Tends to see own unacceptable feelings or impulses in other people instead of in him/herself. [projection]
144	Tends to see self as logical and rational, uninfluenced by emotion; prefers to operate as if emotions were irrelevant or inconsequential. [intellectualization]
78	Tends to express anger in passive and indirect ways (e.g., may make mistakes, procrastinate, forget, become sulky, etc.). [passive aggression]
14	Tends to blame own failures or shortcomings on other people or circumstances; attributes his/her difficulties to external factors rather than accepting responsibility for own conduct or choices. [externalization]
45	Is prone to idealizing people; may see admired others as perfect, larger than life, all wise, etc. [idealization]
165	Tends to distort unacceptable wishes or feelings by transforming them into their opposite (e.g., may express excessive concern while showing signs of unacknowledged hostility, disgust about sexual matters while showing signs of unacknowledged excitement, etc.). [reaction formation]

An illustration: Borderline Personality Pathology

Some clinicians may doubt that a finite set of 200 statements can capture the richness and complexity of clinical case description. However, SWAP statements can be combined in virtually infinite patterns to express subtle clinical concepts. The mathematically inclined reader might note that there are 200 factorial possible orderings of the SWAP statements (an inexpressibly large number). The musically inclined reader might note that all of Western music can be notated using combinations of only 12 tones.

Many clinical theorists consider *splitting, projective identification*, and *identity disturbance* to be hallmarks of borderline personality pathology (see *Personality Patterns and Disorders*, p. 15). Consider, for example, the items reproduced below from the original SWAP-200 item set. The three items, *taken in combination*, convey something of the defensive splitting seen in patients with borderline personality pathology:

SWAP item #	SWAP Item Text
162	Expresses contradictory feelings or beliefs without being disturbed by the inconsistency; has little need to reconcile or resolve contradictory ideas.
45	Tends to idealize certain others in unrealistic ways; sees them as "all good," to the exclusion of commonplace human defects.
79	Tends to see certain others as "all bad," and loses the capacity to perceive any positive qualities the person may have.

The following items, from the SWAP-II, capture some additional meanings of the concept *splitting*.

SWAP item #	SWAP Item Text
9	When upset, has trouble perceiving both positive and negative qualities in the same person at the same time (e.g., may see others in black or white terms, shift suddenly from seeing someone as caring to seeing him/her as malevolent and intentionally hurtful, etc.).
18	Tends to stir up conflict or animosity between other people (e.g., may portray a situation differently to different people, leading them to form contradictory views or work at cross purposes).

The next group of items, *taken in combination*, captures at least one meaning of the term *projective identification*:

SWAP item #	SWAP Item Text
116	Tends to see own unacceptable feelings or impulses in other people instead of in him/herself.
76	Manages to elicit in others feelings similar to those s/he is experiencing (e.g., when angry, acts in such a way as to provoke anger in others; when anxious, acts in such a way as to induce anxiety in others).
154	Tends to draw others into scenarios, or "pull" them into roles, that feel alien or unfamiliar (e.g., being uncharacteristically insensitive or cruel, feeling like the only person in the world who can help, etc.).

The concept *identity disturbance* (or *identity diffusion*) subsumes a wide range of phenomena (Wilkinson-Ryan & Westen, 2000). When the same term has been used in the literature in different ways, or used differently by different theorists, we wrote multiple SWAP items to cover the multiple meanings. The following SWAP-II items illustrate some of the manifestations and facets of identity disturbance:

SWAP item #	SWAP Item Text
15	Lacks a stable sense of who s/he is (e.g., attitudes, values, goals, and feelings about self seem unstable or ever-changing).
151	Appears to experience the past as a series of disjointed or disconnected events; has difficulty giving a coherent account of his/her life story.
90	Is prone to painful feelings of emptiness (e.g., may feel lost, bereft, abjectly alone even in the presence of others, etc.).
172	Seems unable to settle into, or sustain commitment to, identity-defining life roles (e.g., career, occupation, lifestyle, etc.).
150	Tends to identify with admired others to an exaggerated degree, taking on their attitudes, mannerisms, etc. (e.g., may be drawn into the "orbit" of a strong or charismatic personality).
87	Sense of identity revolves around a "cause," movement, or label (e.g., adult child of alcoholic, adult survivor, environmentalist, born-again Christian, etc.); may be drawn to extreme or all-encompassing belief systems.
38	Tends to feel s/he is not his/her true self with others; may feel false or fraudulent.
102	Has a deep sense of inner badness; sees self as damaged, evil, or rotten to the core (whether consciously or unconsciously).

The next group of items helps flesh out a picture of a certain kind of borderline patient, addressing issues of affect regulation, object relations, cognition, and so on:

SWAP item #	SWAP Item Text
191	Emotions tend to change rapidly and unpredictably.
12	Emotions tend to spiral out of control, leading to extremes of anxiety, sadness, rage, etc.
185	Is prone to intense anger, out of proportion to the situation at hand (e.g., has rage episodes).
157	Tends to become irrational when strong emotions are stirred up; may show a significant decline from customary level of functioning.
117	Is unable to soothe or comfort him/herself without the help of another person (i.e., has difficulty regulating own emotions).
98	Tends to fear s/he will be rejected or abandoned.
11	Tends to become attached quickly or intensely; develops feelings, expectations, etc. that are not warranted by the history or context of the relationship.
167	Is simultaneously needy of, and rejecting toward, others (e.g., craves intimacy and caring, but tends to reject it when offered).
153	Relationships tend to be unstable, chaotic, and rapidly changing.
52	Has little empathy; seems unable or unwilling to understand or respond to others' needs or feelings.
176	Tends to confuse own thoughts, feelings, or personality traits with those of others (e.g., may use the same words to describe him/herself and another person, believe the two share identical thoughts and feelings, etc.).
41	Appears unable to describe important others in a way that conveys a sense of who they are as people; descriptions of others come across as two-dimensional and lacking in richness.
29	Has difficulty making sense of other people's behavior; tends to misunderstand, misinterpret, or be confused by others' actions and reactions.

The last group of items includes descriptors that might apply to a more disturbed borderline patient, perhaps one likely to be seen in an inpatient setting (Gunderson, 2001):

SWAP item #	SWAP Item Text
134	Tends to act impulsively (e.g., acts without forethought or concern for consequences).
142	Tends to make repeated suicidal threats or gestures, either as a "cry for help" or as an effort to manipulate others.
109	Tends to engage in self-mutilating behavior (e.g., self-cutting, self-burning, etc.).
188	Work-life and/or living arrangements tend to be chaotic or unstable (e.g., job or housing situation seems always temporary, transitional, or ill-defined).
44	When distressed, perception of reality can become grossly impaired (e.g., thinking may seem delusional).

The items reproduced here are illustrative only and are not intended to describe "the" borderline patient or any particular borderline patient. They are intended only to illustrate that it is possible to describe clinically and psychodynamically important constructs without succumbing to either reductionism or jargon. Further, such descriptions are empirically testable.

A Case Illustration

At present, descriptive psychiatric diagnosis and clinical case formulation are largely independent activities. The former is aimed at classification (a nomothetic approach) whereas the latter is aimed at understanding an individual patient (an idiographic approach). The SWAP bridges these activities. It provides a dimensional diagnosis score for each personality disorder included in DSM-IV (as well as for the additional personality disorders proposed in the DSM-IV appendix). It also provides a richly detailed clinical case narrative relevant to case formulation and treatment planning.

Dimensional personality disorder (PD) scores measure the "fit" or "match" between an individual patient and prototype descriptions representing each personality disorder in its "ideal" or pure form (e.g., a prototype description of paranoid personality disorder). Thus, each personality disorder is diagnosed on a continuum; a low PD score indicates that the patient does not fit or match the personality disorder syndrome and a high PD score indicates that the patient matches it well (with intermediate scores indicating varying degrees of "fit"). PD scores can be graphed to create a personality disorder profile resembling an MMPI profile, as illustrated in Figure 1. Dimensional diagnosis is consistent with clinical thinking and advocated by virtually all contemporary personality researchers (Widiger & Simonsen, 2005). (We are developing web-based software that will allow clinicians to input SWAP scores and receive a computer-generated interpretive report with personality disorder diagnoses, a detailed case description, and treatment recommendations. Visit *www.SWAPassessment.com* to preview the software,).

A clinical case example may best illustrate these diagnostic applications of the SWAP.[5]

Case Background

"Melania" is a 30 year old Caucasian woman. Her presenting complaints included substance abuse and inability to extricate herself from an abusive relationship. The initial assessment included a psychiatric intake interview and administration of both the SCID and SCID-II structured interviews. She met SCID criteria for an Axis I diagnosis of substance abuse and SCID-II criteria for an Axis II diagnosis of borderline personality disorder with histrionic traits. The intake interviewer assigned a score of 45 on the Global Assessment of Functioning (GAF) scale, indicating severe symptoms and impairment in functioning.

Melania's early family environment was marked by neglect and parental strife. A recurring family scenario is illustrative: Melania's mother would scream at her husband, telling him he was a failure and that she was going to leave him; she would then slam the door and lock herself in her room, leaving Melania frightened and in tears. Both parents would then ignore Melania, often forgetting to feed her. Melania's parents divorced when she was 8. After the divorce, Melania lived with her mother, who showed little concern for her needs or welfare.

By adolescence, Melania had developed behavioral problems. She often skipped school and spent her days sleeping or wandering the streets. At age 18, she left home and began what she described as "life on the streets." She engaged in a series of impulsive, chaotic, and rapidly changing sexual relationships which led to three abortions by age 24. She abused street drugs, eventually developing a pattern of cocaine and heroin abuse (snorting). She also engaged in petty criminal activity, including shoplifting and stealing from employers.

Melania held a series of low paying jobs that were not commensurate with her ability or education. She failed to hold any job for more than a few months and was fired from each when she was caught stealing. In her mid-twenties, Melania moved in with her boyfriend, a small-time drug dealer who exploited her financially and abused her physically. He spent his days sleeping or watching television while Melania worked to pay the rent. She often had sex with other men

---

[5] The material presented in this section is adapted from Lingiardi, Shedler, & Gazzillo (2006).

to obtain money or drugs for her boyfriend. He sometimes beat her when he was dissatisfied with what she brought home.

Melania began psychodynamic therapy at a frequency of three sessions per week. The first ten psychotherapy sessions were tape recorded and transcribed. Two clinicians (blind to all other data) reviewed the transcripts and provided SWAP-200 descriptions of Melania, based on the information contained in the session transcripts. The SWAP-200 scores were then averaged across the two clinical judges to obtain a single SWAP-200 description.[6] After two years of psychotherapy, ten consecutive psychotherapy sessions were again recorded and transcribed, and the SWAP assessment procedure was repeated.

Personality Disorder Diagnosis

The solid line in Figure 1 shows Melania's PD scores at the beginning of treatment for the ten personality disorders included in DSM-IV. A "healthy functioning" index is graphed as well, which reflects clinicians' consensual understanding of healthy personality functioning (Westen & Shedler, 1999a). For ease of interpretation, the PD scores have been converted to T-scores (Mean = 50, SD = 10) based on norms established in a psychiatric sample of patients with axis II diagnoses (Westen & Shedler, 1999a). Although the SWAP assesses personality disorders dimensionally and treats each personality disorder diagnosis as a continuum, we have established cutoff scores for "backward compatibility" with DSM-IV. To maintain continuity with the DSM-IV categorical diagnostic system, we have suggested T = 60 as a threshold for making a categorical personality disorder diagnosis, and T = 55 as a threshold for diagnosing "features."[7]

Melania's PD profile shows a marked elevation for borderline personality disorder (T = 65.4, approximately one and a half standard deviations above the sample mean), with secondary elevations for histrionic personality disorder (T = 56.6) and antisocial personality disorder (T = 55.7). Applying the recommended cutoff scores, her axis II diagnosis is borderline personality disorder with histrionic and antisocial features. Also noteworthy is the T-Score of 41 for the "healthy functioning" index, nearly a standard deviation below the mean in a reference sample of patients with Axis II diagnoses. The low score indicates significant impairment in functioning and parallels the low GAF score assigned by the intake interviewer.

---

[6] Averaging across raters enhances the reliability of the resulting scores.
[7] The relatively low thresholds reflect the fact that the reference sample consisted of patients with a diagnosis of personality disorder. Thus, a T-score of 50 indicates "average" functioning among patients with personality disorder diagnoses, and a T-score of 60 represents an elevation of one standard deviation relative to other patients with personality disorder diagnoses.

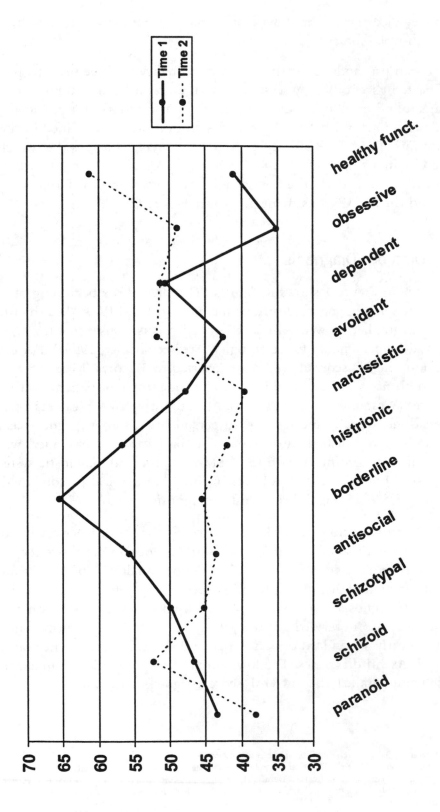

Figure 1: PD score profile

Narrative Case Description

We can generate a narrative case description by listing the SWAP items assigned the highest scores in the patient's SWAP description (e.g., items with scores of 5, 6, and 7). Below is a narrative case description for "Melania" based on the top 30 most descriptive SWAP-200 items. We have grouped together conceptually related items. To aid the flow of the text, we have made some minor grammatical changes and added connecting text. However, the SWAP-200 items are reproduced essentially verbatim. The narrative description is based on the same data used to generate the PD score profile in Figure 1.

Melania experiences severe depression and dysphoria. She tends to feel unhappy, depressed, or despondent, appears to find little or no pleasure or satisfaction in life's activities, feels life is without meaning, and tends to feel like an outcast or outsider. She tends to feel guilty, and to feel inadequate, inferior, or a failure. Her behavior is often self-defeating and self-destructive. She appears inhibited about pursuing goals or successes, is insufficiently concerned with meeting her own needs, and seems not to feel entitled to get or ask for things she deserves. She appears to want to "punish" herself by creating situations that lead to unhappiness, or actively avoiding opportunities for pleasure and gratification. Specific self-destructive tendencies include getting drawn into and remaining in relationships in which she is emotionally or physically abused, abusing illicit drugs, and acting impulsively and without regard for consequences. She shows little concern for consequences in general.

Melania shows many personality traits associated specifically with borderline PD. Her relationships are unstable, chaotic, and rapidly changing. She has little empathy and seems unable to understand or respond to others' needs and feelings unless they coincide with her own. Moreover, she tends to confuse her own thoughts, feelings, and personality traits with those of others, and she often acts in such a way as to elicit her own feelings in other people (for example, provoking anger when she herself is angry, or inducing anxiety in others when she herself is anxious).

Melania expresses contradictory feelings without being disturbed by the inconsistency, and she seems to have little need to reconcile or resolve contradictory ideas. She is prone to see certain others as "all bad," losing the capacity to perceive any positive qualities they may have. She lacks a stable image of who she is or would like to become (e.g., her attitudes, values, goals, and feelings about self are unstable and changing) and she tends to feel empty. Affect regulation is poor: She tends to become irrational when strong emotions are stirred up and shows a noticeable decline from her customary level of functioning. She also seems unable to soothe or comfort herself when distressed and requires the involvement of another person to help her regulate affect. Both her living arrangements and her work life tend to be chaotic and unstable.

Finally, Melania's attitudes toward men and sexuality are problematic and conflictual. She tends to be hostile toward members of the opposite sex (whether consciously or unconsciously) and she associates sexual activity with danger (e.g., injury or punishment). She appears afraid of commitment to a long-term love relationship, instead choosing partners who seem inappropriate in terms of age, status (e.g., social, economic, intellectual), or other factors.

The narrative description provides a detailed portrait of a severely troubled borderline patient. The description helps illustrate the difference between descriptive psychiatry (aimed at establishing a diagnosis) and clinical case formulation (aimed at understanding an individual person). In this instance, however, all findings are derived from the same assessment procedure and grounded in quantitative data.

Assessing Change in Therapy

The case of Melania has a happy ending. After two years of psychotherapy, the SWAP assessment revealed significant personality changes. The changes parallel concrete behavior changes as well as changes in Melania's life circumstances (e.g., ending her drug abuse, getting and keeping a good job, ending her involvement with her abusive boyfriend, no longer engaging in theft, promiscuous sex, or prostitution).

The dotted line in Figure 1 shows Melania's PD scores after two years of psychotherapy. Her scores on the borderline, histrionic, and antisocial dimensions have dropped below $T = 50$ and she no longer warrants a diagnosis of personality disorder. Her score on the healthy functioning index has increased by two standard deviations, from 41.0 to 61.2.

To assess change in an ideographic, more fine-grained manner, we created a change score for each individual SWAP item by subtracting the item score at Time 1 from the score at Time 2. The narrative description of change, below, is comprised of the SWAP items with change scores > 4. Again, we have made some minor grammatical changes and added connecting text to aid the flow of the text, but the SWAP-200 items are reproduced essentially verbatim.

Melania has developed strengths and inner resources that were not evident at the Time 1 assessment. She has come to terms with painful experiences from the past, finding meaning in, and growing from, these experiences; she has become more articulate and better able to express herself in words; she has a newfound ability to appreciate and respond to humor; she is more capable of recognizing alternative viewpoints, even in matters that stir up strong feelings; she is more empathic and sensitive to other's needs and feelings; and she is more likeable.

There is marked improvement in many areas associated specifically with borderline psychopathology. With respect to affect regulation, Melania is less prone to become irrational when strong emotions are stirred up, is more likely to express affect appropriate in quality and intensity to the situation at hand, and is better able to sooth or comfort herself when distressed. She is less prone to confuse her own thoughts and feelings with those of others, less manipulative, and less likely to devalue others and see them as "all bad." She has come to terms with negative feelings toward her parents.

Melania is also less impulsive, more conscientious and responsible, and more aware of the consequences of her actions. Her living arrangements are more stable, as is her work life. Melania's use of illicit drugs has decreased significantly, and she is no longer drawn to abusive relationships.

As the more severe aspects of borderline personality pathology have receded, other conflicts and symptoms have moved to the fore. For example, Melania appears to have developed somewhat obsessional defenses against painful affect. She adheres more rigidly to daily routines and becomes anxious or uncomfortable when they are altered. She is more prone to think in an abstract and intellectualized manner, and tries to see herself as more logical and rational, less influenced by emotion.

Despite her wish to act more logically and rationally, Melania seems engaged in an active struggle to control her affect and impulses. She tends to oscillate between undercontrol and overcontrol of needs and wishes, either expressing them impulsively or disavowing them entirely. She has more difficulty allowing herself to experience strong pleasurable emotions (e.g., excitement, joy). She is more prone to repress, "forget," or otherwise distort distressing events.

Finally, there are changes in Melania's relationships and orientation toward sexuality. Whereas before she presented in a histrionic manner (i.e., with exaggerated feminine traits), she is now more disparaging of traditionally feminine traits, instead emphasizing independence and achievement. Whereas previously she engaged in multiple chaotic sexual relationships, she now seems conflicted about her intimacy needs. She craves intimacy but tends to reject it when offered. She has more difficulty directing both sexual and tender feelings toward the same person, seeing men as either respectable and virtuous, or sexy and exciting, but not both. She is more likely to hold grudges.

We leave it to readers to judge the clinical relevance of the SWAP and the value of the diagnostic profiles and narrative case descriptions that it yields. Note, however, that the standard vocabulary of the SWAP ensures that different clinicians will describe the same patient in much the same way, once they learn to use the SWAP reliably. Had other clinicians described Melania using the SWAP, the narrative descriptions would have been much the same, since the descriptive statements comprising the narrative were taken directly from the SWAP-200 item set.

RELIABILITY AND VALIDITY

Researchers in psychology and psychiatry have often assumed that clinical observation and judgment is unreliable, and a well-established literature documents the limitations of "clinical judgment." Unfortunately, studies of "clinical judgment" have often asked clinicians to make judgments about things that fall well outside their legitimate area of expertise (equally unfortunate, some clinicians have been all too willing to offer such prognostications). More problematic, the studies have typically conflated clinicians' ability to make accurate observations and inferences (which they do well) with their ability to combine and weight variables to derive optimal predictions (a task that is *necessarily* performed better by statistical methods such as regression equations). In fact, a substantial literature documents the reliability and validity of clinical observation and inference *when it is quantified and used appropriately* (see Westen & Weinberger, 2004, for a detailed discussion and literature review).

The SWAP differs from past approaches in that it harnesses clinical judgment using psychometric methods developed specifically for this purpose, then applies statistical and actuarial methods to the resulting variables. In short, it relies on clinicians to do what they do best: making specific behavioral observations and inferences about the individual patients they know well. It relies on statistical algorithms to do what they do best: combining data optimally to derive reliable and valid diagnostic scales and indices.

Inter-rater reliability of SWAP-200 PD scale scores (Figure 1) and other diagnostic scales derived from the SWAP is above 0.80 for all scales in all studies conducted to date (e.g., Westen and Muderrisoglu, 2003, in press) and is often above 0.90 (e.g., Marin-Avellan, McGauley, Campbell, & Fonagy, 2005). These reliability coefficients are at least as high as those typically reported for highly structured research interviews that avoid clinical inference and "just stick to the facts" (i.e., DSM-IV diagnostic criteria). Additionally, the SWAP diagnostic scales correlate highly with a wide range of external criterion measures in both adult and adolescent samples, including, e.g., genetic history variables such as psychosis in first- and second-degree relatives, substance abuse in first- and second-degree relatives, developmental history variables such as childhood sexual and physical abuse, life events such as psychiatric hospitalizations and suicide attempts, ratings of adaptive functioning, and so on (see Shedler & Westen, 2004b; Westen & Muderrisoglu, 2003; Westen & Shedler, 1999a; Westen, Shedler, Durrett, Glass, & Martens, 2003; Westen & Weinberger, 2004).[8]

We will describe some illustrative studies in detail.[9] Westen and Muderrisoglu (2003) interviewed a sample of outpatients using the Clinical Diagnostic Interview (CDI) (Westen, 2002), a systematic interview ($2\frac{1}{2}$ to 3 hours in length) designed to systematize the personality assessment methods employed by knowledgeable clinicians in real-world practice (Westen, 1997). The CDI does not ask patients to describe their own personality traits, but instead elicits narrative descriptions of patients' lives and important relationships. The narrative descriptions allow clinical interviewers to draw reliable inferences about patients' characteristic ways of thinking, feeling, regulating emotions and impulses, relating interpersonally, and so on (much as a sophisticated clinician might do in the first two to four meetings with a new patient).

The primary aims of the study were to (1) assess inter-rater reliability of SWAP diagnostic scales as assessed by independent clinicians who either conducted or observed (on videotape) the CDI interview, and (2) to assess convergent validity between these independent raters and the treating clinicians, whose SWAP scores were based on extensive contact with their patients over time. All of the clinical assessors were blind to the data provided by the others. The study examined the reliability and validity of ten SWAP PD scores plus seven other SWAP diagnostic indices (see Westen & Shedler, 1999b).

Inter-rater reliability between independent interviewers averaged greater than 0.80 for all SWAP scores. Convergent validity coefficients between interviewers and treating clinicians were also above 0.80 for all scores. Discriminant validity coefficients (i.e., correlations between unrelated diagnostic scales) were excellent, hovering near zero. To provide some reference points with which to compare these values, convergent validity between personality disorder diagnoses derived from structured research interviews and diagnoses based on the LEAD standard

---

[8] Interrater reliability of the *overall* SWAP description (versus scales derived from the SWAP) is also high, ranging in prior studies from 0.75 to 0.89 (Marin-Avellan, et al., 2004; Shedler & Westen, 1998; Westen & Muderrisoglu, 2003). Reliability of the overall SWAP description is most relevant to narrative case descriptions derived from the SWAP (such as the narrative description of "Melania"). The overall reliability of a Q-sort personality description refers to agreement between raters regarding the *ordering* of the items or statements, traditionally measured by Pearson's r (Block, 1978). For example, a SWAP-200 description of a patient consists of one column by 200 rows of data (with each row containing the score [0 to 7] for the corresponding SWAP-200 item). Each additional rater adds one additional column of data, and interrater reliability is computed by correlating pairs of columns. Item scores are typically averaged across all available raters to obtain an aggregate Q-sort description. The reliability of the aggregate description is estimated by the Spearman-Brown formula (when there are two raters) or coefficient alpha (when there are multiple raters). The approach is identical to that used to estimate the internal reliability of a psychometric scale, except that the raters are treated as test items and the Q-sort items are treated as cases.

[9] The material presented here is adapted from Westen and Weinberger, 2004.

(Spitzer, 1983) have ranged from 0.00 to 0.40, and discriminant validity has been quite poor (see Pilkonis, Heape, Ruddy, & Serrao, 1991; Pilkonis, et al., 1995). Similarly, a meta-analysis of personality disorder dimensions assessed via self- and informant-report yielded a median correlation of only 0.36 (Klonsky, Oltmanns, & Turkheimer, 2002).

A second study (Bradley & Westen, 2003) examined convergence between SWAP scores and patient self-report data for borderline and antisocial personality disorder (the two personality disorders for which self-report and informant-report data tend to converge). Advanced clinical psychology graduate students used the SWAP–200 to describe 54 outpatients after the fifth clinical contact hour. The patients completed the Personality Assessment Inventory (PAI) (Morey, 1991). Convergent validity was high, with SWAP antisocial and borderline personality disorder scores differentially predicting antisocial and borderline scores on the PAI. Discriminant validity coefficients were desirably low (e.g., the SWAP obsessive-compulsive PD score correlated *negatively* with PAI antisocial and borderline scores), indicating excellent diagnostic specificity. The data provide further evidence for the validity of the SWAP-200 as an assessment tool.

A study from a research group other than our own reported comparable findings (Marin-Avellan, et al., 2005). The investigators applied the SWAP-200 to audiotaped Adult Attachment Interviews (AAI) (Main, Kaplan, & Cassidy, 1985) plus chart records for a sample of inpatients at a maximum security forensic hospital (a method similar to methods for coding psychopathy; Hare, Harpur, Hakstian, Forth, et al., 1990). Interrater reliability for SWAP-200 PD scale provided by independent assessors was high, with a median interrater correlation of r = .91.

Additionally, SWAP PD scores differentiated patients who had committed violent versus nonviolent offenses, whereas SCID–II diagnosis did not. The SWAP-200 also proved superior to the SCID-II in predicting ward behavior, assessed independently by ward nurses (who were blind to all other data) using a 49-item interpersonal rating scale. SWAP antisocial PD scores correlated significantly with dominance behavior and coercive behavior observed on the ward, and correlated negatively with submissive behavior and compliant behavior observed on the ward. In contrast, the SCID-II predicted only dominance behavior. The findings clearly demonstrate incremental validity of the SWAP-200 relative to a widely used instrument for assessing personality disorders that relies substantially on patient self-report.

In summary, experienced clinicians can make highly reliable observations and inferences about personality dynamics, given a suitable technology for harnessing their judgments. The belief that clinicians cannot reliably assess psychodynamic and other complex clinical constructs, is mistaken.

TOWARD DSM-V: AN EMPIRICAL APPROACH TO REVISING AND REFINING DIAGNOSTIC CRITERIA

The approach to personality diagnosis codified by DSM-IV has elicited little enthusiasm from either clinicians or researchers. Ultimately, revisions to the diagnostic categories and criteria over successive editions of the DSM reflect committee decision processes, which can be influenced by group dynamics, the opinions of individual committee members, the sociopolitical *zeitgeist*, and other such factors. Here we describe an alternative, empirical approach to identifying diagnostic criteria of personality disorders.[10]

Identifying Core Features of Personality Disorders

Because the SWAP quantifies clinical case description, it allows investigators to statistically combine case descriptions to obtain a composite description of a particular grouping of patients. This is accomplished by averaging (aggregating) the values assigned to each SWAP item across a relevant patient sample. For example, if we obtain SWAP descriptions for a representative sample of patients diagnosed with paranoid personality disorder, we can average the values for each SWAP items to obtain a composite description of the prototypical paranoid patient.

A fortunate statistical consequence of averaging is that only SWAP items ranked highly for virtually all patients will have a high ranking in the composite description. If a descriptor does not apply to all or most patients in the sample, the item will not achieve a high score. Thus, examination of the highest-ranking items in the composite description for paranoid personality disorder reveals the *core psychological features* shared by paranoid patients treated in the community. This represents a purely empirical procedure for identifying the core features of a personality syndrome.

Method

A national sample of 530 experienced psychiatrists and clinical psychologists recruited from the rosters of the American Psychiatric Association and the American Psychological Association used the SWAP-200 to describe a current patient with a specified personality disorder diagnosis (for a more complete description of the study methods, see Shedler & Westen, 2004a). We aggregated the SWAP descriptions across all patients with a given personality disorder diagnosis to create a *composite description* for each personality disorder included in DSM-IV. The composite descriptions were highly reliable (coefficient alpha > 0.90 for all

---

[10] The material in this section is adapted from Shedler and Westen, 2004a.

descriptions), indicating that the sample sizes were adequate to obtain stable and reproducible personality descriptions.[11]

Results

We will describe the findings for a few personality disorders. (For a more complete account of the study findings for all ten personality disorders, see Shedler & Westen, 2004a.)

Cluster A: The "Odd" Cluster

Tables 1a-1c list the SWAP-200 items that received the highest scores or rankings in each composite description, along with the item's mean score or ranking in the composite (indicating its centrality or importance in defining the personality disorder). Two findings are noteworthy. First, the descriptions differ systematically from the DSM-IV descriptions and include psychological features absent from the DSM criterion sets, especially items addressing inner life or intrapsychic experience. Second, there is considerable overlap in item content between the disorders. Thus, there are psychological features that are central to two or all three of the Cluster A disorders (e.g., difficulty making sense of other people's behavior, problematic reality testing, a propensity to feel misunderstood or mistreated, a tendency toward social isolation). If we consider each composite description as a *whole* (that is, if we consider the "gist" or gestalt of the 15 to 20 most descriptive statements), the descriptions are readily distinguishable. However, if we limit the descriptions to just the first 8 to 9 items—the number included in DSM-IV criterion sets—it is more difficult to distinguish them. This suggests that criterion sets of 8 to 9 items are too small to provide PD descriptions that are both clinically accurate and adequately distinct (Shedler & Westen, 2004b; Westen & Shedler, 2000).

Paranoid Personality Disorder

Empirically observable features of paranoid personality disorder include aggression ("Tends to be angry or hostile") and the defenses of externalization ("tends to blame own one's failures or shortcomings on others") and projection ("tends to see own unacceptable feelings or impulses in other people instead of in him/herself"). The findings are consistent with the psychodynamic hypothesis that projection of aggression is a central dynamic in paranoid personality (i.e.,

---

[11] The reliability of a composite or aggregate personality description is measured by coefficient alpha, which reflects the intercorrelations between the patients (columns of data) included in the aggregate description. The logic is identical to computing the reliability of a psychometric scale, except that patients are treated as scale "items" (columns in the data file) and SWAP-200 items are treated as cases (rows in the data file). See footnote 4 for additional details.

paranoid patients perceive the world as dangerous because they see their own hostility wherever they look). Similar findings emerged when we stratified the data by clinician theoretical orientation and omitted data provided by clinicians who described their theoretical orientation as psychoanalytic or psychodynamic (it is therefore highly unlikely that the reporting clinicians were simply describing their personality theories, rather than the observed characteristics of their patients). Other empirically observable characteristics of paranoid personality disorder absent from DSM-IV include feelings of victimization, difficulties understanding others' actions, hypersensitivity to slights, lack of close friendships and relationships, and the tendency for reasoning to become severely impaired under stress.

Cluster B: The "Dramatic" Cluster

Tables 2a-2d list the SWAP-200 items that received the highest ranking in the composite descriptions for the Cluster B disorders. Again, the descriptions of personality disorders differ systematically from the DSM-IV descriptions and place greater emphasis on inner life. Once again there is significant item overlap, but the disorders are readily distinguishable when the descriptions are considered in total.

Antisocial Personality Disorder

The composite description of antisocial patients includes multiple traits associated with the construct of psychopathy that preceded the current antisocial personality disorder diagnosis (Cleckley, 1941; Patrick & Zempolich, 1998). Included in the composite description, but absent from the DSM-IV criterion set, are items addressing lack of empathy, sadism, emotional manipulativeness, imperviousness to consequences, and externalization of blame. In contrast, DSM-IV emphasizes behaviors associated with criminality (and would therefore miss the more "successful" psychopathic personalities who express their pathology in the world of business or politics).

Cluster C: The "Anxious" Cluster
Avoidant and Dependent Personality Disorder

The empirical portraits of avoidant and dependent personality disorders in Tables 3a and 3b help explain the excessive comorbidity between the disorders observed in virtually every study to date (Millon & Martinez, 1995; Westen & Shedler, 1999a). Patients diagnosed with these disorders share a *depressive* or *dysphoric core* that appears to pervade all areas of functioning. This depression or dysphoria is not captured by the current DSM criteria. Patients diagnosed by their clinicians with avoidant personality disorder attempt to deal with dysphoria by keeping their distance from people, whereas those diagnosed with dependent personality disorder attempt to cope by clinging. However, both groups experience depression and despondency, feelings of inferiority, guilt, shame, anxiety, self-criticism, self-blame, passivity, and inhibitions. Clinicians appear to be using these diagnostic categories to describe patients who might be better conceptualized in terms of depressive personality disorder (see *Personality Patterns and Disorders*, p. 15).

Table 1a: Composite Description of Patients Diagnosed with Paranoid Personality Disorder

Item	Mean
Tends to feel misunderstood, mistreated, or victimized.	6.19
Is quick to assume that others want to harm or take advantage of him/her; tends to perceive malevolent intentions in others' words and actions.	5.97
Tends to be angry or hostile (whether consciously or unconsciously).	5.74
Tends to hold grudges; may dwell on insults or slights for long periods.	5.55
Tends to blame others for own failures or shortcomings; tends to believe his/her problems are caused by external factors.	5.26
Tends to avoid confiding in others for fear of betrayal; expects things she/he says or does will be used against him/her.	5.03
Tends to be critical of others.	5.03
Tends to react to criticism with feelings of rage or humiliation.	4.94
Lacks close friendships and relationships.	4.52
Tends to get into power struggles.	4.48
Has difficulty making sense of other people's behavior; often misunderstands, misinterprets, or is confused by others' actions and reactions.	4.48
Perception of reality can become grossly impaired under stress (e.g., may become delusional).	4.32
Tends to feel like an outcast or outsider; feels as if she/he does not truly belong.	4.26
Tends to express intense and inappropriate anger, out of proportion to the situation at hand.	4.23
Tends to feel helpless, powerless, or at the mercy of forces outside his/her control.	4.16
Tends to see own unacceptable feelings or impulses in other people instead of in him/herself.	4.03

Table 1b: Composite Description of Patients Diagnosed with Schizoid Personality Disorder

Item	Mean
Lacks close friendships and relationships.	5.85
Lacks social skills; tends to be socially awkward or inappropriate.	5.59
Appears to have a limited or constricted range of emotions.	5.44
Tends to feel like an outcast or outsider; feels as if she/he does not truly belong.	5.13
Tends to be inhibited or constricted; has difficulty allowing self to acknowledge or express wishes and impulses.	5.08
Tends to be shy or reserved in social situations.	4.95
Appearance or manner seems odd or peculiar (e.g., grooming, hygiene, posture, eye contact, speech rhythms, etc. seem somehow strange or "off").	4.56
Tends to avoid social situations because of fear of embarrassment or humiliation.	4.46
Has difficulty making sense of other people's behavior; often misunderstands, misinterprets, or is confused by others' actions and reactions.	4.31
Has difficulty acknowledging or expressing anger.	4.28
Tends to feel unhappy, depressed, or despondent.	4.23
Has difficulty allowing self to experience strong pleasurable emotions (e.g., excitement, joy, pride).	4.18
Tends to be passive and unassertive.	4.13
Appears to find little or no pleasure, satisfaction, or enjoyment in life's activities.	4.00
Tends to feel she/he is inadequate, inferior, or a failure.	3.97
Appears to have little need for human company or contact; is genuinely indifferent to the presence of others.	3.92
Appears inhibited about pursuing goals or successes; aspirations or achievements tend to be below his/her potential.	3.90
Tends to be anxious.	3.59

Table 1c: Composite Description of Patients Diagnosed with Schizotypal Personality Disorder

Item	Mean
Lacks close friendships and relationships.	6.17
Appearance or manner seems odd or peculiar (e.g., grooming, hygiene, posture, eye contact, speech rhythms, etc. seem somehow strange or "off").	6.08
Reasoning processes or perceptual experiences seem odd and idiosyncratic (e.g., may make seemingly arbitrary inferences; may see hidden messages or special meanings in ordinary events).	5.17
Tends to feel like an outcast or outsider; feels as if she/he does not truly belong.	4.79
Lacks social skills; tends to be socially awkward or inappropriate.	4.79
Has difficulty making sense of other people's behavior; often misunderstands, misinterprets, or is confused by others' actions and reactions.	4.71
Perception of reality can become grossly impaired under stress (e.g., may become delusional).	4.63
Appears to have a limited or constricted range of emotions.	4.50
Tends to become irrational when strong emotions are stirred up; may show a noticeable decline from customary level of functioning.	4.08
Tens to be shy or reserved in social situations.	4.04
Tends to be anxious.	3.88
Tends to feel unhappy, depressed, or despondent.	3.83
Tends to feel helpless, powerless, or at the mercy of forces outside his/her control.	3.71
Tends to feel misunderstood, mistreated, or victimized.	3.58
Tends to avoid social situations because of fear of embarrassment or humiliation.	3.54
Has little psychological insight into own motives, behavior, etc.; is unable to consider alternate interpretations of his/her experiences.	3.54
Lacks a stable image of who she/he is or would like to become (e.g., attitudes, values, goals, and feelings about self may be unstable and changing).	3.50

Table 2a: Composite Description of Patients Diagnosed with Antisocial Personality Disorder

Item	Mean
Takes advantage of others; is out for number one; has minimal investment in moral values.	5.64
Tends to be deceitful; tends to lie or mislead.	5.50
Tends to engage in unlawful or criminal behavior.	5.36
Tends to be angry or hostile (whether consciously or unconsciously).	5.29
Has little empathy; seems unable to understand or respond to others' needs and feelings unless they coincide with his/her own.	5.04
Appears to experience no remorse for harm or injury caused to others.	4.93
Tends to blame others for own failures or shortcomings; tends to believe his/her problems are caused by external factors.	4.89
Tends to act impulsively, without regard for consequences.	4.89
Tends to show reckless disregard for the rights, property, or safety of others.	4.86
Tries to manipulate others' emotions to get what she/he wants.	4.75
Tends to be unconcerned with the consequences of his/her actions; appears to feel immune or invulnerable.	4.39
Tends to be unreliable and irresponsible (e.g., may fail to meet work obligations or honor financial commitments).	4.32
Has little psychological insight into own motives, behavior, etc.; is unable to consider alternate interpretations of his/her experiences.	4.21
Tends to get into power struggles.	4.07
Appears to gain pleasure or satisfaction by being sadistic or aggressive toward others	4.04
Tends to abuse alcohol.	4.04
Tends to be critical of others.	4.00
Tends to be conflicted about authority (e.g., may feel she/he must submit, rebel against, win over, defeat, etc.).	4.00
Tends to seek power or influence over others (whether in beneficial or destructive ways).	3.93
Has an exaggerated sense of self-importance.	3.75

Table 2b: Composite Description of Patients Diagnosed with Borderline Personality Disorder

Item	Mean
Emotions tend to spiral out of control, leading to extremes of anxiety, sadness, rage, excitement, etc.	5.05
Tends to feel unhappy, depressed, or despondent.	4.88
Tends to feel she/he is inadequate, inferior, or a failure.	4.42
Tends to fear she/he will be rejected or abandoned by those who are emotionally significant.	4.40
Is unable to soothe or comfort self when distressed; requires involvement of another person to help regulate affect.	4.28
Tends to feel helpless, powerless, or at the mercy of forces outside his/her control.	4.19
Tends to be angry or hostile (whether consciously or unconsciously).	4.05
Tends to be anxious.	4.05
Tends to react to criticism with feelings of rage or humiliation.	3.95
Tends to be overly needy or dependent; requires excessive reassurance or approval.	3.93
Tends to feel misunderstood, mistreated, or victimized.	3.79
Tends to become irrational when strong emotions are stirred up; may show a noticeable decline from customary level of functioning.	3.74
Tends to get into power struggles.	3.56
Tends to "catastrophize"; is prone to see problems as disastrous, unsolvable, etc.	3.51
Emotions tend to change rapidly and unpredictably.	3.51
Lacks a stable image of who she/he is or would like to become (e.g., attitudes, values, goals, and feelings about self may be unstable and changing).	3.49
Tends to feel like an outcast or outsider; feels as if she/he does not truly belong.	3.47
Tends to express intense and inappropriate anger, out of proportion to the situation at hand.	3.40

Table 2c: Composite Description of Patients Diagnosed with Histrionic Personality Disorder

Item	Mean
Expresses emotion in exaggerated and theatrical ways.	5.00
Tends to fear she/he will be rejected or abandoned by those who are emotionally significant.	4.66
Tends to be anxious.	4.43
Emotions tend to spiral out of control, leading to extremes of anxiety, sadness, rage, excitement, etc.	4.40
Tends to be overly needy or dependent; requires excessive reassurance or approval.	4.34
Tends to develop somatic symptoms in response to stress or conflict (e.g., headache, backache, abdominal pain, asthma, etc.).	3.77
Tends to get into power struggles.	3.63
Tends to become attached quickly or intensely; develops feelings, expectations, etc. that are not warranted by the history or context of the relationship.	3.60
Tends to be overly sexually seductive or provocative, whether consciously or unconsciously (may be inappropriately flirtatious, preoccupied with sexual conquest, prone to "lead people on," etc.).	3.60
Seeks to be the center of attention.	3.57
Tends to feel misunderstood, mistreated, or victimized.	3.54
Is articulate; can express self well in words.	3.46
Tends to become irrational when strong emotions are stirred up; may show a noticeable decline from customary level of functioning.	3.46
Tends to feel helpless, powerless, or at the mercy of forces outside his/her control.	3.37
Is unable to soothe or comfort self when distressed; requires involvement of another person to help regulate affect.	3.34
Emotions tend to change rapidly and unpredictably.	3.34
Tends to "catastrophize;" is prone to see problems as disastrous, unsolvable, etc.	3.29
Tends to feel unhappy, depressed, or despondent.	3.29
Tends to use his/her physical attractiveness to an excessive degree to gain attention or notice.	3.26
Tends to be angry or hostile (whether consciously or unconsciously).	3.17

Table 2d: Composite Description of Patients Diagnosed with Narcissistic Personality Disorder

Item	Mean
Appears to feel privileged and entitled; expects preferential treatment.	4.95
Has an exaggerated sense of self-importance.	4.68
Tends to be controlling.	4.53
Tends to be critical of others.	4.40
Tends to get into power struggles.	4.28
Tends to feel misunderstood, mistreated, or victimized.	4.28
Tends to be competitive with others (whether consciously or unconsciously).	4.25
Is articulate; can express self well in words.	4.25
Tends to react to criticism with feelings of rage or humiliation.	4.22
Tends to be angry or hostile (whether consciously or unconsciously).	4.15
Has little empathy; seems unable to understand or respond to others' needs and feelings unless they coincide with his/her own.	4.10
Tends to blame others for own failures or shortcomings; tends to believe his/her problems are caused by external factors.	4.00
Seeks to be the center of attention.	3.63
Tends to be arrogant, haughty, or dismissive.	3.63
Seems to treat others primarily as an audience to witness own importance, brilliance, beauty, etc.	3.50
Has fantasies of unlimited success, power, beauty, talent, brilliance, etc.	3.43
Tends to hold grudges; may dwell on insults or slights for long periods.	3.40
Expects self to be "perfect" (e.g., in appearance, achievements, performance, etc.).	3.38

Table 3a: Composite Description of Patients Diagnosed with Avoidant Personality Disorder

Item	Mean
Tends to feel she/he is inadequate, inferior, or a failure.	6.34
Tends to be shy or reserved in social situations.	6.26
Tends to avoid social situations because of fear of embarrassment or humiliation.	5.94
Tends to feel ashamed or embarrassed.	5.71
Tends to be anxious.	5.60
Tends to feel like an outcast or outsider; feels as if she/he does not truly belong.	5.51
Tends to be inhibited or constricted; has difficulty allowing self to acknowledge or express wishes and impulses.	5.31
Tends to be passive and unassertive.	5.29
Tends to feel unhappy, depressed, or despondent.	5.20
Tends to be self-critical; sets unrealistically high standards for self and is intolerant of own human defects.	4.91
Lacks close friendships and relationships.	4.89
Tends to blame self or feel responsible for bad things that happen.	4.86
Tends to fear she/he will be rejected or abandoned by those who are emotionally significant.	4.83
Tends to feel guilty.	4.77
Lacks social skills; tends to be socially awkward or inappropriate.	4.74
Appears inhibited about pursuing goals or successes; aspirations or achievements tend to be below his/her potential.	4.49

Table 3b: Composite Description of Patients Diagnosed with Dependent Personality Disorder

Item	Mean
Tends to be overly needy or dependent; requires excessive reassurance or approval.	6.13
Tends to fear she/he will be rejected or abandoned by those who are emotionally significant.	5.55
Tends to feel she/he is inadequate, inferior, or a failure.	5.47
Tends to feel unhappy, depressed, or despondent.	5.26
Tends to be ingratiating or submissive (e.g., may consent to things she/he does not agree with or does not want to do, in the hope of getting support or approval).	5.24
Tends to feel helpless, powerless, or at the mercy of forces outside his/her control.	5.16
Tends to feel guilty.	4.89
Tends to be passive and unassertive.	4.76
Tends to be anxious.	4.55
Tends to blame self or feel responsible for bad things that happen.	4.53
Has difficulty acknowledging or expressing anger.	4.53
Tends to feel ashamed or embarrassed.	4.39
Is unable to soothe or comfort self when distressed; requires involvement of another person to help regulate affect.	4.37
Has trouble making decisions; tends to be indecisive or to vacillate when faced with choices.	4.26
Appears inhibited about pursuing goals or successes; aspirations or achievements tend to be below his/her potential.	4.21
Tends to express aggression in passive and indirect ways (e.g., may make mistakes, procrastinate, forget, become sulky, etc.).	4.03
Tends to get drawn into or remain in relationships in which she/he is emotionally or physically abused.	3.79

Table 3c: Composite Description of Patients Diagnosed with Obsessive-Compulsive Personality Disorder

Item	Mean
Tends to be conscientious and responsible.	5.83
Tends to be self-critical; sets unrealistically high standards for self and is intolerant of own human defects.	5.20
Has moral and ethical standards and strives to live up to them.	5.17
Tends to be overly concerned with rules, procedures, order, organization, schedules, etc.	4.89
Tends to be anxious.	4.86
Tends to be controlling.	4.80
Tends to become absorbed in details, often to the point that she/he misses what is significant in the situation.	4.74
Expects self to be "perfect" (e.g., in appearance, achievements, performance, etc.).	4.69
Tends to blame self or feel responsible for bad things that happen.	4.49
Tends to feel guilty.	4.43
Tends to adhere rigidly to daily routines and become anxious or uncomfortable when they are altered.	4.29
Is troubled by recurrent obsessional thoughts that she/he experiences as senseless and intrusive.	4.26
Is articulate; can express self well in words.	4.26
Tends to be inhibited or constricted; has difficulty allowing self to acknowledge or express wishes and impulses.	4.14
Is excessively devoted to work and productivity, to the detriment of leisure and relationships.	4.11
Tends to feel unhappy, depressed, or despondent.	4.09
Has difficulty allowing self to experience strong pleasurable emotions (e.g., excitement, joy, pride).	3.97

Discussion of Empirical Findings

Advantages of Expanded Criterion Sets

A consistent theme running through the findings is that DSM-IV criterion sets are too narrow. They do not capture the richness and complexity of the personality syndromes observed empirically in patients treated in the community, nor do they capture the complexity of personality disorders as they are defined by DSM-IV itself. The preamble to Axis II defines personality disorders in terms of multiple domains of functioning including cognition, affectivity, interpersonal relations, and impulse regulation. However, the PD criterion sets do not actually encompass these domains of functioning (Millon, 1990; Millon & Davis, 1997).

DSM-IV limits the number of diagnostic criteria to 8 or 9 criteria (items) per disorder, but it is clinically and psychometrically impossible for such small item sets simultaneously to describe personality syndromes in their complexity, and to describe distinct (non-overlapping) syndromes. Certain traits play central roles in more than one personality disorder (e.g., lack of empathy is characteristic of both narcissistic and antisocial personality disorder; hostility is characteristic of paranoid, antisocial, borderline, and narcissistic personality disorders). Excluding these traits from the PD criterion sets leads to clinically inaccurate descriptions, but including the same items in multiple criterion sets leads to excess comorbidity (i.e., low specificity). As now constituted, Axis II cannot transcend this paradox.

The paradox could be resolved by (1) expanding the size of the criterion sets, and (2) diagnosing personality disorders as configurations or gestalts rather than by tabulating individual symptoms (for discussion of such an approach to diagnosis, which we call "prototype matching," see Shedler & Westen, 2004a; Westen & Shedler, 2000). For example, the composite descriptions of narcissistic and antisocial personality disorder contain numerous overlapping traits, yet they are conceptually distinct and would be difficult to confuse. Expanding the size of the criterion sets would (1) help bridge the gap between science and practice by making the descriptions of personality disorders in the DSM more faithful to clinical reality, (2) make the personality disorder descriptions more faithful to the conceptual definition of *personality disorder* (i.e., multifaceted syndromes encompassing multiple domains of functioning), and (3) reduce comorbidities among personality disorder diagnoses by making the diagnostic categories more distinct from one another.

Addressing Intrapsychic Processes and Inner Experience

DSM-IV tends to underemphasize inner experience or intrapsychic processes that are centrally defining of personality disorders, which limits both its clinical relevance and its empirical fidelity. For example, the data strongly indicate that aggression and the defenses of externalization and projection are defining features of paranoid personality disorder, yet they are not included in the DSM-IV criterion set. The data indicate that hostility, sadism, lack of empathy, lack of insight, self-importance, and power-seeking are defining of antisocial personality disorder. However, these aspects of mental life are absent from the DSM description, which instead emphasizes behavioral markers such as criminality and lack of stable employment. Feelings of inadequacy and inferiority, shame, embarrassment, passivity, depression, anxiety, self-blame, and guilt appear centrally defining of both avoidant and dependent personality disorder (which should probably be subsumed by a diagnosis of depressive personality disorder); instead, DSM-IV emphasizes behavioral indicators of social avoidance in the former and dependency in the latter.

Identifying Optimal Diagnostic Groupings

This chapter has focused on the diagnostic categories currently included in DSM-IV, but the findings raise broader questions about whether these categories are the optimal ones. For example, the composite descriptions of avoidant and dependent personality disorder overlap substantially and contain numerous features that would be better characterized in terms of a depressive personality syndrome (e.g., the tendency to feel unhappy, depressed, despondent; to feel inadequate, inferior, or a failure; to blame themselves for bad things that happen; to be inhibited about pursuing goals or successes; to feel ashamed or embarrassed; to fear rejection and abandonment; etc.). A depressive personality disorder category deserves consideration for DSM-V.

CONCLUSION: INTEGRATING SCIENCE AND PRACTICE

A clinically useful diagnostic system should encompass the spectrum of personality pathology seen in clinical practice and have meaningful implications for treatment. An empirically sound diagnostic system should facilitate reliable and valid diagnoses: Independent clinicians should be able to arrive at the same diagnosis, the diagnoses should be relatively distinct from one another, and each diagnosis should be associated with unique and theoretically meaningful correlates, antecedents, and sequelae (Livesley & Jackson, 1992; Millon, 1991; Robins & Guze, 1970).

One obstacle to achieving this ideal has been an unfortunate schism in the mental health professions between science and practice. Too often, research has been conducted in isolation from the crucial data of clinical observation. The results often strike clinicians as naïve and of dubious clinical relevance. Ultimately, the most empirically elegant diagnostic system will have little impact if clinicians do not find it helpful for understanding their patients (Shedler &

Westen, 2005). On the other hand, clinical theory has too often developed with little regard for questions of falsifiability or empirical credibility. The results have often struck researchers as scientifically naïve.

The SWAP represents an effort to bridge the schism between science and practice by quantifying clinical wisdom and expertise and making clinical constructs accessible to empirical study. It relies on clinicians to do what they do best, namely, making observations and inferences about individual patients they know and treat. It relies on quantitative methods to do what they do best, namely aggregating observations to discern relationships and commonalities, and combining data to yield optimal predictions (cf. Sawyer, 1966). The findings raise possibilities for developing a classification of personality disorders that is both empirically sound and clinically (and psychodynamically) meaningful; for integrating descriptive psychiatric diagnosis with clinical case formulation; for assessing personality change (not just symptom remission) in psychotherapy; and for assessing individual patients in ways that integrate the best features of clinical judgment and psychometric rigor. The SWAP attempts to provide a "language" for case description that is at once clinically rich enough to describe the complexities of the patients we treat, and empirically rigorous enough to meet the requirements of science. There remains a sizeable schism between clinical practitioners and empirical researchers. Perhaps this new language will be a step toward one that all parties can speak.

REFERENCES

Blais, M., & Norman, D. (1997). A psychometric evaluation of the DSM-IV Personality Disorder Criteria. *Journal of Personality Disorders, 11,* 168-176.

Blashfield, R. (1985). Exemplar prototypes of personality disorder diagnoses. *Comprehensive Psychiatry, 26,* 11–21.

Block, J. (1971). *Lives through time.* Berkeley, CA: Bancroft.

Block, J. (1978). *The Q-sort method in personality assessment and psychiatric research.* Palo Alto, CA: Consulting Psychologists Press.

Bradley, R., & Westen, D. (2003). *Validity of SWAP-200 personality diagnosis in an outpatient sample.* Unpublished manuscript. Emory University.

Cantor, N., & Genero, N. (1986). Psychiatric diagnosis and natural categorization: A close analogy. In Contemporary directions in psychopathology. In G.L. Klerman (Ed.), *Toward the DSM-IV* (pp. 233-256). New York: Guilford.

Clark, L. (1992). Resolving taxonomic issues in personality disorders: The value of larger scale analyses of symptom data. *Journal of Personality Disorders, 6,* 360-376.

Cleckley, H. (1941). *The mask of sanity.* St. Louis, MO: Mosby Co.

Davis, R., Blashfield, R., & McElroy, R. (1993). Weighting criteria in the diagnosis of a personality disorder: A demonstration. *Journal of Abnormal Psychology, 102,* 319-322.

First, M., Spitzer, R., Gibbon, M., Williams, J., Davies, J. B., Howes, M., et al. (1995). The Structured Clinical Interview for DSM-III-R Personality Disorders (SCID-II). Part II: Multisite test-retest reliability study. *Journal of Personality Disorders, 9,* 92-104.

Grilo, C. M., Sanislow, C.A., & McGlashan, T. H. (2002). Co-occurrence of DSM-IV personality disorders with borderline personality disorder. *Journal of Nervous and Mental Disease, 190,* 552-553.

Gunderson, J. G. (2001). *Borderline personality disorder: A clinical guide.* Washington, DC: American Psychiatric Publishing, Inc.

Hare, R. D., Harpur, T. J., Hakstian, A. R., Forth, A. E., Hart, S. D., & Newman, J. P. (1990). The revised Psychopathy Checklist: Reliability and factor structure. *Psychological Assessment: A Journal of Consulting and Clinical Psychology, 2,* 338-341.

Harkness, A. (1992). Fundamental topics in the personality disorders: candidate trait dimensions from lower regions of the hierarchy. *Psychological Assessment: A Journal of Consulting and Clinical Psychology, 4,* 251–259.

John, O. (1990). The "big five" factor taxonomy: Dimensions of personality in the natural language and in questionnaires. In L. Pervin (Ed.), *Handbook of personality: Theory and research* (pp. 66-100). New York: Guilford Press.

Kernberg, O. (1975). *Borderline conditions and pathological narcissism.* New York: Jason Aronson.

Kernberg, O. (1984). *Severe personality disorders.* New Haven, CT: Yale University Press.

Kim, N. S., & Ahn, W. (2002). Clinical psychologists' theory-based representations of mental disorders predict their diagnostic reasoning and memory. *Journal of Experimental Psychology, 131(4),* 451-476.

Klonsky, E. D., Oltmanns, T. F., & Turkheimer, E. (2002). Informant-reports of personality disorder: Relation to self-reports and future research directions. *Clinical Psychology: Science and Practice, 9,* 300-311.

Kohut, H. (1971). *The analysis of the self.* New York: International Universities Press.

Linehan, M. M. (1993). *Cognitive-behavioral treatment of borderline personality disorder.* New York: Guilford.

Lingiardi V., Shedler, J., & Gazillo, F. (2006). Assessing personality change in psychotherapy with the SWAP-200: A case study. *Journal of Personality Assessment, 86,* 23-32.

Livesley, W. J. (Ed.). (1995). *The DSM-IV personality disorders.* New York: Guilford Press.

Livesley, W. J., & Jackson, D. N. (1992) Guidelines for developing, evaluating, and revising the classification of personality disorders. *Journal of Nervous and Mental Disease, 180,* 609-618.

Main, M., Kaplan, N., & Cassidy, J. (1985). Security in infancy, childhood, and adulthood: A move to the level of representation. *Monographs of the Society for Research in Child Development, 50*(1-2, Serial No. 209).

Marin-Avellan, L., McGauley, G., Campbell, C., & Fonagy, P. (2005). Using the SWAP-200 in a personality-disordered forensic population: Is it valid, reliable and useful? *Journal of Criminal Behaviour and Mental Health, 15,* 28-45.

McCrae, R., & Costa, P. (1990). *Personality in adulthood.* New York: Guilford Press.

McWilliams, N. (1999). *Psychoanalytic case formulation.* New York: Guilford Press.

Millon, T. (1990). *Toward a new psychology.* New York: Wiley.

Millon, T. (1991). Classification in psychopathology: Rationale, alternatives and standards. *Journal of Abnormal Psychology, 100,* 245-261.

Millon, T., & Davis, R. D. (1997). The place of assessment in clinical science. In T. Millon (Ed.), *The Millon Inventories: Clinical and personality assessment* (pp. 3-20). New York: Guilford Press.

Millon, T. & Martinez, A. (1995). Avoidant personality disorder. In W. J. Livesley (Ed.), *The DSM-IV personality disorders* (pp. 218-233). New York: Guilford Press.

Morey, L. C. (1988). Personality disorders in DSM-III and DSM-III-R: convergence, coverage, and internal consistency. *American Journal of Psychiatry, 145,* 573-577.

Morey, L. C. (1991). *The Personality Assessment Inventory: Professional manual.* Odessa, FL: Psychological Assessment Resources.

Oldham, J., Skodol, A., Kellman, H. D., Hyler, S., Rosnick, L., & Davies, M. (1992). Diagnosis of DSM-III-R personality disorders by two semistructured interviews: Patterns of comorbidity. *American Journal of Psychiatry, 149,* 213-220.

Patrick, C. J., & Zempolich, K. A. (1998). Emotion and aggression in the psychopathic personality. *Aggression and violent behavior, 3(4),* 303-338.

Perry, J. C. (1992). Problems and considerations in the valid assessment of personality disorders. *American Journal of Psychiatry, 149,*1645-1653.

Perry, J. C., & Cooper, S. H. (1987). Empirical studies of psychological defense mechanisms. In J. Cavenar & R. Michels (Eds.), *Psychiatry.* Philadelphia: JB Lippincott.

Pilkonis, P. A., Heape, C. L., Proietti, J. M., Clark, S. W., McDavid, J. D., & Pitts, T. E. (1995). The reliability and validity of two structured diagnostic interviews for personality disorders. *Archives of General Psychiatry, 52,* 1025-1033.

Pilkonis, P. A., Heape, C. L., Ruddy, J., & Serrao, P. (1991). Validity in the diagnosis of personality disorders: The use of the LEAD standard. *Psychological Assessment, 31,* 46-54.

Robins, E., & Guze, S. (1970). The establishment of diagnostic validity in psychiatric illness: Its application to schizophrenia. *American Journal of Psychiatry, 126,* 983-987.

Sawyer, J. (1966). Measurement and prediction, clinical and statistical. *Psychological Bulletin,* 66, 178–200.

Shedler, J. (2002). A new language for psychoanalytic diagnosis. *Journal of the American Psychoanalytic Association, 50(2),* 429-456.

Shedler J., Mayman, M., & Manis, M. (1993). The illusion of mental health. *American Psychologist, 48,* 1117–1131.

Shedler, J., & Westen, D. (1998). Refining the measurement of Axis II: A Q-sort procedure for assessing personality pathology. *Assessment, 5(4),* 333-353.

Shedler, J., & Westen, D. (2004a). Refining DSM-IV personality disorder diagnosis: Integrating science and practice. *American Journal of Psychiatry, 161,* 1350-1365.

Shedler, J., & Westen, D. (2004b). Dimensions of personality pathology: An alternative to the Five Factor Model. *American Journal of Psychiatry, 161,* 1743-1754.

Shedler, J., & Westen, D. (2005). A simplistic view of the Five Factor Model: Drs. Shedler and Westen reply. *American Journal of Psychiatry, 162,* 1551.

Skodol, A., Oldham, J., Rosnick, L., Kellman, D., & Hyler, S. (1991). Diagnosis of DSM-III-R personality disorders: A comparison of two structured interviews. *International Journal of Methods in Psychiatric Research, 1,* 13-26.

Spitzer, R. L. (1983). Psychiatric diagnosis: Are clinicians still necessary? *Comprehensive Psychiatry, 24,* 399–411.

Vaillant, G. (Ed.) (1992*). Ego mechanisms of defense: A guide for clinicians and researchers.* Washington, DC: American Psychiatric Press.

Walker, E., & Lewine, R. J. (1990). Prediction of adult-onset schizophrenia from childhood home movies of the patients. *American Journal of Psychiatry, 147(8),* 1052-1056.

Watson, D., & Sinha, B. K. (1998). Comorbidity of DSM-IV personality disorders in a nonclinical sample. *Journal of Clinical Psychology, 54(6),* 773-780.

Westen, D. (1991). Social cognition and object relations. *Psychology Bulletin, 109,* 429-455.

Westen, D. (1997). Divergences between clinical and research methods for assessing personality disorders: Implications for research and the evolution of Axis II. *American Journal of Psychiatry, 154,* 895-903.

Westen, D. (2002). *Clinical Diagnostic Interview.* Unpublished manual. Emory University. Available from *www.psychsystems.net/lab.* (Accessed 1/30/06.)

Westen, D., & Arkowitz-Westen, L. (1998). Limitations of Axis II in diagnosing personality pathology in clinical practice. *American Journal of Psychiatry, 155,* 1767-1771.

Westen, D., Heim, A.K., Morrison , K., Patterson, M., & Campbell, L. (2002). Classifying and diagnosing psychopathology: A prototype matching approach. In M. Malik (Ed.), *Rethinking the DSM: Psychological perspectives* (pp. 221-250). Washington DC: American Psychological Association Press.

Westen, D., Lohr, N., Silk, K., Gold, L., & Kerber, K. (1990). Object relations and social cognition in borderlines, major depressives, and normals: A TAT analysis. *Psychological Assessment: A   Journal of Consulting and Clinical Psychology, 2,* 355-364.

Westen, D., & Muderrisoglu, S. (2003). Reliability and validity of personality disorder assessment using a systematic clinical interview: Evaluating an alternative to structured interviews. *Journal of Personality Disorders, 17,* 350-368.

Westen, D., & Muderrisoglu, S. (in press). Clinical assessment of pathological personality traits. *American Journal of Psychiatry.*

Westen, D., Muderrisoglu, S., Fowler, C., Shedler, J., & Koren, D. (1997). Affect regulation and affective experience: Individual differences, group differences, and measurement using a Q-sort procedure. *Journal of Consulting and Clinical Psychology, 65,* 429-439.

Westen, D., & Shedler, J. (1999a). Revising and assessing Axis II: I. Developing a clinically and empirically valid assessment method. *American Journal of Psychiatry, 156(2),* 258-272.

Westen, D., & Shedler, J. (1999b). Revising and assessing Axis II: II. Toward an empirically based and clinically useful classification of personality disorders. *American Journal of Psychiatry, 156(2),* 258-272.

Westen D., & Shedler, J. (2000) A prototype matching approach to diagnosing personality disorders toward DSM-V. *Journal of Personality Disorders, 14(2),*109-126.

Westen D., Shedler, J., Durrett, C., Glass, S., & Martens, A. (2003). Personality diagnosis in adolescence: DSM-IV axis II diagnoses and an empirically derived alternative. *American Journal of Psychiatry, 160,* 952-966.

Westen, D., & Weinberger, J. (2004). When clinical description becomes statistical prediction. *American Psychologist, 59,* 595-613.

Widiger, T. A. (1993). The DSM-III-R categorical personality disorder diagnoses: A critique and an alternative. *Psychological Inquiry, 4(2),* 75-90.

Widiger, T. A., & Corbitt, E. M. (1995). Antisocial personality disorder. In J. W. Livesley (Ed.), *The DSM-IV personality disorders. Diagnosis and treatment of mental disorders* (pp. 103-126). New York: Guilford Press.

Widiger, T. A., & Simonsen, E. S. (1995). Alternative dimensional models of personality disorder: Finding a common ground. *Journal of Personality Disorders, 19,* 110-130.

Wilkinson-Ryan, T., & Westen, D. (2000). Identity disturbance in borderline personality disorder: An empirical investigation. *American Journal of Psychiatry, 157,* 528-541.

Zimmerman, M. (1994). Diagnosing personality disorders: A review of issues and research methods. *Archives of General Psychiatry, 51,* 225-245.

Psychic Structure and Mental Functioning: Current Research on the Reliable Measurement and Clinical Validity of Operationalized Psychodynamic Diagnostics (OPD) System*

Reiner W. Dahlbender, MD,[1] Gerd Rudolf, MD,[2] and the OPD Task Force[3]

Editor's Note: Like the two preceding papers, this article describes comprehensively another of the major measures developed in the most recent decades to provide a description of personality structure and an assessment vehicle for psychotherapeutically induced structural change, beyond simply changes in symptoms and manifest behaviors—this measure developed by psychotherapy researchers in Germany (and again also indicated in the review by Wallerstein in his chapter on psychoanalytic therapy research, p. 511).

True to its title, this piece offers a review of both the theoretic conceptualization and the empirical work detailing the psychometric properties of the OPD, similar to the paper by Blatt, et al. on the Object Relations Inventory (ORI), and by Shedler and Westen on the Shedler-Westen Assessment Procedure (SWAP). This article, with even greater detail, describes the manual for the use of the instrument (Operationalized Psychodynamic Diagnostics, OPD) for psychic structure and mental functioning. The authors also present the current thinking about the planned revision, OPD-II. The three articles together represent a significant sampling of the current burgeoning development—and deployment—of this new generation of outcome measures, designed to delineate the kinds of structural changes claimed as the special province of psychoanalytically-based psychotherapies, changes not conceptualized in non-depth psychological therapeutic modalities.

---

* In memory of our colleague and friend Robert Weinryb (Karolinska Institute, Stockholm)
[1] Adjunct Professor, Medical Director, MEDICLIN – Clinic for Psychosomatic Medicine and Psychotherapy, Soltau and Bad Bodenteich; Member of the Medical University of Hannover/University of Ulm, Hannover/Ulm, Germany
[2] Professor Emeritus, Department for Psychosomatic Medicine and Psychotherapy, University of Heidelberg, Heidelberg, Germany
[3] Please see full listing at the end of this article.

ABSTRACT

In the following article, Axis IV of the *Operationalized Psychodynamic Diagnostics* (OPD) system, briefly called "psychic structure," and its theoretical background is introduced. Subsequently, interrater reliability and validity data are presented. Experiences with its application in the current version are reported, and further developments of the structure axis are outlined. Finally, the English translation of the German OPD manual has been reproduced.

The "psychic structure" axis of the OPD is one of four axes of a diagnostic system that defines clinically relevant psychodynamic constructs, as much as possible close to observation and independent of any particular meta-psychological school, in order to complement purely phenomenological diagnostics and descriptive systems like ICD or DSM. The axis, which has been in use for more than 10 years under everyday clinical conditions in different settings as well as in research projects, provides precise guidelines for the assessment of a patient's level of mental functioning and personal integration on the basis of his mental capacities and vulnerabilities. These are displayed in terms of six dimensions which encompass 24 subdimensions that can be detected in past and present interpersonal interactions, in particular with the therapist.

The results of a couple of reliability studies as well as the results of several validity studies underpin the empirical basis of the OPD structure axis and the OPD system in general. Studies showed good reliability in a research context and acceptable reliability for clinical purposes. Validity studies indicate good content, criterion, and construct validity for the axes. Experiences with the OPD system to date show that the "psychic structure" axis is practicable and reliable for clinical use under different treatment conditions and in research. Further developments target more improvements of the clinical applicability, and the planning and conducting of therapies and corresponding treatment research topics.

INTRODUCTION

The diagnosis of mental and psychosomatic disorders is currently dominated by descriptive diagnostic systems, the most important of which are the ICD-10 and DSM-IV. Unfortunately, these purely phenomenology-based classification systems concentrate on surface symptoms and neglect important diagnostic aspects that are meaningful for the planning and guidance of a psychotherapeutic treatment. It would cause immense suffering and personal tragedies if the medical diagnosis of disease would be based only on unspecific superficial symptoms like fatigue, fever, vomiting, or palpable swellings. Beyond superficial symptoms, the diagnosis is always supported by clinical tests and is proved by laboratory results that are interpreted in the light of a fairly thorough understanding of normal physical structure and functioning. Many psychodynamic psychotherapists have criticized the lack of therapeutic relevance of purely descriptive classifications and have called for a multidimensional perspective in the classification of mental disorders, including also not observable intrapsychic conflicts, interpersonal problems, and mental functioning. Similar to the diagnosis of pathological physical conditions, the diagnosis of mental disorders should be based on the psychopathology of a symptomatology and the underlying malfunction, not exclusively on superficial symptoms (see Malik & Beutler, 2002).

Over the last decades in psychodynamic theorizing and therapeutic practice, psychic structure and mental functioning have become a diagnostic core concept besides the evaluation of the patient's typical interpersonal patterns and intrapsychic conflicts (Horowitz, et al., 1993b). Through the lasting contributions of ego-psychologists, object relations theorists, and self psychologists, all major psychoanalytic schools have approved the importance of psychic structure and mental functioning for personal development (Fonagy, & Target, 1997; Fonagy, et al., 2002) and a broader psychodynamic understanding of healthy and malfunctioning personal and interpersonal conditions. The concept of psychic structure and mental functioning describes typical dispositions or patterns of individual experiencing and behavior that mostly become evident in interpersonal interaction. In the genesis of pathological states and diseases, the concept of psychic structure and mental functioning is complementary to the concept of conflict (Schüssler, 2004). While conflict focuses on neurotic triggering events, structure is related to individual vulnerabilities and capacities to adapt to changing conditions. In this sense, psychic structure and mental functioning are to be seen as a backdrop for the unfolding conflicts. As the development of psychic structure and mental functioning is based in early childhood, malfunctioning in adulthood can be conceptualized as deficient growth or regressive merging of mental functions.

Until now, there were some interesting attempts in the psychoanalytic field to operationalize mental functioning and other diagnostic aspects. Anna Freud not only described defense mechanisms, she was also significantly involved in the development of the Hampstead Index which was an early attempt at comprehensive psychoanalytic diagnostics (A. Freud, 1937, 1962). Bellak and Hurvich (1969) operationalized ego functions and developed rating scales to judge them in clinical material. Kernberg (1977) presented the diagnosis of the structural organization of the personality.

Despite these promising early efforts, operationalized diagnostic approaches, at most, remained a matter of empirical psychotherapy research. For example, Gill and Hoffmann's (1982) method for studying the analysis of aspects of the patient's experience in psychoanalysis and psychotherapy originated in clinical issues, but then turned into an almost pure tool for empirical research. Perry (1989, 1990) introduced an operationalization of conflicts to psychotherapy research and Perry and Cooper (1989) presented a rating of defense mechanisms.

Based on psychoanalytic constructs on different levels of abstraction and interference, Weinryb and Rossel (1991) designed the Karolinska Psychodynamic Profile (KAPP) to achieve a comprehensive multidimensional empirical profile of mental functioning and personality traits as they are reflected in a patient's perception of himself and his interpersonal relations. But only those empirical research instruments that assess basic clinical facts close to observation, like cyclic maladaptive interpersonal patterns (Luborsky & Crits-Christoph, 1998; Strupp & Binder, 1993), had impact on clinicians in return, particularly in the conceptualization of the (counter-) transference relationship.

That the outlined approaches did not achieve broader acceptance among psychoanalytic clinicians is due to the fact that psychoanalytic diagnostics, in the stricter sense of the term, has generally remained full of idiosyncratic diagnostic categories and contradictions with regard to the usefulness of a systematic conceptualization and properly operationalized diagnostic process. In their clinical everyday practice, psychotherapists use a multitude of (meta) psychological constructs to describe mental functioning. Many of these were formulated in such an abstract manner that they are more or less detached from clinical phenomena and cannot be applied easily. This led to a confusing heterogeneity of theories and concepts in psychoanalysis and restricted diagnostic developments.

Against this backdrop of a lack of systematic operationalizations in psychodynamic diagnostics, almost 40 German-speaking clinicians and psychotherapy researchers founded a task force called Operationalized Psychodynamic Diagnostics (OPD) in the early 1990s. The goal of this working party was the development of a diagnostic system that would be capable of grasping the main psychodynamically relevant diagnostic features in an easy-to-handle and communicate standardized format. The OPD inventory, first presented in 1996, is a multi-axial operationalized psychodynamic approach based on four axes called "experience of illness and preconditions for treatment," "interpersonal relations," "conflicts," "psychic structure," and the fifth axis, "psychic and psychosomatic disorders," which allows the OPD diagnosis to be related to the descriptive ICD and DSM classifications. The system quickly found broad acceptance, primarily in the German-speaking countries where more than 3500 psychotherapists have been trained. In 2003, a child and adolescent version was published first in German (Arbeitskreis OPD-KJ, 2003). Since various translations became available (English, Italian, Hungarian and Spanish; Turkish and Chinese are in progress), the system is gradually spreading over Europe, South America, and Asia.

OPERATIONALIZATION OF PSYCHIC STRUCTURE AND MENTAL FUNCTIONING IN THE OPD SYSTEM

Over the last decades in psychodynamic theorizing and therapeutic practice, psychic structure and mental functioning have become a diagnostic core concept among others. Through the lasting contributions of ego psychologists, object relations theorists, and self psychologists, all major psychoanalytic schools have approved the importance of psychic structure and mental functioning for a broader psychodynamic understanding of healthy and malfunctioning personal and interpersonal conditions.

def.

The theoretical conceptualization of the OPD Task Force primarily combines object-relational approaches with those from self- and ego-psychology. Psychic structure is determined as a slow-changing developmental process. It is defined as the way the self shapes itself and functions in relations to others. It is assessed by the underlying structural readiness as shown in interpersonal action over the last two years.

The diagnosis of psychic structure and mental functioning is elaborated in Axis IV, briefly called "psychic structure." This OPD axis differentiates four levels of integration of psychic structure: *Good integration* means that an autonomous self possesses a mental internal space in which mental conflicts can be carried out. *Moderate integration* implies lower availability of regulating function and a weaker differentiation of mental substructures. Low integration depicts less developed mental inner space and substructures, so that conflicts are barely mentally worked out, but are mainly worked out in the interpersonal sphere. The *disintegration level* is characterized by fragmentation and psychotic restitution of psychic structure. The patient's level of mental functioning and integration is assessed on the basis of the mental capacities and vulnerabilities displayed in terms of 6 dimensions which encompass 24 subdimensions:

- **Self-Perception**: Self-reflection, self-image, identity, differentiation of affects
- **Self-Regulation**: Tolerance of affects, self-esteem, regulation of instinctual drive, anticipation
- **Defense**: Type, result, stability, flexibility of defense mechanisms
- **Object-Perception**: Subject-object differentiation, empathy, object-perception as a whole, affects concerning objects
- **Communication**: Contact, understanding affects of others, communicating one's own affects, reciprocity
- **Bonding (Attachment)**: Internalization, detachment, variability of attachment

The first 3 dimensions (self-perception, self-regulation, and defense) refer to the patient's self; the second 3 dimensions (object-perception, communication, bonding) focus on the patient's relationship with the objects. In a final assessment, psychic structure and mental functioning is given as a global rating.

The OPD manual provides operationalized diagnostic criteria on these four levels of integration, further descriptions, and clinical examples of the different levels of integration for each structural dimension to determine a structural profile as well as, finally, the total structural level. Additionally, the rating of each item of all subdimensions is facilitated by an extensive checklist which provides short statements for the classification of the integration level (Rudolf, et al., 1998). The 24 subdimensions are contained in the so-called "Heidelberg Focus List," which has been very useful in psychotherapy studies (Grande, et al., 1997).

As psychic structure is conceptualized as shifting slowly, the diagnostic assessment of mental functioning is restricted to the last two years of the patient's history. Reports about the patient's interactions in the last two years and, in particular, the direct encounter between patient and interviewer, are the most important cues for understanding the patient's capacities for mental functioning and the underlying psychic structure under ordinary conditions, as well as under periods of mental disorder. Acute mental disorders may supply indicators for psychic structure and mental functioning, but they do not determine the diagnosis of psychic structure exclusively, as they are often characterized by states of regression and crisis.

During the diagnostic process, the interviewer experiences aspects of the patient's mental functioning and gains a consecutively completing picture from the patient, his daily routine, his life history, etc. Recently published interview guidelines and tools should ensure that relevant information for the axis is obtained during a one to two hour initial interview. These guidelines are flexible enough that the interview can still be conducted as an open psychodynamic interview (Dahlbender, et al., 2004).

RELIABILITY OF THE OPD AXIS "PSYCHIC STRUCTURE/ MENTAL FUNCTIONING"

The OPD system operationalizes central concepts of psychodynamic theory using simple empirical criteria close to observation and exemplifying clinical examples to enable objective and reliable judgments of a patient's functioning. Even though OPD tries not to do this at the expense of essential contents, the use of the system or an axis always demands from the user a critical acceptance of the meaningfully intended simplifications. Only thus does it become possible to meet reliability and validity criteria that are regarded as standard in clinical research.

In a multi-center reliability study, 269 video-recorded diagnostic interviews of one to two hours duration from six mental departments were independently rated by the clinical interviewers and a second judge who was present at each of the interviews (Cierpka, et al., 2001). Interrater reliability was calculated using weighted kappa values (Cohen, 1968). The interrater reliability achieved for the structure axis ranged in the realm of "good" (Landis & Koch, 1977; Fleiss, 1981;

Chicchetti, 1994) and was in the vanguard of all OPD axes. In two departments, the mean weighted kappa values for all six subdimensions were 0.70 and 0.71 respectively and ranged from 0.60 to 0.81 and 0.62 to 0.78 respectively. In summary, the reliability obtained for the axis "interpersonal relations" and the axis "conflicts" were satisfactory and good for the axis "psychic structure," especially when the judgments and the interviews were conducted under more strict research conditions.

For the Karolinska Psychodynamic Profile (KAPP; Weinryb, et al., 1999), for example, the interrater reliability is excellent and ranges between 0.72 and 1.00 but has only been demonstrated for five judges. In two of the six departments in the OPD reliability study, where the interviews were conducted under very pragmatic clinical everyday routine conditions with rather limited time resources, mean weighted kappa values obtained for all four OPD axes ranged between 0.30 and 0.50 and corresponded approximately to the results of an earlier OPD practicability study also conducted under the conditions of clinical routine (Freyberger, et al., 1996, 1998). Compared to these reasonably robust OPD results, the ICD-10 is only moderately reliable under routine clinical conditions (Michels, et al., 2001). The most gratifying clinical practicability and good interrater reliability of the structure axis is mainly due to the fact that its theory of mental functioning is defined within a framework close to observable behavior, and not close to meta-psychological concepts.

The diagnostic system of the OPD Task Force requires complex clinical judgments which demand an intensive clinical education and an OPD training of 60 hours. The results of the OPD reliability study demonstrated this clearly. They suggested that a standard training facilitates the reliable handling of the OPD system, but can not substitute for a lack of basic clinical experience of at least two to three years to enable appropriate clinical conclusions. Apart from an intensive training and the professional experience of a diagnostician, experience shows that the quality of the investigated clinical material plays an important role in the quality of the evaluations as well. The results of the OPD reliability study indicated that diagnostic interviews performed within a research context and ratings using more structured material led to distinctly better values. This finding is also supported by a study which applied the OPD structure axis to the written texts of 118 relationship episodes gathered from a semi-structured interview on relationship episodes. Even though the interviews were conducted by clinicians with only little interviewing practice and the ratings were accomplished by advanced students, a mean intra-class correlation coefficient of 0.70 revealed good interrater reliability (Dahlbender, 2002). Presumably, this was due to the fact that complex mental constructs open up even to clinically less experienced users, through the clear and rather easy-to-apply descriptions offered by the structure axis, especially when using the extensive structure checklist (Rudolf, et al., 1998).

VALIDITY OF THE OPD AXIS "PSYCHIC STRUCTURE/MENTAL FUNCTIONING"

A number of studies deal with concordant validity aspects, that is to say, the agreement between psychic structure evaluation and mental functioning respectively, and other concurrently obtained data.

Nitzgen and Brünger (2000) examined 137 male patients with chronic substance abuse at the start of an in-patient admission and showed that these patients had the poorest values in the area of self-control (Mean = 2.2; 2 corresponds to moderate and 3 to poorly integrated). This result was also to be expected theoretically since this structure area comprises, among others, the aspects, tolerance of affect and impulse control. These findings are confirmed by a study of Reyman, et al. (2000), where structural deficits in self control as well as in object perception were ascertained in 22 alcohol-dependent males on a detoxification ward. Further indications of validity were obtained by the first mentioned study with respect to concordance with ICD-10 diagnoses. Patients who had ICD diagnoses of neuroses (Mean = 1.97) showed higher structured levels of integration than patients with personality disorders (Mean = 2.37, $p < 0.01$). Rudolf, et al. (1996) found that a lower structural level is associated with a longer duration of mental illness (-0.38, $p = 0.06$), which may be due to the poorer mental regulation capacities of these patients. Rudolf, et al. (2002, 2004) demonstrated a statistical association between the two OPD axes "conflict" and "psychic structure." As theoretically expected, the conflict dependency vs. autonomy, as well as the self-esteem conflict, correlated with a low level of mental functioning. Oberbracht (2005) revealed in a study applying the OPD axes "interpersonal relations" and "psychic structure," as well as the IIP (Horowitz, et al., 1993), that a decreasing level of mental functioning goes along with an increasing occurrence of personality disorder diagnoses, and with negative interpersonal capacities on the patient's side, like hostile, aggressive, and separating behavior, as well as negative counter-transference attitudes on the therapist's side.

Other validation studies focused on inner validity aspects. Schauenburg (2000) examined 49 consecutively admitted in-patient psychotherapy patients and found that secure attachment, as determined by the Pilkonis attachment diagnosis (Pilkonis, 1988; -0.30, $p = 0.05$), as well as excessive striving for independence (-0.29, $p = 0.06$), were associated with a better structural level, while borderline traits (0.27, $p = 0.08$), excessive autonomy strivings (0.32, $p = 0.03$), and antisocial traits (0.55, $p = 0.00$) were associated with poorer structural level. In the same sample, Grütering and Schauenburg (2000) compared independent judgments of the Karolinska Psychodynamic Profile (KAPP) with the dimensions of the OPD structure axis and found expected correlations concerning content—the capacity for self-control was associated with the scales, intimacy, and tolerance of frustration. Likewise, there was an association between higher integration and object perception or communication and the capacity to experience intimacy.

Grande, Schauenburg, and Rudolf (2002) compared the Wallerstein Scales of Psychological Capacities (SPC) (Wallerstein, 1988) with mental characteristics measured by the OPD structure axis. Numerous expected associations were found when comparing conceptually similar scales on both sides, e.g., a correlation of $r = 0.30$, $p < 0.05$ between the OPD scale "drive" and the SPC dimension "self-control." Furthermore, there was a significant concordance between low structure level according to OPD and the SPC scale "emotional blunting" ($r = 0.41$, $p < 0.01$) and "rarely able to rely on others" ($r = 0.43$, $p < 0.01$). These two SPC items relate, more than others of this instrument, to the interpersonal capacities of a person and are, therefore, especially close to the theoretical concept of the OPD structure axis, which particularly places the capabilities and vulnerabilities of the "self in its relationship to others" in the center of the examination of mental functioning.

Lange and Heuft (2002) specified an association between psychic structure and mental functioning, respectively, and a score of mental disturbance (Beeintraechtigungsschwere-Score [BSS]; Schepank, 1994). Spitzer, et al. (2002) found associations between mental functioning and demographic aspects, psychopathology and categorical diagnoses. Schneider, et al. (2002) demonstrated a higher level of mental functioning in patients who were recommended to psychotherapy and a lower level in patients who were recommended to psychiatric treatment.

Using the Facial Action Coding System (FACS) and OPD in an experimental design with eight patients, Schulz (2004) found evidence that patients with a higher level of mental functioning had a more comprehensive and more differentiated facial expression than patients with a lower level of integration.

Based on a model of the internalization and actualization of internal representations, Dahlbender (2002) investigated psychodynamic expert-assumptions between the severity of the individual psychopathology and internalized representations of interpersonal patterns, conflicts, defense and mastery mechanisms, and mental functioning. He designed a cross-section study and analyzed relationship interviews of 44 young female patients with a broad spectrum of diagnoses in in-patient psychotherapy with widely used quantitative and qualitative methods. The ratings of independent and reliable judges were analyzed with parametric and non-parametric correlative procedures. The findings showed that the severity of mental illness can be best predicted by the internal representations of interpersonal patterns, intrapsychic conflicts, conflict-defense, conflict-mastery, and specific features of psychic structure and mental functioning. Particularly with regard to different types of psychopathological severity, the results indicated one type with leading problems in mental functioning and psychic structure, respectively, among others with problems predominantly as a result of maladaptive interpersonal relationships, conflicts, and conflict adaptation competences or processing skills. Using the OPD structure axis, he could support expert assumptions and present a hierarchical association model in which mental functioning has a fundamental impact on conflicts and their defense and mastery and, thereby, on interpersonal relationship patterns in turn.

Rudolf, et al. (1996) provided evidence that the level of mental functioning at the beginning of an in-patient treatment was a very good predictor for the success of the further treatment as judged by both patient (0.30) and therapist (0.40, $p < 0.05$). The view of the individual structure dimensions indicates that bonding capability (patient 0.42, therapist 0.46, $p < 0.01$) is particularly relevant for the outcome prediction. It seems that the capacity to imbue others positively over a certain period of time enhances the chance of a successful therapeutic interchange. Strauss, et al. (1997) confirmed in a study with 30 subjects that patients with a higher level of mental functioning benefit more from in-patient psychotherapy than those with a lower level of functioning. Grütering and Schauenburg (2000) found that level of self reflection was a good predictor for the outcome of psychotherapy.

Studies on construct validity indicate that "psychic structure" basically seems to be a one-dimensional construct with various interdependently operating components. A single main factor with a very high eigenvalue arising from a main component factor analysis points in this direction. Internal consistencies of 0.87 for the structure dimensions and of 0.96 for the structure foci respectively underpin this assumption as well. Since structural constitution and mental functioning represent rather stable personal characteristics in the length of time, a pre-post-concordance of 84.4% for structural aspects during a 12-week period of in-patient treatment provides further support for the construct validity of the structure axis (Grande, et al., 2000).

EXPERIENCES WITH THE "PSYCHIC STRUCTURE/MENTAL FUNCTIONING" AXIS OF THE OPD

Since the first edition in 1996, the OPD structure axis has been fruitfully used under clinical circumstances and adapted to a variety of diagnostic, as well as therapeutic, research topics.

Studies that have been conducted have demonstrated the broad scope of psychic structure and mental functioning, mostly in patients with different mental disorders under psychotherapy. They have also revealed a number of clinically relevant findings, especially associations between psychic structure and diagnoses, as well as interpersonal relations and conflicts. The lack of convincing significant associations between OPD axes and ICD-10 diagnosis underlines the concept that the OPD system provides independent psychodynamic diagnostic features and successfully complements purely descriptive classification systems as intended.

As expected, the initial treatment studies conducted by Rudolf and his group (1996) indicated that the diagnostic findings on the OPD axes "conflict" and "psychic structure" did not change noticeably under psychotherapy; neither did the leading conflicts disappear nor did the psychic structure ameliorate substantially. In order to detect sensitively slight changes in these areas, Rudolf and his group picked up this methodological challenge and added a newly invented scale to the family of OPD instruments, the so-called Heidelberg Structural Change Scale (HSCS; Rudolf, et al., 2000; 2002). For the HSCS, interrater agreement of 0.77 (Pearson correlation) was found on the basis of $N = 306$ individual focus ratings. This scale was developed to differentiate therapeutic change in OPD findings above and beyond the simple dichotomy of present vs. not present. Related to the "Assimilation of Problematic Experiences Scales" (APES) (Stiles, et al., 1992), the HSCS operates within a framework of focal changing processes and allows, through its fine gradations, a quantitative weighting of therapeutic change in each individual focus (Grande, et al., 2000, 2001). The HSCS defines dynamically and, therefore therapy-relevant, foci on the OPD axes "interpersonal relations," "conflict," and "psychic structure," and assesses the intensity of the treatment efforts, the degree of awareness, accountability, and integration.

This focus approach enables both therapist and patient to decide which of the patient's particular problems they want to work on, and what therapeutic methods are most convenient to restructure them, namely, at the beginning and at any time in the course of treatment. The restructuring therapy aimed for is not restricted to psychic structure and mental functioning; in fact, it includes verifiable change in the entire personality organization, which means on all OPD operationalizations. To grasp an individual disorder adequately, five foci usually are sufficient (Grande, Rudolf, & Oberbracht, 1997; Grande, Rudolf, Oberbracht, & Pauli-Magnus 2003; Grande, et al., 2004; Rudolf, et al., 2002), in particular if at least one conflict and one structure focus has been chosen.

The definitions provided by the OPD structure axis and the related instruments allow a more accurate identification of a broad variety of alterations and deficiencies of the psychic structural and mental functioning, and direct the clinical attention more selectively towards the psychotherapeutic treatment of these issues. Thus, it becomes possible to complement the traditional emphasis of psychodynamic treatment on the uncovering of conflicts with a structural approach of an OPD-based psychodynamic psychotherapy (Rudolf, 2002a, 2002b, 2002c). The consequent focusing on structural issues, wherever necessary, led to a therapy manual with concrete recommendations for therapeutic work (Rudolf, 2004).

OPD-II: FURTHER DEVELOPMENTS OF THE OPD SYSTEM AND THE "PSYCHIC STRUCTURE/MENTAL FUNCTIONING" AXIS IN PARTICULAR

Since the OPD manual was first published in 1996, many psychotherapists and psychiatrists have become acquainted with and have used the manual. In various psychosomatic clinics, substance abuse clinics, and university departments for psychotherapy and psychosomatics, the OPD is used in day-to-day practice and in several research projects.

Mainly through the work with forensic psychiatric patients, it became apparent that the structure axis needed some differentiations, especially on the disintegrated level of the scale.

Currently, after more then 10 years of clinical and scientific experiences with the diagnostic system of OPD-I, the OPD Task Force is working on a thorough revision. Based on systematic diagnostic findings, according to the well-known OPD-I axes, OPD-II is aiming at criteria for an improved focal treatment planning and processing.

Focusing on four basic capacities, namely perceptive, controlling, communicative, and relating capacities, the structure axis in OPD-II will retain its valuable dichotomous system and evaluate these capacities with regard to the self and to the objects. Because only very few treatment-relevant items have to be supplemented, an easy transformation of OPD-I items into OPD-II items should be possible. As the structural function of defense is a more meta-psychological construct that cannot be described close to observation, this OPD-I subdimension will no longer be part of the axis itself. Defense issues become a separate module in the appendix. Even more clinical applicability in day-to-day practice is the superior goal of all revision efforts. OPD-II will be available in German in 2006 and, shortly after, respectively first in English and then in Spanish.

The English manual, *Operationalized Psychodynamic Diagnostics: Foundations and Manual,* is published under the OPD Task Force (2001). The section below is excerpted with permission from the OPD manual and reflects its numbering scheme.

7   OPD Axis IV: "Psychic Structure/Mental Functioning"

7.1   Structure and Structural Disorder

7.1.1   Prerequisites and Goals of the Diagnostics of Personality Structure

Mental structure is a typical disposition for experience and behavior in the individual. Its patterns become manifest and visible in interaction with others. As to diagnostics, the examiner experiences something of the patient's structure in the direct encounter, gaining a picture from the patient's story about daily routine and life history. The patient's interactions in the diagnostic relationship and the report of past interactions are the material to be structurally examined. The diagnostic assessment of structure need not start from an acute morbid disorder; rather, primary attention should be paid to the underlying structural readiness as revealed in *interactions of the last year or two*. Acute disorders including regressive states and crises do not determine the diagnosis of structure, but are indicators of structural readiness.

Recognizing mental structure is necessarily tied to communication and interaction. The assessment of structural aspects requires a *diagnostic interview* that allows relational diagnostics. This means an interview technique that does not mainly ask questions on single points (e.g., symptoms), but lets patients describe themselves in relation to the investigator. In order to reflect on and to interpret interaction, the investigator must be able to alternate between observation and introspection; he or she must be acquainted with the theory of personality, have acquired diagnostic experience from supervised interviews, and have self-experience.

Structural diagnostics can proceed in one or several interviews. The *primary goal* is to give practical advice for choosing suitable therapies, keeping in mind both the structural possibilities or limitations of the patients (who should not be overburdened) and the aims of therapy (growth of structure as the task of therapy).

7.1.2 The Concept of Structure

Descriptively, structure means the ordered joining of parts into a whole. To explain structures, we use rules on how they function and arise.

In this sense, the concept figures in many different disciplines, e.g., the geological structure of a valley, the molecular structure of a crystal, the age structure of a population, the demographic structure of a society, and the structure of texts, systems of signs, languages, communication.

To see the sense of structures, we usually consider how they developed, i.e., how they came to grow and function in their historical setting. Since we always set up hypotheses, structures that cannot be directly inspected are in fact models and explanatory constructs, formulable only under theoretical assumptions. Such structural models therefore refer to certain theories and their terminology. Dealing with structural concepts therefore needs constant critical review of the underlying assumptions.

Structures can usually be put together from substructures and be taken as parts of a higher order in a network of effective quantities. They constitute a set of information that, in turn, organizes experiences and processes them. This resembles a system stressing dynamic processes of homeostatic balance in terms of sets of recursive rules and the start of nonlinear processes.

7.1.3 The Psychological Concept of Structure

The concept of structure in a psychological sense denotes the set of mental dispositions as a whole. They encompass everything that repeats itself in an individual's experience and behavior (consciously or unconsciously) in accordance with a rule. Structure lies at the basis of long-term personal style (Shapiro, 1965), in that individuals time and again restore their intrapsychic and interpersonal equilibria. A highly integrative structure is flexible and has creative functions that regulate and adapt within and between individuals.

Structure is not rigid and immutable, but dynamic; it develops throughout life, but so slowly that it almost appears to be static. This is where concepts such as identity, character, or personality come into play. To counterbalance too static a view of structure, one must consider arguments suggesting a dynamic view of mental structures, since they grow during life. Although they rest on innate dispositions, they are first shaped during childhood and undergo more or less major changes throughout life. Moreover, mental structures are dispositions, and as such not observable; they are realized only in concrete and present situations, from which one infers back to long-term character traits (dynamic analysis of structures). Such inferences, however, are never exhaustive. The description of personality structures is always provisional and incomplete (logical restriction on the hypothesis of stability). Further, structure implies stability over time, which on the psychological plane is restricted. Assuming that personality can grow and develop throughout one's lifetime, structure contains dynamic aspects of development, though acting slowly (slow-change model). Structures change through new information being integrated, and in this manner set up new rules—which change in turn when further new information is gained.

7.1.4 The Psychoanalytic Concept of Structure

As in other sciences, psychoanalytic literature has no uniform concept of structure. However, several central notions can be distinguished:

- **The topographic model of structure**: Freud, in *The Ego and the Id* (1923), or in the *New Introductory Lectures* speaks of the "structural conditions of mental personality" (1933), describing the interplay of ego, id, and superego. It is not the aim of this model to describe parts of the contents of the mental structure taken singly, but rather their interplay—the set of rules of mental functioning in the topography of the "mental apparatus," e.g., to distinguish the conscious/unconscious systems.

- **Structure of character**: This deals with concepts that succinctly describe types of character attitude. These are based on theory that is derived from metapsychology and developmental psychology (oral personality, anal character, etc.; cf. Abraham, 1925). As a diagnostic category, character neurosis is a countertype to conflict neurosis. There are transitions to what is called personality disorder in contemporary diagnostic systems.

- **Neurotic structure**: In the psychological concept of neurosis by Schultz-Hencke (1951), we speak of hysterical, compulsive, depressive, and schizoid neurotic structure. This concept of instinctual drives describes the consequences for character when certain instincts are repressed. As a rule, clinical diagnosis finds several structural parts in parallel (e.g., depressive hysterical; see Schwidder, 1972a, b).

- **Structure of ego, self, and object relations**: Modern psychoanalysis distinguishes concepts such as the "ego," "the self," and "object relations" more and more in terms of structure, above all as how these develop psychologically, i.e., how the *self in its object relations* becomes more distinct and integrated (see Rudolf, 1993, 55-83). Lately, these notions have been increasingly influenced by observations on infants and small children (see Lichtenberg, 1983; Schüssler and Bertl-Schüssler, 1992; Stern, 1985). They stress the infant's innate object-seeking activity, and its ability, developed early on, to engage the caring adult in social interactions. These pleasurable interactive games involve bodily care and nutrition as well, which classical theory had put in the foreground (e.g., oral or early libidinous relations).

  In these early phases of development, the ego begins to organize itself, shows interest, is ready to act toward the non-ego, i.e., the world of objects (conveying ego intentions, cf. Rudolf, 1977). This is where the self begins to develop, a process completed when the ego comes to see itself as an object, and thus establishes a reflexive relationship. This opens an inner space where conceptual and symbolic representation of experience begins, which is observable from about the 18th month of life onward. In the constant interaction with the world of objects, the guiding and organizing function of the ego becomes more subtle, and pictures of the self and important objects arise (representations of self and of objects).

  Objects are thus experienced apart from the self, recognized, linked with feelings, and internalized. Emotional experiences of important objects, above all affective interactions, between the child and its reference person, affect not only the image of and attitude toward him or her, but also the image and value of the self. The structure of self and object relations matures in a lively mesh; the self grows more coherent, bounded, and able to organize itself, while it also becomes more tied to the others who give security. This in turn favors the growing autonomy of the self, which thus strengthened, learns to detach itself from objects and begins to deal with them. The result of the development is an autonomous self with a sense of identity, always able to adjust its own image and value, and its power to guide and act.

Short definition of some important concepts:

- **The ego**: the central organizer of the psyche, aiming intentionally at objects.

- **The self**: the reflexive mental structure. The ego makes itself the object of perception and thus becomes the self (self-image). The self evaluates itself and feels others evaluating it (self-esteem), and experiences itself as constant and coherent (identity). It conjoins all mental functions and dispositions into a whole, regulating itself and organizing relations to others.

- **Structure**: the way the self shapes itself, and functions, in relations to others.

Structure can be described in several structural aspects. This includes the *ability of self-perception*, *self-regulation*, and the *ability of flexible and "mature" defense*. The self accepts objects as different from itself with their own special properties and rights; this means the ability of *object perception*, of *communication* and *attachment*. This basic growth occurs in the first 5 to 6 years of life. *Structural disorder* in adults can be seen as *deficient growth* or *regressive merging* (see A. Freud, 1977; Heigl-Evers, et al., 1993). In the case of deficient growth, conditions for the maturing self were so adverse, above all the gap between the child's needs and what caregivers offered (or the impact of traumatic experiences so great), that one or more of the structures described above were unable to unfold adequately. The result is an immature, underdeveloped, or disturbed self-structure, able neither to be independent nor to organize itself adequately or be self-reflective. The person is unable to develop reliable bonding with supportive objects—or even perceive them reliably.

In the case of regressive merging, the notion is that the structure was able to develop, but remained too unstable to prevent internal and external stress from habitually triggering regressions that depress structure to a more immature level of tensions and disruptive states. This is not an acute crisis implying illness, but a long-term tendency of the structure toward disorder and regression.

7.1.5 Proposal for Operationalizing Structure for OPD

Psychodynamic diagnostics and indication for therapy demand an assessment of structure. We have much relevant psychoanalytic material here, but there are so many theory-based concepts available that they are hard to apply. We propose an integrative psychodynamic approach that largely avoids traditional psychoanalytic concepts. Instead, staying close to observation, it shows the behavior and experience of patients and therapists in a diagnostic setting. This does not, however, mean an absence of theory.

Our system involves mental structure as that of *self in relation to the other* (see the brief sketch on developmental psychology in the previous section). We mainly combine object relational approaches with those from the psychology of the self and the ego. The concept of the self in any case makes sense only if we consider the other: The self develops through relations, much as it has developed via the other and detachment from the other by internalization (Seidler, 1995a, 1995b; Dahlbender, 2002). This concept of self-structure stresses interpersonal events, not internal ones, though it integrates aspects of ego-psychology.

Of great importance for a diagnostic understanding of structural features is countertransference, which echoes to the examiner what patients put into the relation by virtue of their structure.

The self in relation to the other is described under six aspects that mark *6 observable functions* ("capacities") of the structure concerned.

- **Self-Perception.** Self-reflection, the acquisition of a self-image (provided one can distinguish between self and objects), and the retention of that image over time, coherent in its psychosexual and social aspects (identity); the ability to distinguish internal processes and above all their affective side (differentiation of affects).

- **Self-Regulation.** Organizing oneself so that the self can be experienced as originating competent action, guiding and integrating one's needs and feelings, enduring stress and restoring balance. Especially important is the capacity to assess self-esteem at a realistic level and regulate its fluctuations.

- **Defense.** Using certain means ("defense mechanisms") to maintain or restore balance in the face of internal or external stresses or conflicts.

- **Object Perception.** The ability to distinguish between internal and external reality and hence to perceive others as integral persons with their own aims, rights, and contradictions, and empathizing with them.

- **Communication.** Emotionally addressing others and approaching them, communicating with them, and understanding their affective signals.

- **Bonding/Attachment.** Internal representation of the other (internalizing of objects), and maintaining this over longer periods (constancy of objects). Being able to alternate between bonding and detachment (farewell and grieving). Being able to protect bonding by developing and following rules for interacting with important partners.

These aspects cannot be logically separated from one another; rather, they represent the object of structure (the self in relation to the other) from various perspectives, and capture the complex functional patterns in various connections.

7.1.6   Structure and Structural Disorder: Different Levels of Integration in OPD

In developmental psychology, structure in adults results from maturation with growing differentiation and integration, marked especially by growth in mental aspects. This concerns the internal representation of external objects and the experiences and attitudes of the self in dealing with objects (representation of self and interaction). Structure free from disorder means that the individual has obtained this mental internal space and can regulate it with internal processes, so as to establish and maintain satisfactory interpersonal relations. Structure is *highly individual*, not only in its limitations and weaknesses, but also in the *resources and strengths* the individual has developed.

Structural disorder can mean that certain structural distinctions and integrations have failed to develop *(deficient development)*. The self can neither be autonomous nor organize itself adequately nor reflect upon itself; a reliable bonding with supportive partners did not develop.

In someone who is *structurally vulnerable*, structure has developed though not stably enough, so that regression sets in and structurally anchored functions are lost in the presence of internal or external stress, while feelings of tension and disintegration become active.

In our differential diagnosis we must distinguish between habitual structure and its disorder from striking features that may occur in an *acute crisis*. Conflicts that cause emotional stress (e.g., crises in relations, alterations, or stressful events), when combined with sleeping pills, excessive use of alcohol, nicotine, medicines, drugs, and the like, can set off regressions that become structurally apparent (e.g., loss of self-regulation of feelings and regulation of self-value, doubts as to one's identity, gaps in communication, projective mix-ups between self and objects, etc.). This should be considered exceptional (acute, crisis-linked structural oddity); apart from this, one should consider the long-term structure typical for the person in question for the last one to two years.

To mark the extent and quality of structural disorder or vulnerability, we distinguish *four levels of structural integration* (good, moderate, low, and disintegrated). For a continuum between mature and psychotic structure (well-integrated and disintegrated, respectively), four steps seem too crude, as this would leave out many intermediate cases. However, four steps on six levels of assessment adequately capture the severity of structural disorder and provide a qualitative marker.

The concluding *finding* documents both: the qualitative description of the six assessment levels and a global estimate of the level of integration.

The logic of the different levels of structure is often used in the literature, though on varying theoretical grounds. Kernberg's structural interview (1977, 1981) distinguishes between neurotic, borderline, and psychotic levels, and operationalizes them descriptively, mainly via identity, defense, and reality testing. In a different connection, Kernberg distinguishes four levels (higher, intermediate, lower, psychotic), the criteria being super-ego, ego, ego-identity, reality testing, development of instinct, defense, character traits, object relations, and affects (Kernberg, 1970). An articulated system using a similar psychoanalytic basis is described by Lohmer, et al. (1992). They, too, aim at distinguishing between the neurotic-level, medium-level, and borderline disorders, via assessing the kind and pathology of object relations, ego-structure, defense mechanisms, super-ego development, quality of fear, and doctor-patient relationship. Part of what is described there has entered our manual. The same is true for the scale "Ego/self/object relations," which is used at the Psychosomatic Clinic Heidelberg as a matter of routine for capturing structural levels and their changes during therapy (Rudolf, et al., 1997). Moreover, a psychoanalytic rating device with this aim was used by Engel, et al. (1979). Some assessment scales aim specifically at levels of ego-functions and object relations, e.g., those of Bellak & Hurvich (1969) and Bellak & Goldsmith (1984). These scales were used also in a study with various disorders such as Morbus Crohn and obsession (Davies Osterkamp, et al., 1992). Other possibilities of diagnosis were used by Schüssler, et al. (1990). Weinryb and Rössel in Sweden developed a very subtle psychodynamic profile (KAPP; Weinryb & Rössel, 1991).

Other scales aim only at the level of object relations (e.g., Piper, et al., 1991). Some papers concentrate on partial diagnostic domains, (e.g., the detailed operational account of defense by Ehlers & Czogalik (1984) and Ehlers & Peter (1990), using assessments by self and others (KBAM or SBAK).

Our proposal takes into consideration experiences with such scales and systems. Attendant problems concern above all the objectivity and reliability of highly complex theoretical constructs that are hard to operationalize in behavioral terms. We therefore tried

- to concentrate on *a single theoretical line* (the self and its relation to the other);

- to limit ourselves to a few *criteria for judging structure* (self-perception, self-regulation, defense, object perception, communication and attachment);

- to describe these categories in the *manual* clinically (close to experience, behavior, and observation); and

- To *avoid traditional psychoanalytic concepts* as much as possible (since every concept in its long history of development has acquired various shades of meaning), or to embed such concepts in an explanatory context.

7.2   Manual of the OPD Axis IV: "Psychic Structure/Mental Functioning"

7.2.1   Introduction

The relationship between conflict (axis III) and structure (axis IV) is manifold. Obviously, the two constructs describe distinct aspects of a common reference system. Conflict (also as a repetitive pattern) describes aspects of disease-triggering and of psychodynamics; structure is related more to disposition to disease, vulnerability of personality, and capacity to work things out. This manual describes the general characteristics of the four levels of integration and a thorough operationalized account of the six structural dimensions of assessment with clinical examples.

Basis and Period of Observation

The interaction of the patient with the interviewer during the diagnostic interview and those interpersonal relationships reported by patients from their own lives form the "material" to be examined as to structure. When making a diagnostic assessment of the patient, what is important is not necessarily the current disorder; of primary significance is rather the underlying structural readiness as shown in interpersonal actions over the last year or two. Present disorders, including regressive states and crises, do not on their own determine the structural level, but are indicators of the structural readiness for it.

Finally, we must test which operational measures in the manual apply to the patient. Quite different levels may be described on the six dimensions. The global assessment of structural level is an average value thereof. A checklist of the most important items has been developed (Rudolf, et al., 1998).

7.2.2   Operationalization

7.2.2.1 General Features of the Level of Integration

Good Integration

A good level of integration is marked by internal and interpersonal regulating functions being available to the patient. The patient can keep them going for long periods, or quickly regain them, independently of internal or external stress.

A well integrated mental structure offers inner space in which to decide inner conflicts. These occur between varied needs and attendant feelings, on the one hand, and internalized norms (a mature super-ego) and ideals, on the other hand.

The central fear is that of losing the love of the object.

Countertransference toward such patients is marked by a growing awareness of modulated mutual emotions relating to revival of conflicts actually experienced with persons in the past.

Moderate Integration

Here, the abilities and functions described are still available, but in some situations diminished. Here, too, there are inner conflicts, though different contents are dealt with in a different manner. On the side of needs, there are unconscious feelings of greedy want, taking possession, and submission; on the corrective opposite side, there are strict and rigid punitive norms ("immature super-ego") and covert ideals.

The central fear is that of loss or destruction of the supportive and directing object.

Correspondingly, in countertransference there is an instantaneous and at times almost unbearable experience, which through analysis of countertransference can always be reduced to relevant relational experiences of the patient.

Low Integration

Here, the functions are clearly much less available, either permanently (defective development) or time and again in connection with stress (structural vulnerability). Brief disintegrations are excluded, e.g., posttraumatic stress disorders. In contrast with earlier levels, the inner space is less developed; ideal structure is unrefined, and normative structure (super-ego) is dissociated. Unconscious emotional needs are not internally bound but directed outward. Conflicts are not so much internal as interpersonal (in partnership, profession, and social environment).

The central fear is that of annihilation of the self by the bad object or by loss of the good object.

The tendency to carry out inner conflicts in each interaction corresponds to countertransference as well. It is violent because of abrupt changes in experience; sometimes emotions continue to have an effect even after the patient has left. In their relationship to the other, such patients do not repeat their own past conflicts, but mobilize in the other partial ego-functions they themselves do not have.

Disintegration

Without coherent structure, stress may cause a patient to disintegrate or fragment. Psychotic collapse may be followed by a psychotic restitution.

The patient tries to stabilize this fragile structure by splitting off or denying essential instinctual drives and narcissistic needs. For long periods, these can then no longer be consciously perceived. If the prior unstable balance cannot be kept up, psychotic decompensation projectively digests this. The emotional needs, thus far unconscious, are now experienced as coming from without and not from within: Thoughts are manufactured or inspired, spontaneous sexual excitement is externally contrived, only the others are aggressive and threatening. If a conflict in question is to be settled, there is a danger of fusion with the object against an isolating exclusion, or of narcissistic self-exaltation to compensate for severe self-doubt.

7.2.2.2   Structural Assessment Dimensions

- **Self-Perception:** This describes the ability to gain a picture of one's own self (self-reflection). In addition, the ability to keep this constant over time and coherent as regards psychosexual and social aspects (identity). It also includes a capacity for a refined perception of one's inner processes, in particular, of affects (introspection of affects).

Good Integration

A refined perception of the self is possible; the self-image is basically long-term and coherent (identity, especially the psychosexual kind). Inner processes can be observed with some interest and perceived along with the refined attendant feelings; these include joy, curiosity, pride, fear, anger, contempt, guilt, shame, and grief. The capacities mentioned can be limited by conflicts, but cannot be abolished totally.

Clinical Example: Patients can spontaneously or on request name properties and abilities that illustrate their own self-image, describe what sort of person they are, and possibly also what makes them different from others. They can perceive and communicate different facets of their emotional experience. The investigator gains the impression that the patient has developed a self-reflective interest and can profit from it.

Moderate Integration

Reflexive perception of the self is limited and mainly directed toward the acting ego. The coherence of the self-image is put in question by stress. Introspection as regards one's own feelings (above all tender and aggressive ones) is neurotically stifled. Affective experience centers on anhedonic affects; these include above all anger, fear, disappointment, self-devaluation, and depressiveness.

Clinical Example: When asked, patients cannot really describe who they are, but rather only what they said or did in certain settings. The resultant self-image often seems unstable, flat, or crude, and depends on situation and mood that sweep the patients along. Or they try to remain stable by avoiding feelings.

Low Integration

Reflexive self-perception is impossible, no feeling of psychosexual or social identity has developed, but rather contradictory and dissociated aspects of self co-exist. One's own feelings cannot be perceived in a refined way. Affective experience is marked by chronic contempt, repulsion, and anger. Above all, contempt and repulsion are the affects that are often given expression. Affective experience may be replaced by estrangement, affective void, depressiveness, inward and outward attribution cannot be clearly differentiated.

> **Clinical Example:** Even with help, such patients are unable to draw a full picture of themselves, or give the investigator a testable account of what affects, ideas, and fantasies they have. Such accounts rather vary with external situations and conflicts, and are even contradictory, so that no coherent picture emerges of what is going on in them. "I am many things at once, but nothing genuinely." The self-image looks diffuse, because it is mixed with images of important reference persons. Inner preferences, sexual ones included, remain unclear. Contradictory social roles are assumed. At a later meeting a few days later, the investigator might gain the impression that the person sitting in front of him is a completely different one with a different self-image, expressing utterly different expectations.

Disintegration

Self-characterization is impossible. Depending on the kind of psychosis, social and sexual identities are largely absent (schizophrenia), or there is an over-identification with the social role (manic-depressive psychosis). Outside the psychosis there is perhaps a compensatory narcissistic overrating of one's own person. From within the psychosis a new delusional identity can arise (megalomania, guilt complex, delusion of love, etc.).

> **Clinical Example:** In their self-estimation, patients oscillate between total helplessness as regards their professional goals and a grandiose idea of their professional scope. Since they have no reality-based motivation, they imagine that they might, for example, become the director of a big organization.

- **Self-Regulation:** The dimension of self-regulation describes an integrating aspect of self-reflection and above all the ability to regulate one's own instinctual drives, affects, and self-esteem. This results in the ability to experience oneself as being responsible for originating one's own competent actions. Self-regulation is a bipolar concept: If it is excessive, the ability to act and the scope for communicating with others may be restricted; if it is deficient, so that affects and impulses are insufficiently integrated, the result is unintended or impulsive "acting" out of affects and drives.

To regulate oneself, one must be creative and tolerate wide variations of feelings, especially negative and contradictory ones (tolerance of ambivalence), and one must be able to anticipate feelings. Regulating self-esteem is part of this, too. All this hinges on the ability to deal with inner conflicts, to be described below under "defense."

Good Integration

Instinctual drives do not cause long-term fear and can be tentatively described. Conflicts between one's own desires, the interests of others, and one's own ideas of value can perhaps be reflected upon, and a solution reached through compromise. Ambivalence can be tolerated. Instinctual satisfaction is sought, but may be deferred or displaced. The reaction of the environment can be anticipated. A positive self-esteem, subject to conflict-based limitations, can be maintained. Unpleasant feelings can be tolerated, as well as positive ones. Affects are seen as signals and guides to action.

Clinical Example: In conversation such patients are able to react to the discrepancy the investigator sees between wishes, values, and the interests of the other as described by the patients. They are able to reflect upon this conflict without feeling offended or withdrawing from conversation, and to work on resolving the inner clash.

Moderate Integration

There is a clear reduction in the ability to fulfill instinctual drives in a socially adequate manner, and in accordance with one's own ideas of values. The prevailing tendency is to overregulate. Affects and drives are poorly tolerated consciously and are therefore repulsed; they are not be seen as signals or guides to action. Hence, self-control is strengthened and emotional flexibility is restricted. Alongside overregulation, impulses may break through.

The scope for flexibly dealing with instinctual drives and affects is restricted, since there is great fixation on certain repressed desires. Hence, there is less scope for deferring or displacing instinctual satisfaction. Suppressed aggression can lead to internal self-devaluation, self-punishment, and self-aggression, which look "masochistic." If self-regulation fails, self-aggressive tendencies can emerge. The regulation of self-esteem is clearly subject to disorder, showing grandiosity or self-devaluation.

Clinical Example: Patients might be able to make indirect demands for care and attention; they may stand back and help others (altruism), and not allow their yearning for attention to show. Conversation with them remains stiff, as they are very controlled, externally polite, but still taciturn and lifeless. The interviewer constantly feels that he should do more for such patients and care for and support them better. He discovers rather incidentally that at home, these patients tend to drink excessively when alone.

Low Integration

There is little scope to realize instinctual drives in socially adequate ways and according to one's own ideas of values, or to defer or displace them. This results in impulsive behavior by the person, who at times experiences this as dystonic, overwhelming, and painful—or as something that the environment rejects as inadequate, hostile, or overwhelming. These environmental reactions, however, cannot be foreseen or used as behavioral controls. Lack of empathy with the reactions of objects, which involves lack of sympathy, can lead to a predominance of aggressive impulses. Attempts at regulation are mostly abrupt and ineffective. Tendencies to destroy oneself and others are obvious in fantasies or actions. Guilt feelings are not internally worked on, but lead to self-punishment, sometimes in the form of self-destructive tendencies. Here, in contrast with moderate level of integration, we have underregulation. Impulsive behavior is often triggered by unpleasant feelings that are not internally mastered, and thus lead to sudden changes in behavior. The regulation of self-esteem is very fragile, and shows itself in great touchiness or unrealistic ideas of grandiosity.

> **Clinical Example:** Patients strongly grimace in the first interview, if topics involving emotional stress are mentioned. If a male interviewer points this out, the patient may rebuke him directly and bid him to keep quiet. The patient says he does not want to talk any further, and could in any case not talk to men. Only with great difficulty can the interview proceed, because suddenly patients speak in great detail about their intimate life.

Disintegration

The experience of originating one's own behavior is deficient; outside the psychosis, motivation rests on fantasized grandiosity. If the defense mechanisms are loosened, one comes to perceive one's instinctual drives, and self-regulation becomes grossly disordered (shameless behavior without distance). This is revealed in inadequacy or violence that is too much for the patient and his or her partner. In prepsychotic states these needs become even more intense, so that there is a further loss of regulation. In acute psychosis, drives may break out aggressively to the point of psychotic excitement. Libidinous impulses often crop up unchecked.

> **Clinical Example:** Because of unclear motivation, patients are unable to pursue an objective aim for a long period of time. They break off one line of studies, and turn arbitrarily to quite a different line.

- **Defense:** The dimension of defense is characterized by the fact that patients unconsciously restrict aspects of their cognition with the aim of self-protection.

The dimension of defense describes a specific aspect of mental performance, namely, the particular means used by the ego (defense mechanisms) to keep up mental balance when faced by internal or external stresses or conflicts. These processes cannot be called up deliberately, but occur mostly unconsciously. Their aim is to keep unconscious certain memories and ideas with their attendant contents and affects, especially if they involve stressful, painful, illicit, or unbearable aspects like pleasure, joy, fear, mental pain, grief or depressive feelings, shame, guilt, anger, or aggressive impulses. Defense relates to other structural dimensions such as self-regulation and bonding/attachment. If defense is internal and regulates impulses, desires, and affects, it is an aspect of self-regulation; if defense is interpersonal, involving others in psychosocial arrangements (Mentzos, 1976, 1993) or collusions (Willi, 1975) for regulating mental balance, it has its effects on attachment and object relations. This cannot always be fenced off simply from coping mechanisms that are adopted consciously (Beutel, 1990).

Individual regulating functions are described as defense mechanisms, which can ideally be assigned to various levels, forming a hierarchy from mature defense (good level of integration) to immature defense (level of disintegration) (cf. Vaillant 1971, 1986). However, this is not to say, for example, that, where projection occurs, one has to conclude that the structural level of integration is only moderate.

Criteria for determining levels of defense:

- **Object**: Is it aimed at inner drives and affects, or is the goal the modification of inner images of self and important reference persons?

- **Success**: Does it clearly delimit the self, maintain the relationship to the other? Does it allow adequate fulfillment of goals and desires (scope for satisfying drives or deferring them, etc.)?

- **Stability**: Is it too weak or too strong? Does it always function, or lapse, e.g., in crises?

- **Flexibility**: Are different mechanisms used according to situations that arise, or has the person a severely limited, rigid, and stereotyped pattern of defense at the expense of other dimensions?

- **Form**: What types of mechanism are used? Is it a pattern, the primary function of which is to regulate or inhibit manifest impulses or affects (mature defense, good integrated level)? Or are there defense mechanisms that are no longer able to inhibit them, so that a great proportion of such impulses and affects are uncontrolled and set free (immature defense, low level of integration)?

Good Integration

This defense is directed against inner instinctual drives and affects. Patients' inner images of themselves and others do not undergo changes but remain stable. Defense results in restriction or impossibility of satisfying certain described and conflict-laden instinctual drives, and at the same time to a limitation of mental functions and cognitive performance as well. Dissociation from or relation to others is on the whole untouched by the defense, which remains stable and always available. In described conflicts the flexibility of defense is restricted.

Typical defense mechanisms: repression, rationalization, displacement

- **Repression**: The patient cannot remember certain desires, thoughts, and experiences, so that cognitive ideas remain unconscious. Repression manifests itself in that certain conflictual contents are faded out, forgotten, or overlooked, soon becoming inaccessible to conscious effort. The idea may later recur in consciousness unasked, without the person being able consciously to grasp why.

Clinical Example: The patient forgets an embarrassing experience, with noticeable fading out of a forbidden erotic desire.

- **Rationalization**: Central to defense is expedient and reassuring accounts and justifications, logically and morally acceptable, of one's own or others' behavior. The interviewer sees the patient's story as a pretext, explaining or justifying certain behavior after the event, a sham motive, or an attempt at self-deception about unacceptable reasons for behaving or acting.

Clinical Example: Patient checks his girl friend's mailbox ("it might overflow"), when he clearly suffers from jealousy.

- **Displacement**: The emotional meaning is detached from an idea, and shifts to another initially less intense idea linked to the first one in content. By what they say, patients express their underlying conflictual impulses as a compromise, by turning to a theme they are readier to accept, while for the interviewer this expresses links with the conflictual theme.

Clinical Example: The patient does not speak of his fears of quarrelling with his wife, but of the drawbacks of road anger.

Moderate Integration

Defense is aimed at inner instinctual drives and affects; inner images of self and others remain stable. This means that instinctual satisfactions are more restricted or more difficult. Since at this level defense is directed at dangers from depending too strongly on objects, it helps to delimit the relationships to others. In a way, the defense is too strong (overshooting, inhibiting); but it can temporarily fail in crises and reduce to splitting, idealization, and self-devaluation at the next lower level (low integration).

The pattern of defense is not very flexible and cannot be readily adapted to specific situations. Its inhibiting force is often inadequate, so that it can sometimes lead to underlying impulses breaking through.

Typical defense mechanisms: denial, turning against oneself, reaction formation, isolation, projection.

- **Denial**: Certain aspects of external reality or one's own experience are not acknowledged to oneself or to others, even if such aspects are obvious to others.

    The interviewer notices that patients avoid acknowledging certain areas of their own experience, ideas about themselves and others, and the meanings thereof. They may even deny them, either spontaneously or upon query, trying to steer clear of certain conflictual themes. Faced by real dangers patients sometimes ignore them, though they know better and are aware of them.

Clinical Example: A female patient who clearly suffers from a separation, vigorously denies that she feels any pains about this. During further conversation she completely excludes this topic.

- **Turning against oneself**: An impulse or idea, often of aggressive content, is not directed at another person, but turned back on oneself. Such aggressive impulses result in attacks on oneself (self-debasement, self-aggression, etc.). Fear-inducing aggressive impulses and ideas of this kind are not uttered in words or by the patient's actions, but manifest themselves in depressive moods, self-devaluations or self-hate, and self-destructive impulses, even with masochistic suffering.

Clinical Example: A patient arguing with his work superior reports with outer calm (but clearly under tension) that he repeatedly has doubts about his own performance and ability, just as his boss does. He can find nothing good in himself, and recently he suffered an injury in an avoidable accident at work.

- **Reaction formation**: If impulses or feelings cannot be expressed by the patient because of guilt feelings, they can become replaced by opposite thoughts and feelings. A need of one's own is repressed in favor of socially acceptable modes of behavior, which can function as submission.

Clinical Example: A patient at first describes a delimiting conflict with her younger sister that offended and hurt her. Next, with pointed thoughtfulness for her well-being, she points out that the sister, who lived alone, was helpless and in need of protection. The patient presents herself as "morally superior" to her sister.

- **Isolation**: Cognitive and affective parts of an event are not consciously experienced together; the emotional component is detached from the imagination and kept unconscious. Thoughts appear without appropriate feelings, there seems to be no motivation for thoughts and actions. The patient "uncouples" the link between thoughts and feelings in a conflictual experience, dealing mainly with the cognitive, rational processing of the problem. The patient can feel and name the emotional content only at other times or places.

Clinical Example: Without noticeable feelings, the patient reports that his wife had recently left him. He was now considering how he might keep the lease on their apartment. Only later in the interview does he mention his weeping fits, which he finds inexplicable.

- **Projection**: Feelings and desires are not seen and admitted in oneself, but excluded from one's own experience and attributed to another. Patients cannot experience for themselves what they find unacceptable (thoughts, feelings, desires, impulses), but rather disown them, just as they indignantly recognize them in other people, whom they then regard as clearly and strongly inhibiting them.

Clinical Example: During the account of a female patient, the interviewer notices disguised self-devaluation as part of a long-term stressful conflict with a neighbor, whom she accuses of moral failings and openly aggressive acts. She herself knows no such vice or anger in herself.

Low Integration

At this level, defense against inner instinctual drives and affects is insufficient. What marks this case is the change, i.e., distorted, exaggerated, or devalued shape, of inner images of self and the other (self- and object-representation) through the defense mechanism. Defense here turns interpersonal, as on the next lower level (disintegration).

Delimitation from or relation to the other can no longer be adequately achieved through defense mechanisms, since it changes the borders of self-objects. At this level, it may be stable, but it becomes highly inflexible.

Typical defense mechanisms: Defense at this level is marked by the splitting of images of self from those of objects, which leads to other mechanisms of this level, e.g., projective identification and idealization, or devaluation of external objects.

- **Splitting**: The self and outer objects are not experienced ambivalently, with good and bad features, but one-sidedly as only good or only bad, where the assignment can vary from one person to another, and even within an individual from time to time. Contradictory feelings often uttered with regard to the same person (e.g., idealization and devaluation) stand unlinked side by side, though knowing this does not trigger the corresponding affects or conflictual tension, nor does it lead to a correction or complete reversal of previously expressed feelings and ideas.

Clinical Example: The patient describes his girlfriend in an account the interviewer finds very contradictory: The patient is in a hostile relationship with her, though he has never hurt her. Another time he says that he values her beyond everything, only she could still understand him.

- **Projective identification**: Projection and identification are connected here. The subject experiences split-off parts of self in the other. Unlike in projection, however, this does not create a distance to the other; rather, the other, who "contains" the (threatening) parts of self, appears threatening in his own right and must therefore be constantly watched and controlled. That is how the patient justifies the aggression directed at the other. Projective identification corresponds to incomplete projection as seen from the differentiation of self and object. The interviewer notices that the patient has included the interviewer in a "scenario of perpetrator and victim," with the role of proxy expression of the patient's own unacceptable impulses, so that the patient controls and fears the interviewer. The interviewer feels repeatedly pushed into an otherwise alien role pattern.

Clinical Example: A female patient constantly blames the interviewer for taking no interest in her, and for being indifferent and incompetent. The therapist feels growing anger at her, but notices that despite the blaming and attacking, she does not stop attending her sessions with him regularly and respecting his every impulse and comment. He notices, too, that she relaxes when he controls and integrates his anger.

Disintegration

At this level primitive defense mechanisms come into action. Defense occurs at the expense of further limitation of reality testing. It can be stable here too, i.e., mental balance can be maintained for a long-term at a regressive level, but defense is all but inflexible.

Typical defense mechanisms: splitting, denial, projection, and projective identification

- **Splitting**: In contrast to low integration, where splitting occurs into good and bad images of self and objects, psychotic splitting goes further, because of the marked loss of reality. Here whole areas, such as sexuality, are split off and feelings are withdrawn from it; or delusions seem to stand unrelated to realistic ego parts. In this way irreconcilable parts of the personality are kept apart, so that this kind of splitting has a stabilizing defensive effect. If defense collapses, there is psychotic fragmentation or splintering, e.g., in the form of several delusional identities.

- **Denial**: While this sort of splitting is typical for schizophrenic psychoses, which got their name from the splitting process, denial too is a typical defense mechanism in affective psychoses, e.g., manias. Psychotic denial is marked by failure to perceive evident aspects of reality (e.g., social realities of varied kinds—in partnership, family, profession, and finance).

- **Psychotic projection**: Here, one's own impulses are delusionally externalized and attributed to others. Aggressive or sexual tendencies are experienced as starting from others and caused from outside. The projected part of personality is not defended because of feelings of shame or guilt, but has a strong taboo on it and cannot be recognized as one's own motive, etc.

Clinical Example: In the first interview, the patient, perhaps for the first time ever, entrusts much personal experience to another person, namely, the interviewer. When at the end, a second session is arranged, he gets up anxiously, saying he knows that the interviewer works with the police, that a concealed examination had occurred, that bugs have been installed. The interviewer suggests that the patient must have felt strongly offended at the end of the interview. The patient cannot pick up this interpretation and sees his own emotion as adequate indignation in a criminal situation.

- **Object Perception**: This dimension describes the ability to develop an image of another while distinguishing it from that of oneself (distinguishing internal and external reality, as expression of successful self/object differentiation. For this, one must be able to perceive others' image globally with various facets, and endowed with their own aims and rights (global perception of objects), and keep this image coherent and constant. Moreover, one must be able to empathize with others' inner processes, above all their different feelings (empathy, intuition, and understanding).

Good Integration

On the basis of internalized relations one can perceive others in their varied aspects. The image of others is on the whole constant and coherent. Even in conflictual situations and under pressure from instinctual interests, it remains basically stable. The mental processes of the other can be grasped with interest. Empathy with the other's various feelings is possible. Affectively, care, sympathy, joy, shame, and grief are important. Through conflict one's image of the other may be changed, without endangering the relation as such.

Clinical Example: Requested to draw a picture of a certain important reference person in such a way that the interviewer can imagine for himself what kind of person that is, patients are able to bring to life important persons close to them. A sensitive picture of an important reference person arises, with its limits and scope, weaknesses and strengths. Patients can make clear what they cannot discuss with this concrete other, because a certain topic would go beyond the other's boundaries. But they can also make clear what sort of gift a certain person might particularly like. Moreover, the patient has ideas as to the biographical events that have made this person what he or she is.

Moderate Integration

Stress and the pressure one's own desires imposes on the other, or the pressure the desires of the other puts on the patient, limit the degree of empathy with the other. At times free from conflict, the image of the other can be maintained, but when episodes of conflict occur, it instills fear, the image becomes devalued, and the relation to the other is put in question. However, by conciliation a new relationship may start. Instead of devaluation, there may be depressive clinging, which does not, however, escalate to a breakdown of the relationship, but can restore closeness to the other.

Clinical Example: The patient is able to provide an imaginative picture of the other based on empathy. On being questioned, he states that when approached with strong desires, he might feel rather put under pressure and might speak ill of his girlfriend. Afterwards, he always regretted this and reconciliation followed. The relationship might continue stably. If he approached her with his own desires and she did not want what he wanted, he asked himself whether she was really "right" for him, and he considered ending the relationship. However, as a rule he could distance himself from his violent reactions and a conciliatory discussion would follow. He then regretted that he had made remarks which he knew upset her, regretted frightening her by possibly making her think that he had wanted to put an end to the relationship.

Low Integration

Descriptions of others as given by the patient provoke in the interviewer a feeling that such people could not possibly exist. Everyone must surely have strong and weak sides, but they do not figure in the patient's reports: Patients have no sense for others having a history of their own, with strong and weak points. Either the other must simply match the picture they have painted of them, or the patient can have nothing to do with them. The accounts of others seem flat, patchy, and without depth, and not clearly delineated. On being asked about an ideal partner, a patient describes a super(hu)man with whom everything is possible, but who in turn makes no demands and shows no deficiencies.

Clinical Example: Based on the description the patient gives of others, one is unable to get a lively picture of these people, what they might be like. The patient cannot empathize with them. Seen from without, the reactions of important reference persons look plausible; but when asked, the patient cannot see why his girlfriend behaved as she did in response to a violent remark of his.

Disintegration

It is hard to differentiate aspects of the self from aspects of the object, or to see the object as distinct from the self. Under stress, images of self and other can become confused. Because the symbolization is disordered, individual features of the object stand for the whole (e.g., blue eyes for a pure soul).

> **Clinical Example:** The patient does not correctly recognize the other as an individual (e.g., spouse, business partner), but uses the other as an official badge. The partner is not needed for talking to, but only as a label in life. In this patients cannot differentiate their own needs from those of their partners. They might, for instance, simply adapt themselves to the partners' needs, e.g., in sexual relations or in the remark "we are tired now." In psychosis, patients cease to notice their own needs, experiencing them as induced, inspired, or controlled by the other.

- **Communication:** This dimension describes the ability to take account of others as regards emotions, and to convey to them one's own desires, fantasies, feelings and other contents; and to perceive and differentiate their various mental processes, and to decode their messages. This requires empathy as much as regulation of distance.

Good Integration

Ability to communicate is present, normally without serious breaks. Neurotic conflicts and attendant feelings of fear, shame, and guilt can impair the readiness to communicate and color the content.

> **Clinical Example:** A patient reports that she feels her partner does not understand her regarding certain conflicts (jealousy) and quarrels with him endlessly. The interviewer forms the impression that the partners disagree about certain relational aspects, but otherwise do understand each other.

Moderate Integration

The ability to communicate is in principle present, as a rule without serious disturbances. However, because patients do not completely differentiate their own feelings, whenever disappointment, self-devaluation and depression, or general avoidance of feelings set in, they find it hard to understand themselves and explain themselves to others. They are able to communicate, but their manner of doing so makes it difficult for the others to understand what exactly they are trying to communicate, e.g., by pedantic, rigid, retentive behavior; by being demanding, critical (partly with irritable and irascible reactions); by being apparently modest, reproachful, and demanding; or by behaving in a self-directed way (appearing touchy and vulnerable).

> **Clinical Example:** A patient describes the various things he does to help his wife and put everything in order for her. He cannot understand why she still complains, and he is disappointed that she does not appreciate

his efforts. Discussions tend to end in annoyance and are therefore avoided. The interviewer, too, forms the impression that the patient conveys much indirectly — between the lines, so to speak.

Low Integration

Understanding one's own and others' feelings is a difficult task, as is communicating one's feelings to others. Patients seem uninvolved with the feelings of others, and are hardly able to experience warm and gentle feelings, or to show anger. In extreme cases communication breaks down completely. The relational disorder shows itself in talking past each other and in misunderstandings; the patient tends toward encroachment, manipulation, and lack of distance. Confusion and emptiness are partly concealed by rational argument and as-if communication.

Clinical Example: The interviewer finds it increasingly hard to grasp what the patient wants. He wonders whether he has failed to understand the patient, or whether the patient is unable to express himself adequately. The patient reports that he likes to keep his distance in dealing with people. Above all he cannot show warm and gentle feelings or anger. He seems distant and uninvolved toward the feelings of others. Even in conversation, he shows no emotional link with the interviewer, who feels under pressure from extensive accounts of his symptoms. The interviewer's impulses alternate between overengagement in the patient's presence, and resignation in his absence.

Disintegration

If the internal and external world are not sufficiently differentiated, everything that the patient experiences comes to communicate something. This disorder can produce quite contradictory behavior, such as undistanced or autistic behavior in schizophrenia. Here, patients are either excessively directed toward the environment or typically withdrawn from others, concerned only with themselves via psychotic relational ideas, the contents of which are guilt, hypochondria, and possessions.

Clinical Examples: For years, a patient has avoided getting close to women, for fear of having to submit to their standards and demands. Upon initial intensive contact with a woman he develops a psychosis. Thereafter, he avoids further attempts for quite some time. Therapy widens his scope to enter into relationships with less fear.

A female patient with a manic-depressive psychosis adapts for many years to the role of wife and mother; during mania, she pathologically breaks out of this framework of relationship and role.

- **Bonding/Attachment:** This dimension describes the patient's ability to bond with important attachment figures. Attachment describes the intensity and variability of the interpersonal relationships. It is closely linked with the ability to perceive objects. While the latter describes how others are seen and experienced as separate beings from oneself, attachment describes the relationship patterns occupied by these persons. Disordered attachment is bipolar: Unfruitful efforts at bonding can lead to negatively experienced and painful dependence; an absence of bonding can be experienced as isolation and loneliness.

The dimension of bonding/attachment includes the following categories:

- ability to form inner images of people, so that they need not be present (internalization);
- ability to form stable (long-term and balanced) images of people (object-constancy);
- ability to form a variety of inner images of various people (variability of object relations);
- ability to form bonds and breaks in relations (attachment/detachment); breaks demand ability to grieve;
- ability to create interaction rules and so to protect the interpersonal relationship.

Good Integration

Inner images of important persons are vivid and refined; they appear as individuals, i.e., distinctly different from each other. Although ambivalent feelings are expressed toward these persons, emotional bonding remains fairly constant over time and marked by constant basic feelings.

This constancy of object relations creates security in assessing others. Their world of experience can be at least tentatively empathized with and rehearsed as an independent perspective. They are experienced as people with their own interests, needs, and rights.

Social relations are manifold, and several important people are described. The patient is able to cope with triadic relationships. The relational patterns described are not determined by dependence on objects; rather, conflicts arise because contradictions in bonding with different persons cannot be harmonized, e.g., rivalries, jealousy, contest for affection from a third person, etc. The central fear is of losing the love of the object.

Clinical Example: A female patient suffers from marital conflicts and feels constrained by her husband, because he reacts with jealousy. She can empathize with him, but also delimit herself from his demands. However, she herself fails to notice that her constant flirting gives her partner cause for jealousy.

Moderate Integration

The patient is able to form inner images of important persons, so there is less need of their presence; the images may be stable (long-term and fairly balanced) (object-constancy).

Variability of object relations is, however, restricted: The inner images are not variable, but confined to a few patterns dictated by one's own perspective, desires, and needs. Accordingly, the interests of others are perceived and interpreted from one's own perspective. Important persons are mainly experienced and described in terms of control, care, and stabilization of self-esteem. Conflicts arise because other individuals do not behave as the person concerned would wish. Security in relationships is guaranteed only by the other person entering into a certain desired form of relationship. Patients can hardly or not at all cope with genuine triadic relations, and seek mainly dyadic ones.

In view of strong dependence, the central fear is of being separated from the important supporting object and losing it.

> **Clinical Example:** A patient living in stable social relations, and successful in his profession, vividly describes his relationship with his wife, children, and sisters. The account of relations toward men is dull in comparison: All men, whether father, brother, or business colleagues seem to be the same, being judged only in terms of whether they are better or worse in their achievements and whether they dominate and diminish the patient. The interviewer notices that the patient is constantly on guard against the interviewer slighting or manipulating him.

Low Integration

In contrast to the previous level, the ability to form inner images of people and thus be more independent of them (internalization) is severely disturbed. So, too, is the capacity to form stable (long-term and balanced) ones (object-constancy). Hence, emotional bonding with important people is inconstant over time, and the description thereof is marked by contradictory images. Relational patterns are ambitendent, e.g., oscillating between extreme love and deep hatred, or great distance and intense proximity.

Empathy with the world of others (empathy with objects) is equally disturbed. They become hard to assess, unpredictable; the form in which they are experienced is marked by extremes. The feelings that go along with these object relations are strong and tend toward extremes. Hatred, for instance, is experienced unfiltered and is therefore particularly destructive.

Object dependence is marked by the feeling that one is powerless in relation to the other or is at the mercy of others. The central fear is that the self might be destroyed by the evil object or by the loss of the good object.

> **Clinical Example:** The patient reports rapidly changing, short partnerships. Female friends are described contradictorily and cannot easily be distinguished from each other. Some loving aspects are mentioned, though quite unconnected, and negative accounts are then added. The

patient feels exploited by women and repeatedly deceived. The last one had planned, first, to make him dependent and, then, gradually to leave him. He insists he will never again enter into a relationship and wonders whether he should give up his profession and go to sea.

Disintegration

Close bondings are basically problematic because of the danger of merging oneself with objects and thus losing one's identity. For the sake of self-protection, bondings are often avoided to the point of autistic isolation. If they occur, some desires and needs are often inadequately perceived. In this way stable bondings can be kept up at a very regressive level.

Clinical Example: A female patient, quite able to form bondings, submits over years of therapy to the demands and measures of the female therapist in order to avoid aggressive discussions. Finally, she stops the therapy and after a while becomes psychotic, with acoustic hallucinations corresponding to the therapist's advice. In subsequent therapy, the patient oscillates between anxiously maintaining her autonomy and yielding to the paternalistic provocation of her current therapist.

7.2.2.3   Important Structural Items

In accordance with a structural checklist (Rudolf, et al., 1998), the most important structural items are defined in their relation to the six structural dimensions.

Structural Dimension	Structural Items
1. Self-Perception	Self-reflection, self-image, identity, differentiation of affects
2. Self-Regulation	Tolerance of affects, self-esteem, regulation of instinctual drives, anticipation
3. Defense	Type, result, stability, flexibility of defense mechanisms
4. Object Perception	Subject-object differentiation, empathy, object-perception as a whole, affects concerning objects
5. Communication	Contact, understanding affects of others, communicating one's own affects, reciprocity
6. Bonding/ Attachment	Internalization, detachment, variability of attachment

Synopsis of OPD Axis IV: "Psychic Structure/Mental Functioning"

General features	Level of Integration			
	Good	**Moderate**	**Low**	**Disintegrated**
Self-Perception Ability for self-reflection to gain self-image and identity, for introspection and differen-tiation of affects	Self-reflective ability and identity feeling basically present and sometimes limited by neurotic conflicts; leading affects are joy, pride, fear, guilt, contempt, shame, grief	Gaining a self-image is difficult, as is differentiating affects; identity insecure; leading affects are fear, anger, disappointment, self-devaluation, ambivalence	Self-reflective functions largely absent, identity is diffuse; leading affects are chronic fear, anger, depression, emptiness, alienation	Self-reflective ability absent; social and sexual identity largely missing (schizophrenia) or excessive identification with social roles (manic-depressive psychosis)
Self-Regulation Ability to regulate one's own needs, affects and self-esteem, tolerance for ambivalences and negative affects	Ability to regulate impulses, affects and self-esteem basically present, possibly with neurotic limitations	Overregulation or possible breakthroughs of impulses; emotional flexibility limited; self-devaluating, auto-aggressive tendencies; regulation of self-esteem (easily offended)	Impulsive behavior, self-punishing tendencies, intolerance for negative affects; fragile regulation of self-esteem (very easily offended, grandiosity)	Inadequate idea of causing his/her own actions, possibly strong disorders of self-regulation, (breakthroughs of drives to the point of psychotic excitement)
Defense Ability to maintain or restore mental balance in internal or external conflicts by certain defense mechanisms	Defense stable, effective; directed against drives and affects; repression, rationalizing, displacing	Defense less flexible, excessive or missing; denial, turning against oneself, reaction formation, isolation, projection	Defense by change in self-representation and object-representation; splitting, projective identification, idealization or devaluation	Defense unstable, inflexible; withdrawn from objects; psychotic denial, psychotic projection

(continued)

General features	Level of Integration			
	Good	Moderate	Low	Disintegrated
Object-Perception Ability clearly to differentiate between internal and external reality, perceiving external objects wholly, coherently and with one's own rights and aims; ability to empathize	The image of the other is accurately perceived, though possibly tinged with neurotic conflict; ability for empathy present; object-related affects are possible (care, sympathy, guilt, grief, shame)	Little ability for empathy; conflict-tinged perception of the other. In conflicts, the other can be frightening or there is a threat that the other becomes lost through the conflict	No empathy; the other is not allowed his/her rights and aims; the other as an object that satisfies one's needs or that pursues one	Psychotic confusion of representations; selective perception of single parts of objects
Communication Ability to adapt to others, to communicate with them and grasp their affective signals	Readiness to communicate basically present; need for communication possibly conflictually limited or increased	Ability to communicate can be disordered; readiness for it is limited by offended, aggressive, needy attitude	Ability to communicate impaired; difficulty in grasping the other's affective signals; breakdowns of communication; confusion, mis-understandings	Misinterpretation of affective signals; everything can acquire communicative significance

(continued)

General features	Level of Integration			
	Good	**Moderate**	**Low**	**Disintegrated**
Bonding/ Attachment Ability to set up internal images of the other and deal them affectively over time (internalization, object constancy); variable attachment; alternation between attachment and separation; rules of interaction to protect the relationship	"Good internal objects" are present; different internal objects basically allow triadic relations; possible difficulty to integrate attachment with different people; central fear: loss of the love of the object	Few "good internal objects," images of objects reduced to a few patterns; wishful and dyadic relations predominate; central fear: losing the important object	Few "good internal objects" are internalized; internal objects punish and devalue; dependence on external objects; central fear: the "bad" object or the loss of the "good" one might destroy the self	To protect against feared merging, attachments are shunned, possibly to the point of autistic isolation; on a regressive level stable attachments can be maintained
Global Rating Structure of self in relation to others; available internal and interpersonal regulating functions to maintain autonomy and ability to relate	Largely autonomous self; regulating functions available; internal mental space structured (internal conflict possible); super-ego strict but integrated	Fewer available regulating functions. Inner conflicts more destructive and more archaic; super-ego strict and possibly externalized; exaggerated ego-ideal	Inner mental space and substructures little developed; regulating functions clearly reduced; conflicts are interpersonal rather than internal	No cohesive self is developed; hence risk of disintegration or fragmentation under stress; psychotic collapse may be followed by psychotic restitution

Rating Form of OPD Axis IV: "Psychic Structure/Mental Functioning"

Dimensions	Good (1)	(1.5)	Moder-ate (2)	(2.5)	Low (3)	(3.5)	Disin-tegrated (4)	Unasses-sable (9)
Self-Perception								
Self-Regulation								
Defense								
Object-Perception								
Communication								
Bonding/Attachment								
Global Rating								

REFERENCES

Abraham, K. (1925). Psychoanalytische studien zur charakterbildung. *Int Psychoanal Bibliothek, 16*, 1-64.

Arbeitskreis, OPD. (Ed.) (2003). *Operationalisierte psychodynamische diagnostik im kindes und jugend alter. Grundlagen und manual.* Bern: Huber.

Bellak, L., & Goldsmith, L. A. (1984). *The broad scope of ego function assessment..* New York: John Wiley & Sons.

Bellak, L., & Hurvich, M. (1969). Systematic study of ego functions. *Journal of Nervous Mental Disease, 148*, 569-585.

Beutel, M. (1990). *Coping und abwehr. Zur vereinbarkeit zweier konzepte.* In F. A. Muthny (Ed.), *Krankheitsverarbeitung* (pp. 1-11). Berlin: Springer.

Cicchetti, D. V. (1994). Guidelines, criteria, and rules of thumb for evaluating normed and standardized assessment instruments in psychology. *Psychological Assessment, 6*, 284-290.

Cierpka, M., Grande, T., Stasch, M., et al. (2001). Zur validität der Operationalisierten Psycho-dynamischen Diagnostik (OPD). *Psychotherapeut, 46*, 122-133.

Cohen, J. (1968). Weighted kappa: Nominal scale agreement with provision for scaled dis-agreement or partial credit. *Psychological Bulletin, 70*, 213-220.

Dahlbender, R. W. (2002). *Schwere psychischer erkrankungen und meisterung internalisierter Bezie-hungskonflikte.* Ulm: Profund.

Dahlbender, R. W., Grande, T., Buchheim, A., Schneider, G., Perry, J. C., Oberbracht, C., et al. (2004) *Qualitätssicherung im OPD-interview: Entwicklung eines interviewleitfadens.* In R. W. Dahl-bender, P. Buchheim, & G. Schüssler (Eds.), *Lernen an der praxis. OPD und die qualitätssicher-ung in der psychodynamischen psychotherapie* (pp. 41-66). Bern: Huber.

Davies-Osterkamp, S., Hartkamp, N., Heigl-Evers, A., & Standke, G. (1992). Zur diagnostik von ich-funktionen und objektbeziehungen. *Zschr Psychosom Med, 38*, 17-30.

Ehlers, W., & Czogalik, D. (1984). Dimensionen der klinischen beurteilung der abwehr. *Prax Psychother Psychosom, 29*, 129-138.

Ehlers, W., & Peter, R. (1990). Entwicklung eines psychometrischen verfahrens zur selbstbeur-teilung von abwehrkonzepten (SBAK). *PPmP Disk Journal, Stuttgart, 1*, 1-19.

Engel, K., Haas, E., von Rad, M., Senf, W., & Becker, H. (1979). Zur einschätzung von behandlungen mit hilfe psychoanalytischer konzepte (Heidelberger Rating). *Med Psychol, 5,* 253-268.

Fleiss, J. L. (1981). *Statistical methods for rates and proportions.* New York: John Wiley & Sons.

Fonagy, P., Gergely, G., Jurist, E. L., & Target, M. (2002). *Affect regulation, mentalization and development of the self.* New York: Other Press.

Fonagy, P., & Target, M. (1997). Attachment and reflective function: The role in self-organization. *Development and Psychopathology, 9,* 679-700.

Freud, A. (1937). *The ego and the mechanisms of defense.* New York: International University Press.

Freud, A. (1962). Assessment of childhood disturbances. *Psychoanalytic Study of the Child, 17,* 149-158.

Freud, A. (1977). *Assessment of childhood disturbances.* In *Psychoanalytic assessment: The diagnostic profile* (pp. 1-10). New Haven/London: Yale University Press.

Freud, S. (1923). The ego and the id. *Standard Edition, 19,* 1-66.

Freud, S. (1933). New introductory lectures on psycho-analysis. *Standard Edition, 22,* 5-182.

Freyberger, H., Dierse, B., Schneider, W., Strauss, B., Heuft, G., Schauenburg, H., et al. (1996). Operationalisierte Psychodynamische Diagnostik (OPD) in der erprobung—Ergebnisse einer multizentrischen Anwendungs—und Praktikabilitätsstudie. *Psychother Psychosom Med Psychol, 46,* 356-365.

Freyberger, H., Schneider, W., Heuft, G., Schauenburg, H., & Seidler, G. H. (1998). Zur anwendbarkeit, praktikabilität, reliabilität und zukünftigen forschungsfragen der OPD. In H. Schauenburg, H. J. Freyberger, M. Cierpka, & P. Buchheim (Eds.), *OPD in der Praxis* (pp. 105-120). Huber: Bern.

Gill, M. M., & Hoffmann, I. Z. (1982). A method for studying the analysis of aspects of the patient's experience in psychoanalysis and psychotherapy. *Journal of the American Psychoanalytic Association, 30,* 137-167.

Grande, T., Rudolf, G., Oberbracht, C., & Jakobsen, T. (2001). Therapeutische Veränderungen jenseits der Symptomatik. Wirkungen stationärer Psychotherapie im Licht der Heidelberger. *Umstrukturierungsskala, 47,* 213–233.

Grande, T., Rudolf, G., Oberbracht, C., Jakobsen, T., & Keller, W. (2004). Investigating structural change in the process and outcome of psychoanalytic treatment: The Heidelberg-Berlin Study. In P. Richardson, H. Kächele, & C. Renlund (Eds.), *Research on psychoanalytic psychotherapy with adults* (pp. 35-61). London: Karnac.

Grande, T., Rudolf, G., & Oberbracht, C. (1997). Die praxisstudie analytische langzeittherapie. Ein projekt zur prospektiven untersuchung struktureller veränderungen in psychoanalysen. In M. Leuzinger-Bohleber, & U. Stuhr (Eds.) *Psychoanalysen im rückblick* (pp. 415-431). Frankfurt: Psychosozial-Verlag.

Grande, T., Rudolf, G., & Oberbracht, C. (2000). Veränderungsmessung auf OPD-Basis: Schwierigkeiten und ein neues konzept. In W. Schneider, & H. Freyberger (Eds.) *Was leistet die OPD? Empirische Befunde und klinische Erfahrungen mit der Operationalisierten Psychodynamischen Diagnostik* (pp. 148-161). Bern: Huber.

Grande, T., Rudolf, G., Oberbracht, C., & Pauli-Magnus, C. (2003). Progressive changes in patients' lives after psychotherapy: Which treatment effects support them? *Psychotherapy Research, 13,* 43-58.

Grande, T., Schauenburg, H., & Rudolf, G. (2002). Zum begriff der "struktur" in verschiedenen operationalisierungen. In G. Rudolf, T. Grande, & P. Henningsen (Eds.) *Die struktur der persönlichkeit: Vom theoretischen verständnis zur therapeutischen anwendung des psychodynamischen strukturkonzepts* (pp. 177-196). Stuttgart: Schattauer.

Grütering, T., & Schauenburg, H. (2000). Die erfassung psychodynamisch relevanter persönlich-keitsmerkmale: Vergleich zweier klinisch relevanter instrumente. Karolinska Psycho-dynamic Profile (KAPP) und OPD-Strukturachse. In M. Bassler (Ed.), *Leitlinien in der stationären psychotherapie: Pro und kontra* (pp. 115-136). Giessen: Psychosozial-Verlag.

Heigl-Evers, A., Heigl, F., & Ott, J. (1993). *Lehrbuch der psychotherapie.* Stuttgart/Jena: Fischer.

Horowitz, L. M., Strauss, B., & Kordy, H. (1993a). *Manual zum inventar zur erfassung interperso-naler probleme (IIP-D).* Weinheim: Beltz.

Horowitz, M. J., Kernberg, O. F., & Weinshel, E. M. (1993b). *Psychic structure and psychic change. Essays in honor of Robert S. Wallerstein, M. D.* Madison: International University Press.

Kernberg, O. F. (1970). A psychoanalytic classification of character pathology. *Journal of the American Psychoanalytic Association, 18,* 800-822.

Kernberg, O. F. (1977). The structural diagnosis of borderline personality organization. In P. Hartocollis (Ed.), *Borderline personality disorder.* New York: International University Press.

Kernberg, O. F. (1981). Structural interviewing. *Psychiatric Clinics of North America, 4,* 169-195.

Landis, J. R., & Koch, G. G. (1977). The measurement of observer agreement for categorical data. *Biometrics, 33,* 159-174.

Lange, C., & Heuft, G. (2002). Die beeinträchtigungsschwere in der psychosomatischen und psychiatrischen qualitätssicherung: Global assessment of functioning scale (GAF) versus beeinträchtigungsschwere-score (BSS). *Z Psychosomat Med Psychother, 3,* 256-269.

Lichtenberg, J. D. (1983). *Psychoanalysis and infant research.* Hillsdale/London: Analytic Press.

Lohmer, M., Klug, G., Herrmann, B., Pouget, D., & Rauch, M. (1992). Zur diagnostik der früh-störung: Versuch einer standortbestimmung zwischen neurotischem niveau und border-line-störung. *Prax Psychother Psychosom, 37,* 243-255.

Luborsky, L., & Crits-Christoph, P. (1998). *Understanding transference: The core conflictual relation-ship theme method.* New York: Basic Books.

Malik, M. L., & Beutler, L. (2002). Rethinking the DSM. A psychological perspective. Washing-ton: APA Books.

Mentzos, S. (1976). *Interpersonelle und institutionalisierte abwehr.* Frankfurt: Suhrkamp.

Mentzos, S. (1993). Abwehr. In W. Mertens (Ed.), *Schlüsselbegriffe der psychoanalyse* (pp. 191-199). Stuttgart: Verlag Internationale Psychoanalyse.

Michels, R., Siebel, U., Freyberger, H. J., Schönell, H., & Dilling, H. (2001). Evaluation of the multiaxial system of ICD-10 (preliminary draft): Correlations between multiaxial assess-ment and clinical judgments of aetiology, treatment indication and prognosis. *Psycho-pathology, 34,* 69-74.

Nitzgen, D., & Brünger, M. (2000). Operationalisierte psychodynamische diagnostik in der rehabilitationsklinik birkenbuck: Einsatz und befunde. In W. Schneider, & H. Freyberger (Eds.), *Was leistet die OPD? Empirische befunde und klinische erfahrungen mit der operationalisier-ten psychodynamischen diagnostik* (pp. 238-252). Bern: Huber.

Oberbracht, C. (2005). *Psychische struktur im spiel der beziehung: Klinische anwendung und empir-ische prüfung der strukturachse der operationalisierten psychodynamischen diagnostik bei stationären psychosomatischen patienten.* Inaugural dissertation, Medizinische Fakultät Universität Heidel-berg.

OPD Task Force (Ed.) (2001). *Operationalized psychodynamic diagnostics (OPD): Foundations and manual.* Göttingen: Kirkland, Hogrefe & Huber.

Perry, J. C. (1989). Scientific progress in psychodynamic formulation. *Psychiatry, 52,* 245-249.

Perry, J. C. (1990). *The psychodynamic conflict rating scales.* Cambridge, MA: The Cambridge Hos-pital.

Perry, J. C., & Cooper, S. H. (1989). An empirical study of defense mechanism. *Archives of General Psychiatry, 46,* 444-452.

Pilkonis, P. A. (1988). Personality prototypes among depressives: Themes of dependency and autonomy. *Journal of Personality Disorders, 2,* 144-152.

Piper, W. E., Azim, H. F., Joyce, A. S., McCallum, M., Nixon, G. W., & Segal, P. S. (1991). Quality of object relations versus interpersonal functioning as predictors of therapeutic alliance and psychotherapy outcome. *Journal of Nervous and Mental Disease, 179,* 432-438.

Reymann, G., Zbikowski, A., Martin, K., Tetzlaff, M., & Janssen, P. L. (2000). Erfahrungen mit der anwendung von operationalisierter psychodynamischer diagnostik bei alkoholkranken. In W. Schneider, & H. Freyberger (Eds.), *Was leistet die OPD? Empirische befunde und klinische erfahrungen mit der operationalisierten psychodynamischen diagnostik* (pp. 229-237). Bern: Huber.

Rudolf, G. (1977). Krankheiten im grenzbereich von neurose und psychose: Ein beitrag zur psychopathologie des ich-erlebens und der zwischenmenschlichen Beziehungen. Göttingen: Vandenhoeck & Ruprecht. (Nachdruck Deutscher Studienverlag 1987).

Rudolf, G. (1993). Die struktur der persönlichkeit. In G. Rudolf (Ed.), *Psychotherapeutische Medizin* (pp. 55–83). Stuttgart: Enke.

Rudolf, G. (2002a). Konfliktaufdeckende und strukturfördernde zielsetzungen in der tiefenpsychologisch fundierten psychotherapie. *Zsch Psychosom Med Psychother, 28,* 163-173.

Rudolf, G. (2002b). Struktur als psychodynamisches konzept der persönlichkeit. In G. Rudolf, T. Grande, & P. Henningsen (Eds.), *Die struktur der persönlichkeit: Vom theoretischen verständnis zur therapeutischen anwendung des psychodynamischen strukturkonzepts* (pp. 2-48). Stuttgart: Schattauer.

Rudolf, G. (2002c). Strukturbezogene psychotherapie. In G. Rudolf, T. Grande, & P. Henningsen (Eds.), *Die struktur der persönlichkeit* (pp. 249-271). Stuttgart: Schattauer.

Rudolf, G. (2004). *Strukturbezogene psychotherapie. Leitfaden zur psychodynamischen therapie struktureller störungen.* Stuttgart: Schattauer.

Rudolf, G., Grande, T., & Oberbracht, C. (2000). Die heidelberger umstrukturierungsskala. Ein modell der veränderung in psychoanalytischen therapien und seine operationalisierung in einer schätzskala. *Psychotherapeut, 45,* 237-246.

Rudolf, G., Grande, T., Dilg, R., et al. (2002). Structural changes in psychoanalytic therapies—the Heidelberg-Berlin Study on long-term psychoanalytic therapies (PAL). In M. Leuzinger-Bohleber, & M. Target (Eds.), *Outcomes of psychoanalytic treatment: Perspectives for therapists and researchers* (pp. 201-222). London: Whurr Publishers.

Rudolf, G., Grande, T., Jakobsen, T., Krawietz, B., Langer, M., & Oberbracht, C. (2004). Effektivität und effizienz psychoanalytischer langzeittherapie: Die praxisstudie analytische langzeitpsychotherapie. In A. Gerlach, A. M. Schlösser, & A. Springer (Eds.), *Psychoanalyse des glaubens* (pp. 515-528). Giessen: Psychosozial-Verlag.

Rudolf, G., Grande, T., Oberbracht, C., & Jakobsen, T. (1996). Erste empirische untersuchungen zu einem neuen diagnostischen system: Die operationalisierte psychodynamische diagnostik (OPD). *Z Psychosom Med Psychoanal, 42,* 343-357.

Rudolf, G., Laszig, P., & Henningsen, C. (1997). Dokumentation im dienste von klinischer forschung und qualitätssicherung. *Psychotherapeut, 42,* 145-155.

Rudolf, G., Oberbracht, C., & Grande, T. (1998). Die struktur-checkliste—Ein umweltfreundliches hilfsmittel für die strukturdiagnostik nach OPD. In H. Schauenburg, H. J. Freyberger, M. Cierpka, & P. Buchheim (Eds.), *OPD in der praxis—Konzepte, anwendungen, ergebnisse der operationalisierten psychodynamischen diagnostik.* Bern: Huber.

Schauenburg, H. (2000). Zum verhältnis zwischen bindungsdiagnostik und psychodynamischer diagnostik. In W. Schneider, & H. Freyberger (Eds.), *Was leistet die OPD? Empirische befunde und klinische erfahrungen mit der operationalisierten psychodynamischen diagnostik* (pp. 196-217). Bern: Huber.

Schepank, H. (1994). *Der beeinträchtigungsschwere-score (BSS): Ein instrument zur bestimmung der schwere einer psychogenen erkrankung.* Hogrefe: Göttingen.

Schneider, G., Lange, C., & Heuft, G. (2002). Operationalized psychodynamic diagnostics and differential therapy indication in routine diagnostics at a psychosomatic outpatient department. *Psychotherapy Research, 12,* 159–178.

Schultz-Hencke, H. (1951). Lehrbuch der analytischen psychotherapie. Stuttgart: Thieme.

Schulz, S. (2004). Affektive indikatoren struktureller störungen. Ergebnisse einer empirischen studie. In R. W. Dahlbender, P. Buchheim, & G. Schüssler (Eds.), *Lernen an der Praxis. OPD und die qualitätssicherung in der psychodynamischen psychotherapie* (pp. 207-217). Bern: Huber.

Schüssler, G., & Bertl-Schüssler, A. (1992). Neue ansätze zur revision der psychoanalytischen entwicklungstheorie. *Zschr Psychosom Med, 38,* 77-87, 101-114.

Schüssler, G., Leibing, E., & Rüger, U. (1990). Multiaxiale diagnostik in der psychosomatik. *Zschr Psychosom Med, 36,* 343-354.

Schüssler, G. (2004). Innerpsychischer konflikt und struktur: Wo steht das unbewusste heute? In R. W. Dahlbender, P. Buchheim, & G. Schüssler (Eds.), *Lernen an der praxis. OPD und die qualitätssicherung in der psychodynamischen psychotherapie* (pp. 181-192). Bern: Huber.

Schwidder, W. (1972a). Klinik der neurosen. In K. P. Kisker, J. E. Meyer, M. Müller, & E. Strömgren (Eds.), *Psychiatrie der gegenwart II/1* (pp. 351-477). Berlin/Heidelberg/New York: Springer.

Schwidder, W. (1972b). Neopsychoanalyse. In G. Bally (Ed.), *Grundzüge der neurosenlehre* (Vol. 2, pp. 563-612). Berlin/Wien: Urban & Schwarzenberg.

Seidler, G. H. (1995a). Narziss, Teiresias und Φdipus: Internalisierungsschritte von der "interaktionellen unbewusstheit des gegenübers" zur "Verinnerlichung der Urszene." In G. Schneider, & G. H. Seidler (Eds.), *Internalisierung und Strukturbildung. Theoretische perspektiven und klinische anwendungen in psychoanalyse und psychotherapie* (pp. 95-115). Opladen, Westdeutscher: Verlag.

Seidler, G. H. (1995b). *Der blick des anderen. Eine analyse der scham.* Stuttgart: Internationale Psychoanalyse.

Shapiro, D. (1965). *Neurotic styles.* New York/London: Basic Books.

Spitzer, C., Michels-Lucht, F., Siebel, U., & Freyberger, H. J. (2002). Die strukturachse der operationalisierten psychodynamischen diagnostik (OPD): Zusammenhänge mit soziodemographischen, klinischen und psychopathologischen merkmalen sowie kategorialen diagnosen. *Psychotherapie, Psychosomatik, Medizinische Psychologie, 52,* 392-397.

Stern, D. (1985). *The interpersonal world of the infant. A view from psychoanalysis and developmental psychology.* New York: Basic Books.

Stiles, W. B., Meshot, C. M., Anderson, T. M., & Sloan, W. W. (1992). Assimilation of problematic experiences: The case of John Jones. *Psychotherapy Research, 2,* 81-101.

Strauss, B., Hüttmann, B., & Schulz, N. (1997) Kategorienhäufigkeit und prognostische bedeutung einer operationalisierten psychodynamischen diagnostik. Erste erfahrungen mit der "OPD-1" im stationären rahmen. *Psychother Psychosom Med Psychol, 47,* 58-63.

Strupp, H. H., & Binder, J. L. (1993). *Kurzpsychotherapie.* Stuttgart: Klett-Cotta.

Vaillant, G. E. (1971). Theoretical hierarchy of adaptive ego mechanisms. *Archives of General Psychiatry, 24,* 107-118.

Vaillant, G. E. (1986). *Werdegänge. Ergebnisse der lebenslaufforschung.* Reinbek: Rowohlt.

Wallerstein, R. S. (1988). Assessment of structural change in psychoanalytical therapy and research. *Journal of the American Psychoanalytic Association, Suppl. 36,* 241-261.

Weinryb, R. M., & Rössel, R. J. (1991). Karolinska Psychodynamic Profile KAPP. *Acta Psychiatr Scand, 83,* 1–23.

Weinryb, R. M., Rössel, R. J., & Schauenburg, H. (1999). Eine deutsche version des "Karolinska Psychodynamic Profile—KAPP." *Psychotherapeut, 44,* 227-233.

Willi, J. (1975). *Die zweierbeziehung.* Reinbek: Rowohlt.

OPD TASK FORCE

Speaker	Manfred Cierpka[1]
Secretary	Reiner W. Dahlbender,[2] Michael Stasch[1]
Coordinators	Peter Buchheim,[3] Manfred Cierpka,[1] Reiner W. Dahlbender,[2] Harald J. Freyberger,[4] Tilman Grande,[5] Gereon Heuft,[6] Paul L. Janssen,[18] Gerd Rudolf,[5] Henning Schauenburg,[5] Wolfgang Schneider,[7] Gerhard Schüssler,[8] Michael Stasch,[1] Matthias von der Tann[9]
Speaker of the Axis	Axis I: Wolfgang Schneider,[7] Axis II: Manfred Cierpka,[1] Axis III: Gerhard Schüssler,[8] Axis IV: Gerd Rudolf,[5] Axis V: Harald J. Freyberger[4]

Working Groups

Axis I	Reiner W. Dahlbender,[2] Matthias Franz,[10] Karsten Hake,[7] Thomas Klauer,[7] Reinholde Kriebel,[11] Doris Pouget-Schors,[12] Wolfgang Schneider[7]
Axis II	Manfred Cierpka,[1] Reiner W. Dahlbender,[2] Tilman Grande,[5] Henning Schauenburg,[5] Michael Stasch,[1] Matthias von der Tann[9]
Axis III	Markus Burgmer,[6] Reiner W. Dahlbender,[2] Gereon Heuft,[6] Sven Olaf Hoffmann,[19] Paul L. Janssen,[18] Elmar Mans,[13] Gudrun Schneider,[6] Gerhard Schüssler[8]
Axis IV	Stephan Doering,[14] Tilman Grande,[5] Thorsten Jakobsen,[17] Marianne Junghan,[20] Joachim Küchenhoff,[15] Doris Pouget-Schors,[12] Claudia Oberbracht,[21] Gerd Rudolf[5]
Axis V	Harald J. Freyberger,[4] Wolfgang Schneider[7]
Interview	Reiner W. Dahlbender,[2] Cord Benecke,[16] Stephan Doering,[14] Tilman Grande,[5] Paul L. Janssen,[18] Gudrun Schneider[6]

---

[1] Universitätsklinikum Heidelberg, Institut für Psychosomatische Kooperationsforschung und Familientherapie
[2] Klinik für Psychosomatische Medizin und Psychotherapie am Zentrum für Rehabilitative Medizin Soltau und Seepark Klinik, Bad Bodenteich / Medizinische Hochschule Hannover
[3] Technische Universität München, Klinik für Psychiatrie und Psychotherapie
[4] Universitätsklinikum Greifswald, Klinik und Poliklinik für Psychiatrie und Psychotherapie
[5] Universitätsklinikum Heidelberg, Klinik für Psychosomatische und Allgemeine Klinische Medizin
[6] Universitätsklinikum Münster, Klinik und Poliklinik für Psychosomatik und Psychotherapie
[7] Universitätsklinikum Rostock, Klinik und Poliklinik für Psychosomatik und Psychotherapeutische Medizin
[8] Universitätsklinikum Innsbruck, Klinik für Medizinische Psychologie und Psychotherapie
[9] Portman Clinic London, Tavistock & Portman NHS Trust
[10] Universitätsklinikum Düsseldorf, Klinisches Institut für Psychosomatische Medizin und Psychotherapie
[11] Gelderland-Klinik, Fachklinik für Psychotherapie und Psychosomatik, Geldern
[12] Technische Universität München, Institut und Poliklinik für Psychosomatische Medizin, Psychotherapie und Medizinische Psychologie
[13] Psychosomatische Fachklinik St. Franziska-Stift, Bad Kreuznach
[14] Universitätsklinikum Münster , Poliklinik für Zahnärztliche Prothetik, Bereich Psychosomatik in der Zahnheilkunde
[15] Universitätsklinikum Basel, Abteilung Psychotherapie und Psychohygiene der psychiatrischen Universitätsklinik
[16] Universität Innsbruck, Institut für Psychologie
[17] Institut für Psychotherapieforschung und Qualitätssicherung, Heidelberg
[18] Professor emeritus, Dortmund
[19] Professor emeritus, Hamburg
[20] Private practice, Thun
[21] Private practice, Frankfurt am Main

Overview of Empirical Support for the DSM Symptom-Based Approach to Diagnostic Classification

Abby Herzig, PsyD[1] and Jodi Licht, PsyD[2]

Editor's Note: This section, by Abby Herzig and Jodi Licht, is a detailed exposition of the problems involved in the DSM effort to establish an ostensibly atheoretical nosology for mental health disorders, based on categorization into defining symptom clusters. The DSM was designed to provide discrete homogeneous symptom and illness categories that would be reliable and valid for a range of purposes: diagnosis, and treatment planning, epidemiological survey, research cooperation across sites, and reimbursement formulae established by insurance carriers.

Through study of the accumulated empirical data concerning some of the most widely used and most important DSM categories, the authors reveal impressively the difficulty in reaching adequate reliability and validity for these important rubrics, and the problems and controversies generated around them, which have led to ever increasing refinement and accommodation efforts.

What this increasingly buttresses for us is the necessity to develop a complemental, individualized, and dimensional depth psychological approach to personality assessment and treatment planning, as exemplified, for example, in Sidney Blatt's Object Relations Inventory (ORI), p. 511; Shedler and Westen's Shedler-Westen Assessment Procedure (SWAP), p. 573; and in the OPD Task Force's Operationalized Psychodynamic Diagnostics (OPD), p. 615. The following three articles, from the United States, the United Kingdom, and Germany, respectively, are efforts to present how much empirical support for nosological classification efforts can, nonetheless, be found in psychotherapy outcome studies, even within the limitations of the DSM framework in most of the studies surveyed, with varying attention in the three following articles to the cautions expressed in this article.

INTRODUCTION

The DSM offers many advantages to both researchers and clinicians, including facilitating communication among mental health professionals, developing a

[1] George Washington University Psychoanalytic Candidate, NYU Psychoanalytic Institute at NYU Medical Center
[2] Postdoctoral Candidate in Psychoanalysis and Psychotherapy, Adelphi University

foundation for theories of psychopathology, promoting research activity and ongoing discussions about the validity of the diagnoses, and providing information about prognosis, clinical course, and the further refinement of treatment (Blashfield & Livesley, 1999; Mezey & Robbins, 2001).

The current diagnostic system has great limitations, however, particularly with respect to its ability to translate from research to clinical practice and to help clinicians in their work. Over the past 30 years, the mainstream psychiatric approach to diagnosis of mental health disorders has focused on surface symptom patterns in the hopes of achieving enhanced reliability and validity for diagnostic categories. Nonetheless, many argue that in the effort to devise a more objective, reliable, and operationalizable system, the validity of the diagnostic criteria has been questionable. In this chapter, we will review these arguments as they apply to selective diagnostic categories and highlight a number of the challenges that have emerged from focusing on surface symptom patterns.

The constructs of reliability and validity evolved out of psychometric theory and methodology within the field of psychology. The four main types of validity—construct, content, concurrent, and predictive—emerged as critical to the assessment of the validation of psychological tests. There is no certainty that the criteria implicit within these types of validity are applicable outside of psychometrics, where they were originally generated (Jablensky & Kendell, 2002). Furthermore, many argue that few psychiatric diagnoses meet the very stringent criteria that define the four types of validity.

Since the development of the DSM-III, the emphasis has been on improving diagnostic reliability and concurrent and descriptive validity, as well as on maximizing sensitivity and specificity (Widiger, Frances, Pincus, & First, 1991). Prior to the development of the DSM-IV, the major focus was on reliability (Nelson-Gray, 1991; Widiger, et al., 1991). With respect to its application to the DSM, reliability refers to the consistency with which diagnoses are assigned (Nelson-Gray, 1991). Its components include internal consistency, inter-rater or inter-diagnostician reliability, and temporally consistent or test-retest reliability (Nelson-Gray, 1991). The improved reliability in the DSM was achieved at the expense of greater validity (Nelson-Gray, 1991).

Unlike reliability, there is no set measure by which one can assess the validity of a diagnosis (Gleaves, May, & Cardeña, 2001). In the absence of a simple measure, several methods for establishing the validity of psychiatric diagnoses have been created (see Andreasen, 1995; Blashfield, Sprock, & Fuller, 1990; Kendler, 1980; Robins & Guze, 1970; and Spitzer & Williams, 1985). Jablensky and Kendell (2002) point out, however, that the problem with these methods is their inherent assumption that mental illness is comprised of distinct diagnostic entities, which do not overlap within the large spectrum of psychological disorders. For example, for a disorder to have diagnostic validity, the Robins and Guze

(1970) criteria heavily emphasize diagnostic homogeneity over (1) time and (2) familial aggregation (Rounsaville, Alarcón, Andrews, Jackson, Kendell, & Kendler, 2002). Comparing these two validating criteria, if we were to select individuals with schizophrenia whose symptoms had been chronic for many years, we would likely satisfy the first Robins and Guze validating criterion of homogeneity and stability over time. If, on the other hand, we were to gather a sample of patients with schizophrenia based on familial aggregation, the sample would include a much broader range of psychotic disorders (Rounsaville, et al., 2002). Thus, we would still not have established the critical validators for that diagnosis. Consequently, we do not always specify the subtype of validity measured in a study, or still lacking for a disorder, since validity itself, as it pertains to psychiatric nosology, lacks specificity, remains poorly defined, and has yet to be properly adapted in its application to the study of psychiatric disorders (Rounsaville, et al., 2002).

Despite the complications and imperfections inherent in definitions of validity and methods for assessing it, there are more global diagnostic issues that strain both reliability and validity as they apply to a diagnostic category. Problems with methodologies (Nelson-Gray, 1991; Regier, Kaelber, Rae, Farmer, Knauper, & Kessler, 1998); high rates of comorbidity (Brown, Antony, & Barlow, 1995); and classification debates surrounding categorical versus threshold models (Grayson, 1987; Jablensky & Kendell, 2002) all affect the results and conclusions on reliability and validity obtained by different studies.

An assessment of the controversies surrounding reliability and validity in the DSM would be incomplete without addressing the topic of diagnostic threshold cutoffs. Requirements for a diagnosis include not only the presence of various symptoms in an individual but also the stipulation that the symptoms meet DSM standards for intensity and duration. For example, a diagnosis of dysthymic disorder requires that that individual has been depressed for at least two years. Similarly, for an individual to receive a diagnosis of ADHD, he or she must have been experiencing at least six out of a list of nine symptoms for inattention and six out of nine symptoms for hyperactivity-impulsivity, and must display impairment in at least two settings. Thresholds, and studies that aim to authenticate them, have been established to purify and refine the homogeneity of the samples that comprise a disorder. But while such attempts have enhanced the reliability of a diagnosis, they inadvertently diminish its validity. Consequently, some people who are suffering are sequestered from research samples and given inadequate treatment because their subthreshold presentations preclude accurate identification of the nature of their distress. A concrete indication of this problem is the growing number of disorders in the DSM each year. While the category "not otherwise specified" has been added to capture individuals who do not meet threshold levels, suggestions for new diagnoses increase with every edition. According to Pincus, McQueen, and Elinson (2003), 150 new diagnoses were proposed for the fourth edition of the DSM.

Exploring the limitations of the existing diagnostic system not only clarifies areas for further research, it also emphasizes the need for a complementary framework—one that looks at larger patterns within which specific symptoms occur. Such an in-depth psychological framework focuses both on individual variations and unifying psychological processes. Now that many of these processes can be reliably measured (see the articles by Blatt, Auerbach, Zuroff, and Shahar, by Dahlbender, Rudolf and the OPD-Task Force, by Shedler and Westen; and by Wallerstein on Psychoanalytic Therapy Research in this section), it is important to address limitations of the current diagnostic system, so that a complementary approach can help strengthen our understanding of complex clinical phenomena.

Efforts to improve the empirical foundation of the DSM-IV included three interactive stages: literature reviews, data reanalysis, and field trials (Widiger, et al., 1991). Below we address some of the findings and conclusions that emerged from this collaborative effort, incorporating studies that assessed changes to the DSM-IV subsequent to its publication. This chapter will explore some of the clinical problems posed by the current diagnostic system for a number of selected disorders, including major depressive disorder, dysthymic disorder, general anxiety disorder, ADHD, conduct disorder, and oppositional defiant disorder. The reader will observe that the quantity of research on each of these disorders is highly variable.

Mood Disorders

Mood disorders, especially depressive conditions, are the most studied, discussed, and debated of the 365 disorders identified by the American Psychiatric Association (Westen, Heim, Morrison, Patterson, & Campbell, 2002). In the transition from the DSM-III-R to the DSM-IV, changes were made to the diagnostic criteria for the mood disorders, based mainly on large-scale studies examining reliability (Brown, Di Nardo, Lehman, & Campbell, 2001b). Below we elaborate upon some of the diagnostic dilemmas surrounding major depressive disorder and dysthymia.

Major Depressive Disorder
I. Reliability

The DSM-IV work group for mood disorders assessed the inter-rater reliability of both current and lifetime diagnosis of DSM-III-R major depression. Investigators obtained one measure of intrasite reliability (concordance between assessment of interviewer and co-rater at one site); two measures of intersite relia-bility (concordance between assessments of interviewer and off-site rater, and con-cordance between assessments of co-rater at original site and those of the off-site rater); and one measure for the six-month test-reliability, using the kappa statis-tic. Intrasite inter-rater reliability was good (k = 0.72) for current and excellent (k = 0.77) for lifetime major depression first; intersite reliability was (k = 0.68) good for current and fair (k = 0.57) for lifetime major depression, and second intersite reliability was fair (k = 0.52) for current and good (k = 0.52) for lifetime major depression. Six-month test-retest reliability was fair (k = 0.43) for current and poor (k = 0.36) for lifetime diagnoses of major depression.[3]

The authors of the mood disorders field trial (Keller, Klein, Hirschfeld, Kocsis, McCullough, Miller, et al., 1998) recommended that the DSM would more accurately represent the clinical presentation of major depression with a course-based classification system rather than one based solely on symptoms, as the authors found major depression to be more chronic and unremitting than previously believed. They tested the reliability for six different course patterns for major depression and concluded that the inter-rater reliability ranged from poor to excellent. Overall, the median kappa for the six course patterns was 0.55. The six-month test-retest reliability of the six patterns ranged from poor to good with a median kappa of 0.56.

Since changes were made to major depression in the DSM-IV, researchers have made efforts to assess the reliability and validity of the revised diagnostic criteria. Brown, Di Nardo, Lehman, and Campbell (2001b), measured the reliabil-ity of current and lifetime anxiety and mood disorders (in the DSM-IV) using the semistructured Anxiety Disorders Interview Schedule for DSM-IV: Lifetime ver-sion (ADIS-IV-L). The inter-rater reliability for major depression was evidenced by a kappa value of 0.67 (as opposed to 0.65 in the DSM-III-R). Inter-rater agree-ment was also assessed for the course and onset specifiers. The course and onset specifiers for Manic-Depressive Disorder (MDD) were associated with fair to good reliability (ks = 0.46 to 0.67), whereas the severity specifier had poor reliability (ks = 0.30 and 0.36).

According to Brown, et al. (2001b), sources of unreliability involved boundary issues with dysthymia, anxiety disorder Not Otherwise Specified (NOS), and depressive disorder NOS. Thus, even if a clinician recognized the presence of a disorder, a formal diagnosis was not always assigned because a patient's self-report (e.g., number or duration of symptoms) fell below the threshold for DSM. Similar problems occurred with respect to categorical specifiers (e.g., single or recurrent; mild, moderate, or severe; or chronic or nonchronic) for major

---

[3] Note: 0.75 or greater = excellent beyond a chance; 0.60-0.74 = good agreement; 0.40-0.59 = fair agreement; under 0.40 = poor agreement – see Keller et al., 1998)

depressive disorder. Highlighting the fact that the dimensional ratings for the severity of MDD had good reliability, whereas the categorical specifiers of MDD severity evidenced poor reliability, the authors emphasize the limitations of the categorical approach to diagnostic classification (Brown, et al., 2001b). Several authors (e.g., Brown, et al., 2001b; McCullough, Klein, Borian, Howland, Riso, Keller, et al. [2003]) call for continued research, which they hope will establish a firm evidentiary basis for a dimensionally based classification system.

II. Controversies

First, Frances and Pincus (2004, p. 186) describe a major depressive episode as "one of the oldest and best studied criteria sets in DSM-IV-TR," adding that the criteria for diagnosing it have undergone relatively few changes since it was first formulated in the early 1970s. They note, however, that despite its strong empirical grounding, the criteria set for major depressive disorder have their limitations, including the heterogeneity of clinical presentations to which the criteria may apply. The thresholds for severity and duration are too high to capture all those with clinically significant symptoms, yet too low to avoid false-positive diagnoses. In addition, the criteria are difficult to apply to medically ill patients.

Furthermore, it has become clearer that mood disorders do not follow a (previously assumed) standard pattern, characterized by a severe episode with an acute onset and a remitting course (Keller, Klein, Hirschfeld, Kocsis, McCullough, Miller, et al., 1995). Rather, there is increasing evidence that individuals with mood disorders experience a more chronic and unremitting disturbance that spans the full spectrum of severity (Keller, et al., 1995, 1998). As previously mentioned, the DSM-IV Mood Disorders Field Trial (Keller, et al., 1995, 1998) identified as one of its goals the achievement of a better understanding of variations in the severity and course of mood disorders. According to Westen, Heim, Morrison, Patterson, & Campbell (2002) the two most salient problems with the current classification of mood disorders in the DSM are the issues of subthreshold and comorbidity. Thresholds in diagnostic criteria were included for the first time in the DSM-III with the hope of improving reliability. While some say this strategy proved effective, others (e.g., Brown, et al., 2001b) argue that unreliability is a problem not in making the decision of whether a symptom exists, but rather in deciding to what degree or at what level of severity it exists. That is, there are problems in reliability vis-à-vis whether or not symptoms meet clinical threshold criteria. Is there sufficient distress or impairment to constitute a disorder, and, if so, of what magnitude?

According to Pincus, McQueen, and Elinson (2003), the samples used in studies to establish criteria thresholds were mainly collected from mental health care settings, and are not necessarily representative of the full spectrum of individuals who suffer from depression. As previously mentioned, "Not Otherwise Specified" was created to account for those individuals whose symptoms are clinically significant but which do not meet threshold levels. This emendation has evidently not prevented a demand for more diagnoses to account for those not represented in the primary categories. Because of their high prevalence rate (approximately 24%), clinical significance, and cost (Pincus, McQueen, & Elinson, 2003), there has been an ongoing discussion about subthreshold levels of depressive conditions. In the DSM-IV-TR, subthreshold depressions have been included in the category of depression NOS. There is immense confusion surrounding subthreshold depression, however, manifested in a myriad of names for the same phenomena, varying symptoms, and other defining criteria depending on the study, population, and setting. Pincus, et al. (2003) regard the studies that have presented subthreshold depression as methodologically weak.

With respect to subthreshold symptoms and major depressive disorder, there is ongoing debate as to whether the diagnosis represents a single clinical disorder that encompasses a continuum of different subtypes and levels of symptoms, or whether major depressive disorder is a distinct entity with unique qualities, characteristics and biological origins. The results from the Mood Disorders Field Trial (Keller, et al., 1998) indicate that in fact major depression is often characterized by major, minor, and subthreshold levels of depressive symptoms, which alternate during the course of the illness. An implication of this finding is that higher levels of MDD symptoms represent only the tip of the depressive iceberg. It is clear that there is still a great deal to understand about the nature of depression and whether the imposition of thresholds and cutoffs improves or decreases the validity and reliability of the diagnosis of major depressive disorder.

III. Validity

One of the more debated areas regarding the validity of the diagnosis of major depression is how to categorize the variations and fluctuations within the disorder. At present, there is limited data available on the validity of the subtypes currently used to characterize the variations within major depression (McCullough, et al., 2000). Whereas some conceive of depression as a continuum ranging from mild to severe forms (Kendell, 1982; Zimmerman, Coryell, & Pfohl, 1986), others propose that depression is heterogeneous and consists of discrete subtypes (Schotte, Maes, Cludydts, & Cosyns, 1997).

In a study examining the stability over time of the nine criterion symptoms of MDD within the course of a depressive episode, Minor, Champion, and Gotlib (2005) concluded that patients' symptoms remained stable over time and that fluctuations were the result of changes in severity rather than alterations in type or profile of symptom(s). In a two-part study, using two distinct samples and altered methods, McCullough, et al. (2000) and McCullough, Klein, Borian, Howland, Riso, Keller, et al. (2003) first measured the validity of the chronic depression subtypes in the DSM-III-R and, later, in the DSM-IV. Through a comparison of clinical features, family history, and response to treatment, McCullough and her colleagues (2000, 2003) challenge the validity of the distinctions among the various subtypes of major depression. They report finding minimal differences between demographic variables, symptomatology, comorbidity, social adjustment, family history of psychopathology, and response to antidepressant medication. As opposed to the distinct forms and types of major depression described in the DSM, the authors of these studies advocate for a single, broad category representing chronic depression, which can be expressed in a variety of symptom patterns and clinical course configurations.

Alternatively, using data obtained using cluster analytic techniques, Schotte, et al. (1997) gave support to the construct validity of the DSM-III melancholic subtype of major depression. Their research supports an integration of categorical and dimensional views on melancholia, which the authors refer to as the integrated threshold model. They note the existence of a continuum of severity (from melancholic to non-melancholic depression) and add that as severity increases, distinct symptom clusters emerge. Thus, Schotte, et al. (1997) supports the construct validity of the DSM-III's classification of melancholic and non-melancholic subtypes of depression.

Citing studies which found that different types of depressions respond differently to different medications, Quitkin (2002) asserts that depressive subtypes are in fact biologically distinct ("distinct neuropathology") and thus support a categorical approach to classifying depression. Specifically, based on psychopharmacologic and genetic studies of depressive syndromes, Quitkin supports the validity of the diagnosis of depression with atypical features as a discrete entity with its own neuropathophysiology.

Similarly, Angst, Gamma, Sellaro, Zhang, and Merikangas (2002) concluded that the atypical subtype of depression is a valid disorder with adequate indicators of validity such as inclusion criteria, discrimination from other disorders, clinical severity, course, and stability. Angst, et al. (2002) noted that more research is needed to establish its reliability, to understand better its high comorbidity with bipolar II disorder, and to justify the hierarchical classification of specific features. The authors noted, however, that two of the more salient defining features of atypical depression, namely, mood reactivity and leaden paralysis, have not been systemically studied to confirm their reliability and validity as inclusion criteria.

Dysthymic Disorder

There has been a long history of controversy surrounding the addition of dysthymic disorder into the DSM (Han, Schmaling, & Dunner, 1995; Kocsis &

Frances, 1987). The DSM-IV mood disorder field trial (Keller, et al., 1998) recognized several problematic areas remaining in the diagnosis of DSM-III-R dysthymia. First, there is a paucity of data on inter-rater reliability; second, the criteria used to define dysthymia in the DSM-III-R was not reflective of the patients seen in clinical practice; third, the overlap and boundaries between dysthymia and MDD remain unclear (Kocsis & Frances, 1987); and finally, there is a need to address additional categories to capture other forms of minor depression (Keller, et al., 1998).

I. Reliability

The work group assessed the inter-rater reliability of both current and lifetime diagnosis of DSM-III-R dysthymia. Investigators obtained one measure of intrasite reliability (concordance between assessment of interviewer and co-rater at one site); two measures of intersite reliability (concordance between assessments of interviewer and off-site rater, and concordance between assessments of co-rater at original site and off-site rater); and one measure for the six-month test-reliability, using the kappa statistic. Intrasite inter-rater reliability was excellent (k = 0.82 and k = 0.81) for current and lifetime dysthymia, respectively; first intersite reliability was fair (k = 0.44 and k = 0.57) for current and lifetime dysthymia, respectively; and second intersite reliability was fair (k = 0.59) for current and good (k = 0.65) for lifetime dysthymia. Six-month test-retest reliability was fair (k = 0.56 and k = 0.53) for current and lifetime diagnoses of dysthymia.

Measuring the diagnostic reliability of DSM-IV mood and anxiety disorders, Brown, et al. (2001b), found good to excellent inter-rater agreement for all principal diagnostic categories except dysthymia. Diagnostic reliability for dysthymia was k = 0.22 using DSM-IV criteria versus k = -0.05 using DSM-III-R criteria. The majority of disagreements about the diagnosis of dysthymia involved other mood disorders, although differentiating between dysthymia and general anxiety disorder also posed an occasional diagnostic dilemma. Interestingly, when major depressive disorder and dysthymia were collapsed into one category, rather than analyzed as two separate diagnoses, a higher reliability (0.72) was obtained, perhaps implying the limitations of a categorical classification system, particularly with such inherently dimensional illnesses (Brown, et al., 2001b).

II. Controversies

Challenges to the validity of this diagnosis have focused on the overlap between dysthymic disorder and both major depression and depressive personality disorder (Brown, et al., 2001b; Han, et al., 1995). Han, et al. (1995) noted that while differentiating these disorders is contingent upon developing more accurate criteria, dysthymic disorder and major depressive disorder may not be qualitatively different. Han, et al. (1995) assessed the stability of the field trial's proposed criteria for dysthymia in the DSM-IV. The authors concluded that the new criteria had good sensitivity, reliability, and stability over time. Finally, the authors encouraged further research in the inconclusive area of additional diagnoses for milder depressive disorders.

III. Validity

The Mood Disorders Work Group (Keller & Russell, 1996) addressed the poor content validity of DSM-III-R dysthymic disorder. Results from the field trial indicated that dysthymic disorder would be more aptly defined and have improved content validity with a greater emphasis on cognitive and affective symptoms (e.g., social withdrawal, loss of interest, and irritability) and less emphasis on vegetative symptoms, the latter being a more predominant feature in major depressive disorder. Nonetheless, the Mood Disorders Work Group felt that there is not yet sufficient empirical evidence to warrant a change in the diagnostic criteria (Rush, 1998).

Furthermore, the field trial addressed the issue of diagnostic overlap and high rate of comorbidity between DSM-III-R dysthymia and major depression. The authors concluded that since there were no criteria unique to dysthymia, it is difficult to enhance discriminant validity. They noted, however, that a greater emphasis on somatic/vegetative symptoms for major depression might help in establishing it, given that these symptoms are more characteristic of major depression than dysthymia.

Anxiety Disorders

Generalized Anxiety Disorder

I. Reliability

Generalized Anxiety Disorder (GAD) has historically generated very low diagnostic agreement (Brown, Barlow, & Liebowitz, 1994). Studies of reliability on DSM-III-R GAD have reported kappa coefficients of 0.57 (Dinardo, Moras, Barlos, Rapee, & Brown, 1993) and 0.27 (Manuzza, 1989). One possible source of this low reliability is that GAD, unlike other disorders, does not have clear behavioral markers to enable its identification and distinction from other mood and anxiety disorders (Brown, et al., 1994). Its notoriously high rate of comorbidity has generated great concern as to whether it should be retained as a diagnostic category in the DSM-IV (Brown, et al., 1994).

Based on the Work Group's literature review, reliability for DSM-III GAD was determined to be low, particularly as compared with the other anxiety disorders (Moras, Borkovec, DiNardo, Rapee, Riskind, & Barlow, 1996). The findings on the reliability of GAD for DSM-III-R varied from poor (k=0.27) to good (k=0.64) depending on the nature of the study. Sources of unreliability included the difficulty of distinguishing worry related to GAD from worry associated with other Axis I disorders. The Task Force also reported that literature reviews on the reliability of the criterion that 16 of 18 symptoms be present found it to be poor (.08 to .48 and .05 to .63).

Since the publication of DSM-IV, several studies have investigated the diagnostic criteria for GAD. For example, Brown, et al. (2001b) found an improvement in the reliability of the diagnosis of GAD in DSM-IV (k=0.67) over the reliability of the same diagnosis as described in DSM-III-R (k=0.57). Diagnostic disagreements for DSM-IV GAD most often involved boundaries with mood disorders, which pose more of a boundary threat to GAD than to other anxiety disorders (Brown, et al., 2001b). A secondary source of unreliability in diagnosing GAD was patient report, perhaps indicative of the vagueness of diagnostic features and patients' difficulty differentiating GAD from other disorders (Brown, et al., 2001b). Brown, et al. (1994) contend that individuals with GAD should have a specific presentation that differentiates their disorder from other diagnostic categories, and recommend future studies to assess discriminant validity between GAD and other mood disorders.

Sources of threats to the validity of GAD include its high rate of comorbidity (approximately 80%, according to Brown, Campbell, Lehman, Grisham, and Mancill [2001a] and Brown, et al. [2001b]), a lack of family studies, and the observation that anxiety and mood disorders are erroneously differentiated, rather than existing along a continuum (Brown, et al., 1994; 2001b). It remains unclear whether GAD is in fact a disorder or a trait or a vulnerability to the development of other emotional disorders.

II. Validity

The GAD Task Force (Moras, et al., 1996) conducted a literature review to assess the reliability and discriminant validity of GAD, particularly from dysthymia, somatoform disorders, and psychophysiological disorders. The task force concluded that GAD as described in the DSM-III was so close to depression that the two disorders were indistinguishable. Studies that compared the DSM-III-R version of GAD with major depression noted significant differences between the two disorders. The more difficult distinction, however, has been between GAD and dysthymia, on which there is a conspicuous lack of empirical research. Similarly, no well-controlled studies were found comparing GAD to hypochondriasis or to psychophysiological disorders such as irritable bowel syndrome.

In response to suggestions from the GAD Work Group and information from the field trials, the diagnostic criteria for GAD were substantially revised. In an effort to increase the reliability and discriminant validity of GAD, changes included a reduction in criterion symptoms from 18 to 6, with more focus on somatic symptoms, and the new criterion that the afflicted person describes the worry as uncontrollable (Brown, Di Nardo, Lehman, & Campbell, 2001b).

In consideration of such factors as age of onset, response to treatment, and distinct criteria involving anhedonia and somatic symptoms, other studies have concluded that GAD can be distinguished from disorders such as Obsessive Compulsive Disorder (OCD) (Brown, Moras, Zinbarg, & Barlow, 1993) and MDD (Brown, et al., 1994; Zimmerman & Chelminski, 2003).

Mood and Anxiety Disorders

Problems with Comorbidity and Subthreshold

The complexities of questions of comorbidity between mood and anxiety disorders and the issues involved in attempts to create new diagnoses, such as mixed anxiety and depression, go beyond the scope of this chapter. It is important to acknowledge these diagnostic dilemmas, however, as they are inherent consequences of the current classification system. The evolution of the DSM has been heavily influenced by the perspective that diagnoses are discrete syndromes with specific longitudinal courses, prevalence rates, symptom profiles, and responses to treatment (Rivas-Vasquez, Saffa-Biller, Ruiz, Blais, & Rivas-Vasquez, 2004). Despite improvements in the reliability of DSM diagnosis (largely owing to more objective and operationalized measures), the DSM threshold criteria preclude detection of large proportions of psychopathology (Rivas-Vasquez, et al., 2004).

Contributing to this concern is the finding in both research and clinical settings that diagnoses such as mood and anxiety disorders often co-occur (Brown, et al., 2001a; Rivas-Vasquez, et al., 2004). Many contend that both high comorbidity between mood and anxiety disorders and the addition of more disorders and disorder types, in efforts to increase precision, have compromised the discriminant validity of DSM disorders (Brown, et al., 2001a). Furthermore, it has been suggested that these comorbid conditions are variations of an underlying and broader syndrome—a greater middle ground—which has yet to be officially incorporated into the current classification system(s) (Rivas-Vasquez, et al., 2004).

Comorbid anxiety and depression and mixed anxiety and depression, as well as subthreshold presentations of these disorders, remain unrecognized and understudied. Rivas-Vasquez, et al. (2004) contend that the prevalence of individuals with depression and anxiety whose symptoms cause great psychosocial impairment despite not meeting DSM thresholds, is much higher than previously suspected. If they are right, there is a substantial danger of misdiagnoses and improper treatment.

The DSM Task Force addressed this ongoing dilemma but, after reviewing criteria sets for mixed anxiety and depression, concluded that there was not yet enough empirical evidence to create an official disorder (Rivas-Vasquez, et al., 2004). Zinbarg, et al. (1998), reporting on the DSM-IV Field Trial for Mixed Anxiety-Depression, recommends more research on inter-rater reliability and more specificity with symptom thresholds, as well as the establishment of validity criteria, such as associated features, age at onset, family patterns, and treatment response before a distinct diagnostic entity is established. In the meantime, the task force suggested including a mixed anxiety-depression category in the DSM-IV appendix to generate further study.

Disorders Usually First Diagnosed in Infancy, Childhood, or Adolescence

Diagnosing mental illnesses in young children is difficult given their communicative limitations, the unreliability or absence of parental reports, and the impact of rapid developmental changes in the early years (Boris, et al., 2004). Despite these unique challenges, many argue that the DSM-IV is a vast improvement over the first edition, particularly with respect to reliability. Others contend that many of the childhood mental disorders in the DSM have not been studied extensively enough to warrant their existence as separate entities (Achenbach, 1991; Gadow, Sprafkin, & Nolan, 2001; Scheeringa, Peebles, Cook, & Zeanah, 2001; Spence, 1997). Their reliability has, not surprisingly, also been questioned (Boris, et al., 2004).

This section addresses several of the disorders of infancy, childhood, and adolescence that evoke controversy and confusion among clinicians and researchers. While many of the disorders excluded from this section engender less confusion and debate, it is not the intention of the authors to communicate that they are less worthy of close scrutiny. The purpose of this chapter is to provide some examples of the ongoing inquiry into the empirical soundness of the DSM.

Attention Deficit Hyperactive Disorder (ADHD)

The conceptualization of ADHD has changed with the evolution of the DSM, from motoric disinhibition in DSM-II (hyperkinetic reaction), to inattention in DSM-III (attention deficit disorder, ADD), to inattention and hyperactivity in both DSM-III-R and DSM-IV (attention deficit/hyperactivity disorder, ADHD). Based upon a review of the literature, data reanalysis, and a field trial, the DSM-IV Task Force recommended subtyping the condition into three homogeneous areas rather than conceptualizing the disorder as a unitary construct. The three ADHD subtypes now include: predominately inattentive (ADHD-I); predominately hyperactive/impulsive (ADHD-HI); and a combined presentation

(ADHD-C). Interestingly, since these changes to the classification of ADHD in the DSM-IV, there have been significantly more children diagnosed with, and prescribed medication for, ADHD (Woo & Rey, 2005).

I. Reliability

Very few studies have researched the reliability of ADHD as it is described in the DSM-IV or as it was described in previous editions of the DSM (Morgan, Hynd, Riccio, & Hall, 1996; Woo & Rey, 2005). Morgan, Hynd, Riccio and Hall (1996) assessed children who received retrospective diagnoses (ADHD-I and ADHD-C) according to the DSM-IV but whose original diagnoses were obtained using DSM-III and DSM-III-R criteria. ADHD-I was diagnosed in 30 children, a kappa of 0.87. ADHD-C was diagnosed in 26 children with a kappa of 0.85. Morgan, et al. (1996) concluded that ADHD-HI and ADHD-C can be reliably diagnosed. Based on their own literature review, Woo and Rey (2005) reported that kappa values for ADHD assessed using structured interviews have ranged from fair (e.g., 0.48) to good (e.g., 0.91). The authors note that the disparities in results have been a function of choice of informant. Specifically, disagreements between parents and teachers (see below regarding the requirement that symptoms be present in multiple settings) reduce test-retest reliability.

Reliability of the DSM-IV subtypes has also been questioned based on evidence that children shift between or develop into different subtypes, particularly from ADHD-I to ADHD-C (Lahey, Pelham, Loney, Lee, & Willcutt, 2005). This finding supports the claim that such subgroupings do not remain discrete categories over time (Lahey, et al., 2005). More research is needed on the reliability of the new ADHD subtypes as defined in the DSM-IV, particularly the inattention and hyperactive-inattention subtypes (Woo & Rey, 2005).

II. Controversies

While the DSM-IV's use of more empirically derived criteria for ADHD have been recognized, the integrity of the disorder still remains in question (Barkley, 2003). In the DSM-III, a diagnosis of ADHD required a number of symptoms from the following three groups: inattention, impulsivity, and hyperactivity. In the DSM-III-R these three groups were collapsed, and a diagnosis required the presence of 8 out of 14 possible symptoms (McBurnett, 1997). One controversy about ADHD is whether the diagnosis should be represented and conceptualized multi-dimensionally, as in the DSM-III, or unidimensionally, as in the DSM-III-R. McBurnett (1997) highlighted that the unidimensional model, which is comprised of a single symptom list, elicited heterogeneous symptom presentations, lacking in any core component. Such an approach to ADHD conflicts with current research that supports at least two separate clusters of symptoms (e.g., inattention-disorganization and impulsivity-hyperactivity) (Shaffer, Widiger, & Pincus, 1998). Research remains inconclusive as to whether ADHD as defined in the DSM-III-R lacks specific diagnostic criteria, resulting in heterogeneous samples (Lahey, Carlson, & Frick, 1997; Morgan, et al., 1996) or whether it is more accurately conceptualized as less static, developmentally influenced, and more inherently dimensional (Barkley, 2003).

The question of what exactly constitutes ADHD remains a salient area for research and clinical practice. Whereas previous conceptualizations of the disorder had focused on inattentive, impulsive, and overactive behavior, more recent theories have conceptualized ADHD as reflecting poor inhibition, problems with self-regulation, and deficient executive functioning (Barkley, 2003). Similarly, it remains unclear as to whether ADHD is a disorder primarily of inattention or of hyperactivity, as reflected in the changing definitions of ADHD (First, Frances, & Pincus, 2004; Shaffer, et al., 1998).

The issue of threshold criteria is an area of controversy throughout the DSM, and ADHD is no exception. A low threshold occasions the risk of false-positive diagnoses and the consequent prescribing of stimulants to children who do not need them. A high threshold risks the possibility that many individuals will go undiagnosed, leaving them vulnerable to ambiguous and misleading labels such as "spacey," "unintelligent," and "unmotivated" (First, et al., 2004).

The diagnostic criteria for ADHD in the DSM-III-R were highly criticized for leading to over-diagnosis of unimpaired children (Shaffer, et al., 1998). In response to these concerns, the ADHD category in the DSM-IV now requires that the symptoms occur often and in multiple settings, on the assumption that if it is a disorder, ADHD will be evident in a variety of circumstances. Barkley (2003) argues, however, that the criterion that symptoms exist in two of three environments implicitly confounds settings (home and school) with sources of information (parents and teachers). Sources vary in their judgments, and children's behavior can vary across settings (Mota & Schachar, 2000; Woo & Rey, 2005). Furthermore, Barkley contends that the criterion that symptoms persist for at least six months is not only too short, but is also arbitrarily selected, with no supporting empirical research. He, therefore, recommends that the criterion for duration of symptoms should be 12 months or more.

Concerns regarding the boundary between what constitutes a disorder and what is age-appropriate distractibility and over-activity abound throughout the literature (First, et al., 2004). For example, the diagnostic criteria may not be applicable to all age groups; at some points in development, normative conflicts are more accountable for problems with attention and impulsivity. Hyperactivity, for example, may be more prevalent in younger populations, whereas inattention may have a wider developmental applicability to older populations (Barkley, 2003). Likewise, a child suffering from anxiety may appear inattentive because of internal distractions, but may not have ADHD (Newcorn, et al., 2001). False positive diagnoses can thus be a consequence of not taking into account other developmental variables and internal struggles within the child. Furthermore, Barkley (2003) highlights that the field trials (Lahey, et al., 1994) looked only at ADHD in children from 4 to 10, thus calling into question the applicability of the diagnostic threshold for ADHD to those outside this age range.

Finally, since ADHD often coexists with other psychiatric disorders (Newcorn, et al., 2001; Volk, Neuman, & Todd, 2005), Barkley (2003) argues that the DSM provides little guidance to clinicians making the differential diagnosis. Following the section on conduct and oppositional defiant disorders, we will address the rate of comorbidity between ADHD and these other behavioral disturbances.

III. Validity

Despite the controversy and lack of research prior to the DSM-IV, there were still numerous studies which, based upon longitudinal follow-up information (Gittelman, Mannuzza, Shenker, & Bonagura, 1985), family-genetic data (Biederman, et al., 1992), and treatment studies (Barkley, 1977), purported to support the concurrent and predictive validity of the diagnosis of ADHD—at least as it was defined in the DSM-III and DSM-III-R. Such studies have been few and far between, however, leaving ADHD insufficiently validated. Since the publication of the DSM-IV, some standardized psychometric data has been obtained on individual subtypes in epidemiologically representative samples (Faraone, Biederman, & Friedman, 2000a; Lahey, et al., 2005; Willcutt, Pennington, Chhabildas, Friedman, & Alexander, 1999). Below we review areas relevant to the question of whether ADHD is a valid diagnostic entity.

While findings have often been contradictory, support for the validity of the ADHD subtypes has included data from genetic research (Faraone, et al., 2000a; Hudziak, et al., 1998; Todd, et al., 2001; Volk, et al., 2005) as well as from factor analytic studies of symptom patterns (Hudziak, et al., 1998; Woo & Rey, 2005). There appears to be contradictory evidence as to whether any or all of the subtypes are associated with ADHD. For example, it is assumed by many that inattention is the core of ADHD (Woo & Rey, 2005). But it has yet to be proven that ADHD-HI is not more closely related to the behavioral disorders, to ADHD (Woo & Rey, 2005). Findings from studies assessing comorbidity (Newcorn, et al., 2001; Willcutt, Pennington, Chhabildas, Friedman, & Alexander, 1999) and neuropsychological deficits (Chhabildas, Pennington, & Willcutt, 2001; Lahey, Loeber, et al., 1998) also raise this diagnostic quandary. Alternatively, ADHD-I has been singled out as a symptom pattern, a disorder that stands alone (e.g., a learning disability), embodying unique academic and cognitive difficulties (Barkley, 2003; Lahey, et al., 2005). Further adding to the confusion are studies purporting to show that ADHD-C has higher rates of comorbidity (Baumgaertel, Wolraich, & Dietrich, 1995; Faraone, et al., 2000a) and is in fact more indicative of impairment and of future psychopathology (Lahey, et al., 1994; Morgan, et al., 1996). Longitudinal research is still needed to assess whether these subtypes actually reflect different stages of the same disorder, manifesting at different ages, and how these subtypes develop into adulthood (Woo & Rey, 2005).

In a study which evaluated each subtype of ADHD in children ages 4 through 6, Lahey, Pelham, et al. (1998) concluded that when diagnosed by a structured protocol, all three subtypes of ADHD in the DSM-IV are valid. Lahey, Pelham, et al. (1998) emphasize their finding that independent reports of the children's behavior (i.e., from observers other than parents and teachers) correlated with other reports (i.e., reports from the children themselves and from other school personnel), indicating that the criteria for ADHD were perceived by various sources. This stands in contrast to Barkley's (2003) argument, mentioned above, that such a requirement falsely assumes that children are consistent within all settings.

The DSM-IV requires that for a diagnosis of ADHD, the symptoms must cause impairment. Mota and Schachar (2000) question the validity of the DSM-IV's definition of ADHD because of the ambiguity surrounding the word "impairment." The authors argue that the DSM does not provide a means by which to distinguish whether or not a child is in fact impaired. They consequently recommend limiting the diagnostic criteria of ADHD to symptoms that reliably predict impairment.

Very few studies have investigated the DSM-IV criterion for onset (that symptoms be present and cause impairment before the age of 7) (Willoughby, Curran, Costello, & Angold, 2000). Researchers who have attempted to do so have produced contradictory findings. These studies have mostly defined ADHD as a unitary construct rather than as a 2-dimensional disorder as currently characterized in the DSM-IV (Applegate, et al., 1997; Willoughby, et al., 2000). In an analysis of validity of age of onset, Applegate, et al. (1997) concluded that there is variation in when symptoms from each of the subtypes begins to emerge. More specifically, the authors found that many youths with symptoms representing ADHD-C and ADHD-I experienced impairment after 6 years. Thus, the DSM-IV age-of-onset requirement precludes accurate identification of youths who experience the same symptoms after age 6. This study also found that clinicians often ignore the age of onset criterion and diagnose children with ADHD regardless of when the impairment appears.

The validity of ADHD has also been challenged on the grounds that there is less empirical data on the disorder in females (Faraone, Biederman, & Monuteaux, 2000b). The population sample for the DSM field trials was comprised mainly of boys, raising skepticism of its applicability to females.

Oppositional Defiant Disorder and Conduct Disorder

Oppositional Defiant Disorder (ODD) is defined as a recurrent pattern of negativistic, defiant, irritable, and hostile behavior, usually towards authority figures. Conduct Disorder (CD) is a persistent pattern of more serious violations of the rights of others and defiance of age-appropriate and societal norms. ODD and CD are commonly diagnosed in juvenile delinquent populations and are of great concern because of their potential to develop into adult psychopathology, such as antisocial personality disorder (Loeber, Burke, Lahey, Winters, & Zera, 2000). ODD and CD are also among the most common diagnoses assigned to children and adolescents (Wakefield, Pottick, & Kirk, 2002).

In the DSM-III-R, the diagnostic threshold for ODD (oppositional disorder in the DSM-III) was raised (Angold & Costello, 1996), resulting in confusion and a blurring of boundaries between it and the related but more severe CD. In response to recommendations by the Work Group, attempts were made to address this diagnostic predicament (Shaffer, et al., 1998). Similarly, research conducted subsequent to the publication of the DSM-IV has set out to decipher whether these disorders are discrete entities or manifestations of the same underlying disorder.

I. Reliability

Results from the field trial (Lahey, et al., 1994) suggest that the DSM-IV definitions of ODD and CD have better internal consistency and test-retest agreement than those in the DSM-III-R. Angold and Costello (1996) have raised concerns, however, with those conclusions on reliability. First, good reliability was achieved when three symptoms were identified, rather than four, as required in the DSM-IV. Angold and Costello (1996) thus recommend reducing the number of criterion symptoms for ODD to two or three to prevent misdiagnosing impaired children who might otherwise be overlooked. Another concern with the findings of the field trial is that the conclusions were derived using a biased sample, one composed of subjects who were clinically referred and who might not accurately represent the heterogeneity and complexity of ODD (Angold & Costello, 1996). Despite an exhaustive and comprehensive literature search, the authors of this chapter were unable to find additional data on the reliability of ODD and CD.

II. Controversies

While changes to ODD and CD in the DSM-IV sought to clarify the boundary between these two disorders, questions remain as to whether ODD is a milder variant of, a precursor to, or a prodromal syndrome of CD (Biederman, et al., 1996; First, et al., 2004; Werry, Reeves & Elkind, 1987), or whether ODD and

CD are discrete disorders (Loeber, Burke, Lahey, Winters, & Zera, 2000). Contributing to the obstacles in deciphering how related or unrelated these two disorders are is the fact that the majority of studies that have investigated behavioral disorders have lumped CD and ODD together, reflecting the assumption that they are similar enough to combine (Lahey, Loeber, Quay, Frick, & Grimm, 1997). The DSM-IV Task Force concluded that separate categories should be maintained because not all children with ODD go on to develop CD (Abikoff & Klein, 1992; Lahey, et al., 1997b). Similarly, based on differences on comorbidity rates, symptom patterns, and types of aggression, for example, many researchers contend that the two disorders are distinct diagnostic entities (Cohen & Flory, 1998; Loeber, et al., 2000).

Given the heterogeneity within CD, along with concerns about distinguishing youths who will outgrow such symptoms from those who will escalate to more severe levels of antisocial behavior (Biederman, et al., 1996; Loeber, et al., 2000), questions remain as to whether the disorder would be more accurately captured by dividing the diagnosis into subtypes (Loeber, et al., 2000). Based on the finding that youths who exhibited aggressive behavior in childhood later engaged in more aggressive behavior than those who developed CD in adolescence, the field trial concluded that maintaining subtypes based on age of onset is valid. The Task Force for DSM-IV decided to include three subtypes for CD–childhood-onset (symptoms appear before the age of 10), adolescent-onset (symptoms appear after the age of 11), and unspecified onset (age of onset is unknown), as well as three severity specifiers (American Psychiatric Association, 2000). Therefore, the DSM-IV reflects the theory that those who go on to develop antisocial personality disorder typically manifest symptoms in childhood rather than in adolescence (Lahey, Loeber, et al., 1998; Loeber, et al., 2000).

Because of a lack of research on these disorders in preschool children (Keenan & Wakschlag, 2002), however, age of onset has been criticized as a marker of psychopathology. The unreliability of memory and the lack of empirical data on age of onset for females have also been raised as problems (Lahey, Loeber, et al., 1998; Loeber, et al., 2000). The data used as evidence for making revisions in the DSM-IV have been questioned because they were obtained from a limited sample made up of school-age male children and adolescents (Keenan & Wakschlag, 2002; Lahey, Loeber, et al., 1998). Currently, research remains inconclusive as to whether late-onset CD is more common in females than in males (Lahey, Loeber, et al., 1998).

The scarcity of empirical data on the disruptive behavioral disorders in females has further called into question the validity of these diagnoses (Lahey, Loeber, Quay, Frick, & Grimm, 1997; Lahey, Pelham, et al., 1998). There are concerns that the criteria for CD reflect a gender bias, which might explain the preponderance of diagnoses in boys over girls (First, et al., 2004; Loeber, et al.,

2000). The DSM-IV made attempts to rectify this problem by including in the text a discussion of differences in the manifestations of CD in boys and girls. Non-confrontational defiant behaviors (e.g., lying, truancy, running away, substance use, and prostitution) are more common in girls.

III. Validity

As with the other disorders reviewed in this chapter, the validity of CD and ODD await empirical grounding (Angold, et al., 1996; Lahey, Loeber, et al., 1997). Yet several studies provide data suggesting that there is some validity to these diagnoses. For example, according to Cohen and Flory (1998), despite the overlap between CD and ODD (e.g., common negative outcomes), there is evidence of both discriminate and predictive validity of these disorders based on differences in comorbid disorders, symptom patterns, and certain negative outcomes. These results were obtained using DSM-III-R criteria, however. Similarly, the Work Group addressed other external factors, such as differences in family history, greater impairment in CD than ODD, and variety in age of onset, as possible indicators that the two disorders in fact represent two levels of severity within the same disorder. Nevertheless, the Work Group concluded that these disorders should remain distinctly classified for three reasons: (1) not all children with ODD go on to develop CD; (2) children who do transition from ODD into CD do not always escalate in levels of impairments; and (3) youths who develop CD in adolescence present a less aggressive pattern of symptoms with a better prognosis (Lahey, Loeber, et al., 1997).

Furthermore, many argue that some instances of CD and ODD reflect not a mental disorder but rather "a lack of personal responsibility" (First, et al., 2004, p. 383). Addressing the concern of false positive diagnoses, Richters and Cicchetti (1993) point out that Tom Sawyer and Huckleberry Finn would have qualified for a DSM diagnosis of conduct disorder. In the same vein, it is not always clear when ODD and CD would be more accurately seen as a means of coping with harsh life circumstances. Oppositional behavior in a child may be, for example, a means of getting attention from a neglectful father or a way to disguise a learning disability.

Scotti, Morris, McNeil, and Hawkins (1996) emphasize the lack of clinical utility of CD and ODD diagnoses as defined by the DSM. The authors indicate that identifying a child who meets the ODD criteria for "a pattern of negativistic, hostile, and defiant behavior" (e.g., loses temper, argues with adults, actively defies rules, is angry and spiteful) does not inform the clinician as to the functions of these behaviors. Therefore, little guidance is provided with regard to how to treat such a child. Two children with the same diagnosis and similar symptoms might require completely different treatments. Whether such behavioral symptoms are reflective of a biological vulnerability to frustration and anxiety (Jellinek & McDermott, 2004) or of a means of coping with an abusive home is important to consider. No matter how valid or reliable a diagnosis is, its statistical measure reveals little of the meaning behind the symptom(s). A more in-depth look into symptoms goes back at least to the writings of Anna Freud (1965), who recognized the importance of inferring the meaning of each child's behavior. She wrote:

> Some children run away from home because they are maltreated, or because they are not tied to their families by the usual emotional bonds . . . Here, the cause of the deviant behavior is rooted in the external conditions of the child's life and is removed with improvement of the latter. In contrast to this simple situation, there are other children who wander or are truant not for external but for internal reasons. (p. 111)

In response to such criticisms, the text of the DSM-IV-TR now states that a diagnosis of CD should be given only when it is the result of a psychological dysfunction and not a reaction to a negative environment: " . . . the Conduct Disorder diagnosis should be applied only when the behavior in question is symptomatic of an underlying dysfunction within the individual and not simply a reaction to the immediate social context" (American Psychiatric Association, 2000, p. 96). The diagnostic criteria do not include this exclusion criterion, however, and it is the criteria and not the text which clinicians use to identity patients and that researchers use to identify samples for a particular disorder (Wakefield & First, 2003).

Wakefield, Pottick, and Kirk (2002) found that clinicians' judgments about whether a disorder is present are more consistent with the text than with the diagnostic criteria. Also of importance was their finding that clinicians recommended treatment regardless of whether the symptoms were attributed to an internal dysfunction or a negative environment (Wakefield, et al., 2002). The findings from this study implied that for CD to be a valid diagnosis, an inference of whether an internal dysfunction exists should be included in the criteria. Furthermore, Wakefield and his colleagues call into question the generalizability and validity data obtained from studies that rely upon flawed diagnostic criteria (Wakefield, et al., 2002). Adding to the controversy as to whether CD and ODD are discrete or more closely linked disorders, interest and inquiry have similarly centered around the commonly occurring overlap between the behavioral disorders and ADHD (Drabick, Gadow, Carlson, & Bromet, 2004; Faraone, Biederman, & Monuteaux, 2000b). As the Work Group noted, investigation into comorbidity between ADHD and other disorders has been hampered by the dearth of empirical data to support the validity of ADHD itself as a discrete clinical entity (Biederman, et al., 1997).

Attempts to research comorbidity among these disorders have primarily focused upon the relationship between ADHD and CD (Biederman, Newcorn, &

Sprich, 1997; Faraone, et al., 2000b; Schachar & Tannock, 1995). Investigation into the comorbidity between ADHD and ODD has been relatively minimal (Biederman, et al., 1996, 1997; Loeber, et al., 2000). Results from the DSM-IV field trials suggest that ODD and ADHD are discrete disorders (Frick, Lahey, Applegate, Kerdyck, Ollendick, Hynd, et al., 1994). Since the addition of subtypes to ADHD in the DSM-IV, there has been contradictory evidence as to whether comorbidity with the behavioral disorders is more prevalent with ADHD-C (Willcutt, et al., 1999) or with ADHD-HI (Woo & Rey, 2005). There is evidence that individuals with ADHD plus a comorbid disorder not only respond differently to various treatments, but are also at a higher risk of developing more severe psychopathology (Biederman, Newcorn, & Sprich, 1997). This diagnostic dilemma illustrates the larger concern regarding the implications of accurately classifying related, overlapping and co-occurring disorders.

As a consequence of the co-occurring behavioral and attentional disorders, many studies have been unable to make clear distinctions between children with ODD, CD, and ADHD behaviors (Drabick, Gadow Carlson, & Bromet, 2004; Biederman, et al., 1996; Abikoff & Klein, 1992). According to Abikoff and Klein (1992) studies have found estimates of co-occurrence of ODD and CD among children with ADHD ranging from 20% to 60%, and the rate of ADHD can be as high as 90% among children referred for conduct disorders.

Furthermore, it is not clear whether a disorder such as ADHD in pure form is the same as when it coexists with another syndrome, such as CD (Abikoff & Klein, 1992). Put differently, questions remain as to whether the co-occurrence of ADHD and CD would be more accurately conceptualized as two commonly coexisting yet separate disorders or as a completely separate and discrete disorders (Faraone, Biederman, & Monuteaux, 2000b; Taylor, 1994). Faraone, et al. (2000a) concluded that ADHD with and without CD may be two distinct disorders, based on different etiologies. More specifically, the authors stated that ADHD + CD is a familial distinct subtype, characterized by different risk factors and clinical course, although further work is needed to determine whether the family etiology is genetic or environmental or both. Others have argued, based upon similarities in outcome, treatment responses, and intercorrelations of symptoms, and the lack of differences in psychosocial and neurodevelopmental factors between children with ADHD and CD, that ADHD and CD are indistinguishable (Biederman, Newcorn, & Sprich, 1997). Alternatively, studies have provided data highlighting differences in family backgrounds, cognitive deficits and performances, and responses to treatment (Biederman, et al., 1992, 1997), to support the independence of ADHD and CD from each other.

Based on their own review of the literature, the DSM-IV Work Group concluded that external factors such as outcome (cognitive dysfunction in ADHD versus aggression, substance abuse, and anti-social behaviors in CD); etiology (family aggregation); and psychosocial and developmental correlates contribute to the validation of ADHD and CD as discrete clinical entities (Biederman, et al., 1997).

CONCLUSION

This chapter has aimed to illuminate the limitations of our current classification system by examining some controversies surrounding reliability and validity. Although this concern applies to all diagnoses in the DSM, we have chosen to focus upon disorders that are commonly diagnosed, that are often believed to be empirically grounded, and that have spawned controversy leading to investigative attention. We have explored the issues of reliability and validity within the context of related diagnostic concerns such as comorbidity and threshold cutoffs. At the heart of this exploration is the question of whether diagnoses can be so precisely defined and squarely categorized as they are currently, or whether mental illnesses are broader and more fluid phenomena, which merge imperceptibly into one another.

Advocates for a dimensional model insist that the wide variation of symptom patterns, the indistinct boundaries between diagnoses, and the range of levels of intensity experienced by people with the same disorder are not properly captured in the discrete and artificially reified diagnostic categories upon which we currently rely. Despite the arguments of advocates of change to a dimensional representation, no well-researched and widely accepted dimensional model currently exists (Rounsaville, et al., 2002). The PDM represents an initial effort to provide one. We hope that integrating the PDM into our assessment of mental illness will enrich our understanding and enhance our treatment of psychological problems.

REFERENCES

Abikoff, H., & Klein, R. G. (1992). Attention-deficit hyperactivity and conduct disorder: Comorbidity and implications for treatment. *Journal of Consulting and Clinical Psychology, 60*(6), 881-892.

Achenbach, T. M. (1991). "Comorbidity" in child and adolescent psychiatry: Categorical and quantitative perspectives. *Journal of Child and Adolescent Psychopharmacology, 1,* 271-278.

American Psychiatric Association. (2000). *Diagnostic and statistical manual of mental disorders* (4th ed. Text revision.). Washington DC: Author.

Andreasen, N. C. (1995). The validation of psychiatric diagnosis: New models and approaches. *American Journal of Psychiatry, 152,* 161-162.

Angold, A., & Costello, J. (1996). Toward establishing an empirical basis for the diagnosis of oppositional defiant disorder. *Journal of the American Academy of Child and Adolescent Psychiatry, 35*(9), 1205-1212.

Angst, J., Gamma, A., Sellaro, R., Zhang, H., & Merikangas, K. (2002). Toward validation of atypical depression in the community: Results of the Zurich cohort study. *Journal of Affective Disorders, 72,* 125-138.

Applegate, B., Lahey, B. B., Hart, E. L., Biederman, J., George, W., Barkley, R. A., et al. (1997) Validity of the age-of-onset criterion for ADHD: A report from the DSM-IV field trials. *Journal of the American Academy of Child and Adolescent Psychiatry, 36,* 1211-1221.

Barkley, R. A. (1977). A review of stimulant drug research with hyperactive children. *Journal of Child Psychology and Psychiatry, 18,* 137-165.

Barkley, R. A. (2003). Issues in the diagnosis of attention-deficit/hyperactivity disorder in children. *Brain and Development, 25,* 77-83.

Baumgaertel, A., Wolraich, M., & Dietrich, M. (1995). Comparison of diagnostic criteria for ADHD in a German elementary school sample. *Journal of the American Academy of Child and Adolescent Psychiatry, 34,* 629-638.

Biederman, J., Faraone, S. V., Keenan, K., Benjamin, J., Krifcher, B., Moore, C., et al. (1992). Further evidence for family-genetic risk factors in attention deficit hyperactivity disorder (ADHD): Patterns of comorbidity in probands and relatives in psychiatrically and pediatrically referred samples. *Archives of General Psychiatry, 49,* 728-738.

Biederman, J., Faraone, S. V., Milberger, S., Jetton, J. G., Chen, L., Mick, E., et al. (1996). Is childhood oppositional defiant disorder a precursor to adolescent conduct disorder? Findings from a four-year follow study of children with ADHD. *Journal of the American Academy of Child and Adolescent Psychiatry, 35*(9)1193-1204.

Biederman, J., Newcorn, J. H., & Sprich, S. (1997). Comorbidity of attention-deficit/ hyperactivity disorder. In T. A. Widiger, A. J. Frances, H. A. Pincus, R. Ross, M. B. First, & W. Davis (Eds.), *DSM-IV Sourcebook* (Vol. 3, pp. 145-162). Washington DC: American Psychiatric Association.

Blashfield, R. K, & Livesley, W. J. (1999). Classification. In T. Millon, P. H. Blaney, & R. D. Davis (Eds.), *Oxford textbook of psychopathology* (pp. 3-28). New York: Oxford University Press.

Blashfield, R. K., Sprock, J., & Fuller, A. K. (1990). Suggested guidelines for including or excluding categories in the DSM-IV. *Comprehensive Psychiatry, 31,* 15-19.

Boris, N. W., Hinshaw-Fuselier, S. S., Smyke, A. T., Scheeringa, M. S., Heller, S. S., & Zeanah, C. H. (2004). Comparing criteria for attachment disorders: Establishing reliability and validity in high-risk samples. *Journal of the American Academy of Child and Adolescent Psychiatry, 43*(5), 568-577.

Brown, T. A., Antony, M. M., & Barlow, D. H. (1995). Diagnostic comorbidity in panic disorder: Effect on treatment outcomes and course of comorbid diagnoses following treatment. *Journal of Consulting and Clinical Psychology, 63,* 408-418.

Brown, T. A., Barlow, D. H., & Liebowitz, M. R. (1994). The empirical basis of generalized anxiety disorder. *The American Journal of Psychiatry, 151*(9), 1272-1280.

Brown, T. A., Campbell, L. A., Lehman, C. L., Grisham, J. R., & Mancill, R. B. (2001a). Current and lifetime comorbidity of the DSM-IV anxiety and mood disorder in a large clinical sample. *Journal of Abnormal Psychology. 110*(4), 585-599.

Brown, T. A., Di Nardo, P. A., Lehman, C. L., & Campbell, L. A. (2001b). Reliability of DSM-IV anxiety and mood disorders: Implications for the classification of emotional disorders. *Journal of Abnormal Psychology, 110*(1), 49-58.

Brown, T. A., Moras, K., Zinbarg, R. E., & Barlow, D. H. (1993). Diagnostic and symptom distinguishability of generalized anxiety disorder and obsessive-compulsive disorder. *Behavior Therapy, 24,* 227-240.

Chhabildas, N., Pennington, B. F., & Willcutt, E. G. (2001). A comparison of the neuropsychological profiles of the DSM-IV subtypes of ADHD. *Journal of Abnormal Psychology, 29*(6), 529-540.

Cohen, P., & Flory, M. (1998). Issues in the disruptive behavior disorders: Attention deficit disorder without hyperactivity and the differential validity of oppositional defiant and conduct disorders. In T. A. Widiger, A. J. Frances, H. A. Pincus, R. Ross, M. B. First, W. Davis, et al. (Eds.), *DSM-IV Sourcebook* (Vol. 4, pp. 455–463). Washington DC: American Psychiatric Association.

Dinardo, P. A., Moras, K., Barlow, D. H., Rapee, R. M., & Brown, T. A. (1993). Reliability of DSM-III-R anxiety disorder categories using the Anxiety Disorders Interview Schedule–Revised (ADIS-R). *Archives of General Psychiatry, 50,* 2251-2256.

Drabick, D. A. G., Gadow, K. D., Carlson, G. A., & Bromet, E. J. (2004). ODD and ADHD symptoms in Ukrainian children: External validators and comorbidity. *Journal of the American Academy of Child and Adolescent Psychiatry, 34*(6), 735-743.

Faraone, S. V., Biederman, J., & Friedman, D. (2000a). Validity of DSM-IV subtypes of attention-deficit/hyperactivity disorder: A family study perspective. *Journal of the American Academy of Child and Adolescent Psychiatry, 39,* 300-307.

Faraone, S. V., Biederman, J., & Monuteaux, M. C. (2000b). Attention-deficit disorder and conduct disorder in girls: Evidence for a familial subtype. *Biological Psychiatry, 48,* 21-29.

First, M. B., Frances, A., & Pincus, H. A. (2004). *DSM-IV-TR Guidebook.* Washington DC: American Psychiatric Association.

Freud, A. (1965). *The writings of Anna Freud, Volume 4: Normality and pathology in childhood: Assessments of development.* New York: International Universities Press.

Frick, P. J., Lahey, B. B., Applegate, B., Kerdyck, L., Ollendick, T., Hynd, et al. (1994). DSM-IV field trials for the disruptive behavior disorders: Symptoms utility estimates. *Journal of the American Academy of Child and Adolescent Psychiatry, 33*(4), 529-539.

Gadow, K. D., Sprafkin, J., & Nolan, E. E. (2001). DSM-IV symptoms in community and clinic preschool children. *Journal of the American Academy of Child and Adolescent Psychiatry, 40*(12) 1383-1392.

Gittelman, R., Manuzza, S., Shenker, R., & Bonagura, N. (1985). Hyperactive boys almost grown up. 1. Psychiatric status. *Archives of General Psychiatry, 42,* 937-947.

Gleaves, D. H., May, M. C., & Cardeña, E. (2001). An examination of the validity of dissociative identity disorder. *Clinical Psychology Review, 21*(4), 577-608.

Grayson, D. A. (1987). Can categorical and dimensional views of psychiatric illness be distinguished? *British Journal of Psychiatry, 26,* 57-63.

Han, L., Schmaling, K. B., & Dunner, D. L. (1995). Descriptive validity and stability of diagnostic criteria for dysthymic disorder. *Comprehensive Psychiatry, 36,* 338-343.

Hudziak, J. J., Heath, A. C., Madden, P. F., Reich, W., Bucholz, K. K., Slutske, W., et al. (1998). Latent class and factor analysis of DSM-IV ADHD: A twin study of female adolescents. *Journal of the American Academy of Child and Adolescent Psychiatry, 37*(8), 848-857.

Jablensky, A., & Kendell, R. E. (2002). Criteria for assessing a classification in psychiatry. In M. Maj, W. Gaebel, J. J. Lopez-Ibor, & N. Sartorius (Eds.), *Psychiatric diagnosis and classification* (pp. 1-24). West Sussex, UK: John Wiley & Sons, Ltd.

Jellinek, M. S., & McDermott, J. F. (2004). Formulation: Putting the diagnosis into a therapeutic context and treatment plan. *Journal of the American Academy of Child and Adolescent Psychiatry, 43*(7), 913-916.

Keenan, K., & Wakschlag, L. S. (2002). Can a valid diagnosis of disruptive behavior disorder be made in preschool children? *American Journal of Psychiatry, 159,* 351-358.

Keller, M. B., Klein, D. N., Hirschfeld, R. M. A., Kocsis, J. H., McCullough, J. P., Miller, I., et al. (1995). Results of the DSM-IV mood disorders field trial. *American Journal of Psychiatry, 152,* 843-849.

Keller, M. B., Klein, D. N., Hirschfeld, R. M. A., Kocsis, J. H., McCullough, J. P., Miller, I., et al. (1998). Results of the DSM-IV mood disorder field trial. In T. A. Widiger, A. J. Frances, H. A. Pincus, R. Ross, M. B. First, W. Davis, & M. Kline (Eds.), *DSM-IV sourcebook* (Vol. 4, pp. 717-732). Washington DC: American Psychiatric Association.

Keller, M. B., & Russell, C. W. (1996). Dysthymia. In T. A. Widiger, A. J. Frances, H. A. Pincus, R. Ross, M. B. First, & W. W. Davis (Eds.) *DSM-IV Sourcebook* (Vol. 2, pp. 21-35). Washington DC: American Psychiatric Association.

Kendell, R. E. (1982). The choice of diagnostic criteria for biological research. *Archives of General Psychiatry, 39,* 1334-1339.

Kendler, K. S. (1980). The nosologic validity of paranoia (simple delusional disorder). A review. *Archives of General Psychiatry, 37,* 699-706.

Kocsis, J. H., & Frances, A. J. (1987). A critical discussion of DSM-III dysthymic disorder. *American Journal of Psychiatry, 144,* 1534-1542.

Lahey, B. B., Applegate, B., Barkley, R. A., Garfinkel, B., McBurnett, K., Kerdyk, L., et al. (1994). DSM-IV field trials for oppositional defiant disorder and conduct disorder in children and adolescents. *American Journal of Psychiatry, 151,* 1163-1171.

Lahey, B. B., Carlson, C. L., & Frick, P. F. (1997). Attention-deficit disorder without hyperactivity. In T. A. Widiger, A. J. Frances, H. A. Pincus, R. Ross, M. B. First, & W. Davis (Eds.), *DSM-IV Sourcebook* (Vol. 3, p. 163-188). Washington, DC: American Psychiatric Association.

Lahey, B. B., Loeber, R., Quay, H. C., Applegate, B., Shaffer, D., Waldman, I., et al. (1998). Validity of DSM-IV subtypes of conduct disorder based on age of onset. *Journal of the American Academy of Child and Adolescent Psychiatry, 37,* 435-442.

Lahey, B. B., Loeber, R., Quay, H. C., Frick, P. J., & Grimm, J. (1997). Oppositional defiant disorder and conduct disorder. In T. A. Widiger, A. J. Frances, H. A. Pincus, R. Ross, M. B. First, & W. Davis (Eds.), *DSM-IV Sourcebook* (Vol. 3, p. 189-209). Washington, DC: American Psychiatric Association.

Lahey, B. B., Pelham, W. E., Loney, J., Lee, S. S., & Wilcutt, E. (2005). Instability of the DSM-IV subtypes of ADHD from preschool through elementary school. *Archives of General Psychiatry, 62,* 896-902.

Lahey, B. B., Pelham, W. E., Stein, M. A., Loney, J., Trapani, C., Nugent, K., et al. (1998). Validity of DSM-IV attention–deficit/hyperactivity disorder for younger children. *Journal of the American Academy of Child and Adolescent Psychiatry, 37,* 695-702.

Loeber, R., Burke, J. D., Lahey, B. B., Winters, A., & Zera, M. (2000). Oppositional defiant and conduct disorder: A review of the past ten years. Part 1. *Journal of the American Academy of Child and Adolescent Psychiatry, 39(12),* 1468-1484.

Manuzza, S., Fyer, A., Martin, L. Y., Gallops, M. S., Endicott, J., Gorman, J. M., et al. (1989). Reliability of anxiety assessment: I. Diagnostic agreement. *Archives of General Psychiatry, 46,* 1093-1101.

McBurnett, K. (1997). Attention-deficit/hyperactivity disorder: A review of diagnostic issues. In T. A. Widiger, A. J. Frances, H. A. Pincus, R. Ross, M. B. First, W. Davis, et al. (Eds.), *DSM-IV Sourcebook* (Vol. 3, pp. 111–143). Washington, DC: American Psychiatric Association.

McCullough, J. P., Klein, D. N., Borian, F. E., Howland, R. H., Riso, L. P., & Keller, M. B., et al. (2003). Group comparisons of DSM-IV subtypes of chronic depression: Validity of the distinctions. Part 2. *Journal of Abnormal Psychology, 112(4),* 614-622.

McCullough, J. P., Klein, D. N., Keller, M. B, Holzer, C. E., Davis, S. M., Kornstein, S. G., et al. (2000). Comparison of DSM-III-R chronic major depression and major depression superimposed on dysthymia (double depression): Validity of the distinction. *Journal of Abnormal Psychology, 109(3),* 419-427.

Mezey, G., & Robbins, I. (2001). Usefulness and validity of post-traumatic stress disorder as a psychiatric category. *British Medical Journal, 323,* 561-563.

Minor, K. L., Champion, J. E., & Gotlib, I. H. (2005). Stability of DSM-IV criterion symptoms for major depressive disorder. *Journal of Psychiatric Research, 39,* 415-420.

Moras, K., Borkovec, T. D., DiNardo, P. A., Rapee, R., Riskind, J., & Barlow, D. H. (1996). General anxiety disorder. In T. A. Widiger, A. J. Frances, H. A. Pincus, R. Ross, M. B. First & W. W. Davis (Eds.), *DSM-IV Sourcebook* (Vol. 2, pp.607-621). Washington DC: American Psychiatric Association.

Morgan, A. E., Hynd, G. W., Riccio, C. A., & Hall, J. (1996). Validity of DSM-IV ADHD predominantly inattentive and combined types: Relationship to previous DSM diagnoses/subtype differences. *Journal of the American Academy of Child and Adolescent Psychiatry, 35*(3), 325-333.

Mota, V. L., & Schachar, R. J. (2000). Reformulating attention-deficit/hyperactivity disorder according to signal detection theory. *Journal of the American Academy of Child and Adolescent Psychiatry, 39*(9), 1144-1151.

Nelson-Gray, R. O. (1991). DSM-IV: Empirical guideline from psychometrics. *Journal of Abnormal Psychology, 100*(3), 308-315.

Newcorn, J. H., Halperin, J. M., Jensen, P. S., Abikoff, H. B., Arnold, L. E., Cantwell, D. P., et al. (2001). Symptom profiles in children with ADHD: Effects of comorbidity and gender. *Journal of the American Academy of Child and Adolescent Psychiatry, 40*(2), 137-146.

Pincus, H. A., McQueen, L. E., & Elinson, L. (2003). In K. A. Philips, M. A. First, & H. A. Pincus (Eds.), *Advancing the DSM: Dilemmas in psychiatric diagnosis* (pp. 129-144). Washington DC: American Psychiatric Association.

Quitkin, F. M. (2002). Depression with atypical features: Diagnostic validity, prevalence, and treatment. *Journal of Clinical Psychiatry—Primary Care Companion, 4*(3), 94-99.

Regier, D. A., Kaelber, C. T., Rae, D. S., Farmer, M. E., Knauper, B., & Kessler, R. C., et al. (1998). Limitations of diagnostic criteria and assessment instruments for mental disorders. *Archives of General Psychiatry, 55*, 109-115.

Richters, J. E., & Cicchetti, D. (1993). Mark Twain meets DSM-III-R: Conduct disorder, development, and the concept of harmful dysfunction. *Developmental Psychopathology, 5*, 5-29.

Rivas-Vasquez, R. A., Saffa-Biller, D., Ruiz, I., Blais, M. A., & Rivas-Vasquez, A. (2004). Current issues in anxiety and depression: comorbid, mixed, and subthreshold disorders. *Professional Psychology: Research and Practice, 35*(1), 74-83.

Robins, E., & Guze, S. B. (1970). Establishment of diagnostic validity in psychiatric illness: Its application to schizophrenia. *American Journal of Psychiatry, 126*, 983-987.

Rounsaville, B. J., Alarcó, R. D., Andrews, G., Jackson, J. S., Kendell, R. E., & Kendler, K. (2002). Basic nomenclature issues for DSM-V. In D. J. Kupfer, M. B. First, & D. A. Regier (Eds.), *A research agenda for DSM-V* (pp. 1-29). Washington DC: American Psychiatric Association.

Rush, A. J. (1998). DSM-IV mood disorders: Final overview. In T. A. Widiger, A. J. Frances, H. A. Pincus, R. Ross, M. B. First, W. Davis, et al. (Eds.), *DSM-IV Sourcebook* (Vol. 4, pp. 1019-1033), Washington DC: American Psychiatric Association.

Schachar, R., & Tannock, R. (1995). Test of four hypotheses for the comorbidity of attention-deficit hyperactivity disorder and conduct disorder. *Journal of the American Academy of Child and Adolescent Psychiatry, 35*(5), 639-648.

Scheeringa, M. S., Peebles, C. D., Cook, C. A., & Zeanah, C. H. (2001). Toward establishing procedural, criterion, and discriminant validity for PTSD in early childhood. *Journal of the American Academy of Child and Adolescent Psychiatry, 40*(1), 52-60.

Schotte, C. K. W., Maes, M., Cludydts, R., & Cosyns, P. (1997). Cluster analytic validation of the DSM melancholic depression: The threshold model. Integration of quantitative and qualitative distinctions between unipolar depressive subtypes. *Psychiatry Research, 71*, 181-195.

Scotti, J. R., Morris, T. L., McNeil, C. B., & Hawkins, R. P. (1996). DSM-IV and disorders of childhood and adolescence: Can structural criteria be functional? *Journal of Consulting and Clinical Psychology, 64*(6), 1177-1191.

Shaffer, D., Widiger, T. A., & Pincus, H. A. (1998). DSM-IV child disorders. Part II: Final Overview. In T. A. Widiger, A. J. Frances, H. A. Pincus, R. Ross, M. B. First, W. Davis, et al. (Eds.), *DSM-IV Sourcebook* (Vol. 4, pp. 963-977). Washington DC: American Psychiatric Association.

Spence, S. (1997). Structure of anxiety symptoms among children: A confirmatory factor-analytic study. *Journal of Abnormal Psychology, 106*(2), 280-297.

Spitzer, R. L., & Williams, J. B. W. (1985). Classification in psychiatry. In H. I. Kaplan, & B. J. Sadock (Eds.), *Comprehensive textbook of psychiatry 4th edition* (pp. 591-612). Baltimore: Williams Wilkins.

Taylor, E. (1994). Similarities and differences in DSM-IV and ICD-10 diagnostic criteria. *Child and Adolescent Psychiatry Clinics of North America, 3*, 209-226.

Todd, R. D., Rasmussen, E. R., Neuman, R. J., Reich, W., Hudziak, J. J., Bucholz, K. K., et al. (2001). Familiality and heritability of subtypes of attention deficit hyperactivity disorder in a population sample of adolescent female twins. *American Journal of Psychiatry, 158*, 1891-1898.

Volk, H. E., Neuman, R. J., & Todd, R. D. (2005). A systematic evaluation of ADHD and comorbid psychopathology in a population-based twin sample. *Journal of the American Academy of Child and Adolescent Psychiatry, 44*(8), 768-775.

Wakefield, J. C., & First, M. B. (2003). Clarifying the distinction between disorder and nondisorder: Confronting the overdiagnosis (false-positives) problem in the DSM-V. In K. A. Phillips, M. B. First, H. A. Pincus (Eds.), *Advancing DSM: Dilemmas in psychiatric diagnosis* (pp. 23-55). Washington DC: American Psychiatric Association.

Wakefield, J. C., Pottick, K. J., & Kirk, S. A. (2002). Should the DSM-IV diagnostic criteria for conduct disorder consider social context? *American Journal of Psychiatry, 159*, 380-386.

Werry, J. S., Reeves, J. C., & Elkind, G. S. (1987). Attention deficit, conduct, oppositional and anxiety disorders in children: I. A review of research on differentiating characteristics. *Journal of the American Academy of Child and Adolescent Psychiatry, 26*, 133-143.

Westen, D., Heim, A. K., Morrison, K., Patterson, M., & Campbell, L. (2002). Simplifying diagnosis using a prototype-matching approach: Implications for the next edition of the DSM. In L. E. Beutler, & M. L. Malik (Eds.), *Rethinking the DSM: A psychological perspective* (pp. 221-250). Washington, DC: American Psychological Association.

Widiger, T. A., Frances, A. J., Pincus, H. A., Davis, W. W., & First, M. B. (1991). Toward an empirical classification for the DSM-IV. *Journal of Abnormal Psychology, 100*(3), 280-288.

Willcutt, E. G., Pennington, B. F., Chhabildas, N. A., Friedman, M. C., & Alexander, J. (1999). Psychiatric comorbidity associated with DSM-IV ADHD in a nonreferred sample of twins. *Journal of the American Academy of Child and Adolescent Psychiatry, 38*(11), 1355-1362.

Willoughby, M. T., Curran, P. T., Costello, E. J., & Angold, A. (2000). Implications of early versus late onset of attention-deficit/hyperactivity disorder symptoms. *Journal of the American Academy of Child and Adolescent Psychiatry, 39*(12), 1512-1519.

Woo, B. S. C., & Rey, J. M. (2005). The validity of the DSM-IV subtypes of attention-deficit/hyperactivity disorder. *Australian and New Zealand Journal of Psychiatry, 39*, 344-353.

Zimmerman, M., Coryell, W., & Pfohl, B. (1986). Melancholic subtyping: A qualitative or quantitative distinction? *American Journal of Psychiatry, 143*, 98-100.

Zimmerman, M., & Chelminski, I. (2003). Generalized anxiety disorder in patients with major depression: Is DSM-IV's hierarchy correct? *The American Journal of Psychiatry, 160*(3), 504-512.

Zinbarg, R. E., Barlow, D. H., Liebowitz, M. R., Street, L., Broadhead, E., Katon, W., et al. (1998). The DSM-IV field trial for mixed anxiety-depession. In T. A. Widiger, A. J. Frances, H. A. Pincus, R. Ross, M. B. First, W. Davis, et al. (Eds.), *DSM-IV Sourcebook* (Vol. 4, pp. 735-760). Washington DC: American Psychiatric Association.

Reprinted with the permission of American Psychological Association
Psychological Bulletin
2004, Vol. 130, No. 4, 631-663

The Empirical Status of Empirically Supported Psychotherapies: Assumptions, Findings, and Reporting in Controlled Clinical Trials

Drew Westen, PhD,[1] Catherine M. Novotny, PhD,[2]
Heather Thompson-Brenner, PhD[3]

Editor's Note: This article (reprinted here by permission), does not portray the development and deployment of a particular instrument, or a particular investigative approach, for personality diagnosis or for treatment assessment, but is instead a meta-analysis of a large array of reported studies of psychotherapy outcome research across the entire spectrum of therapeutic approaches, psychodynamic, behavioral and cognitive-behavioral, humanistic or existential, etc., including both general studies over the range of psychopathology, as well as discrete studies focused on the treatment of specific syndromes and disorders.

The authors focus on elucidating the assumptions as well as the findings used to establish psychotherapies as empirically supported, and they demonstrate impressively how the attempt to establish the randomized control trial (RCT) methodology as the so-called "gold standard" for psychotherapy research rests on particular assumptions that may indeed be valid enough for some disorders and treatments, but are substantially violated for others. This severely constrains the actual clinical and scientific usefulness of those findings when generalizing to naturalistic effectiveness studies or to individual clinical usefulness. The authors propose procedures to significantly reduce these discrepancies to the scientific and clinical usefulness of psychotherapy research studies.

[1] Professor, Department of Psychology and Department of Psychiatry and Behavioral Sciences, Emory University
[2] Clinical Psychologist, Department of Veterans Affairs Medical Center, San Francisco
[3] Director, Eating Disorders Program, Center for Anxiety and Related Disorders and Department of Psychology, Boston University

This article provides a critical review of the assumptions and findings of studies used to establish psychotherapies as empirically supported. The attempt to identify empirically supported therapies (ESTs) imposes particular assumptions on the use of randomized controlled trial (RCT) methodology that appear to be valid for some disorders and treatments (notably exposure-based treatments of specific anxiety symptoms) but substantially violated for others. Meta-analytic studies support a more nuanced view of treatment efficacy than implied by a dichotomous judgment of supported versus unsupported. The authors recommend changes in reporting practices to maximize the clinical utility of RCTs, describe alternative methodologies that may be useful when the assumptions underlying EST methodology are violated, and suggest a shift from validating treatment packages to testing intervention strategies and theories of change that clinicians can integrate into *empirically informed therapies*.

When the results of scientific studies are applied to new and important questions that may directly or indirectly affect clinical training, clinical treatment, and financial decisions about how to treat, it is useful for us to return to our roots in empirical science and to carefully consider again the nature of our scientific methods and what they do and do not provide in the way of possible conclusions relevant to those questions. (Borkovec & Castonguay, 1998, p. 136)

Robert Abelson (1995) has argued that the function of statistics is not to display "the facts" but to tell a coherent story—to make a principled argument. In recent years, a story has been told in the clinical psychology literature, in graduate programs in clinical psychology, in psychiatry residency programs, and even in the popular media that might be called "The Tale of the Empirically Supported Therapies (ESTs)." The story goes something like this.

Once upon a time, in the Dark Ages, psychotherapists practiced however they liked, without any scientific data guiding them. Then a group of courageous warriors, whom we shall call the Knights of the Contingency Table, embarked upon a campaign of careful scientific testing of therapies under controlled conditions.

Along the way, the Knights had to overcome many obstacles. Among the most formidable were the wealthy Drug Lords who dwelled in Mercky moats filled with Lilly pads. Equally treacherous were the fire-breathing clinician-dragons, who roared, without any basis in data, that their ways of practicing psychotherapy were better.

After many years of tireless efforts, the Knights came upon a set of empirically supported therapies that made people better. They began to develop practice guidelines so that patients would receive the best possible treatments for their specific problems. And, in the end, Science would prevail, and there would be calm (or at least less negative affect) in the land.

In this article we tell the story a slightly different way, with a few extra twists and turns to the plot. Ours is a sympathetic but critical retelling, which goes something like this.

Once upon a time, psychotherapists practiced without adequate empirical guidance, assuming that the therapies of their own persuasion were the best. Many of their practices were probably helpful to many of their patients, but knowing which were helpful and which were inert or iatrogenic was a matter of opinion and anecdote.

Then a group of clinical scientists developed a set of procedures that became the gold standard for assessing the validity of psychotherapies. Their goal was a valorous one that required tremendous courage in the face of the vast resources of the Drug Lords and the nonempirical bent of mind of many clinician-dragons, who tended to breathe some admixture of hot air, fire, and wisdom. In their quest, the Knights identified interventions for a number of disorders that showed substantial promise. The treatments upon which they bestowed Empirical Support helped many people feel better—some considerably so, and some completely.

In the excitement, however, some important details seemed to get overlooked. Many of the assumptions underlying the methods used to test psychotherapies were themselves empirically untested, disconfirmed, or appropriate only for a range of treatments and disorders. And although many patients improved, most did not recover, or they initially recovered but then relapsed or sought additional treatment within the next 2 years. Equally troubling, the Scientific Method (Excalibur) seemed to pledge its allegiance to whosoever had the time and funding to wield it: Most of the time, psychotherapy outcome studies supported the preferred position of the gallant knight who happened to conduct them (Sir Grantsalot).

Nevertheless, clinical lore and anecdotal alchemy provided no alternative to experimental rigor, and as word of the Knights' crusade became legendary, their tales set the agenda for clinical work, training, and research throughout the land. Many graduate programs began teaching new professionals only those treatments that had the imprimatur of Empirical Validation, clinicians seeking licensure had to memorize the tales told by the Knights and pledge allegiance to them on the national licensing examination, and insurance companies used the results of controlled clinical trials to curtail the treatment of patients who did not improve in 6 to 16 sessions, invoking the name of Empirical Validation.

This is a very different version of the story, but one that is, we hope to show, at least as faithful to the facts. The moral of the first, more familiar version of the story is clear: Only science can distinguish good interventions from bad ones. Our retelling adds a second, complementary moral: Unqualified statements and dichotomous judgments about validity or invalidity in complex arenas are unlikely to be scientifically or clinically useful, and as a field we should attend more closely to the conditions under which certain empirical methods are useful in testing certain interventions for certain disorders.

Let us be clear at the outset what we are not arguing. We are not advocating against evidence-based practice, looking to provide refuge for clinicians who want to practice as they have for years irrespective of empirical data. A major, and well-justified, impetus for the attempt to develop a list of ESTs was the literal Babble in the field of psychotherapy, with little way of distinguishing (or helping the public distinguish) useful therapeutic interventions from useless or destructive ones. And although we argue for a more nuanced story about efficacy and treatment of choice than sometimes seen in the scientific literature, we are not claiming our own narrative to be bias free (see Westen & Morrison, 2001). None of us is capable of being completely dispassionate about topics we are drawn to study, truth be told, by passionate beliefs. We have endeavored to present a balanced argument and have been aided in that endeavor by a number of colleagues, including several whose inclination might have been to tell a somewhat different tale. Fortunately, where our own critical faculties failed us, others' usually did not. What we are suggesting, however, is that the time has come for a thoroughgoing assessment of the empirical status of not only the data but also the methods used to assign the appellations empirically supported or unsupported.

We now tell our story in the more conventional language of science, beginning with an examination of the empirical basis of the assumptions that underlie the methods used to establish empirical support for psychotherapies. We then reexamine the data supporting the efficacy of a number of the treatments currently believed to be empirically supported.[4] We conclude by offering suggestions for reporting hypotheses, methods, and findings from controlled clinical trials and for broadening the methods used to test the clinical utility of psychosocial interventions for particular disorders. Throughout, we argue from data because ultimately the future of psychotherapy lies not in competing assertions about whose patients get more help but in replicable data. The question is how to collect and interpret those data so that, as a field, we maximize our chances of drawing accurate inferences.

RETELLING THE STORY: THE ASSUMPTIONS UNDERLYING ESTs

The idea of creating a list of empirically supported psychosocial treatments was a compelling one, spurred in part by concerns about other widely

---

[4] A number of researchers have pointed to important caveats in the enterprise of establishing a list of ESTs using randomized controlled trial (RCT) methodology, whose work we draw on here (Borkovec & Castonguay, 1998; Goldfried & Wolfe, 1996, 1998; Ingram & Ritter, 2000; Kazdin, 1997; Seligman, 1995).

disseminated practice guidelines that gave priority to pharmacotherapy over psychotherapy in the absence of evidence supporting such priority (Barlow, 1996; Beutler, 1998, 2000; Nathan, 1998). The mandate to use, and train professionals exclusively in the use of, empirically validated therapies (now often called *empirically supported therapies*, or ESTs; Kendall, 1998) gained powerful momentum in 1995 with the publication of the first of several task force reports by the American Psychological Association (Task Force on Psychological Intervention Guidelines, 1995). This report, and others that followed and refined it, distinguished ESTs from the less structured, longer-term treatments conducted by most practicing clinicians. Since that time, many advocates of ESTs have argued that clinicians should be trained primarily in these methods and that other forms of treatment are "less essential and outdated" (Calhoun, Moras, Pilkonis, & Rehm, 1998, p. 151; see also Chambless & Hollon, 1998; Persons & Silberschatz, 1998).

ESTs, and the research methods used to validate them, share a number of characteristics (see Chambless & Ollendick, 2000; Goldfried & Wolfe, 1998; Kendall, Marrs-Garcia, Nath, & Sheldrick, 1999; Nathan, Stuart, & Dolan, 2000). Treatments are typically designed for a single Axis I disorder, and patients are screened to maximize homogeneity of diagnosis and minimize co-occurring conditions that could increase variability of treatment response. Treatments are manualized and of brief and fixed duration to minimize within-group variability. Outcome assessment focuses primarily (though not necessarily exclusively) on the symptom that is the focus of the study. In many respects, these characteristics make obvious scientific sense, aimed at maximizing the internal validity of the study—the "cleanness" of the design. A valid experiment is one in which the experimenter randomly assigns patients, manipulates a small set of variables, controls potentially confounding variables, standardizes procedures as much as possible, and hence is able to draw relatively unambiguous conclusions about cause and effect.

What we believe has not been adequately appreciated, however, is the extent to which the use of RCT methodologies to validate ESTs requires a set of additional assumptions that are themselves neither well validated nor broadly applicable to most disorders and treatments: that psychopathology is highly malleable, that most patients can be treated for a single problem or disorder, that psychiatric disorders can be treated independently of personality factors unlikely to change in brief treatments, and that experimental methods provide a gold standard for identifying useful psychotherapeutic packages. Psychotherapy researchers can put RCT methodology to different uses, some of which (hereafter referred to as *EST methodology* or *the methodology of ESTs*) entail all of these assumptions. Other uses of RCT methodology, such as those focused on testing basic theoretical postulates about change processes (Borkovec & Castonguay, 1998; Kazdin, 1997), mediators and moderators of outcome, or specific interventions (rather than entire treatments), entail only some of these assumptions some of the time. Here we focus on the assumptions of EST methodology rather than RCT methods more broadly and describe each of these assumptions and the extant data bearing on them. As the discussion below makes clear, we are not arguing that these assumptions are never valid. Rather, we are arguing that they are not *generally* valid—that is, that they apply to some instances but not others—and that researchers and consumers of research need to be more cognizant about the conditions under which their violation renders conclusions valid only with substantial qualification.

Psychological Processes Are Highly Malleable

The assumption of malleability is implicit in the treatment lengths used in virtually all ESTs, which typically range from about 6 to 16 sessions. As Goldfried (2000) has observed, historically the exclusive focus on brief treatments emerged less from any systematic data on the length of treatment required to treat most disorders effectively than from pragmatic considerations, such as the fact that if psychotherapy researchers were to compare their psychotherapies with medications, they needed to avoid the confound of time elapsed and hence tended to design treatments of roughly the length of a medication crossover design.[5] Equally important in determining the length of clinical trials was a simple, unavoidable fact of experimental method as applied to psychotherapy, the wide-ranging impact of which has not, we believe, drawn sufficient attention: The longer the therapy, the more variability within experimental conditions; the more variability, the less one can draw causal conclusions. As we argue, the preference for brief treatments is a natural consequence of efforts to standardize treatments to bring them under experimental control. Even 16 to 20 carefully controlled hour-long sessions pose substantial threats to internal validity. Indeed, we are aware of no other experiments in the history of psychology in which a manipulation intended to constitute a single experimental condition approached that length.

Given the centrality of the malleability assumption, one would expect that it rests on a strong evidentiary foundation; and for some disorders, brief, focal treatments do produce powerful results (see Barlow, 2002; Roth & Fonagy, 1996). However, a substantial body of data shows that, with or without treatment, relapse rates for all but a handful of disorders (primarily anxiety disorders with

---

[5] Other considerations have influenced the near-exclusive focus on brief treatments as well, such as considerations of cost, funding, and feasibility of research. Another is that most psychotherapy research is behavioral or cognitive-behavioral. Theorists from Skinner through Bandura have argued that human behavior is under substantial environmental control and that one system of responses can readily be changed without worrying about broader systems in which they may be embedded (see, e.g., Bandura, 1977; Skinner, 1953). Although this assumption was most strenuously advanced in the early days of behavior therapy, and many cognitive-behavioral therapy (CBT) researchers no longer explicitly endorse it, this assumption is now implicit in the design of virtually all clinical trials of psychotherapy.

very specific therapeutic foci) are high. For example, data on the natural course of depression suggest that the risk of repeated episodes following an initial index episode exceeds 85% over 10 to 15 years (Mueller, et al., 1999), and on average, individuals with major depressive disorder will experience four major depressive episodes of approximately 20 weeks duration each as well as a plethora of other depressive symptoms during periods of remission from major depressive episodes (Judd, 1997).

The malleability assumption is also inconsistent with data from naturalistic studies of psychotherapy, which consistently find a dose-response relationship, such that longer treatments, particularly those of 1 to 2 years and beyond, are more effective than briefer treatments (Howard, Kopta, Krause, & Orlinsky, 1986; Kopta, Howard, Lowry, & Beutler, 1994; Seligman, 1995). Of particular relevance is the finding from naturalistic samples that substantial symptom relief often occurs within 5 to 16 sessions, particularly for patients without substantial personality pathology; however, enduring "rehabilitation" requires substantially longer treatment, depending on the patient's degree and type of characterological impairment (Howard, Lueger, Maling, & Martinovich, 1993; Kopta, et al., 1994). For example, Kopta, et al. (1994) found that patients with characterological problems required an average of 2 years of treatment before 50% showed clinically significant change.

Although one might raise many legitimate methodological concerns about naturalistic designs, perhaps the most compelling data on the malleability assumption come from controlled trials themselves. As we discuss below, meta-analytic data on ESTs for a range of disorders using outcome intervals longer than 6 months suggest that most psychopathological vulnerabilities studied are in fact highly resistant to change, that many are rooted in personality and temperament, and that the modal patient treated with brief treatments for most disorders (other than those involving specific associations between a stimulus or representation and a highly specific cognitive, affective, or behavioral response) relapses or seeks additional treatment within 12 to 24 months.

Suggestive findings also come from research using implicit and other indirect measures (e.g., Gemar, Segal, Sagrati, & Kennedy, 2001; Hedlund & Rude, 1995), such as emotional Stroop tasks (in which participants are presented, for example, with neutral and depressive words in randomly varying colors and have to ignore the content of the word to report the color as quickly as possible; see Williams, Mathews, & MacLeod, 1996) or audio presentations of homophones associated with anxiety or depression (e.g., weak-week; see Wenzlaff & Eisenberg, 2001). Patients whose depression has remitted often show continued attentional biases toward depressive words, indexed by longer response latencies in Stroop tests and greater likelihood of choosing the depressive spelling of homophones. Research using implicit measures often finds continued biases toward depressive words and thematic content among people who are no longer depressed, suggesting that changes in state may or may not be accompanied by changes in diatheses for those states encoded in implicit networks and raising questions about the durability of change. A. T. Beck (1976) described similar studies decades ago on the dream content of patients with remitted depression in his classic book on cognitive therapy for emotional disorders. These findings make sense in light of contemporary research in cognitive neuroscience (and social psychology) on implicit associational networks, which reflect longstanding regularities in the individual's experience, can be resistant to change, and likely provide a diathesis for many psychological disorders (Westen, 1998b, 1999, 2000). Although this is a frontier area of research, suggestive findings are beginning to emerge on prediction of future behavior, outcome, or relapse from indirect measures such as these (e.g., Segal, Gemar, & Williams, 1999; Wiers, van Woerden, Smulders, & De Jong, 2002).

Most Patients Have One Primary Problem or Can Be Treated as if They Do

The assumption that patients can be treated as if they have one primary, discrete problem, syndrome, or disorder—and the correlative assumption that if they have more than one disorder, the syndromes can be treated sequentially using different manuals (e.g., Wilson, 1998)—again reflects an admixture of methodological constraints and theoretical meta-assumptions. Perhaps most important are two features of the pragmatics of research. First, including patients with substantial comorbidities would vastly increase the sample size necessary to detect treatment differences if comorbidity bears any systematic relation to outcome. Thus, the most prudent path is arguably to begin with relatively "pure" cases, to avoid confounds presented by co-occurring disorders. Second, the requirement that research proposals be tied to categories defined by the *Diagnostic and Statistical Manual of Mental Disorders* (*DSM*; 4th ed.; *DSM–IV*; American Psychiatric Association, 1994) to be considered for funding has virtually guaranteed a focus on single disorders (or at most dual diagnosis, such as posttraumatic stress disorder [PTSD] and substance abuse).

If we examine more carefully the empirical basis of this assumption, however, we find that, as a general rule, it fares no better than the malleability assumption. We focus here on three issues: the empirical and pragmatic limits imposed by reliance on *DSM–IV* diagnoses, the problem of comorbidity, and the way the different functions of assessing comorbidity in controlled trials and clinical practice may place limits on generalizability.

The Pragmatics of DSM–IV Diagnosis

Linking treatment research to *DSM*-defined categories has many benefits, the most important of which are the ability to generalize across different settings and the link between understanding psychopathology and identifying processes that might alter it. We note here, however, three costs.

First, *DSM* diagnoses are themselves created by committee consensus on the basis of the available evidence rather than by strictly empirical methods (such as factor analysis or latent class analysis), and in many cases they are under serious empirical challenge. For example, whether major depression is a distinct disorder or whether it simply represents the more severe end of a depressive continuum is unknown; nor is it known the extent to which the high comorbidity of major depressive disorder and generalized anxiety disorder (GAD) is an artifact of the way the two disorders are defined (overlapping criterion sets) or of a common diathesis for negative affect (see Brown, Chorpita, & Barlow, 1998; Westen, Heim, Morrison, Patterson, & Campbell, 2002). To the extent that some of the *DSM–IV* categories are themselves not empirically well supported, hitching our therapeutic wagons to these disorders may commit us to a range of empirically unsupported assumptions about psychopathology.

Second, the implicit assumption that patients typically present with symptoms of a specific Axis I diagnosis and can identify at the start of treatment precisely which one it is (with, perhaps, the aid of a telephone screen and a structured interview) is not generally valid.[6] For historical rather than rational or scientific reasons, treatment research has proceeded independently of any kind of systematic needs assessment of the reasons the average patient presents for psychotherapy in clinical practice. Instead, *DSM* (typically Axis I) categories have largely guided the psychotherapy research agenda in the past 20 years (Goldfried, 2000). Whether most patients seek treatment complaining primarily of Axis I disorders, either clinical or subclinical; whether most patients present primarily with interpersonal concerns (or with depression or anxiety in the context of interpersonal concerns, such as problematic relationship patterns, difficulties at work, etc.); or whether the average patient presents with a diffuse picture that requires more extensive case formulation than counting up diagnostic criteria is unknown (see Persons, 1991; Westen, 1998a). However, the best available data from both naturalistic and community (catchment) studies suggest that between one third and one half of patients who seek mental health treatment cannot be diagnosed using the *DSM* because their problems do not fit or cross thresholds for any existing category (see Howard, et al., 1996; Messer, 2001). As Goldfried (2000) has observed, the requirement by funding agencies that researchers focus treatment research on *DSM*-defined psychiatric conditions has virtually eliminated research on problems that once dominated psychotherapy research, such as public speaking anxiety, interpersonal problems, or problems often associated

---

[6] This assumption is, we suspect, rarely challenged in the treatment literature because of sampling techniques commonly used in psychotherapy research that render the problem opaque: Researchers typically establish specialty clinics for particular disorders and draw patients who self-identify as suffering primarily from those disorders. This is an area in which clinical observation may provide an important corrective to observation in the laboratory.

with anxiety and depression both between and during episodes such as problematic self-esteem regulation.

A third problem in linking treatment research to Axis I categories is a pragmatic one. As several commentators have pointed out (e.g., Beutler, Moleiro, & Talebi, 2002; Weinberger, 2000), the sheer number of disorders in the *DSM–IV* renders the notion of clinicians learning disorder-specific manuals for more than a handful of disorders unrealistic. Given that 40% to 60% of patients do not respond to a first-line EST for most disorders (e.g., major depression or bulimia nervosa), clinicians would need to learn at least two or three manuals for each disorder. If researchers then start developing manuals for other disorders—including "atypical," "not otherwise specified," and subthreshold diagnoses—the number of manuals required for competent practice would be multiplied even further. This is a good example of a problem that is not inherent in the use of RCTs (e.g., for testing specific interventions, such as exposure, or theories of change) but that is inherent in the effort to identify *treatment packages* appropriate for a particular patient population and in the shift from manuals as tools for standardizing treatment in the laboratory to tools for standardizing treatment in clinical practice, a point to which we return.

The Problem of Comorbidity

Aside from the problem of linking treatment manuals to *DSM*-defined disorders is the question of whether, in fact, patients in clinical practice typically present with one primary disorder. The literature on comorbidity in both clinical and community samples suggests that single-disorder presentations are the exception rather than the rule. (We use the term *comorbidity* here only to imply co-occurrence, given the multiple potential meanings of the term; see Lilienfeld, Waldman, & Israel, 1994). Studies consistently find that most Axis I conditions are comorbid with other Axis I or Axis II disorders in the range of 50% to 90% (e.g., Kessler, et al., 1996; Kessler, Stang, Wittchen, Stein, & Walters, 1999; Newman, Moffitt, Caspi, & Silva, 1998; Oldham, et al., 1995; Shea, Widiger, & Klein, 1992; Zimmerman, McDermut, & Mattia, 2000).

The data on comorbidity are troublesome in light of the fact that the methodology underlying the identification of ESTs implicitly commits to a model of comorbidity that most psychotherapy (and psychopathology) researchers would explicitly disavow, namely that comorbidity is random or additive (i.e., that some people just happen to have multiple disorders, rather than that their symptoms might be interrelated). It may well be, as many advocates of ESTs have argued (e.g., Wilson, 1998), that the best way to approach a polysymptomatic picture is to use sequential manuals, one for depression, one for PTSD, one for GAD, and so forth. However, sequential symptom targeting may not be an optimal treatment strategy under conditions in which (a) seemingly distinct Axis I symptoms reflect common underlying causes, such as anxiety and depression that both stem from rejection sensitivity or a tendency to experience negative affect; (b) Axis I symptoms arise in the context of enduring personality patterns that create psychosocial vulnerabilities to future episodes; or (c) the presence of multiple symptoms can have emergent properties not reducible to the characteristics of each symptom independently.

As we argue below, the available data suggest that each of these conditions is frequently met. For example, depressed patients with a lifetime history of panic-agoraphobia spectrum symptoms not only show less response to interpersonal psychotherapy (IPT) in controlled clinical trials but also take substantially longer to respond to a sequential treatment strategy including selective serotonin reuptake inhibitors if they fail to respond to psychotherapy (Frank, et al., 2000). This is not to say that such findings are universal; RCTs for some treatments and disorders have found just the opposite, that comorbidity has little impact on treatment outcome or that treatment of the target disorder leads to reduction of comorbid symptomatology (e.g., Borkovec, Abel, & Newman, 1995; Brown & Barlow, 1992). The point is simply that one cannot routinely assume that psychopathology is additive or can be treated as such.

The Function of Comorbidity Assessment and Generalizability to Everyday Clinical Practice

What is perhaps less obvious than the problem of comorbidity for treatments designed for single disorders is that the function of assessing for co-occurring conditions differs in research and practice in a way that can affect the generalizability of ESTs. Researchers typically begin by soliciting patients with a particular disorder, either through direct advertising or by informing clinicians in a treatment setting (usually a university clinic or medical center) about the kinds of patients suitable for the study. Respondents undergo a brief initial screen (often by telephone) to determine whether they are potentially appropriate for the treatment protocol, followed by a structured interview or set of interviews to make a final determination about their appropriateness for the study and to obtain pretreatment diagnostic data. Following this assessment, those admitted to the study arrive at the research therapist's office, and the treatment begins. Clinicians in studies assessing the efficacy of ESTs usually do not conduct their own evaluation and proceed on the assumption that the diagnosis is accurate and primary.

The point to note here is the function of assessing comorbid conditions in the laboratory, which is generally to eliminate patients who do not meet study criteria. The treating clinician may not even know whether the patient received a secondary diagnosis, which is typically immaterial to the treatment. Indeed, the clinician usually is kept blind to secondary diagnoses if one goal of the study is to assess their potential role as moderators of outcome.

In clinical practice, the situation is very different. Unless the patient has specifically sought out a specialist who works with a particular population, clinicians typically do not assume that one symptom or syndrome is primary. Rather than starting with one symptom or syndrome in mind, clinicians are likely to inquire broadly about the patient's symptoms, history, and so forth. Even for the unknown percentage of patients in clinical practice who identify a primary concern, the aim of inquiring about co-occurring conditions is not to decide whether to refer them elsewhere but to understand them better. This generally entails developing a tentative case formulation that cuts across symptoms and is likely to be substantially more varied than the standardized formulations about maladaptive schemas, interpersonal role transitions, and so forth that are essential in research to minimize within-group variation in interventions (see Persons & Tompkins, 1997; Westen, 1998a). We are not arguing here about the validity of clinicians' formulations, an issue addressed elsewhere (see Westen & Shedler, 1999a; Westen & Weinberger, 2003). Rather, we are simply noting the extent to which the requisites of experimental control in EST methodology limit the extent of variation permitted in case formulation, if variation in formulation is potentially related to variation in treatment delivered.

In clinical practice, symptoms initially identified as primary may not remain the focus of treatment over time, even if the clinician is appropriately responding to the patient's concerns. For example, many young people struggling with sexual orientation suffer from depression, anxiety, or suicidality (Harstein, 1996), and these psychiatric symptoms may be their primary complaint. In these cases, weeks or months of treatment may pass before the patient is able to recognize or acknowledge the source of distress. To what extent issues of this sort are responsible for some or most symptomatology in everyday practice is unknown, but the methodology of ESTs commits to the assumption of their irrelevance, for two reasons. First, testing treatments brief enough to maintain experimental control and prescribing the number of sessions in advance to maximize comparability of treatments within and across conditions places a premium on rapid identification of treatment targets. Second, manualization presupposes that the same techniques (e.g., challenging dysfunctional cognitions, addressing problems in current relationships) should work for the same Axis I symptom or syndrome regardless of etiology, the circumstances that elicited it, the patient's personality, and so forth. This is one of many possible assumptions about the relationship between interventions and symptoms, but it is an untested one, and it should not be built into the structure of hypothesis testing for all forms of treatment for all disorders. It seems unlikely on the face of it, for example, that the same techniques useful for helping a depressed patient with situationally induced feelings of inadequacy (e.g., after a job loss) will always be optimal for treating someone with *chronic* feelings of inadequacy, let alone someone with the same symptom (depression) who is struggling with unacknowledged homosexuality, adult sequelae of childhood sexual abuse, aging in the context of a narcissistic personality style, or gene expression in the context of a family history of major depression.

Psychological Symptoms Can Be Understood and Treated in Isolation from Personality Dispositions

The assumption that psychological symptoms can be understood and treated in isolation from the personality of the person who bears them is essential to the methodology of ESTs, in large measure because of the brief, focal nature of treatment required to maximize experimental control and in part because of the focus on syndromes rather than processes or diatheses. Although treatments such as CBT and IPT target dysfunctional schemas or interpersonal patterns with roots in personality, neither treatment was intended to change enduring personality processes, and we know of no theory of personality or data suggesting that enduring personality processes or traits can typically be changed in 6 to 16 hour-long sessions. The only treatment considered an EST for personality disorders, Linehan's (1993) dialectical behavior therapy (DBT) for borderline personality disorder (BPD), takes roughly a year to complete what is essentially the first of several stages (M. M. Linehan, personal communication, May 2002). Research testing the efficacy of this first phase of DBT has found substantial behavioral change in parasuicidal behaviors (e.g., cutting) by 12 months along with a number of other clinically important outcomes (e.g., reduction in the number of days of hospitalization). However, personality variables such as feelings of emptiness showed little decline with even a year of treatment, and the enduring effects of DBT over years are unknown (Scheel, 2000).

The assumption that Axis I conditions can be treated as if they were independent of enduring personality dispositions has two complications, one empirical and one methodological, which we address in turn. The first is that, empirically, most Axis I syndromes are not independent of personality, and personality often moderates treatment response. The second is that, pragmatically, including patients who share a diagnosis such as depression but vary considerably in personality would require using sample sizes that are substantially larger than either customary or tenable for establishing ESTs.

Independence of Symptoms and Personality Processes

Accumulating evidence suggests that the first part of this assumption, that Axis I symptoms or syndromes can be understood apart from personality processes, is inaccurate for most disorders. Studies using factor analysis, latent class analysis, and structural equation modeling suggest that Axis I anxiety and mood disorders are systematically related to variables long considered personality variables, notably high negative and low positive affect (Brown, et al., 1998; Krueger, 2002; Mineka, Watson, & Clark, 1998; Watson & Clark, 1992; Watson, et al., 1994; Zinbarg & Barlow, 1996). Other research has found that different kinds of personality diatheses, such as vulnerability to loss versus vulnerability to failure, predispose different individuals to become depressed under different circumstances (e.g., Blatt & Zuroff, 1992; Hammen, Ellicott, Gitlin, & Jamison, 1989; Kwon & Whisman, 1998). The prevalence of comorbid Axis I conditions in patients treated for disorders such as depression, GAD, PTSD, and bulimia may actually provide an index of the prevalence of underlying personality diatheses. Studies using both adult (Newman, et al., 1998) and adolescent (Lewinsohn, Rohde, Seeley, & Klein, 1997) samples suggest that the presence of multiple Axis I conditions is essentially a proxy for the presence of an Axis II condition, with the more Axis I symptoms present, the greater the likelihood of Axis II pathology.

Furthermore, a growing body of data suggests that the same Axis I symptom or syndrome may have different functions or implications in the presence of certain kinds of personality disturbance. Research on adolescents and adults with BPD has found differences on dozens of variables between patients diagnosed with major depressive disorder with and without BPD. A case in point is the way these patients experience, express, and attempt to regulate their distress. Borderline depression is not only quantitatively but qualitatively distinct from non-borderline depression, with markedly different correlates (Westen, et al., 1992; Westen, Muderrisoglu, Fowler, Shedler, & Koren, 1997; Wixom, Ludolph, & Westen, 1993). For example, for people with both major depressive disorder and BPD, severity of depression is strongly correlated with a latent variable that includes abandonment fears, diffuse negative affectivity, an inability to maintain a soothing and constant image of significant others, and feelings of self-loathing and evilness. For people who have major depressive disorder without BPD, the same qualities are negatively correlated with severity of depression.

As noted above, data from many disorders and treatments (but not all; see, e.g., Hardy, et al., 1995; Kyuken, Kurzer, DeRubeis, Beck, & Brown, 2001) suggest that patients treated for Axis I conditions often fare less well if they also have certain personality disorders, particularly BPD (e.g., Johnson, Tobin, & Dennis, 1991; Steiger & Stotland, 1996). Although this is typically described in terms of comorbidity as a moderator variable, the concept of comorbidity may be misleading because it implies that personality variables are an add-on to a symptom picture that is essentially distinct from them. This may be analogous to studying aspirin as a treatment for fever and viewing "comorbid" meningitis, influenza, or appendicitis as moderating the relation between treatment (aspirin) and outcome (fever reduction). From a treatment perspective, the high correlations between trait anxiety and depression, and the substantial comorbidity between major depression and virtually every anxiety disorder, suggest that researchers might do well to develop treatments for negative affectivity and emotional dysregulation rather than focusing exclusively on *DSM*-defined syndromes.

The Paradox of Pure Samples

The prevalence of personality diatheses for psychopathology presents a methodological paradox. If researchers include patients with substantial personality pathology in clinical trials, they run the risk of ambiguous conclusions if these variables moderate outcome, unless sample sizes are sufficiently large to permit covariation or moderator analyses. If instead they exclude such patients (which, as we later note, is the norm, either explicitly or de facto through use of exclusion criteria such as suicidal ideation or substance abuse), one cannot assume generalizability to a target population that is rarely symptomatically pure.

The reader may object that starting with relatively pure cases is just the beginning of the enterprise: The appropriate way to develop and test a treatment is to begin with relatively circumscribed efficacy trials and then to move to community settings, where researchers can test experimental conditions that have already demonstrated efficacy in the laboratory. This sequential progression from pure to impure cases is probably an appropriate strategy for testing some therapies for some disorders (e.g., simple phobia or panic disorder, which may present as relatively discrete symptom constellations even within a polysymptomatic picture), but with two important caveats.

First, this approach commits de facto to many of the assumptions adumbrated here, most importantly the assumption that the polysymptomatic conditions seen in the community have no emergent properties that might call for different types of interventions. Interventions to address such emergent properties will, as a simple result of methodological preconditions, never be identified if investigators routinely start with less complex cases and focus studies in the community on interventions previously validated in RCTs. For example, a primary focus on eating symptoms may well be appropriate for some or many patients with bulimia nervosa; however, for others, such as those who are more impulsive, eating symptoms may need to be addressed within the context of broader problems with impulse and affect regulation, of which bingeing and purging may be one clinically salient example (Westen & Harnden-Fischer, 2001). The exclusion criteria frequently used in controlled clinical trials for bulimia nervosa, including substance abuse and suicidality (which exclude patients with substantial emotional dysregulation) and abnormally low weight (which excludes patients with anorexic symptoms) may be systematically constraining the phenomena seen in the laboratory and the interventions consequently chosen for examination (for empirical data, see Thompson-Brenner, Glass, & Westen, 2003).

The second caveat is that as researchers, educators, administrators, and clinicians, we need to exercise considerable circumspection in attempting to draw conclusions for training or public policy while we await data that could provide us with a fuller understanding of the conditions under which treatments developed in the laboratory are likely to be transportable to everyday clinical practice. It is one thing to say that cognitive therapy and IPT are the best treatments tested thus far in the laboratory for patients with major depression who pass rigorous screening procedures and that we do not know yet how these or other treatments will fare in naturalistic settings with more polysymptomatic patients. It is another to say that existing laboratory data already have demonstrated that we should stop teaching, and third-party payers should stop reimbursing, longer term, often more theoretically integrative treatments widely practiced for these disorders in the community. One can argue one or the other, but not both. As we suggest later, for some disorders and some treatments, existing laboratory data do appear to have strong implications for training and practice. For others, including several treatments widely viewed as ESTs, the empirical data support greater restraint in drawing conclusions until considerably more is known about the parameters within which these treatments are likely to operate effectively.

Controlled Clinical Trials Provide the Gold Standard for Assessing Therapeutic Efficacy

Perhaps the most central assumption underlying the enterprise of establishing ESTs is that RCT methodology provides the gold standard for assessing the efficacy of psychotherapeutic interventions. In this section we address a series of subassumptions or corollary assumptions central to assessing the validity of this assumption. These assumptions regard the functions of manualization, the pragmatics of dismantling, the independence of scientific conclusions from the processes used to select treatments to test, and the compatibility of the requisites of good science and good practice.

The Functions of Manualization

A key component of the assumption that experimental methods provide a gold standard for establishing ESTs is the corollary assumption that the elements of efficacious treatment can be spelled out in manualized form and that the interventions specified in the manual are the ones that are causally related to outcome. This corollary assumption is central to the rationale for the experimental study of psychotherapy because the aim of manualization is standardization of the intervention across participants and the control of potential confounding variables (see Wilson, 1998). Here we examine the logic of this assumption and the empirical data bearing on it.

The logic of manualization. There can be no question that some form of manualization, whether in the form of specific prescriptions or in the form of more general "practice guidelines" for therapists in RCTs, is essential in psychotherapy research, for multiple reasons. Manualization is essential to minimize variability within experimental conditions, to insure standardization across sites, and to allow consumers of research to know what is being tested. One cannot test experimental manipulations one cannot operationalize. We argue, however, that EST methodology imposes constraints on the ways manualization can be implemented that limit its flexibility and utility in generating scientifically and clinically useful data.

From the standpoint of experimental methodology, the best manual is one that can standardize the "dose," the timing of the dose, and the specific ingredients delivered in each dose. This is the only way to minimize within-group variation and hence to be certain that all patients in a given treatment condition are really receiving the same treatment. The ideal manual from an experimental point of view would thus specify not only the number of sessions but precisely what is to happen in each session or at least within a narrow band of sessions. The more a manual deviates from this ideal, the less one can draw causal conclusions about precisely what caused experimental effects.

This simple methodological desideratum has broad implications, the most important of which is as follows: The extent to which a treatment requires a competent clinical decision maker who must decide how and where to intervene on the basis of principles (even principles carefully delineated in a manual) is the extent to which that treatment will not be able to come under experimental control in the laboratory. This places a premium on development of treatment packages that minimize clinical judgment because such treatments are the only ones that allow researchers to draw firm causal conclusions. If clinicians are then to use these treatments in everyday practice, the most empirically defensible way to do so is to adhere closely to the manual. This simple logical entailment of scientific method as applied to ESTs has led to a significant shift in training goals in many clinical psychology programs, away from training clinicians who can intervene with patients on the basis of their knowledge of relatively broad, empirically supported principles of change (e.g., efforts at response prevention must include attention to covert forms of avoidance that prevent extinction or habituation) toward training clinicians who can competently follow one manual for depression, another for BPD, another for social phobia, and so forth.

Historically, manuals did not arise as prescriptions for clinical practice. Manualization was simply a method for operationalizing what investigators were trying to study. The goal of manual development was to obviate the need for the kinds of secondary correlational analyses that are becoming increasingly common in psychotherapy research as researchers address the limits of experimental control in complex treatments (e.g., predicting outcome from therapist competence or adherence). Secondary analyses of this sort shift the nature of the question from a causal one (does this treatment produce better results than another treatment or a control condition?) to a correlational one (are these particular intervention strategies associated with positive outcome?). The more researchers must ask the second question, the less valuable manualization becomes (and indeed, the more problematic it becomes, because it artificially restricts the range of interventions tested to those predicted to be useful a priori and hence limits what might be learned about mechanisms of change).

The reader may object that manualization is a broad construct, and one that is currently undergoing considerable discussion and revision (see, e.g., Carroll & Nuro, 2002). However, as argued above, the logic of EST methodology requires a very particular form and use of manualization, one that many of its advocates may explicitly reject. As RCT methodology has metamorphosed into EST methodology, a shift has occurred from a view of experimental manipulations as *exemplars* of specific constructs to a view of experimental conditions as *constitutive* of those constructs. Put another way, a reversal of means and ends is taking place whereby manuals are not just convenient ways of operationalizing treatments in the laboratory but are the defining features of the treatments themselves. In the former approach to experimentation, as in most psychological research, the investigator sees the experimental intervention as drawn from a sample of possible interventions instantiating a particular construct. Just as a researcher studying the impact of positive affect on problem solving can operationalize induction of positive affect by having participants eat a candy bar, think about pleasant memories, or receive positive feedback, a researcher studying the impact of exposure on specific social phobia can operationalize exposure in dozens of ways. The goal in these cases is to generalize about the impact of positive affect or exposure on the dependent variables of interest, not about the impact of receiving a candy bar or performing a particular set of role-plays in a group. In the latter approach, in contrast, the researcher views the intervention not as an example of how one might proceed but as how one actually should proceed. Viewed this way, deviation from the package is just as problematic in everyday practice as in the laboratory because it renders the intervention different from the one that has been tested.

The difference between these two approaches to manualization is subtle, but the implications are enormous. Consider the case of IPT for depression. The IPT manual was originally devised simply as an attempt to operationalize, for research purposes, the kinds of interventions dynamically informed psychopharmacologists of the late 1960s used with their patients, particularly as a complement to acute medication treatment (see Frank & Spanier, 1995). Within a short span of years, however, researchers were exhorting clinicians to practice IPT but not the kinds of treatments it was attempting to approximate because the latter, unlike the former, had never been empirically validated.

Along with this shift in means and ends has come a shift from the study of treatment principles to the validation of treatment packages and a corresponding shift in the function of manuals from a descriptive one (allowing researchers to describe their experimental manipulations precisely) to a prescriptive one (standardization of clinical activity in everyday practice, so that clinicians carry out interventions in the precise ways they have been tested). In a prior era, clinicians who kept abreast of the empirical literature might have tried an exposure-based technique with a patient who manifested some form of avoidance, regardless of whether the patient carried a particular diagnosis. Today, an empirically minded clinician faces a dichotomous choice when confronted with a patient who meets certain diagnostic criteria: either to implement an empirically supported treatment package as a whole or to disregard psychological science. The clinician cannot, in good empirical faith, pick and choose elements of one treatment package or another because it is the package as a whole, not its specific components or mechanisms that have been validated. Any divergence from the manual represents an unfounded belief in the validity of one's clinical judgment, which the clinician has learned is likely, on average, to produce worse outcomes.

What has not, we believe, been adequately appreciated is the extent to which a particular view of clinicians is an unintended but inexorable consequence of EST methodology. Any exercise of clinical judgment represents a threat to internal validity in controlled trials because it reduces standardization of the experimental manipulation and hence renders causal inferences ambiguous. A good clinician in an efficacy study (and, by extension, in clinical practice, if practitioners are to implement treatment manuals in the ways that have received empirical support) is one who adheres closely to the manual, does not get sidetracked by material the patient introduces that diverges from the agenda set forth in the manual, and does not succumb to the seductive siren of clinical experience. The more researchers succeed in the scientifically essential task of reducing the clinician to a research assistant who can "run subjects" in a relatively uniform (standardized) way, the more they are likely to view psychotherapy as the job of paraprofessionals who cannot—and should not—exercise clinical judgment in selecting interventions or interpreting the data of clinical observation.

The logic of experimental method in ESTs actually dictates not only the kind of therapist interventions that can be tested or permitted (those that can be rigorously manualized) but also the kind of patient activity. The scientific utility of treatment manuals is maximized in treatments in which the therapist sets the agenda for each session. Where patients have a substantial degree of control over the content or structure of treatment hours, therapists by definition have less control. Where therapists have less control, standardization is diminished and within-group variance attributable to sources other than standardized technique is correspondingly increased. The paradox of manualization for disorders such as depression and GAD is that the patient's active involvement in the treatment is likely to be essential to good outcome but destructive of experimental control. Modeled after dosing in medication trials (an analogy explicit in dose-response curves in psychotherapy research; see Stiles & Shapiro, 1989), manualization commits researchers to an assumption that is only appropriate for a limited range of treatments, namely that therapy is something done to a patient—a process in which the therapist applies interventions— rather than a transactional process in which patient and therapist collaborate. As we note below, within the range of cognitive- behavioral treatments, those that require genuine collaboration and creative problem solving on the part of the patient, such as A. T. Beck's (1976) cognitive therapy for depression (which explicitly aims at a "collaborative empiricism" between therapist and patient), have proven most recalcitrant to experimental control and require the most secondary correlational analyses to understand what is curative.

Empirical data on manualization. We have argued thus far that the logic of manualization is problematic for many disorders and treatments. So too are the empirical data bearing on assumption that the interventions specified in treatment manuals are causally linked to change. For many brief treatments for many disorders, the lion's share of the effect emerges before the patient has been administered the putatively mutative components of the treatment. For example, most of the treatment effects demonstrated in studies of cognitive therapy for depression occur by the fifth session, with treatment effects leveling off asymptotically after that (Ilardi & Craighead, 1994). Although researchers have challenged these findings (Tang & DeRubeis, 1999), studies using CBT to treat bulimia nervosa similarly have found that patients who do not reduce purging by 70% by the sixth session (prior to most of the interventions aimed at cognitive restructuring) are unlikely to respond to treatment (Agras, et al., 2000; see also Wilson, 1999), and recent research with a different treatment, supportive-expressive therapy, has similarly found that sudden gains tend to occur around the fifth session (Asay, Lambert, Gregersen, & Goates, 2002). Similar findings have also emerged repeatedly in naturalistic samples of psychotherapy for patients with a range of problems, who tend to experience a "remoralization" process that restores hope and reduces symptomatology after a handful of sessions (Howard, et al., 1993).

Furthermore, therapist adherence to manuals has proven only variably associated with outcome—sometimes positively correlated, sometimes negatively, and sometimes not at all (e.g., Castonguay, Goldfried, Wiser, Raue, & Hayes, 1996; Feeley, DeRubeis, & Gelfand, 1999; Henry, Strupp, Butler, Schacht, & Binder, 1993; Jones & Pulos, 1993)—and correlational analyses have sometimes identified important but unexpected links between process and outcome, such as the finding that focusing on parental issues may be associated with positive outcome in cognitive therapy for depression (Hayes, Castonguay, & Goldfried, 1996). In one study (Ablon & Jones, 1998), researchers used the Psychotherapy Process Q Set (Jones, 2000; Jones & Pulos, 1993) to measure process variables from psychotherapy transcripts of both cognitive and psychodynamic short-term therapies for depression. Not only did therapists of both persuasions use techniques from the other approach (a finding similar to that reported by Castonguay, et al., 1996), but in both forms of treatment, positive outcome was associated with the extent to which the treatment matched the empirical prototype of psychodynamic psychotherapy. In this study, the extent to which cognitive therapists used cognitive techniques was actually unrelated to outcome.

In a second study (Ablon & Jones, 1999, 2002), the investigators used the Psychotherapy Process Q Set to study the process of psychotherapy in the National Institute of Mental Health (NIMH) Treatment of Depression Collaborative Research Program (Elkin, et al., 1989). They found that both treatments, as actually practiced, strongly resembled the empirical prototype of cognitive therapy, and neither resembled the psychodynamic prototype, even though IPT was derived from the work of theorists such as Sullivan (1953; see also Frank & Spanier, 1995) and is frequently described as a brief psychodynamic variant. Ablon and Jones (1999, 2002) suggested that despite careful efforts at manualization and adherence checks, the NIMH Collaborative Research Program may have compared two cognitive therapies. In this study, adherence to the cognitive therapy prototype was most predictive of change, regardless of which treatment the clinician was attempting to practice.

Another study, using an instrument designed specifically to distinguish CBT and IPT, did find small but significant mean differences between the CBT and IPT conditions on factors designed to distinguish them (Hill, O'Grady, & Elkin, 1992). However, both treatments were best characterized by items designed to assess two nonspecific aspects of treatment characteristic of the control condition, labeled *explicit directiveness* and *facilitative directiveness*.

To what extent similar findings would emerge for other disorders is unknown. We suspect that for specific anxiety disorders, such as simple phobia, specific social phobia, and obsessive-compulsive disorder (OCD), different treatments would be more readily distinguishable. The point, however, is that, as a general assumption, the assumption that the interventions specified in treatment manuals are causally linked to change is not well supported and needs to be demonstrated empirically for a given set of treatments rather than assumed.

Dismantling and the Scientific Testing of Treatment Packages

Another corollary to the assumption that experimental methods provide a gold standard for establishing the validity of therapeutic interventions is that the elements of efficacious treatment are dissociable and hence subject to dismantling. Again, as with the other assumptions and corollary assumptions described here, this one is likely applicable to varying degrees to different treatments and disorders. Dismantling is most readily applied to brief treatments with highly specific procedures, where therapists can adhere closely to a manual and either include or exclude a particular set of interventions, such as cognitive restructuring in exposure-based treatments for OCD or PTSD.

The dismantling assumption is appropriate for RCT methodology (and is indeed one of the advantages of that methodology), but it is invalid as a general rule for EST methodology. The reason lies again in what is being tested, namely treatment packages rather than specific interventions or classes of intervention. Consider, for example, the manual for CBT for bulimia nervosa (Fairburn, Marcus, & Wilson, 1993), which has received considerable empirical support. The manual prescribes that clinicians begin with psychoeducational and behavioral interventions, then move to cognitive interventions, and conclude with interventions aimed at maintenance of change over time. But would treatment as prescribed by this manual as currently configured be superior to the same treatment delivered without the behavioral interventions, or with the order of interventions inverted (cognitive first, behavioral second), or with an initial 5 sessions devoted to alliance building, or with an additional module aimed at addressing interpersonal problems or affect regulation, or simply with the exact same treatment extended to 60 sessions? No one has ever tested, or will ever likely test, any of these variations, even though each of them could be equally justified by theory and might well be more efficacious. The process of selecting the particular package of interventions the investigators selected is, in the philosopher of science Karl Popper's (1959) terms, a *pre*scientific process (i.e., prior to hypothesis testing), and one that has set the agenda for the subsequent scientific process of testing this manual against other treatments and control conditions. Or to use the language of Paul Meehl (1954), it is a prime example of *clinical prediction* (nonquantitative, synthetic judgments about what might work).

The reality is that researchers generally solidify treatment packages (manuals) so early and on the basis of so little hard data on alternative strategies, even within the same general approach, that clinicians have to accept *on faith* that the treatment as packaged is superior to the myriad variants one could devise or improvise with a given patient. It is difficult enough to conduct one or two methodologically rigorous clinical trials with a single manual. To expect researchers to test one or more of the infinite variants of it that could potentially have better efficacy is simply untenable. As we suggest below (see also Beutler, 2000), investigators may do better to focus RCT methodology on the testing of interventions, intervention strategies, and processes of change rather than putatively complete treatments and to strive for guidelines that foster the practice of empirically informed rather than empirically validated psychotherapies.

Science and Prescience: Selection of Treatments to Test as a Source of Bias

Another significant caveat to the assumption that experimental methods provide a gold standard for testing treatments is the problem of determining which treatments to test. One can only separate lead from gold by testing the properties of both. If, as a field, we choose to study only certain kinds of treatments, we cannot draw conclusions about treatment of choice except within the (small) universe of treatments that have received empirical attention. Because of its requirement of brevity and experimenter control, the methodology of ESTs has precluded the testing of treatments widely used in the community, leading to the conclusion that such treatments are empirically unsupported. This conclusion, however, is logically entailed by the method, not determined empirically. Treatments that cannot be tested using a particular set of methods by definition cannot be supported using those methods. Given the powerful allegiance effects documented in psychotherapy research, in which the treatment favored by the investigator tends to produce the superior outcome (Luborsky, et al., 1999),[7] perhaps the best predictors of whether a treatment finds its way to the empirically supported list are whether anyone has been motivated (and funded) to test it and whether it is readily testable in a relatively brief format.

Lest the reader object that this is an unfair characterization, consider a recent monograph commissioned by the American Psychological Society (APS) on the treatment of depression (Hollon, Thase, & Markowitz, 2002). As the authors noted, numerous studies have shown that CBT and IPT (and a number of lesser-known brands) produce initial outcomes comparable with those obtained with medications. Over the course of 3 years, however, patients who receive these 16-session psychotherapies relapse at unacceptably high rates relative to patients in medication conditions if the latter are maintained on medication during the follow-up period (Hollon, et al., 2002). These findings have prompted researchers to test maintenance psychotherapy, which essentially extends brief manualized treatments into long-term treatments.

The results have been promising. As the authors suggested, although monthly IPT maintenance treatment over 3 years does not fare as well as continuous provision of medication, studies testing it have compared low-dose IPT with high-dose imipramine (Hollon, et al., 2002), and IPT might do considerably better if provided continuously for 3 years on a more frequent basis. At the end of the monograph, the authors reiterated that CBT and IPT are the psychotherapies

---

[7] Luborsky, et al. (1999) found that by measuring allegiance in multiple ways, they could account for over 69% of the variance in outcome across a large set of studies by allegiance alone. If one converts their multiple correlation (R) of .85 to a binomial effect size (Rosenthal, 1991), the implication is that 92.5% of the time, they could predict which treatment will be most successful based on investigator allegiance alone. Although this may be a liberal estimate, even an estimate one third of this magnitude would have tremendous consequences for the enterprise of testing psychotherapies.

of choice for depression but suggested that the wave of the future may be long-term maintenance CBT and IPT:

> Despite real progress over the past 50 years, many depressed patients still do not respond fully to treatment. Only about half of all patients respond to any given intervention, and only about a third eventually meet the criteria for remission . . . . Moreover, most patients will not stay well once they get better unless they receive ongoing treatment. (Hollon, et al., 2002, p. 70)

The authors likened depression to chronic disorders such as diabetes, suggested that depression "may require nearly continuous treatment in order to ensure that symptoms do not return," and concluded with the familiar lamentation that "too few patients have access to empirically supported treatments" (Hollon, et al., 2002, p. 70).

If one steps back for a moment, however, the argument appears circular. Thirty years ago, a group of researchers, convinced that the therapies practiced by most clinicians were needlessly long and unfocused, quite reasonably set about to use experimental methods to test more focal treatments aimed at changing explicit thoughts and feelings and current interpersonal circumstances contributing to depression. After an initial 20 years or so of enthusiasm, counterevidence began to amass, first and most importantly from the NIMH Collaborative Research Program (Elkin, et al., 1989). The NIMH Collaborative Research Program had an enormous sample size relative to prior studies, and it eliminated two confounds that had rendered interpretation of prior findings difficult: common factors (a confound eliminated by incorporating a rigorous "medical management" placebo control group) and allegiance effects (eliminated by employing investigators at all three sites with allegiance to each of the treatments under investigation). Despite a promising initial response, by 18 months post treatment, the outcome of brief psychotherapy was indistinguishable from a well-constructed placebo. Subsequent studies (see Hollon, et al., 2002) found that 16 weeks of IPT or CBT could not compare in efficacy with a continuous course of medication.

Placed in their broader context, these studies appear to provide a definitive disconfirmation of the central hypothesis that motivated this line of research, namely that depression is amenable to brief psychotherapies, specifically those focusing on explicit cognitive processes or current interpersonal patterns. Yet the authors of the monograph came to a very different conclusion. On the basis of data showing that extending short-term interventions by several months substantially improves outcome, they concluded that only long-term versions of these short-term treatments are empirically supportable (Hollon, et al., 2002). This conclusion makes sense of the available data, but the available data were predicated on a set of methodological assumptions that presume the disconfirmed hypothesis, that depression is malleable in the face of brief interventions. These methods precluded from the start the testing of the kind of long-term psychotherapies the researchers had set out to show 30 years ago were unnecessarily lengthy, and these methods continue today to preclude the testing of integrative treatments that might address current states and diatheses, explicit and implicit processes, current and enduring interpersonal problems, and so forth (see Westen, 2000).[8] This is not to say that such treatments would turn out to be more effective. That is an unknown. But it will remain unknown as long as treatments are required to fit the requisites of methods rather than vice versa.[9]

Can hypothesis testing be isolated from hypothesis generation?

What we are suggesting here is that the influence of prescientific processes can lead to scientifically invalid conclusions despite the safeguards of scientific method imposed at the level of hypothesis testing. Consider again the example of psychotherapy for depression and what might have happened if the NIMH Collaborative Research Program had compared CBT not with IPT but with psychodynamic psychotherapy, which at that time was the most widely practiced psychotherapy in the community. Given the ultimate convergence of the findings from the NIMH Collaborative Research Program with the results of decades of psychotherapy research indicating that brief psychotherapies for depression tend to show similar results as long as they are tested by investigators invested in them (Luborsky, et al., 1999; Wampold, et al., 1997), what would probably be taught today is that CBT and psychodynamic psychotherapy are the psychotherapeutic treatments of choice for depression.

This example highlights the extent to which the conclusions reached in the EST literature depend on a highly problematic tenet of Popper's (1959) philosophy of science that as a field we have implicitly embraced: that the essence of science lies in hypothesis testing (the context of scientific justification) and that

---

[8] The reader may object, with some justification, that clinical experience should not dictate the treatments that are tested. We suspect, however, that the failure to test treatments widely used in clinical practice is imprudent, given that clinicians, like other organisms subject to operant conditioning, are likely to learn something useful, if only incidentally, when they peck at a target long enough. They may also develop all kinds of superstitious behavior (as well as false beliefs, illusory correlations, and all the other biases and heuristics that inflict information processors, including clinical information processors), but one should not assume that expertise in clinical work or any other domain leads only to such biases and errors.

[9] One could, in fact, tell a very important story from the data summarized by the authors of the APS monograph (Hollon, et al. 2002): that helping patients in an acute depressive episode problem solve, recognize ways they may be inadvertently maintaining their depression, and get moving again behaviorally and interpersonally can, in the context of a supportive relationship, be extremely useful in reducing the severity and duration of depressive episodes (and that some patients can remember and mobilize these resources the next time they become severely depressed). Ellen Frank, who has been one of the most productive contributors to the IPT literature, reached a similar conclusion in one of the most balanced presentations of the results of RCT's of CBT and IPT for depression we have seen (Frank & Spanier, 1995, p. 356). Such a conclusion is, we believe, justified by the available data and is in fact a variation on the theme of the story the authors told. But it requires a substantial shift in aims, from using RCT's to validate treatment packages for depression to using RCT's to assess intervention strategies that may prove useful to clinicians at particular junctures with patients for whom depressive symptoms are clinically significant.

where one finds one's hypotheses (the context of discovery) is one's own business. There can be no more powerful way to create a gulf between clinical practice and research than to compare laboratory derived interventions with everything but what clinicians practice in the community. The paradoxical effect of doing so is that it places empirically minded clinicians in the position of having to guess, without data, how their own ways of intervening might fare relative to laboratory-based treatments.

The reader may object that a host of studies have compared established therapies with "treatment as usual" (TAU). Unfortunately, TAU comparison groups virtually all consist of low-budget, low-frequency treatments with minimally trained paraprofessionals struggling to cope with enormous caseloads (see, e.g., Scheel, 2000). The use of this kind of TAU comparison is not likely to change the mind of many clinicians and in fact should not do so if they understand scientific method, because such conditions do not control for several obvious confounds that render causal inference impossible (e.g., treatment frequency, caseload size, commitment of clinicians to the treatment, and level of training and supervision; see Borkovec & Castonguay, 1998). As suggested below, as researchers, we should exercise more caution in using terms such as *treatment as usual*, *traditional therapy*, or treatment as practiced *in the community* (e.g., Weiss, Catron, & Harris, 2000) if what we really mean is treatment as practiced by masters-level clinicians in community mental health centers (CMHCs) with low-income patients, where notoriously difficult treatment populations intersect with notoriously limited care.

Empirically unvalidated and empirically invalidated

The failure to apply scientific methods to the selection of treatments to subject to empirical scrutiny has contributed to a widespread confusion in the literature, sometimes explicit and sometimes implicit, between empirically untested and empirically disconfirmed, or empirically *un*validated and empirically *in*validated, psychotherapies (Roth & Fonagy, 1996; Weinberger, 2000; Westen & Morrison, 2001). Consider, for example, the following statement from the chapter on CBT for bulimia nervosa in the *Handbook of Treatment for Eating Disorders*:

> Many patients will be somewhat symptomatic at the end of the 19-session manual-based treatment. In our clinical experience, patients in the United States, with its ready availability of different forms of psychological therapy and a tradition of largely open-ended treatment, will often wish to seek additional therapy at the end of the 19 sessions of CBT. We reiterate the caveat issued by Fairburn, Marcus and Wilson . . . about the inadvisability of a rush into further therapy. Patients should be encouraged to follow through on their maintenance plans and to "be their own therapists" as CBT has emphasized. If after a period of some months

their problems have not improved, or possibly deteriorated, they can then seek additional treatment. (Wilson, Fairburn, & Agras, 1997, p. 85)

What is clear from this quotation is that the authors do not take an agnostic attitude toward empirically untested treatments practiced in the community. They clearly view the absence of evidence for efficacy of treatments practiced in the community as evidence for absence of efficacy and hence feel confident informing non- or partial-responders (who constitute more than half of patients who undergo CBT or any other brief treatment for bulimia nervosa) that other treatments are unlikely to help them.[10] The authors of the APS monograph on treatment of depression similarly equated untested treatments with inadequate treatments when they concluded that "the empirically supported psychotherapies are still not widely practiced. *As a consequence* [italics added], many patients do not have access to adequate treatment" (Hollon, et al., 2002, p. 39).

Incompatibilities between the Requisites of Experimental Design and Practice

A final problem with the assumption that experimental methods provide a gold standard for separating the clinical wheat from the chaff is the extent to which the requisites of experimental research aimed at identifying ESTs can diverge from the requisites of good treatment, leading to a state of affairs in which the methodological tail wags the clinical dog. Consider again the case of IPT as an empirically supported treatment for bulimia. (We hope readers do not interpret our occasional oversampling of research on bulimia nervosa, which has produced some of the most impressive findings in the treatment literature, as indicative of anything other than our familiarity with it.) When Fairburn, Kirk, O'Connor, and Cooper (1986) conducted their first RCT for bulimia, their explicit goal was to test a cognitive-behavioral treatment previously piloted in an uncontrolled study against a nondirective, nonspecific comparison treatment with some putative credibility (Fairburn, 1997). Thus, they designed a short-term focal comparison treatment, intended as a psychodynamic treatment, in which the therapist first assessed "underlying difficulties" that precipitated the bulimia and then focused on these issues for the remainder of the treatment (Fairburn, et al., 1986, p. 632). In their next trial, Fairburn, et al. (1991) substituted IPT for the original short-term focal psychotherapy because "it was similar to it in style and focus, but had the advantages of being better known and having a treatment manual available" (Fairburn, 1997, p. 280). In the first four sessions, the role of the IPT therapist was to analyze the interpersonal context in which the eating

---

[10] This example is not unusual. The national licensing examination in psychology now includes a series of questions about the "correct" treatment for disorders such as depression. Indeed, in an oral examination for licensure, one colleague who indicated that his theoretical orientation was other than CBT was asked why he practiced "an outmoded form of treatment."

disorder occurred. Thereafter, "no attention was paid to the patients' eating habits or attitudes to shape and weight" (Fairburn, et al., 1991, pp. 464-465). The reason for this injunction was to avoid any overlap with CBT, because the aim of the study was to test the effects of the specific interventions prescribed in the CBT manual.

The results of this second study were unexpected: CBT initially showed the predicted superiority to IPT, but patients in the IPT condition caught up in outcome over the months following termination (Fairburn, 1997; Fairburn, et al., 1991, 1993). As a result of the apparent success of IPT in this trial (recently replicated by Agras, et al., 2000), Klerman and Weissman (1993) published the IPT manual for treatment of bulimia nervosa. The practice of IPT for bulimia nervosa as summarized by Fairburn (1997) faithfully mirrors the manual designed for experimental use, including "little emphasis on the patient's eating problem as such, except during the assessment stage" (p. 281). The therapist explains to the patient this paradoxical injunction against discussing the symptoms that brought her in for treatment as follows: "This is because focusing on the eating disorder would tend to distract the patient and therapist from dealing with the interpersonal difficulties" (Fairburn, 1997, p. 281).

In fact, the developers of IPT for bulimia did not proscribe discussion of food, body image, eating behavior, or eating attitudes because they or their colleagues had noticed that doing so seemed to be effective. Nor did they do so because they had reason to believe, theoretically or empirically, that talking about eating behavior should be counterproductive or distracting. Indeed, their own prior controlled trials of CBT had demonstrated just the opposite. The reason the IPT manual proscribes any focus on the symptoms is that doing so made for a clean experiment, in which the effects of the two experimental conditions could be readily distinguished. And when, by accident, IPT turned out to be helpful to many patients, suddenly an experimental manipulation never intended as anything but a credible-enough control found its way into review articles as an EST for bulimia, despite the lack of any empirical evidence for one of its key components (or noncomponents), the counterintuitive injunction against discussing one of the main things the patient came in to talk about.

This example is not an anomaly. It reflects a confusion of two uses of RCT methodology, one reflecting the goal of discovering what kinds of interventions work, and the other reflecting the goal of distinguishing valid from invalid treatment packages. The latter goal becomes particularly problematic in light of the common factors problem (the repeated finding that common factors account for much of the variance in RCTs; see Lambert & Bergin, 1994; Luborsky, Barton, & Luborsky, 1975; Wampold, et al., 1997; Weinberger, 1995). A researcher testing a novel intervention in an RCT needs to control for common factors (either by eliminating them from the experimental treatment or using a rigorous control condition that includes them) to test its incremental efficacy, but this does not mean clinicians should do so. Controlling for common factors is essential for causal inference in RCTs but would be counterproductive in clinical practice, given their powerful effects on outcome. As RCTs metamorphosed into tests of the utility of treatment packages taken as a whole, however, researchers had to maximize the purity of their treatments to distinguish them from other treatments or credible controls, leading them to minimize common factors in manuals intended for use by practicing clinicians.

The case of IPT for bulimia (and the fact that CBT for bulimia places limited emphasis on interpersonal problems, reflecting the same effort to minimize treatment overlap with IPT; Wilson, et al., 1997, p. 87) is an example of what might be called the *uncommonly differentiated factors paradox* (Westen, 2002): To maximize detection of clinically and statistically significant between groups effects for ESTs, researchers need to design treatments that are maximally differentiable. Doing so, however, renders them vulnerable to developing treatments that lack precisely the factors that produce much of the effect of brief psychotherapies for many disorders. To put it another way, the demands of experimental investigation in the real world, where researchers cannot easily collect samples of several hundred patients that might help them assess the incremental effects of specific over common factors, often conflict with the demands of clinical practice in the real world. Just as experimenters cannot afford the loss of statistical power that invariably follows from implementation of *impure* treatments, clinicians cannot afford the loss of therapeutic power that follows from implementation of *pure* treatments, particularly where common factors play a role in outcome or where more than one treatment has shown incremental efficacy beyond common factors. If clinicians tend to prefer eclectic or integrative treatments for disorders such as bulimia or depression over treatments that fail to address aspects of their patients' pathology that are obvious to the naked eye but proscribed by one manual or another to maximize their distinctiveness in experiments, they are probably exercising both common sense and good clinical judgment.

Summary: The Assumptive Framework of ESTs

The question of what works for who is an empirical question that can only be addressed using empirical methods. Yet the effort to identify ESTs has led to the parallel evolution of "practice guidelines" for the conduct of psychotherapy research whose assumptions need to be carefully examined. These assumptions— that psychopathology is highly malleable, that most patients can be treated for a single problem or disorder, that personality is irrelevant or secondary in the treatment of psychiatric disorders, and that a straightforward application of experimental methods as used in other areas of psychology and in research in psychopharmacology provides the primary if not the only way to identify therapeutically useful interventions strategies—appear to be applicable to some degree to some treatments for some disorders. However, when applied indiscriminately, they are likely to lead to substantial error because they are only applicable with substantial qualification and under particular conditions. A central task ahead, and a focus of the final section of this article, is to examine more systematically the conditions under which these assumptions are likely to be accurate or inaccurate, or violated in ways that do or do not produce systematic error.

Retelling the Story: A Reexamination of the Data Supporting ESTs

Thus far we have examined the assumptions underlying the methodology widely assumed to provide the best answers to the question of what works for whom. We now turn to a reconsideration of the empirical findings using this methodology.

Consider a study of cognitive therapy for depression, which illustrates a well-designed investigation of an exemplary EST. Thase, et al. (1992) screened 130 patients with depression, of whom 76 were suitable for the treatment protocol, for an inclusion rate of 58%. Of the 76 patients included, 64 (81%) completed the treatment. Of these 64, 23 were described as fully recovered and 27 as partially recovered at the end of treatment, for a full recovery rate of roughly 36% and a partial recovery rate of slightly greater magnitude (42%). At 1-year follow-up, 16 of these 50 fully to moderately successful cases had fully relapsed, leaving 34 at least partially successful treatments at follow-up. When the definition of *relapse* was relaxed to include not only those who developed a subsequent major depressive episode but also those who developed a diagnosable mood disorder short of major depression or who required further treatment, the number who remained improved or recovered fell to 38% of those who entered treatment, or 29 of the 130 who originally sought treatment.

Whether this is the story of an empirically supported or an empirically disconfirmed therapy depends on where one puts the asterisk. In our laboratory we are in the process of completing a series of multidimensional meta-analyses of data from RCTs for a range of disorders, which provide a set of indices yielding information on both outcome and generalizability that we believe are essential for drawing scientifically and clinically meaningful conclusions from the literature (Westen & Morrison, 2001).[11] We first briefly describe those variables and then examine the findings with respect to five disorders: major depressive disorder, panic disorder, GAD, bulimia nervosa, and OCD. Next, we place these find-

---

[11] See also McDermut, Miller, and Brown (2001) for an example of the creative application of meta-analytic techniques to a range of metrics important for drawing inferences about efficacy.

ings in the context of naturalistic studies recently completed that bear on the external validity of RCTs used to establish treatments as empirically supported. Finally, we consider recent research attempting to address concerns about the external validity of ESTs.

Multidimensional Meta-Analysis: Aggregating a Range of Indicators of Outcome

The most common way of assessing the value of a treatment is to compare mean outcome of treatment, usually (but not always or exclusively) focusing on the symptom or syndrome deemed primary, with pretreatment scores, outcome obtained in a placebo or control conditions, or outcome obtained using another treatment. This method leads to a significance test, which is useful but can be misleading because statistical significance is a joint function of effect size and sample size, so that varying sample size can produce substantial fluctuations in significance values for treatments with equal effects; and to a quantifiable effect size estimate (e.g., Cohen's d) that provides a relatively straightforward measure of central tendency that can be readily summarized meta-analytically.

Effect size estimates are essential in evaluating the efficacy of a psychotherapy; however, they have certain limits. Pre-post effect size estimates, though widely reported, are difficult to interpret because passage of time, regression to the mean, spontaneous remission in disorders with fluctuating course, tendency to present for treatment (and hence for research) when symptoms are particularly severe, and other variables not specific to a given treatment can lead to symptomatic change over time. Treatment-control effect size estimates, which do not share these limitations, provide a better estimate of the extent to which a treatment is useful for the average patient. However, they do not provide information on clinically meaningful variation in treatment response. A treatment that has an enormous effect in 20% of patients can appear superior to another treatment that has a smaller but clinically meaningful impact on 90% of patients. These caveats are not meant to "demean the mean," or to devalue probability statistics, only to suggest that mean differences and their corresponding significance values and effect size estimates provide only one measure of efficacy.

A second common index of outcome, readily available in most published reports but rarely aggregated meta-analytically, is percentage improved or recovered. This metric, which we believe is an essential meta-analytic complement to effect size estimates, has a number of variations that need to be distinguished. One variation depends on the numerator (i.e., the number of patients who improved): How does one define clinically significant improvement or recovery? One could, for example, require that patients be symptom free, that their scores on outcome measures fall one or two standard deviations below their original means or within one to two standard deviations of published norms of nonclinical samples, or that they fall below a predetermined cutoff (e.g., the cut-off for major depressive disorder or panic disorder). A considerable body of literature on clinical significance has emerged to attempt to address these issues but has not yet led to any consensus (see, e.g., Jacobson, Roberts, Berns, & McGlinchey, 1999; Jacobson & Truax, 1991; Kendall, et al., 1999).[12] From a meta-analytic standpoint, the best one can usually do in aggregating across studies is to adopt "local standards" for a given disorder (e.g., rely on the most widely used definitions of improvement in the literature for a particular disorder) and care-fully distinguish between improvement and complete recovery. A treatment could, for example, lead to substantial declines in symptoms for most patients but leave all patients symptomatic. That may or may not be an indictment of an experimental treatment, depending on the severity of the disorder, the disability it imposes, and the availability of other treatments.

A second variation in estimating the percentage of patients improved or recovered involves the denominator (the number improved in relation to whom, i.e., success rates divided by what number?). Percentage improved can be calcu-lated relative to the number of patients who complete treatment or the number who entered treatment (intent-to-treat sample). If dropout rates are as high as even 20%—which they usually are—these metrics can yield very different esti-mates of improvement or recovery.

A third metric that can be readily obtained from most published reports but is rarely noted in reviews is the average level of symptomatology after treatment. A treatment may be highly efficacious in reducing symptoms in the average patient or even in most patients but still leave the vast majority of patients symp-tomatic. Thus, another way to describe outcome is to look at mean scores on widely used outcome measures or face-valid measures, such as number of panic episodes per week, to assess the absolute value of symptomatology at the end of treatment.

The question of when to measure outcome is as important as how. A key dis-tinction in this regard is between initial response and sustained efficacy. Most nonpsychotic psychiatric conditions show an initial response to a very wide range of psychosocial interventions. Fifteen percent of patients improve signifi-cantly after making the initial call to a therapist's office, before attending the first session (see Kopta, et al., 1994), and as mentioned above, much of the change seen in many brief therapies occurs within the first few sessions. Whether changes that occur by the fifth of sixth session are durable, and whether they bear any relation to long-term efficacy, is a crucial question.

---

[12] For an example of the use of clinically significant change indices in meta-analytic investigations, see McDermut et al. (2001).

Thus, a fourth set of indices assess outcome at long-term follow-up intervals. An important distinction at follow-up is between percentage improved or recovered at follow-up, and the percentage that *remained* improved or recovered at follow-up. Many psychiatric disorders are characterized by a course of multiple periods of remission and relapse or symptom exacerbation over many years; hence, knowing whether a patient is better 1, 2, or 5 years later is not the same as knowing that he or she got better as a result of treatment and remained better. Major depression, for example, is an episodic disorder, with an average duration of roughly 20 weeks if left untreated (Judd, 1997). Thus, patients who did not respond to therapy are likely, a year later, to appear improved, recovered, or no longer meeting the diagnostic threshold for major depression, but this says nothing about efficacy, particularly since patients in control conditions are rarely followed for comparison. Data on the percentage of patients who seek additional treatment in the 1 or 2 years following a controlled clinical trial can also be useful in painting a clear portrait of what works for whom. Although treatment seeking can be evidence that patients found a treatment helpful (see Kendall, et al., 1999), healthy people typically do not seek further treatment; thus, treatment seeking can provide useful information on incomplete outcomes.

A final set of indices bear on generalizability. One simple metric is the percentage of potential participants excluded at each step of screening (usually once after a phone screen and then again after a structured interview). A second way to provide research consumers with data on the kinds of patients to whom the results of a study can be assumed to generalize is to count the number of exclusion criteria and compile a list of prototypical exclusion criteria across studies. Aside from using this index as a potential moderator variable, researchers can also apply these prototypical exclusion criteria to naturalistic samples to assess the extent to which patients included in RCTs resemble patients with the same disorder treated in clinical practice (and whether comorbid conditions that lead to exclusion of patients from controlled trials are associated in everyday practice with variables such as treatment length and outcome).

Meta-analysis, like any procedure, has its advantages and limits (see Eysenck, 1995; Feinstein, 1995; Rosenthal, 1991; Rosenthal & DiMatteo, 2000), and we do not believe that our approach is without limitations. For example, because we were interested in reexamining conclusions drawn from the published literature, we did not attempt to address the "file drawer" problem by tracking down unpublished studies that might have had null findings, and hence our results are likely to be biased slightly toward positive outcomes. Similarly, too little is written about investigator bias in meta-analysis and the importance of maintaining investigator blindness in making determinations that can substantially affect the findings (Westen & Morrison, 2001). On the other hand, as a field we have known since Meehl's (1954) classic work about the advantages of actuarial over informal, synthetic (in his terms, *clinical*) judgments, and this applies as much to literature reviews as to diagnostic judgments. The best one can do is to present a range of statistics that summarize the data as comprehensively as possible and let readers study the tables and draw their own conclusions.

Efficacy of ESTs for Common Psychological Disorders: A Meta-Analytic Reassessment

In our laboratory, we have thus far completed multidimensional meta-analyses of controlled clinical trials of psychotherapy for five disorders (Eddy, Dutra, & Westen, 2004; Thompson-Brenner, et al., 2003; Westen & Morrison, 2001) and are in the process of completing similar analyses for four others. We begin with the take-home message: Empirical support is a matter of degree, which varies considerably across disorders. A dichotomous judgment of empirically supported versus not supported (implicit in the enterprise of constructing a list of ESTs) provides a very crude assessment of the state of the art.

Efficacy of Treatments for Depression, Panic, and GAD

In a first set of studies, Westen and Morrison (2001) examined all studies of ESTs for depression, panic, and GAD published in the major high-quality journals that publish controlled outcome studies of psychotherapy during the 1990s. With the partial exception of treatments for depression, effect sizes for these treatments (in standard-deviation units) were generally impressive, similar to the findings of meta-analyses of psychotherapy published since the pioneering study by Smith and Glass (1977). At termination of treatment, the median effect sizes for depression, panic, and GAD relative to placebo or control conditions were .30, .80, and .90, respectively. Data on percentage of patients improved painted a more variable picture than effect size estimates, depending on the number used as the denominator. Of those who completed treatment, success rates (defined variably across studies, but including patients who improved as well as those who recovered) ranged from 63% for panic to 52% for GAD. Of those who entered treatment (intent-to-treat analysis), improvement rates ranged from 37% for depression to 54% for panic.

Although the average patient improved substantially in active treatment conditions, the average patient also remained symptomatic (Westen & Morrison, 2001). For example, depressed patients completed the average EST with a Beck Depression Inventory (A. T. Beck, Ward, Mendelson, Mock, & Erbaugh, 1961) score above 10, which is above the cutoff for clinically significant pathology using Jacobson and Truax's (1991) criteria for clinical significance (Bouchard, et al., 1996). The average panic patient continued to panic about once every 10 days and had slightly over four out of the seven symptoms required for a *DSM–IV* panic disorder diagnosis, enough to qualify for limited-symptom attacks. This is not to diminish the very powerful effects of many of these treatments, especially for panic, given that the average patient began with frequencies of attacks that substantially affected their possibility for life satisfaction. It is simply to suggest that empirical support of validation comes in shades of gray.

For all three disorders, long-term follow-up data were almost nonexistent, and where they did exist, they tended to support only treatments for panic. Across all disorders, by 2 years post treatment, roughly half of patients in active treatment conditions had sought further treatment. Of those treated for depression, only one third had improved and remained improved over 2 years. For panic, the success rates were higher. Roughly half of patients who entered or completed treatment improved and remained improved. Even for treatments for panic, however, the investigators found that many of the patients who were symptom free at 2 years were not symptom free at 1 year, and vice versa, suggesting a variable course of waxing and waning symptoms for many whose outcomes were generally positive (Brown & Barlow, 1995). For GAD, the authors could locate no data on efficacy at 2 years or beyond.

One question that is difficult to answer because of ethical limitations of keeping patients treatment free for long periods is how treated versus untreated patients fare at extended follow-up. The only study reporting follow-up data at 18 months or longer for both treatment and control conditions was the NIMH Treatment of Depression Collaborative Research Program, which included a relatively active control condition (see Shea, Elkin, et al., 1992). In this study, 78% to 88% of those who entered treatment completely relapsed or sought further treatment by 18 months. Shea, Elkin, et al. (1992) found no significant differences on any outcome measure among any of the active treatments (cognitive therapy, IPT, and imipramine) and controls at follow-up.

Finally, with respect to generalizability, exclusion rates in Westen and Morrison's (2001) meta-analysis ranged from 65% for GAD to 68% for depression. Thus, the average study excluded two thirds of patients who presented for treatment. Researchers studying all three disorders appropriately excluded patients with psychotic, bipolar, and organic mental disorders; medical conditions that might affect interpretability of results; and those in imminent danger of suicide. However, additional exclusion criteria that were common across studies render generalizability for many of these treatments difficult to deduce. The prototypical study of depression excluded patients if they had suicidal ideation or comorbid substance use disorders, both of which are common symptoms in patients with depression. For panic, prototypical exclusion criteria were moderate to severe agoraphobic avoidance, any concurrent Axis I or Axis II disorder in need of immediate treatment, major depression deemed primary, and recent previous therapy. Prototypical GAD exclusion criteria included major depression, substance use disorders, and suicidality. The fact that such a high percentage of patients had to be excluded across all three disorders suggests that comorbidities of the types excluded may be the rule rather than the exception. Exclusion criteria for all three disorders also tended to eliminate many of the more troubled, comorbid, difficult-to-treat patients, such as patients with borderline features, who are likely to be suicidal and to have substance use disorders.

Efficacy of Treatments for Bulimia Nervosa and OCD

This first set of studies led, we believe, to some important incremental knowledge about the strengths and limitations of treatments currently described as empirically supported, using the best available published studies as data sources. Nevertheless, the meta-analyses of these three disorders had two primary limitations. First, to maximize the quality of the sample and to make the task manageable, Westen and Morrison (2001) included only studies published in major journals with relatively rigorous methodological standards (except for GAD, for which a broader computer search was conducted because of the dearth of studies) and focused on data published in the 1990s to capitalize on methodological advances since the 1980s. Second, because preliminary analyses showed only minor differences in outcome across types of treatment for most of the disorders when enough studies were available to meta-analyze, and because allegiance effects tend to yield higher effect sizes for investigators' preferred treatments (Luborsky, et al., 1999), Westen and Morrison did not report findings for specific treatments (e.g., cognitive, cognitive-behavioral, and strictly behavioral treatments for depression). Thus, in subsequent studies, our research team has broadened criteria to include all published studies meeting methodological criteria (experimental methods and randomization of patients) published since publication of the third edition of the *DSM* in 1980 (American Psychiatric Association, 1980). Here we briefly describe the results of the first two such studies, of RCTs for bulimia nervosa and OCD.

Treatments for bulimia nervosa

For bulimia nervosa (Thompson-Brenner, et al., 2003), mean effect sizes of treatments compared with controls were substantial (0.88 and 1.01 for binge eating and purging, respectively). However, most patients continued to be symptomatic at the end of treatment. Of those who completed treatment, 40% recovered; of those who entered treatment, 33% recovered. The average patient continued to binge 1.7 times per week and purge 2.3 times per week at the end of treatment. Although this still comes close to the diagnostic threshold for bulimia nervosa in the *DSM–IV*, it nevertheless represents a very substantial improvement from baseline. Findings at 1-year follow-up, though hard to come by, were similar to post treatment data, with the average patient across treatments showing substantial improvement over pretreatment baseline but also substantial residual symptomatology. However, only one third of patients across treatments or in individual CBT (which tended to fare slightly better than other treatments, particularly group CBT) showed sustained recovery at 1 year (i.e., recovered at termination and remained recovered at 1 year).

With respect to exclusion rates and criteria, the average study excluded 40% of the patients screened. Approximately half the studies excluded patients for either low or high weight (excluding patients with both anorexic symptoms and obesity) or suicide risk, and an additional one third excluded patients for substance abuse or dependence (31%). A large number of studies also excluded patients who had "major psychiatric illness," "serious comorbidity," or similar nonspecific exclusion criteria.

Treatments for OCD

For OCD (Eddy, et al., 2004), as reported in previous meta-analyses (e.g., Cox, Swinson, Morrison, & Paul, 1993; Kobak, Greist, Jefferson, Katzelnick, & Henk, 1998; van Blakom, van Oppen, Vermeulen, van Dyck, & Harne, 1994), effect sizes were very high, averaging 1.50 to 1.89 depending on the outcome measure, and were uniformly high across treatment conditions (behavioral, cognitive, and cognitive-behavioral). Approximately two thirds of patients who completed treatment improved (defined variously as 30% to 50% reduction in symptoms), and one third recovered. Among the intent-to-treat sample, about one half improved and one fourth recovered. Post treatment scores on standardized instruments suggested that the average patient experienced substantial improvement but also remained symptomatic.

Eddy, et al. (2004) intended to meta-analyze follow-up data as in the previous studies, but only two studies included follow-up at or beyond 1 year, and both of these reported data using the last observation carried forward, which does not allow readers to distinguish between data collected at 12 weeks and 12 months for patients who were inaccessible for follow-up. With respect to generalizability, few studies reported on the percentage of patients screened out, but among those that did, the average study excluded 62% of patients. The most common exclusion criteria were substance abuse and a variety of co-occurring disorders that varied across studies.

A counterpoint: Randomized trials of psychopharmacology for bulimia and OCD

One useful way of contextualizing these findings is to apply the same metrics to pharmacological interventions for the same disorders, which our laboratory has done thus far for both bulimia and OCD. Psychopharmacology for bulimia appears to be useful in many cases as an adjunctive treatment, but outcomes obtained using medication alone do not compare with the results of psycho-therapies such as CBT (Nakash-Eisikovits, et al., 2002). The average effect sizes for bulimia nervosa were 0.64 for binge episodes and 0.59 for purge episodes, slightly over half the effect sizes for psychotherapy. Although many patients improved, few recovered (slightly over 20%). On average, at termination patients binged 4.3 times a week and purged 6.2 times weekly, which represents roughly twice the post treatment means for CBT.

The data on psychopharmacological treatments for OCD are much more encouraging, with outcomes that rival behavioral and cognitive-behavioral inter-ventions for the same disorder (Eddy, et al., 2004). Treatment-control effect sizes in this study, as in prior meta-analyses of the same literature, were large (e.g., for clomipramine, which outperformed the other medications, $d = 1.35$). Almost two thirds of patients who completed and half of those who entered a medica-tion trial improved. As in the psychotherapy studies, however, recovery is a rare event, and high exclusion rates and the absence of follow-up data at clinically meaningful intervals rendered clinically meaningful conclusions more difficult to come by in this and virtually every other psychopharmacological literature we have examined.

In many respects, meta-analysis of the results of medication trials, like psy-chotherapy trials, underscores the problems inherent in making dichotomous determinations of empirical support or nonsupport when the data call for more nuanced appraisals. Medication for bulimia is useful, but only in certain ways for certain patients. The data on medication for OCD are much stronger in terms of effect size, but medication rarely leads to cure for OCD. Whether to call pharma-cological treatments for one of these disorders empirically supported and the other empirically unsupported is unclear because they are each efficacious and inefficacious in their own ways, if to differing degrees.

Comparing ESTs and Naturalistic Studies of Psychotherapy

Naturalistic studies of treatment in the community provide another useful context for assessing the findings of RCTs for ESTs (see, e.g., Asay, et al., 2002; Kopta, et al., 1994; Seligman, 1995). Our research team recently followed up the meta-analyses described above with naturalistic studies of several disorders designed to shed light on external validity. Naturalistic studies as implemented thus far (including our own) tend to have a number of methodological short-comings, such as nonrandom assignment of patients and lack of experimental control. However, they provide a window to phenomena not readily observed in the laboratory and can be particularly useful both for hypothesis generation and for providing a context within which to interpret data from RCTs, particularly data bearing on external validity.

Morrison, Bradley, and Westen (2003) began with a simple naturalistic study involving 242 clinicians randomly selected from the registers of the American Psychiatric and American Psychological Associations as participants. Approximately 20% of clinicians contacted (1/3 psychiatrists and 2/3 psychologists) returned completed materials, for which they received no compensation. (Despite their differential response rates, psychologists and psychiatrists provided highly similar data, suggesting that response rates do not likely account for the bulk of the findings.) The clinicians tended to have multiple institutional affiliations: 31% worked in hospitals at least part time, 20% worked in clinics, 82% worked in private practice, and 11% worked in forensic settings. Respondents were a highly experienced group, with 18 years of post training experience being the median.

As a follow-up to our research team's first set of multidimensional meta-analyses, Morrison, et al. (2003) asked responding clinicians to describe their last completed psychotherapy with three patients: one who presented with clinically significant depressive symptoms, one who presented with clinically significant panic symptoms, and one who presented with clinically significant anxiety symptoms other than panic. (The decision was made to widen the diagnostic net to include patients with clinically significant depression, panic, and anxiety because the emphasis was on generalizability to the clinical population.) Clinicians provided information about length of treatment, Axis I comorbidity, and Axis II comorbidity. They also completed a checklist of other clinically significant personality variables found in previous research to be frequent targets of therapeutic attention, such as problems with intimacy, relatedness, or commitment in close relationships; difficulty with assertiveness or expression of anger or aggression; authority problems; problems with separation, abandonment, or rejection; and so forth (Westen & Arkowitz-Westen, 1998).

Two findings are of particular relevance from the present point of view. First, median treatment length ranged from 52 sessions for panic to 75 sessions for depression. When Morrison, et al. (2003) stratified clinicians by theoretical orientation (psychodynamic, cognitive-behavioral, and eclectic, which were the primary orientations in the sample), the briefest treatments, not surprisingly, were cognitive-behavioral. Even these treatments, however, were almost twice as long on the average as manualized CBTs for the same disorders. It may be the case, of course, that these therapies were long relative to ESTs because clinicians were inefficient or influenced by monetary incentives to retain patients longer than necessary. However, the consistent finding in RCTs for these disorders that the average patient remains symptomatic at the end of a trial of brief psychotherapy and seeks further treatment suggests that clinicians were likely responding to the fact that patients continued to manifest clinically significant symptoms.

Second, comorbidity was the norm rather than the exception. As in previous community and clinical samples, roughly half of patients for each disorder had at least one comorbid Axis I condition, and slightly less than half had an Axis II disorder. The data on depression are illustrative: Half of patients had at least one comorbid Axis I condition, half had at least one comorbid Axis II disorder, and virtually no clinician reported treating any patient exclusively for depression when completing the personality problems checklist. For example, 67% of clinicians described their patients diagnosed with depression as suffering from clinically significant problems with intimacy, relatedness, or commitment in relationships that the patient and clinician agreed was causing substantial distress or dysfunction, and 77% of clinicians reported clinically treating the patient for clinically significant problems with assertiveness or expression of anger. These percentages were invariant across therapeutic orientations, appearing with virtually identical frequencies regardless of clinicians' theoretical preconceptions, and were systematically related to treatment length. Across disorders and theoretical orientations, average treatment length doubled when patients had any form of Axis I comorbidity or Axis II comorbidity, and the presence of clinically significant personality problems also predicted treatment length. For example, presence of externalizing pathology (an aggregate variable from the personality problem checklist) was strongly associated with treatment length ($r \_ 0.40$).

This first set of studies (Morrison, et al., 2003), though providing useful data on common comorbidity and on current practices in the community, had several limitations. It focused only on successful treatments, so we could not assess the relation between comorbid conditions and outcome; it provided no data on the interventions used by clinicians, so that we could not rule out the possibility that clinicians were simply using inefficient strategies; it was retrospective, leaving open the possibility of reporting bias; and the treating clinician was the only source of data.

Thompson-Brenner and Westen (2004a, 2004b) addressed the first two of these problems in a subsequent study in which they asked a random national sample of clinicians to describe their most recently terminated patient with clinically significant bulimic symptoms, including treatment failures. The demographics of the clinicians were similar to the first study. Patients in the study averaged 28 years of age, and were, like the population from which they were drawn (women with eating disorders), primarily middle class and Caucasian.

Although most clinicians described their patients as improved over the course of treatment, only 53% of patients completely recovered (a percentage that was similar across all theoretical orientations). Once again, clinicians of all theoretical orientations reported treating patients for much longer than the 16 to 20 sessions prescribed in the most widely tested and disseminated manuals. Although CBT treatments were of shorter duration than eclectic/integrative and psychodynamic treatments, the average CBT treatment lasted 69 sessions on average, substantially longer than the 19 prescribed in the manual.

Comorbidity was also the rule rather than the exception, and both Axis I and Axis II comorbidity were negatively associated with treatment outcome. Over 90% of the sample met criteria for at least one comorbid Axis I diagnosis other than an eating disorder. Axis II comorbidity was also high: One third of the sample met criteria for at least one Cluster B (dramatic, erratic) diagnosis, and the same proportion met criteria for at least one Cluster C (anxious) diagnosis. Several comorbid Axis I disorders (notably major depressive disorder, PTSD, and substance use disorders) and Axis II disorders (borderline, dependent, and avoidant) commonly seen in patients with eating disorders were positively correlated with treatment length and negatively correlated with outcome, with small to medium effect sizes. When Thompson-Brenner and Westen (2004a) applied four common exclusion criteria from RCTs to the naturalistic sample (substance use disorder, weight 15% or more over ideal, weight 15% or more below ideal, and bipolar disorder), they found that approximately 40% of the naturalistic sample would have been excluded (the same percentage excluded in the average RCT). Two thirds of the patients with BPD would have been excluded on the basis of these criteria, and the 40% of patients who would have been excluded (whether or not they had BPD) showed worse treatment outcome across a number of indices.

Finally, Thompson-Brenner and Westen (2004a, 2004b) measured intervention strategies by asking clinicians to complete an interventions questionnaire adapted from Blagys, Ackerman, Bonge, and Hilsenroth (2003). Factor analysis of the interventions questionnaire yielded three factors: Psychodynamic, Cognitive-Behavioral, and Adjunctive interventions (e.g., pharmacotherapy, hospitalization). Across the entire sample, greater use of CBT interventions was associated with more rapid remission of eating symptoms, whereas greater use of Psychodynamic interventions was associated with larger changes in global outcome, such as Global Assessment of Functioning (American Psychiatric Association, 1994) scores. Clinicians of all theoretical backgrounds reported using more Psychodynamic interventions when treating patients with comorbid pathology, which is perhaps not surprising given that these interventions are more oriented toward personality. Psychodynamic clinicians reported using more CBT interventions (such as structuring the therapy hours) with emotionally constricted patients. In contrast, CBT clinicians reported using more Psychodynamic interventions (e.g., exploring patterns in relationships, exploring sexuality, and exploring unconscious processes) when treating emotionally dysregulated patients (i.e., those with borderline features, substance use disorders, etc.). These data suggest that clinicians of all theoretical orientations attend to personality and comorbid symptomatology and adjust their intervention strategies accordingly. An important point of note is that clinicians did not appear reluctant to describe unsuccessful cases or to self-report the use of interventions explicitly associated with their nonpreferred theoretical orientation, suggesting that the data cannot simply be reduced to clinician bias.

We do not consider the data from these naturalistic studies by any means definitive. The exclusive reliance on clinicians as respondents, the retrospective design, and the use of a brief therapy process measure completed by the clinician without independent verification by external observers impose severe constraints on what we can conclude. We also do not know whether the patients in these naturalistic studies fared better or worse than patients in the ESTs examined in Thompson-Brenner, et al.'s (2003) meta-analysis, except by clinicians' own report (slightly greater than 50% recovery from bulimia nervosa at termination). That question can only be answered by comparing outcome in naturalistic and manualized treatments for similar patients and including shared outcome measures. The data are consistent, however, with the dose-response relationship found in virtually all naturalistic studies, which shows that patients tend to show greater improvement with more extensive treatment, particularly when they have characterological problems (Howard, et al., 1986; Kopta, et al., 1994; Seligman, 1995). Perhaps most important, the data suggest limitations in manualized treatments designed to address specific Axis I syndromes that do not address enduring personality dispositions relevant to these syndromes to which clinicians of all theoretical orientations attend and which are not readily explained in terms of sampling or response bias.

Studies Testing the Transportability of ESTs

A critic might object that the data presented thus far do not address the amassing literature on the transportability of ESTs to more naturalistic settings. Reading the contemporary literature, one is indeed impressed with how rapidly and successfully researchers have responded to the clarion call for research addressing critics' concerns about the generalizability of treatments tested in the laboratory (e.g., Persons & Silberschatz, 1998). Within a short span of years, a number of effectiveness and benchmarking studies have found manualized treatments to be highly transportable, with little if any decrement in effect size or response rates (see, e.g., Chambless & Ollendick, 2000). This emerging consensus is somewhat surprising, given that researchers have presumably been imposing relatively stringent exclusion criteria in RCTs for 20 years for a reason. We have no doubt that many manualized treatments (and, more broadly, many interventions tested in RCTs) will ultimately show substantial transportability. However, at this juncture, we suspect that the best way to advance knowledge of what works for whom would be to begin testing in a systematic way the conditions under which particular treatments or interventions are likely to be useful in everyday practice, rather than to try to make dichotomous judgments about transportability.

Consider some of the studies now widely cited as evidence for transportability. One showed an impressively low relapse rate at 1-year follow-up for patients treated with CBT for panic in a community mental health setting (Stuart, Treat, & Wade, 2000). Another examined patients excluded from RCTs conducted at the same site (a superb comparison sample to address the question) to assess the transportability of exposure-based treatment for OCD (Franklin, Abramowitz, Levitt, Kozak, & Foa, 2000). This study produced outcomes (average pre-post effect sizes above 3.00) that exceeded the mode in the investigators' own table of benchmark RCTs. Although we suspect that these are indeed two of the most portable of all the ESTs—and the data may well reflect the robustness of these treatments—both studies suffered from a substantial limitation that has not been noted in any review of which we are aware, namely non-blind assessment.[13]

Another recent study, designed to test the hypothesis that CBT for depression in children and adolescents is superior to treatment in the community, used a creative benchmarking design to compare treatment response among child and adolescent patients with depression treated at what appear to have been six inner-city CMHCs with the average response of patients of similar age and severity of depression treated in RCTs (Weersing & Weisz, 2002). Patients in the RCTs showed much more rapid improvement, although outcome converged by 1-year follow-up. The authors concluded that the treatment trajectories of CMHC-treated youth "more closely resembled those of control condition youth than youth treated with CBT" in RCTs, and drew implications about the transportability and benefits of manualized treatments relative to "the effectiveness of community psychotherapy for depressed youth" (Weersing & Weisz, 2002, p. 299). They noted that the "CMHC services were predominantly psychodynamic, whereas therapists in clinical trials provided a pure dose of CBT" (Weersing & Weisz, 2002, p. 299) and suggested that these treatment differences likely accounted for much of the difference in outcome.

Several features of Weersing and Weisz's (2002) study, however, suggest caution in drawing even preliminary conclusions about transportability of manualized therapies or about their superiority to therapies practiced in the community. Although the authors reported no data on socioeconomic status of the CMHC sample, their description of the sample suggests that they compared a low-socioeconomic status CMHC sample with a set of benchmark studies of primarily Caucasian, presumably less socioeconomically disadvantaged, patients.

---

[13] In the panic study, follow-up assessment was conducted by graduate research assistants who knew that all patients being followed up had been in the active treatment condition. In the OCD study, the sole OCD outcome measure reported was a semistructured interview, with the interviewers presumably aware both that all patients had been treated with the same therapy and that the purpose of the study was to demonstrate ecological validity of this treatment. In both studies, secondary measures such as the Beck Depression Inventory, which are less likely to be contaminated by experimenter expectancy effects, provided promising corroborating data but unfortunately did not directly address the target symptom. Surprisingly, however, the rival explanation of experimenter bias, which rendered both studies perhaps more comparable to open label trials than controlled clinical trials, was not discussed as a potential limitation in either research report, and both have been cited frequently as evidence for the transportability of manualized treatments to clinical practice.

The authors noted that mood disorder diagnoses did not differ substantially between the CMHC and benchmark samples, nor did severity of depression, suggesting equivalence of the samples. However, our calculations from data provided in tabular form in their article indicate very different rates of comorbid conditions known to influence outcome in children and adolescents. Frequency of conduct disorder and oppositional defiant disorder averaged only 11% in benchmark studies that either reported or excluded these diagnoses but averaged 61% in the CMHC sample. Rates of anxiety disorders were 25% and 58%, respectively. Whereas some investigators studying generalizability from RCTs to clinical practice have maximized comparability of samples by applying the same inclusion and exclusion criteria to the community sample (e.g., Humphreys & Weisner, 2000; Mitchell, Maki, Adson, Ruskin, & Crow, 1997; Thompson-Brenner & Westen, 2004a, 2004b), Weersing and Weisz (2002) excluded patients only if they "were unable to complete study measures as a result of psychosis or developmental disability" (p. 301). Although the intent appears to have been to maximize external validity (which would have been appropriate if the goal were to compare CBT in the laboratory with CBT in a CMHC sample), we are unaware of any RCT for depression in either adults or children with comparable inclusion criteria. Thus, any obtained results could reflect differences in the samples, differences in the treatments delivered, or both.

Sampling issues aside, of particular note was Weersing and Weisz's (2002) conclusion that patients treated in RCTs not only did better than those treated in the community but that the CMHC patients actually looked more like patients in the control conditions than in experimental conditions in controlled trials. The authors rested this conclusion on an extrapolation from the slope of change in RCT control conditions from pretreatment to 3 months, arguing that by 12 months, continuation of this slow but steady reduction of symptoms would have yielded data indistinguishable from the treated CMHC patients (i.e., return to normalcy). Such a procedure, however, would dissolve any treatment effect ever documented at 1 year for any EST for child or adult depression of which we are aware. The authors explained the convergence in outcome at 1 year between benchmark and CMHC patients by suggesting that improvement in the CMHC group likely reflected the natural course of the illness (i.e., gradual waning of a depressive episode), which it may well have. However, this explanation is notably different from the conclusion typically drawn from the same finding when obtained in RCTs, for which converging outcomes at 1 year for IPT and CBT for bulimia, for example, have been interpreted as demonstrating a delayed treatment effect for IPT.

Our point here is not to criticize particular studies or investigators but simply to note the danger of confirmatory biases when a community of scientists feels some urgency to respond to published critiques with creative demonstration projects that enter into the empirical lore as disconfirmations of the critiques. At this point, we believe the most scientifically appropriate way to resolve the question of generalizability of ESTs is a moratorium on exclusion criteria in RCTs other than those a reasonable clinician might apply in everyday practice (e.g., reliably documented organic brain disease) or that are medically or ethically necessary and the use of correlational analyses to identify moderators of outcome worth studying in future investigations. Either exclusion criteria are necessary, and generalizability from RCTs is correspondingly limited, or exclusion criteria are unnecessary, and studies using them have a serious sampling flaw and should not be published in first-tier journals or cited without substantial qualification. The near-universal exclusion of patients with suicidality from clinical trials is no exception: If, as a field, we truly believe that the state of our science justifies the kinds of distinctions between empirically supported and unsupported treatments for disorders such as depression that are leading to massive shifts in training, practice, and third-party payment, it is neither scientifically nor ethically justifiable to relegate suicidal patients to unvalidated treatments, at least in studies that could randomly assign patients with suicidal ideation to two or more active interventions.

Summary: How Valid Are Empirically Validated Psychotherapies?

The data from RCTs of treatments widely described as empirically supported for depression, panic, GAD, bulimia nervosa, and OCD over the past decade suggest that these treatments do indeed lead to substantial initial reductions in painful mood states and pathological behaviors that substantially affect life satisfaction and adaptive functioning. The treatments we have studied meta-analytically have proven as or more effective than pharmacotherapies that have had the advantage of billions of dollars of industry support for testing and marketing. At the same time, the existing data support a more nuanced and, we believe, empirically balanced view of treatment efficacy than implied by widespread use of terms such as *empirically supported, empirically validated,* or *treatment of choice.*

As a discipline we have clearly identified a set of techniques that can be helpful to many patients suffering from many disorders. However, the effects of brief manualized psychotherapies are highly variable across disorders, with some findings justifying claims of empirical support and others reminding us that in science, empirical support is usually not a dichotomous variable. With the exception of CBT for panic, the majority of patients receiving treatments for all the disorders we reviewed did not recover. They remained symptomatic even if they showed substantial reductions in their symptoms or fell below diagnostic thresholds for caseness; they sought further treatment; or they relapsed at some point within 1 to 2 years after receiving ESTs conducted by clinicians who were expert in delivery of the treatment, well supervised, and highly committed to the success of their treatment of choice.

The extent to which even the more qualified conclusions offered here can be generalized to the population of patients treated in the community is largely unknown because of high, and highly variable, exclusion rates and criteria that render the findings from different studies difficult to aggregate and apply to the treatment seeking population. In the modal efficacy study, somewhere between 40% and 70% of patients who present for treatment with symptoms of the disorder are excluded (not including the unknown percentage of patients who are screened by referring clinicians who know the study's exclusion criteria), and patients treated in everyday clinical practice who resemble those excluded tend to take longer to treat and to have poorer outcomes.[14] The data from naturalistic studies suggest that, in fact, most patients are polysymptomatic, and the more co-occurring conditions with which the patient suffers, the longer and more wide-ranging the treatment appears to be—a conclusion similarly reached in a qualitative review by Roth and Fonagy (1996). The correlation between treatment length and comorbidity is one of the few generalizations that appears to apply across treatments and disorders. The polysymptomatic nature of patient pathology in clinical practice suggests that a primary or exclusive clinical focus on a single Axis I syndrome does not appear to be appropriate in the majority of cases, particularly if polysymptomatic cases have any emergent properties that cannot be reduced to variance accounted for by each symptom or syndrome in isolation.

A striking gap in the literature is the relative absence of follow-up studies that span the length of time during which relapse is known to be common in untreated patients for the disorders in question. More encouraging findings are on the horizon for some treatments, such as data suggesting that CBT can help prevent relapse and recurrence of panic following discontinuation of alprazolam several years after treatment (Bruce, Spiegel, & Hegel, 1999) or that cognitive therapy for depression may help prevent relapse in a subset of patients (see Hollon, et al., 2002). However, the limited data on long-term outcome of ESTs suggest that initial response may or may not bear a relationship to efficacy at 2- to 5-year follow-up (e.g., Shea, Elkin, et al., 1992; Snyder, Wills, & Grady, 1991). Treatments that differ in initial response may yield highly similar efficacy estimates at 2 years, and treatments that appear similar in initial response may have very different outcomes at 5 years.

REWRITING THE STORY: IMPLICATIONS FOR EVIDENCE-BASED PRACTICE

Although the story we have told thus far has been critical of many of the uses and interpretations of controlled clinical trials, we are not arguing against

---

[14] These findings do not appear to be limited to the disorders we have studied thus far. Humphreys and Weisner (2000) recently applied the prototypical exclusion criteria taken from alcohol treatment studies to two large community samples to assess the external validity of efficacy trials for alcoholism. The resulting samples were highly unrepresentative, heavily composed of Caucasian, stable, higher functioning patients with less substantial comorbidity—the kinds of patients who, empirically, are likely to respond more favorably to treatment.

the utility of RCTs or experimental methods more generally in psychotherapy research. This final section has two goals. The first is to suggest standards for reporting aspects of design and findings in RCTs to maximize their clinical utility and applicability. The second is to examine ways researchers might design rigorous studies of interventions that do not violate the assumptions outlined in the first part of this article.

Maximizing the Efficacy of Clinical Trials

In reviewing hundreds of studies over the course of several meta-analyses, we have observed a number of common problems in reporting that limit the impact and applicability of many controlled trials to everyday clinical practice. Here we describe some of these problems and potential solutions. Most of the suggestions we offer may appear obvious, and many have been detailed elsewhere (e.g., Chambless & Hollon, 1998) but are not yet normative in practice.

Describing the Hypotheses and Experimental Conditions

A central issue that has received little attention in the literature involves the framing and reporting of hypotheses. Because the interpretation of most statistical tests depends on whether the analysis is planned or post hoc, it is essential that researchers clearly label their hypotheses as primary, secondary, a priori, post hoc, one-tailed, or two-tailed. Nothing is wrong with unexpected findings, but readers need to know which hypotheses were predicted. Of particular relevance in this regard is the clear labeling of comparison and control groups. Researchers need to specify clearly and a priori whether a condition is intended as an active, credible treatment; a dismantled component of a treatment that may or may not prove useful; a credible control that is likely to be superior to no treatment because of common factors; a weak control that largely controls for number of sessions and some very nonspecific factors; or a simple wait-list or similar group that controls only for the passage of time.

The frequent use of wait-list and TAU controls in RCTs for many disorders can lead to substantial problems of data interpretation (Borkovec, 1994; Borkovec & Castonguay, 1998). Given that virtually any 10- to 20-session intervention will produce an initial response in most patients if carried out by a clinician who expects it to be effective (Luborsky, McLellan, Diguer, Woody, & Seligman, 1997), the only scientifically valid conclusion one can draw from observed differences between experimental and waitlist control conditions is that doing something is better than doing nothing, yet it is remarkable how many literatures rely primarily on such comparisons and how many investigators draw much more specific conclusions (see Kazdin, 1997).

As noted earlier, TAU conditions are often interpreted as demonstrating the superiority of experimental treatments to everyday clinical practice, but this is only a valid conclusion if control therapists are well paid, motivated, and see the patients on a regular basis. This is seldom the case. The literature on DBT, for example, has relied almost exclusively on TAU comparisons (Scheel, 2000), but DBT therapists (who are available around the clock, provide several hours a weeks of group and individual therapy, undergo weekly supervision, etc.) and community mental health practitioners differ on so many variables that it is difficult to draw causal conclusions from such comparisons. Our own suspicion is that DBT is a highly efficacious treatment for many aspects of borderline pathology, but the frequent use of TAU conditions renders confidence in this conclusion weaker than it likely need be.

Researchers should also exercise caution in labeling control treatments not constructed to maximize their efficacy (what Wampold, et al., 1997, described as *non-bona fide* treatments, or what might be called *intent-to-fail* conditions) with brand names that are readily confused with genuine treatments and create sleeper effects in the literature. For example, as described earlier, to test the efficacy of CBT for bulimia, Garner, et al. (1993) developed a treatment they called *supportive-expressive therapy*, an abbreviated treatment described as nondirective and psychodynamically inspired, in which clinicians were forbidden to discuss the target symptoms with the patient and were instead instructed to reflect them back to the patient. Such a practice is not in fact characteristic of psychodynamic therapies for eating disorders (e.g., Bruch, 1973) and is analogous to a researcher creating a cognitive therapy comparison condition in which the therapist is instructed to say, "That's irrational," every time a patient tries to discuss the symptom. Unfortunately, this study is frequently cited in review articles as demonstrating that CBT is superior to psychodynamic psychotherapy for bulimia nervosa (e.g., Compas, Haaga, Keefe, & Leitenbert, 1998).

A similar example can be seen in the graph on the cover of the APS monograph on the treatment of depression (Hollon, et al., 2002), which was adapted from a practice guidelines document published almost a decade earlier (a document whose purported biases had in fact contributed to the movement among psychologists to construct a list of ESTs). The graph showed response rates above 50% for IPT, CBT, and medication, compared with response rates hovering slightly above 30% for placebo and psychodynamic therapy. Given the absence of any manual for psychodynamic psychotherapy for depression (at least ca. 1993, the publication date of the practice guidelines), it is unclear what treatments one would include in such a graph. As best we could ascertain from the authors' thorough (and very balanced) review in the text of the monograph, the treatments summarized in the graph for psychodynamic therapy were largely intent-to-fail controls. By the methodological standards used elsewhere in the monograph and in the EST literature more generally, the most appropriate conclusion to draw (and the one the authors in fact drew in the text) is that there are no credible data either way on psychodynamic therapy for depression and certainly none for the longer term therapies most commonly denoted by that term. Unfortunately, the message all but the most careful readers are likely to take away from the monograph is that psychodynamic therapy for depression is empirically invalidated, not unvalidated.

Reporting, Justifying, and Interpreting the Data in the Context of Inclusion and Exclusion Criteria

Another important issue pertains to the reporting, justification, and interpretation of findings in light of inclusion and exclusion criteria. As we argued earlier, as a field we would do well to stop using exclusion criteria other than those that are medically necessary or similar to those a clinician might be expected to apply in everyday practice (e.g., brain damage) if our goal is to guide practice. If researchers impose criteria other than those that are obviously necessary, they should routinely provide the following information. In the Method section, they need to describe and justify precisely what the criteria were and whether they made these decisions prior to the study, prior to examining the data, after noticing that certain kinds of patients had anomalous results, and so forth. In the Results section, they should describe how many patients were excluded at each step (e.g., both at initial phone screen and upon interview) and for what reasons. In the Discussion section, they should describe the precise population to which they expect the results to generalize. The abstract should also be qualified if the study excluded patients a reader might readily assume were included, such as depressed patients with suicidal ideation. As noted earlier, only a minority of research reports describes the number of patients excluded at each level of screening and how and when decisions were made, and fewer still carefully limit their conclusions to what is usually a subpopulation. By the time the results find their way into reviews or meta-analyses, qualifications about patients excluded tend to disappear.

Describing the Clinicians

Another aspect of reporting that requires greater attention regards the clinicians who conducted the treatments. Investigators need to describe clearly the number and characteristics of the treating clinicians in each condition and to describe and justify any choices that could bear on interpretation of the results. Given the small number of clinicians who can participate in any RCT, there are no right answers to the question of how to select therapists. For example, having different therapists in two treatment conditions creates the possibility of uncontrolled therapist effects, whereas using the same therapists in two conditions raises questions about allegiance effects. Crits-Christoph and Mintz (1991) reviewed 140 clinical trials of psychosocial treatments and found that 26 used only one therapist, one pair of therapists working together, or one therapist per treatment, which rendered treatment effects and therapist effects confounded. Seventy-seven studies made no mention of therapist effects; and 32 conducted one-way analyses of variance to rule out therapist effects but set the significance level at the conventional .05, which left the analyses seriously underpowered to detect even substantial effects.

In a large percentage of the studies we reviewed, it was difficult or impossible to ascertain precisely how many therapists conducted the treatments, who these therapists were, and whether they had commitments to one approach or another. Frequently (especially in smaller studies) the first author, who was expert in and committed to the treatment approach under consideration, appeared to be the therapist in the active treatment condition, but the report provided no data on whether the clinician or clinicians in other conditions were similarly expert and motivated. As Luborsky and others have noted (e.g., Luborsky, et al., 1999), differing levels of expertise and commitment provide one of the likely mediators of allegiance effects. Protecting against this threat to validity would probably require multi-allegiance research teams to become the norm in treatment research.

Assessing Psychopathology and Outcome

The reliability and validity of assessment is obviously crucial in treatment studies and extends to the way investigators assess the primary diagnosis required for inclusion in the study, the diagnosis of comorbid conditions, and outcome. With respect to reliability and validity of diagnosis for inclusion, clinical trials for many anxiety disorders are exemplary (e.g., J. G. Beck, Stanley, Baldwin, Deagle, & Averill, 1994; Borkovec & Costello, 1993; Bouchard, et al., 1996; Shear, Pilkonis, Cloitre, & Leon, 1994). Less optimal reporting, however, is common in clinical trials for many other disorders. For example, of 26 studies reviewed for a meta-analysis of psychotherapies for bulimia, many reported data on the reliability and validity of the assessment instrument in general (e.g., as used by its developers), but none that used a structured interview reported data on inter-rater reliability in the study being reported (Thompson-Brenner, et al., 2003).

Even when researchers establish the primary diagnosis carefully, they generally pay less attention to the diagnosis or reporting of comorbid conditions or exclusion criteria (see Strupp, Horowitz, & Lambert, 1997). This is understandable given that diagnosis of other conditions is generally considered secondary to the point of the study. Because exclusion of patients on the basis of comorbid diagnoses or other criteria is crucial to generalizability, however, assessment of exclusion criteria can be just as important as reliable assessment of the target syndrome. For example, many studies require that patients have a primary diagnosis of the index disorder to be included in the clinical trial. However, researchers virtually never describe how, how reliably, and when in the screening process they made that determination of primacy. This is again a potential avenue for unnoticed allegiance effects and threats to generalizability that cannot be detected from reading published reports, as interviewers or screeners may determine that the problems of more difficult patients are primary and hence lead to their exclusion. Because comorbid conditions can have implications for treatment outcome, even studies that do not exclude patients for common forms of comorbidity need to provide reliability data on diagnosis of comorbid conditions that might bear on clinical utility outside of the laboratory.

With respect to the measurement of outcome, the primary focus of most outcome studies is outcome vis-à-vis the syndrome under investigation, and appropriately so. At the same time, outcome studies should always supplement assessment of primary symptom measures in four ways, some of which are becoming more common (e.g., measures of high end-state functioning or global adaptation) and some of which are rarely used. First, because most patients have multiple problems that affect their adaptation and life satisfaction, studies should routinely include measures of other Axis I conditions, adaptive functioning, and quality of life. Second, given the strong links between Axis I conditions and personality, efficacy studies should routinely include measures of relevant personality variables, particularly where data are available suggesting that these variables may be diatheses that render the patient vulnerable to future episodes. Third, given the growing evidence distinguishing implicit from explicit processes (and linking implicit processes to underlying vulnerabilities; e.g., Segal, et al., 1999), studies should routinely include measures designed to assess implicit networks or implicit attentional biases (e.g., emotional Stroop tasks) that may indicate the likely durability of changes. Finally, studies that include extended follow-up should implement reliable and systematic ways of assessing post-termination treatment seeking. Given the demand characteristics inherent in participating in a controlled trial (e.g., wanting to please the therapist by reporting feeling better at the end), behavioral indices are crucial to supplement self-reports, and one of the most useful such indices is whether the patient seeks further treatment (and whether he or she seeks it from the investigators or from someone else).

In the studies we reviewed, the reliability, validity, and demand characteristics of outcome measures for even the symptoms considered primary was highly variable. Many studies of anxiety and eating disorders, for example, use symptom diaries as primary outcome measures (Arntz & van den Hout, 1996; Ost & Westling, 1995; Shear, et al., 1994). The benefits of diary-type recording are clear: Patients can observe and record panic or eating behavior as it occurs, rather than relying on memory during an interview that may occur weeks or months after the fact. At the same time, diaries impose a number of problems that are rarely controlled or addressed. Because diaries are often used as treatment tools in cognitive-behavioral treatments, the accuracy and calibration of diary reports are likely to differ across conditions if one condition repeatedly uses diaries throughout treatment and the other does not. Furthermore, in many treatments, patients and clinicians use diaries to chart progress, leading to demand characteristics as the treatment draws to an end if the diary is used as a primary outcome measure. How diaries are collected is another relevant issue. In several studies we reviewed, the final outcome diary appears to have been collected directly by the therapist, which could obviously influence patients' symptom reports.

Diaries are not the only measures subject to potentially differential calibration or demand characteristics across conditions. In several studies we reviewed, psychoeducational components of the treatment could well have biased the way respondents used self-report measures. For example, when clinicians provide education on the precise meaning of *panic attack* or *binge* in one experimental condition, patients' assessment of the frequency of these events is likely to change irrespective of behavioral change, particularly if clinicians are motivated to see improvement and subtly bias the severity required to "count" as an episode. Bouchard, et al. (1996) addressed this potential problem in a creative way by explicitly educating all participants on the definition of a panic attack before they began keeping diaries. Such practices should be standard. At the very least, researchers need to report explicitly how and when patients in each condition are provided information that might impact the way they respond to outcome questionnaires for symptoms whose definition is at all ambiguous.

Tracking Relevant Ns

As suggested earlier, tracking precisely how many patients have come through each stage of a study is essential for assessing both efficacy and generalizability (see Table 1). In this respect, psychotherapy researchers should follow the lead of medical researchers, who have recently developed consolidated standards for the reporting of trials that provide guidelines for reporting sample sizes at each stage, including providing flow diagrams (Egger, Juni, & Bartlett, 1999). For the modal study, in which the investigators use both an initial telephone screen and a subsequent, more extensive screen via structured interview, research reports need to describe the percentage excluded at each step and the reasons for exclusion. Rarely do researchers provide data on exclusion at both of these two points (indeed, the majority of studies we have reviewed did not include either), which is essential for assessing generalizability. Many exemplary cases of reporting exist in the literature, however, that should serve as models for standard practice (e.g., Barlow, Gorman, Shear, & Woods, 2000; Fairburn, et al., 1991; Ost & Westling, 1995).

Definitions of dropout and completion also deserve greater attention. A large number of published reports use idiosyncratic definitions of completion, and it is often unclear whether these definitions were set a priori. This is another potential locus for intrusion of allegiance effects, as researchers may, with no conscious intention of deception, select definitions of completion that tell the best

Table 1. The Complex Meanings of N: Indispensable Data for Interpreting the Results of Clinical Trials

Stage of patient participation	Necessary to report
Participants assessed for eligibility	Estimated N in the community or treatment center who were likely to have seen recruitment or referral advertisements or notices
	N who responded and received phone screen
	N who passed initial phone screen and received a subsequent interview
Participants excluded	N who failed to meet each specific inclusion criterion
	N who met inclusion criteria but met each specific exclusion criterion
Participants included	N randomized to each condition
	N who began each condition; reasons, if known, why any patients randomized did not enter treatment
	N who completed each condition; reasons, if known, why any patients did not complete each intervention
	N who completed each condition but did not participate in assessments; reasons, if known, why patients were not available for assessment
	N analyzed, for each analysis
	N excluded from each analysis and reasons, including exclusion of outliers

story for one condition or another. Including relatively early dropouts as *completers*, for example, can bias results in either a positive or a negative direction, depending on whether the last observation carried forward is high or low. Consider a comparison of cognitive therapy, applied relaxation, and imipramine for depression by Clark, et al. (1994). Although the intended length of the psychosocial treatments was 15 sessions, the investigators defined *dropouts* as those who completed no more than 3 sessions; thus, patients who attended only 4 out of 15 sessions would be considered completers. This could be a very conservative way of analyzing the data, retaining the last observation carried forward of patients who did not find the treatment useful or tolerable. Alternatively, it could inflate completion rates or include data from patients who made immediate improvements that had little to do with any specific treatment components. Decisions such as this are rarely discussed or justified in published reports. Many of the reports we reviewed across disorders not only failed to explain decisions about completer definitions but used different definitions in different analyses. The only reason we even noticed this problem was that we were meta-analyzing data that required us to record Ns, and noticed different Ns in different tables or discrepancies between the Ns reported in the tables and the text.

Reporting and Interpreting Results

One of our primary conclusions in this article has been the importance of reporting a range of outcome statistics and indicators of generalizability that allow readers, reviewers, and meta-analysts to draw more accurate and nuanced conclusions. As a number of researchers have persuasively argued, primary research reports should always supplement tests of statistical significance with effect size estimates such as Cohen's d or Pearson's r (see, e.g., Rosenthal, 1991). Others have noted, however, that even these effect size estimates can sometimes fail to represent clinical significance (e.g., Jacobson & Truax, 1991). The investigation that demonstrated the value of aspirin in reducing heart attacks so clearly that the study had to be discontinued for ethical reasons produced an r of only .03—and an $R2$ less than .01. Although seemingly minimal to null, this effect size translates to 15 people out of 1,000 who will live or die depending on whether they take aspirin (Rosenthal, 1995). The debate about how to measure clinical significance is an important one that will likely continue for some time. In the meantime, we recommend that all published RCTs report, at minimum, each of the metrics described earlier.

Several other data reporting and interpretation issues also require attention. One involves pretreatment group differences in symptom levels that occur despite randomization. Much of the time, researchers call attention to and report attempts at controlling for accidental pretreatment group differences (e.g., J. G. Beck, et al., 1994; Ost & Westling, 1995). However, particularly in studies with small samples, researchers need to be careful to note and address potentially important pretreatment differences that may exceed one to two standard deviations but not cross conventional significance thresholds (e.g., Wolf & Crowther, 1992).

An additional set of reporting issues seems obvious but represents such a widespread problem in the literature for both psychotherapy and psychopharmacology that it requires vigilance by reviewers and editors, namely the clear reporting of sample and subsample sizes, treatment of outliers, and appropriate measures of central tendency. In reviewing studies across disorders, it was surprising how frequently we had difficulty ascertaining which subgroups of the sample were used in different analyses (e.g., intent-to-treat vs. completer samples). When researchers present intent-to-treat analyses, they should also state whether the analyses used the last observation carried forward, particularly in follow-up analyses. More generally, tables and analyses reported in the text should always include the N or degrees of freedom and indicate whether participants were excluded and for what reasons. If outliers are deleted, investigators need to state explicitly whether (and why or why not) they deleted the corresponding outliers at the other end of the distribution or the same number of participants from the other treatment conditions. Similarly, researchers should always report means and standard deviations where appropriate, and if they switch to medians in some analyses, they should justify the reasons for doing so. A surprisingly large number of reports did not include pretreatment and post treatment means for the primary outcome measures. In some cases research reports included only figures or charts without the raw numbers, which makes meta-analysis of findings difficult. In other cases, researchers reported means without standard deviations, which are impossible to interpret, except if the investigators also provided all the relevant F values, p values, degrees of freedom, and so forth that could allow a motivated reader to calculate the size of the effect.

Finally, several issues concerning reporting of follow-up data deserve attention. As noted earlier, the dearth of follow-up data for ESTs over extended periods is a serious problem with the existing literature, as it is for the medication literature for the same disorders. Researchers routinely refer to treatments that show short-term effects in multiple studies as empirically supported, when they know only about initial response and effects at brief follow-up intervals (e.g., 3 to 9 months). Including a plan for maintaining contact with patients after treatment should be a prerequisite for funding.

When researchers conduct follow-ups at multiple intervals (e.g., at 3, 6, and 12 months post treatment), they need to report their data with and without non-completers and with and without the last observation carried forward. A typical practice is to follow up only the completers (or responders) and to carry forward the last follow-up observation (e.g., at 3 months) if the patient is no longer available to the researchers at later intervals such as 12 months (e.g., Foa, et al., 1999). Unfortunately, doing so renders the 12-month data uninterpretable because these data are contaminated by 3-month data on what is often a sizeable proportion of patients. Researchers also need to be very cautious in the way they summarize follow-up findings in abstracts and reviews. If they follow up only completers or responders, this needs to be clearly stated in summarizing follow-up findings in the abstract.

Not only is the interval between termination and follow-up important, but so is the timeframe patients are asked to consider in follow-up assessments

(Brown & Barlow, 1995). Most long-term follow-up studies ask patients to report whether they experienced the target symptoms over a very brief span of the recent past, usually 1 to 4 weeks. This is likely to be an unreliable sample of behavior over the course of a 12- to 24-month period and can lead to the mistaken impression that a treatment shows sustained efficacy. The problem is exacerbated by the lack of comparison to controls, which are usually not assessed at long-term follow-up for ethical reasons (e.g., they have received treatment in the interim).

To maximize both reliability of reporting (e.g., because patients may not accurately recall precisely how many times they purged per week over the past 6 months) and comprehensiveness, the most sensible course may be for researchers to assess both the immediate past (e.g., symptoms in the past month) as well as the entire period since termination or the last follow-up assessment. Dimensional symptom assessment and assessment of related diagnoses (e.g., not-otherwise-specified diagnoses) should also be standard, given that many patients may no longer meet threshold for a disorder but still show residual symptoms that are clinically meaningful and bear on genuine efficacy.

Selecting an Appropriate Design: RCTs and Their Alternatives

We have suggested that reporting changes could maximize the utility of controlled trials of psychotherapy. Better reporting, however, can only address some of the problems we have outlined. To the extent that the assumptions underlying efficacy trials are violated in ways that threaten the robustness of the conclusions, researchers need to turn to other methods, or at least to triangulate on conclusions using multiple methods. We focus here, first, on the conditions under which RCTs are likely to be useful and second, on strategies that may prove useful when RCTs are not.

When RCT Designs Are Useful

Throughout this article, we have suggested a distinction between RCT methodology and EST methodology, the latter denoting a particular use of the former. An important question regards the conditions under which researchers can use RCT designs without making the assumptions that derail many EST designs relying on RCT methodology. We note here two such conditions.

First, the assumptions of EST methodology are only minimally violated for particular kinds of symptoms and particular kinds of interventions. (In these cases EST methodology and RCT methodology are for all intents and purposes identical.) The symptoms or syndromes that least violate the assumptions of EST methodology involve a link between a specific stimulus or representation and a specific cognitive, affective, or behavioral response that is not densely interconnected with (or can be readily disrupted despite) other symptoms or personality characteristics. Prime examples are simple phobia, specific social phobia, panic symptoms, obsessive-compulsive symptoms, and PTSD following a single traumatic experience (particularly one that does not lead to disruption of foundational beliefs about the world, such as its safety, beneficence, etc.; see Janoff-Bulman, 1992). In each of these instances, patients should, theoretically, be able to obtain substantial relief from an intervention aimed at breaking a specific associative connection, regardless of whatever other problems they may have, presuming that these problems do not interfere with compliance or other aspects of the treatment. Empirically, exposure-based treatments of such disorders have in fact produced many of the most impressive results reported over decades of psychotherapy research (see Roth & Fonagy, 1996). Syndromes that involve *generalized* affect states, in contrast, violate virtually all of the assumptions of EST methodology: They are highly resistant to change, they are associated with high comorbidity, they are strongly associated with (if not constitutive of) enduring personality dispositions, and efficacy trials testing treatments for them have typically required secondary correlational analyses to make sense of the findings. Perhaps not coincidentally, empirically, brief manualized treatments for these disorders tend to fail to produce sustained recovery at clinically meaningful follow-up intervals for any but a fraction of the patients who receive them.[15]

With respect to treatments, those that readily lend themselves to parametric variation (and hence to genuine dismantling) and to the degree of within-condition standardization required for causal inference in RCTs are least likely to violate the assumptions of EST methodology. Such treatments are brief, highly prescriptive, and comprise only a small number of distinct types of intervention (e.g., exposure, or exposure plus cognitive restructuring). Any treatment that (a) requires principle-based rather than intervention-based manualization, (b) prescribes a large set of interventions from which clinicians must choose on the basis of the material the patient presents, or (c) allows the patient to structure the session will introduce too much within-condition variability to permit the optimal use of EST designs. A convergence of theory and data should now be apparent: The studies that have yielded the best results in the psychotherapy literature are those that have targeted syndromes that least violate the assumptions regarding comorbidity and personality inherent in EST methods, applying treatments that least violate the requisites of experimental design as applied in EST methodology.

Second, even where many of the assumptions of EST methods are violated, researchers can still make considerable use of RCT designs to assess specific inter-

---

[15] In retrospect, the reasons for this seem clear: Neither two decades of psychotherapy research nor any other data of which we are aware suggest that any treatment is likely to change lifelong patterns ingrained in neural networks governed by Hebbian learning principles in a brief span of hours, particularly when these patterns are highly generalized or serve affect-regulatory functions. The neural networks governing these disorders likely extend so far and wide that models and methods appropriate for targeting specific associative links are likely to be a poor fit.

vention strategies or principles, general approaches to treatment, and moderators of outcome. Rather than assuming the burden of demonstrating that they have developed a complete package for treating depression that is superior to any other package for the heterogeneous population of patients who become depressed, investigators might address the more modest goal of testing whether a specific intervention strategy (e.g., challenging dysfunctional explicit beliefs) is associated with a clinically significant reduction in depressed mood, and if so, for how long. The goal of establishing a list of "approved" treatments has led to a primary focus on main effects (e.g., "cognitive therapy is an empirically sup-ported treatment for depression"), with the assumption that once researchers have done the hard work of identifying main effects, they can turn their atten-tion to studying moderators and interactions (i.e., the conditions under which the effect holds or does not hold). Although sensible from one point of view, this strategy poses serious dilemmas for clinicians, who need to know today, rather than 10 or 20 years from now, whether they should try a given treatment for depression with patients who are acutely suicidal, have BPD, have chronic low-level depression rather than major depression, and so forth.

In contrast, a focus on testing specific interventions allows researchers to move more quickly from main effects to clinically meaningful questions. For example, does the intervention produce effects that last for hours, days, weeks, or months? Does it work for patients who are mourning a specific loss? Does it work for individuals who have recently become unemployed and suffered a loss in self-esteem? Does it work for patients with various forms of comorbidity? The goal of a study of this sort is not to test a complete treatment package for a spe-cific disorder that would need to be modified and tested in modified form with every new subpopulation. Rather the goal is to isolate intervention strategies that clinicians can integrate into their practice when working with a patient for whom depression is a prominent symptom.

Perhaps one of the most important uses of RCTs would be to establish, empirically, the length of a given treatment required to produce a clinically mean-ingful response, a relatively enduring change, and so forth, vis-à-vis a particular set of outcome variables. For example, consider what might have happened if, in the 1980s, having found cognitive interventions to be useful in the first two or three studies, researchers had systematically compared outcome at 1, 2, and 5 years of 16, 52, 100, and 200 sessions of cognitive therapy for depression. This question, of course, reflects the benefits of hindsight, but it points to important implications for the ways researchers could maximize the use of clinical trials in the future.

The use of RCT designs we are advocating here is clearly more limited than the use propounded in the EST literature, although several prominent RCT meth-odologists have come to very similar conclusions (Borkovec & Castonguay, 1998;

Kazdin, 1997). If the goal is to study specific interventions or mechanisms of change, RCT designs may be more limited still if the disorder is one for which the malleability assumption does not apply and if the goal is to address diatheses for disorders as well as current states or episodes. For example, RCT methods can be very useful in identifying interventions designed to curtail (or perhaps forestall) a depressive episode, because effects of the intervention on target symptoms are proximal (within weeks or months), and natural variation in patients (if exclusion criteria are minimized) should allow for testing of moderators of treatment response (e.g., presence of comorbid conditions). If, however, the goal is to test interventions useful for treating depression over the long run or treating psychological diatheses for depression (e.g., negative affectivity, emotional dysregulation, or deficits in self-esteem regulation), it is unlikely that any small set of relatively brief, readily operationalizable procedures will produce a large enough signal to be detected across several subsequent years of noise (except, perhaps, through secondary correlational analyses), particularly given the likelihood that patients will seek other forms of treatment in the interim. Matters are even more complicated for polysymptomatic presentations with substantial personality diatheses, which are unlikely to show enduring change in response to brief, targeted interventions. In such cases, psychotherapy researchers will need to supplement RCTs with alternative designs or to tailor experimental methods to real-world clinical problems in ways that go beyond adding an extra 6-session module to a 12- or 16-session treatment.

Alternatives to RCT Designs

The question, then, is how to supplement RCT designs to converge on findings that are both scientifically rigorous and clinically relevant (see also Beutler, 2000; Lambert, Hansen, & Finch, 2001; Seligman, 1995). We argue that doing so requires a rethinking of the relation between science and practice in clinical science and a reconsideration of ways researchers and clinicians may be able to collaborate to spin clinical yarn(s) into empirical gold.

A transactional approach to knowledge generation in clinical science

Designing treatments and methodologies to match the clinical complexities of polysymptomatic patients, personality diatheses, and symptoms that are resistant to change requires, we believe, rethinking some pervasive assumptions not only about methodology in psychotherapy research but also, more broadly, about the relation between science and practice. Perhaps most important is the need to reconsider the top-down, unidirectional model of science and practice that has become increasingly prevalent in recent years, which assumes that knowledge flows primarily from researchers to clinicians. This assumption is implicit in the EST movement, in frequently voiced concerns about the need for better dissemination or marketing of well-tested manuals that clinicians do not seem to use (e.g., Addis, Wade, & Hatgis, 1999; Wilson, 1998), in clinical scientist models that are rapidly replacing scientist-practitioner models in the most prestigious clinical psychology graduate programs (e.g., McFall, 1991), and in the prevailing view of effectiveness research as a second stage of research in which laboratory-proven treatments are implemented in the community. The implicit metaphor underlying this view is essentially a biomedical one (see Stiles & Shapiro, 1989), in which researchers develop new medications, which pharmaceutical companies then market to physicians, who are perceived as consumers.

In some cases this is an appropriate metaphor, as when developments in basic science lead to novel therapeutic procedures. Perhaps the best example can be seen in exposure-based treatments that emerged from research on classical conditioning. In other cases, however, as a field we might be better served by a more transactional philosophy of clinical science, in which the laboratory and the clinic are both seen as resources for hypothesis generation and testing, albeit with different strengths and limitations. As researcher-clinicians, we can some-times capitalize on our knowledge of relevant basic and applied literatures as well as our clinical observation, and those who happen to be talented clinical observers as well as talented researchers (names like Barlow, Borkovec, and Linehan come to mind) are likely to generate novel approaches to treatment that few who live on only one side of the mountain would have been likely to develop. On the other hand, those of us who practice both research and psycho-therapy (or just research) cannot, over time, match the sheer number of hours full-time clinicians spend with their patients that allows them greater opportuni-ties for uncontrolled observation, innovation, and the kind of trial and error that constitutes the most scientific aspect of clinical practice.

The reality is that many, if not most, of the major clinical innovations in the history of our field have come from clinical practice. Cognitive therapy did not emerge in the laboratory. It emerged from the practice of a psychoanalyst, Aaron T. Beck (and from converging observations of another psychoanalyst, Albert Ellis), whose clinical data convinced him that the psychoanalytic methods of the time were too inefficient and whose *clinical empiricism* —that is, trial and error and careful assessment of the results—led him to develop a set of more struc-tured, active procedures that he and others subsequently put to more formal experimental test. What has perhaps distinguished A. T. Beck over the course of his career has been his ability to integrate what he and others have seen in the consulting room with both basic and applied research and his willingness, in a true scientific spirit, to change his theories and techniques when the available data—clinical and empirical—suggest the importance of doing so.

Using practice as a natural laboratory

We argued earlier that a failure to use systematic procedures to determine which treatments to test ultimately undermines any conclusions reached, however rigorously one tests interventions of interest. One way of selecting treatment strategies more systematically is to use clinical practice as a natural laboratory. Thus, as investigators, we might take advantage of the wide variation that exists in what clinicians do in practice and use correlational analyses to identify intervention strategies associated with positive outcome, initially and at multiple-years follow-up. Instead of requiring individual investigators to predict, on the basis of their best guesses and theoretical preferences, which treatments are most likely to work, this approach allows us to extend scientific method to the context of discovery. Once we have identified potentially useful interventions (and moderators) correlationally, we can then set our experimental sights on the interventions that appear most likely to pay off *as well as* on experimentally derived interventions that have received support in the laboratory.

Consider what such a design might look like in practice. An investigative team enlists the support of a large sample of clinicians who agree to participate and enlist participation of their next 3 patients with a given problem or disorder (e.g., clinically significant depression, bulimia nervosa, substance abuse, low self esteem, narcissistic personality disorder, negative affectivity, emotional dysregulation), irrespective of comorbid conditions or whether one disorder or another appears primary. The researchers may choose to study a random sample of clinicians, or they may use a peer nomination procedure to select clinicians whose peers (within or across theoretical orientations) consider master clinicians.

At the beginning of treatment and at periodic intervals thereafter, the investigators obtain data on symptoms, personality, and adaptive functioning from clinicians, patients, and independent interviewers. To assess what is happening in the treatment, clinicians audiotape two consecutive sessions at regular intervals until the treatment is over, which the investigators code for process-intervention variables using an instrument such as the Psychotherapy Process Q Set (Jones & Pulos, 1993). For each of the next 5 years, the investigators examine the process-intervention profiles of patients in the upper and lower 25th percentile on important outcome measures to see which items, singly and in combination, are predictive of success or failure. They may develop a single prototype of what effective treatment looks like (by simply aggregating data across all treatments in the upper 25th percentile), or use techniques such as Q-factor analysis to identify prototypes of successful treatments (on the assumption that more than one strategy may be effective and that mean item ratings may conceal two or more effective ways of working with patients that are very different or even polar opposites). If the sample is large enough, the investigators may develop different prototypes for different kinds of patients (e.g., those with particular personality styles, levels of severity of depression) or different profiles for different points in the treatment (e.g., the use of more structured interventions early, when depressive or bulimic symptoms are most acute, and the use of more exploratory interventions later). Clinicians would treat patients as they normally do, with no limits on number of sessions or type of interventions.

To move to an experimental phase that permits the testing of causal hypotheses, the investigators then use a similar design, but this time they add an experimental condition in which a group of randomly selected clinicians from the same sample is supervised to match the prototype of a successful treatment derived from the correlational phase of the study. Thus, clinicians in this condition might receive regular feedback on audio taped hours, including identification of items from the Psychotherapy Process Q Set on which they diverged by at least one standard deviation from the empirically generated prototype and consultation on how they might alter their technique to approximate the prototype. Aside from a no-supervision condition, an additional comparison group might receive regular feedback on the Q-sort profile of their treatment without comparison to any prototype, or supervision by a master clinician of their theoretical orientation. The investigators could then compare outcomes in these conditions to see whether clinicians supervised to match the empirical prototype were able to do so and whether doing so was associated with greater success. In so doing, researchers could use clinical practice not only to generate hypotheses but to test them using experimental methods. They could also take specific interventions associated with positive outcomes in the correlational phase of the research, particularly interventions with relatively proximal correlates, back to the laboratory to refine and test.

This approach represents an inversion of the relation between efficacy and effectiveness designs as currently understood. Rather than starting with pure samples and treatments in the laboratory and then taking only those with proven efficacy into the community, this strategy works in precisely the opposite direction: It begins with unselected samples in the community and then turns to experimental designs, in the community, in the laboratory, or both. This strategy essentially retains the advantages of relatively open-ended case studies in the process of scientific discovery but reduces their disadvantages by aggregating across cases from the start. Westen and colleagues have applied a similar approach to basic science research on psychopathology by quantifying clinicians' observations of their patients and then aggregating across cases to generate ways of classifying disorders empirically (e.g., Westen & Shedler, 1999a, 1999b; Westen, Shedler, Durrett, Glass, & Martens, 2003). For both basic and applied practice network research of this sort (see also, e.g., Asay, et al., 2002; Borkovec, Echemendia, Ragusea, & Ruiz, 2001; West, Zarin, Peterson, & Pincus, 1998), the goal is not to survey clinical opinion (e.g., about what works or how to classify psychopathology) but to quantify data from clinical practice in such a way as to derive scientifically valid generalizations across cases. Using this approach does not assume the wisdom of any given clinician's clinical experience. Rather, it assumes that variability among clinicians will allow the investigator to identify and distill clinical wisdom empirically.

Summary: Maximizing the Efficacy of Psychotherapy Research

To summarize, we are not arguing against the use of controlled clinical trials to assess the efficacy of psychotherapies. We are arguing, rather, that as a field, we need to make better use of them, and to triangulate on conclusions with other methods for which RCT designs are not optimal. For disorders and treatments for which the use of RCTs is appropriate, we need to apply standards of reporting with which most scientists would agree in theory but are not routinely implemented in practice. For disorders and treatments for which the assumptions of EST methodology are violated, we need not abandon scientific method. We can make better use of RCT designs if we focus on intervention strategies and change processes rather than treatment packages, and if we focus on target symptoms likely to change within relatively brief intervals. Where RCT designs provide only limited information, we should take advantage of one of the greatest resources at our disposal, clinical practice, which can and should serve as a natural laboratory for both generating and testing hypotheses. Correlational designs can extend the reach of scientific method into the context of discovery, identifying promising interventions that can then be tested experimentally, both in the community and the laboratory.

CONCLUSION: TOWARD EMPIRICALLY INFORMED PSYCHOTHERAPY

A reconsideration of both the assumptions and the findings of RCTs generally interpreted as evidence for the validity of a specific set of brief manualized treatments suggests the need for both a more nuanced view of outcome and a reexamination of the enterprise of compiling a list of empirically supported psychotherapies. Inherent in the methodology that has been shaping the agenda for clinical training, practice, licensing, and third-party reimbursement is a series of assumptions that are violated to a greater or lesser degree by different disorders and treatments. These assumptions include symptom malleability, incidental comorbidity, dissociation between symptoms and personality dispositions, and a one-size-fits-all model of hypothesis testing. For disorders characterized by readily identifiable, maladaptive links between specific stimuli or representations and specific responses, and treatments capable of a kind of manualization that allows genuine experimental control, these conditions are minimally violated. Not coincidentally, these are the disorders and treatments that have generated the clearest empirical support using RCT methodology: exposure-based treatments for specific anxiety symptoms (as well as many behavioral treatments of the 1960s and

1970s, which focused on specific problems such as speech anxiety and assertiveness).

For most disorders and treatments, however, the available data suggest that the need to rethink the notion of empirical support as a dichotomous variable, a notion on which practice guidelines comprising a list of validated treatments is implicitly predicated. The average RCT for most disorders currently described as empirically supported excludes between one third and two thirds of patients who present for treatment, and the kinds of patients excluded often appear both more representative and more treatment resistant in naturalistic studies. For most disorders, particularly those involving generalized symptoms such as major depression or GAD, brief, largely cognitive-behavioral treatments have demonstrated considerable efficacy in reducing immediate symptomatology. The average patient for most disorders does not, however, recover and stay recovered at clinically meaningful follow-up intervals.

Reporting practices in the psychotherapy literature also require substantial changes to maximize the benefits of RCT designs. Frequently consumers cannot obtain details essential for assessing the internal and external validity of even high-quality studies. These details, particularly relating to external validity, tend to be absent from qualitative and quantitative reviews as well, leading to conclusions that are often under qualified and over generalized.

Despite frequent claims in the literature about treatment of choice, few data are available comparing manualized treatments with treatment as usual for patients with the financial resources to obtain treatment from experienced professionals in private practice, who may or may not provide as good or better care. What *is* known is that treatments in the community tend to be substantially longer than treatments in the laboratory, regardless of the therapist's theoretical orientation, and that in naturalistic samples, more extensive treatments tend to achieve better results according to both patient and clinician reports. To what extent this is a methodological artifact is unknown. For the polysymptomatic patients who constitute the majority of patients in the community, researchers and clinicians need to collaborate to make better use of natural variations in clinical practice to identify interventions associated empirically with good outcomes and to subject correlationally identified intervention strategies to experimental investigation to assess their potential causal impact.

Rather than focusing on treatment packages constructed in the laboratory designed to be transported to clinical practice and assuming that any single design (RCTs) can answer all clinically meaningful questions, as a field we might do well to realign our goals, from trying to provide clinicians with step-by-step instructions for treating decontextualized symptoms or syndromes to offering them empirically tested interventions and empirically supported theories of change that they can integrate into *empirically informed treatments*. This realignment would require a very different conception of the nature of clinical work, and of the relation between science and practice, than is current in our discipline, where researchers and clinicians often view each other with suspicion and disrespect (see Goldfried & Wolfe, 1996). Perhaps most important, it would require the assumption of clinically competent decision makers (rather than paraprofessionals trained to stay faithful to a validated manual) who have the competence to read and understand relevant applied *and* basic research, as well as the competence to read people—competencies we suspect are not highly correlated. Learning how to create such clinicians will, we suspect, prove at least as challenging as designing treatments for them to conduct.

REFERENCES

Abelson, R. (1995). *Statistics as principled argument*. Hillsdale, NJ: Erlbaum.

Ablon, J. S., & Jones, E. E. (1998). How expert clinicians' prototypes of an ideal treatment correlate with outcome in psychodynamic and cognitive behavioral therapy. *Psychotherapy Research, 8,* 71–83.

Ablon, J. S., & Jones, E. E. (1999). Psychotherapy process in the National Institute of Mental Health Treatment of Depression Collaborative Research Program. *Journal of Consulting and Clinical Psychology, 67,* 64–75.

Ablon, J. S., & Jones, E. E. (2002). Validity of controlled clinical trials of psychotherapy: Findings from the NIMH Treatment of Depression Collaborative Research Program. *American Journal of Psychiatry, 159,* 775–783.

Addis, M. E., Wade, W. A., & Hatgis, C. (1999). Barriers to dissemination of evidence-based practices: Addressing practitioners' concerns about manual-based psychotherapies. *Clinical Psychology: Science and Practice, 6,* 430–441.

Agras, W. S., Crow, S. J., Halmi, K. A., Mitchell, J. E., Wilson, G. T., & Kraemer, H. C. (2000). Outcome predictors for the cognitive behavior treatment of bulimia nervosa: Data from a multisite study. *American Journal of Psychiatry, 157,* 1302–1308.

American Psychiatric Association. (1980). *Diagnostic and statistical manual of mental disorders* (3rd ed.). Washington, DC: Author.

American Psychiatric Association. (1994). *Diagnostic and statistical manual of mental disorders* (4th ed.). Washington, DC: Author.

Arntz, A., & van den Hout, M. (1996). Psychological treatments of panic disorder without agoraphobia: Cognitive therapy versus applied relaxation. *Behaviour Research and Therapy, 34,* 113–121.

Asay, T. P., Lambert, M. J., Gregersen, A. T., & Goates, M. K. (2002). Using patient-focused research in evaluating treatment outcome in private practice. *Journal of Clinical Psychology, 58,* 1213–1225.

Bandura, A. (1977). *Social learning theory*. Englewood Cliffs, NJ: Prentice-Hall.

Barlow, D. (1996). The effectiveness of psychotherapy: Science and policy. *Clinical Psychology: Science and Practice, 1,* 109–122.

Barlow, D. (2002). *Anxiety and its disorders* (2nd ed.). New York: Guilford Press.

Barlow, D. H., Gorman, J. M., Shear, M. K., & Woods, S. W. (2000). Cognitive–behavioral therapy, imipramine, or their combination for panic disorder: A randomized controlled trial. *Journal of he American Medical Association, 283,* 2529–2536.

Beck, A. T. (1976). *Cognitive therapy and the emotional disorders*. New York: International Universities Press.

Beck, A. T., Ward, C. H., Mendelson, M., Mock, J. E., & Erbaugh, J. K. (1961). An inventory for measuring depression. *Archives of General Psychiatry, 4,* 561–571.

Beck, J. G., Stanley, M. A., Baldwin, L. E., Deagle, E. A., & Averill, P. M. (1994). Comparison of cognitive therapy and relaxation training for panic disorder. *Journal of Consulting and Clinical Psychology, 62,* 818–826.

Beutler, L. E. (1998). Identifying empirically supported treatments: What if we didn't? *Journal of Consulting and Clinical Psychology, 66,* 113–120.

Beutler, L. E. (2000). David and Goliath: When empirical and clinical standards of practice meet. *American Psychologist, 55,* 997–1007.

Beutler, L. E., Moleiro, C., & Talebi, H. (2002). How practitioners can systematically use empirical evidence in treatment selection. *Journal of Clinical Psychology, 58,* 1199–1212.

Blagys, M., Ackerman, S., Bonge, D., & Hilsenroth, M. (2003). *Measuring psychodynamic-interpersonal and cognitive–behavioral therapist activity: Development of the Comparative Psychotherapy Process Scale*. Unpublished manuscript.

Blatt, S., & Zuroff, D. (1992). Interpersonal relatedness and self-definition: Two prototypes for depression. *Clinical Psychology Review, 12,* 527–562.

Borkovec, T. D. (1994). Between-group therapy outcome design: Design and methodology. In L. S. Onken & J. D. Blaine (Eds.), *NIDA Research Monograph No. 137* (pp. 249–289). Rockville, MD: National Institute on Drug Abuse.

Borkovec, T. D., Abel, J. L., & Newman, H. (1995). Effects of psychotherapy on comorbid conditions in generalized anxiety disorder. *Journal of Consulting and Clinical Psychology, 63,* 479–483.

Borkovec, T. D., & Castonguay, L. G. (1998). What is the scientific meaning of empirically supported therapy? *Journal of Consulting and Clinical Psychology, 66,* 136–142.

Borkovec, T. D., & Costello, E. (1993). Efficacy of applied relaxation and cognitive–behavioral therapy in the treatment of generalized anxiety disorder. *Journal of Consulting and Clinical Psychology, 61,* 611–619.

Borkovec, T. D., Echemendia, R. J., Ragusea, S. A., & Ruiz, M. (2001). The Pennsylvania practice research network and future possibilities for clinically meaningful and scientifically rigorous psychotherapy effectiveness research. *Clinical Psychology: Science and Practice, 8,* 155–167.

Bouchard, S., Gauther, J., Laberge, B., French, D., Pelletier, M., & Godbout, C. (1996). Exposure versus cognitive restructuring in the treatment of panic disorder with agoraphobia. *Behaviour Research and Therapy, 34,* 213–224.

Brown, T. A., & Barlow, D. H. (1992). Comorbidity among anxiety disorders: Implications for treatment and *DSM–IV*. *Journal of Consulting and Clinical Psychology, 60,* 835–844.

Brown, T. A., & Barlow, D. H. (1995). Long-term outcome in cognitive–behavioral treatment of panic disorder: Clinical predictors and alternative strategies for assessment. *Journal of Consulting and Clinical Psychology, 63,* 754–765.

Brown, T. A., Chorpita, B. F., & Barlow, D. H. (1998). Structural relationships among dimensions of the *DSM–IV* anxiety and mood disorders and dimensions of negative affect, positive affect, and autonomic arousal. *Journal of Abnormal Psychology, 107,* 179–192.

Bruce, T. J., Spiegel, D. A., & Hegel, M. T. (1999). Cognitive-behavioral therapy helps prevent relapse and recurrence of panic disorder following alprazolam discontinuation: A long-term follow-up of the Peoria and Dartmouth studies. *Journal of Consulting and Clinical Psychology, 67,* 151–156.

Bruch, H. (1973). *Eating disorders: Obesity, anorexia nervosa, and the person within*. New York: Basic Books.

Calhoun, K. S., Moras, K., Pilkonis, P. A., & Rehm, L. (1998). Empirically supported treatments: Implications for training. *Journal of Consulting and Clinical Psychology, 66,* 151–162.

Carroll, K. M., & Nuro, K. F. (2002). One size cannot fit all: A stage model for psychotherapy manual development. *Clinical Psychology: Science and Practice, 9,* 396–406.

Castonguay, L. G., Goldfried, M. R., Wiser, S., Raue, P., & Hayes, A. M. (1996). Predicting the effect of cognitive therapy for depression: A study of unique and common factors. *Journal of Consulting and Clinical Psychology, 64,* 497–504.

Chambless, D., & Hollon, S. (1998). Defining empirically supported therapies. *Journal of Consulting and Clinical Psychology, 66,* 7–18.

Chambless, D., & Ollendick, T. (2000). Empirically supported psychological interventions: Controversies and evidence. *Annual Review of Psychology, 52,* 685–716.

Clark, D. M., Salkovskis, P. M., Hackmann, A., Middleton, H., Anastasiades, P., & Gelder, M. (1994). A comparison of cognitive therapy, applied relaxation and imipramine in the treatment of panic disorder. *British Journal of Psychiatry, 164,* 759–769.

Compas, B. E., Haaga, D. A. F., Keefe, F. J., & Leitenbert, H. (1998). Sampling of empirically supported psychosocial treatments from health psychology: Smoking, chronic pain, cancer, and bulimia nervosa. *Journal of Consulting and Clinical Psychology, 66,* 89–112.

Cox, B. J., Swinson, R. P., Morrison, B. L., & Paul, S. (1993). Clomipramine, fluoxetine, and behavior therapy in the treatment of obsessive-compulsive disorder: A meta-analysis. *Journal of Behavior Therapy and Experimental Psychiatry, 24*(2), 149–153.

Crits-Christoph, P., & Mintz, J. (1991). Implications of therapist effects for the design and analysis of comparative studies of psychotherapies. *Journal of Consulting and Clinical Psychology, 59,* 20–26.

Eddy, K. T., Dutra, L., & Westen, D. (2004). *A multidimensional metaanalysis of psychotherapy and pharmacotherapy for obsessive- compulsive disorder.* Unpublished manuscript. Emory University, Atlanta, GA.

Egger, M., Juni, P., & Bartlett, C. (1999). Value of flow diagrams in reports of randomized controlled trials. *Journal of the American Medical Association, 285,* 1996–1999.

Elkin, I., Shea, T., Watkins, J., Imber, S., Sotsky, S., Collins, J., et al. (1989). National Institute of Mental Health Treatment of Depression Collaborative Research Program. *Archives of General Psychiatry, 46,* 971–982.

Eysenck, H. J. (1995). Meta-analysis squared—Does it make sense? *American Psychologist, 50,* 110–111.

Fairburn, C. G. (1997). Interpersonal psychotherapy for bulimia nervosa. In D. M. Garner & P. E. Garfinkel (Eds.), *Handbook of treatment for eating disorders* (2nd ed., pp. 278–294). New York: Guilford Press.

Fairburn, C. G., Jones, R., Peveler, R., Carr, S. J., Solomon, R. A., O'Connor, M., et al. (1991). Three psychological treatments for bulimia nervosa: A comparative trial. *Archives of General Psychiatry, 48,* 463– 469.

Fairburn, C. G., Kirk, J., O'Connor, M., & Cooper, P. J. (1986). A comparison of two psychological treatments for bulimia nervosa. *Behaviour Research and Therapy, 24,* 629–643.

Fairburn, C. G., Marcus, M. D., & Wilson, G. T. (1993). Cognitive behaviour therapy for binge eating and bulimia nervosa: A comprehensive treatment manual. In C. G. Fairburn & G. T. Wilson (Eds.), *Binge eating: Nature, assessment, and treatment* (pp. 361–404). New York: Guilford Press.

Feeley, M., DeRubeis, R. J., & Gelfand, L. (1999). The temporal relation of adherence and alliance to symptom change in cognitive therapy for depression. *Journal of Consulting and Clinical Psychology, 67,* 578– 582.

Feinstein, A. R. (1995). Meta-analysis: Statistical alchemy for the 21st century. *Journal of Clinical Epidemiology, 48,* 71–79.

Foa, E. B., Dancu, C. V., Hembree, E. A., Jaycox, L. H., Meadows, E. A., & Street, G. P. (1999). A comparison of exposure therapy, stress inoculation training, and their combination for reducing posttraumatic stress disorder in female assault victims. *Journal of Consulting and Clinical Psychology, 67,* 194–200.

Frank, E., Shear, M. K., Rucci, P., Cyranowski, J., Endicott, J., Fagiolini, A., et al. (2000). Influence of panic-agoraphobic spectrum symptoms on treatment response in patients with recurrent major depression. *Archives of General Psychiatry, 157,* 1101–1107.

Frank, E., & Spanier, C. (1995). Interpersonal psychotherapy for depression: Overview, clinical efficacy, and future directions. *Clinical Psychology: Science and Practice, 2,* 349–369.

Franklin, M. E., Abramowitz, J. S., Levitt, J. T., Kozak, M. J., & Foa, E. B. (2000). Effectiveness of exposure and ritual prevention for obsessive–compulsive disorder: Randomized compared with nonrandomized samples. *Journal of Consulting and Clinical Psychology, 68,* 594–602.

Garner, D. M., Rockert, W., Davis, R., Garner, M. V., Olmstead, M. P., & Eagle, M. (1993). A comparison of cognitive–behavioral and supportive–expressive therapy for bulimia nervosa. *American Journal of Psychiatry, 150,* 37–46.

Gemar, M. C., Segal, Z. V., Sagrati, S., & Kennedy, S. J. (2001). Mood-induced changes on the Implicit Association Test in recovered depressed patients. *Journal of Abnormal Psychology, 110,* 282–289.

Goldfried, M. R. (2000). Consensus in psychotherapy research and practice: Where have all the findings gone? *Psychotherapy Research, 10,* 1–16.

Goldfried, M. R., & Wolfe, B. (1996). Psychotherapy practice and research: Repairing a strained relationship. *American Psychologist, 51,* 1007–1016.

Goldfried, M. R., & Wolfe, B. E. (1998). Toward a more clinically valid approach to therapy research. *Journal of Consulting and Clinical Psychology, 66,* 143–150.

Hammen, C., Ellicott, A., Gitlin, M., & Jamison, K. R. (1989). Sociotropy/autonomy and vulnerability to specific life events in patients with unipolar depression and bipolar disorders. *Journal of Abnormal Psychology, 98,* 154–160.

Hardy, G. E., Barkham, M., Shapiro, D. A., Stiles, W. B., Rees, A., & Reynolds, S. (1995). Impact of Cluster C personality disorders on outcomes of contrasting brief psychotherapies for depression. *Journal of Consulting and Clinical Psychology, 63,* 997–1004.

Harstein, N. B. (1996). Suicide risk in lesbian, gay, and bisexual youth. In R. P. Cabaj, T. S. Stein, et al. (Eds.), *Textbook of homosexuality and mental health* (pp. 819–837). Washington, DC: American Psychiatric Press.

Hayes, A. M., Castonguay, L. G., & Goldfried, M. R. (1996). Effectiveness of targeting the vulnerability factors of depression in cognitive therapy. *Journal of Consulting and Clinical Psychology, 64,* 23–627.

Hedlund, S., & Rude, S. S. (1995). Evidence of latent depressive schemas in formerly depressed individuals. *Journal of Abnormal Psychology, 104,* 517–525.

Henry, W., Strupp, H., Butler, S., Schacht, T., & Binder, J. (1993). Effects of training in time-limited dynamic psychotherapy: Changes in therapist behavior. *Journal of Consulting and Clinical Psychology, 61,* 434–433.

Hill, C. E., O'Grady, K. E., & Elkin, I. (1992). Applying the Collaborative Study Psychotherapy Rating Scale to rate therapist adherence in cognitive–behavior therapy, interpersonal therapy, and clinical management. *Journal of Consulting and Clinical Psychology, 60,* 73–79.

Hollon, S. D., Thase, M. E., & Markowitz, J. C. (2002). Treatment and prevention of depression. *Psychological Science in the Public Interest, 3,* 39–77.

Howard, K. I., Cornille, T. A., Lyons, J. S., Vessey, J. T., Lueger, R. J., & Saunders, S. M. (1996). Patterns of mental health service utilization. *Archives of General Psychiatry, 53,* 696–703.

Howard, K. I., Kopta, S. M., Krause, M. S., & Orlinsky, D. E. (1986). The dose-effect relationship in psychotherapy. *American Psychologist, 41,* 159–164.

Howard, K. I., Lueger, R., Maling, M., & Martinovich, Z. (1993). A phase model of psychotherapy: Causal mediation of outcome. *Journal of Consulting and Clinical Psychology, 54,* 106–110.

Humphreys, K., & Weisner, C. (2000). Use of exclusion criteria in selecting research subjects and its effects on the generalizability of alcohol treatment outcome studies. *American Journal of Psychiatry, 157,* 588–594.

Ilardi, S. S., & Craighead, W. E. (1994). The role of nonspecific factors in cognitive–behavior therapy for depression. *Clinical Psychology: Science and Practice, 1,* 138–156.

Ingram, R. E., & Ritter, J. (2000). Vulnerability to depression: Cognitive reactivity and parental bonding in high-risk individuals. *Journal of Abnormal Psychology, 109,* 588–596.

Jacobson, N. J., Roberts, L. J., Berns, S. B., & McGlinchey, J. B. (1999). Methods for defining and determining the clinical significance of treatment effects: Description, application, and alternatives. *Journal of Consulting and Clinical Psychology, 67,* 300–307.

Jacobson, N. J., & Truax, P. (1991). Clinical significance: A statistical approach to defining meaningful change in psychotherapy research. *Journal of Consulting and Clinical Psychology, 59,* 12–19.

Janoff-Bulman, R. (1992). *Shattered assumptions: Towards a new psychology of trauma.* New York: Free Press.

Johnson, C., Tobin, D. L., & Dennis, A. (1991). Differences in treatment outcome between borderline and nonborderline bulimics at one-year follow-up. *International Journal of Eating Disorders, 9,* 617–627.

Jones, E. E. (2000). *Therapeutic action.* Northvale, NJ: Aronson.

Jones, E. E., & Pulos, S. M. (1993). Comparing the process in psychodynamic and cognitive–behavioral therapies. *Journal of Consulting and Clinical Psychology, 61,* 306–316.

Judd, L. (1997). The clinical course of unipolar major depressive disorders. *Archives of General Psychiatry, 54,* 989–991.

Kazdin, A. E. (1997). A model for developing effective treatments: Progression and interplay of theory, research, and practice. *Journal of Clinical Child Psychiatry, 26,* 114–129.

Kendall, P. C. (1998). Empirically supported psychological therapies. *Journal of Consulting and Clinical Psychology, 66,* 3–6.

Kendall, P. C., Marrs-Garcia, A., Nath, S. R., & Sheldrick, R. C. (1999). Normative comparisons for the evaluation of clinical significance. *Journal of Consulting and Clinical Psychology, 67,* 285–299.

Kessler, R. C., Nelson, C. B., McGonagle, K. A., Liu, J., et al. (1996). Comorbidity of DSM-III—R major depressive disorder in the general population: Results from the US National Comorbidity Survey. *British Journal of Psychiatry, 168*(Suppl. 30), 17–30.

Kessler, R. C., Stang, P., Wittchen, H. U., Stein, M., & Walters, E. (1999). Lifetime comorbidities between social phobia and mood disorders in the US National Comorbidity Survey. *Psychological Medicine, 29,* 555–567.

Klerman, G. L., & Weissman, M. M. (1993). *New applications of interpersonal psychotherapy.* Washington, DC: American Psychiatric Press.

Kobak, K. A., Greist, J. A., Jefferson, J. W., Katzelnick, D. J., & Henk, H. J. (1998). Behavioral versus pharmacological treatments of obsessive compulsive disorder: A meta-analysis. *Psychopharmacologia, 136,* 205–216.

Kopta, S., Howard, K., Lowry, J., & Beutler, L. (1994). Patterns of symptomatic recovery in psychotherapy. *Journal of Consulting and Clinical Psychology, 62,* 1009–1016.

Krueger, R. F. (2002). The structure of common mental disorders. *Archives of General Psychiatry, 59,* 570–571.

Kwon, P., & Whisman, M. A. (1998). Sociotropy and autonomy as vulnerabilities to specific life events: Issues in life event categorization. *Cognitive Therapy and Research, 22,* 353–362.

Kyuken, W., Kurzer, N., DeRubeis, R. J., Beck, A. T., & Brown, G. K. (2001). Response to cognitive therapy in depression: The role of maladaptive beliefs and personality disorders. *Journal of Consulting and Clinical Psychology, 69,* 560–566.

Lambert, M. J., & Bergin, A. E. (1994). The effectiveness of psychotherapy. In A. E. Bergin & S. L. Garfield (Eds.), *Handbook of psychotherapy and behavior change* (4th ed., pp. 143–189). New York: Wiley.

Lambert, M. J., Hansen, N. B., & Finch, A. E. (2001). Patient-focused research: Using patient outcome data to enhance treatment effects. *Journal of Consulting and Clinical Psychology, 69,* 159–172.

Lewinsohn, P., Rohde, P., Seeley, J. R., & Klein, D. N. (1997). Axis II psychopathology as a function of Axis I disorders in childhood and adolescence. *Journal of the American Academy of Child and Adolescent Psychiatry, 36,* 1752–1759.

Lilienfeld, S. O., Waldman, I., & Israel, A. C. (1994). A critical examination of the use of the term and concept of comorbidity in psychopathology research. *Clinical Psychology: Science and Practice, 1,* 71–83.

Linehan, M. M. (1993). *Cognitive-behavioral treatment of borderline personality disorder.* New York: Guilford Press.

Luborsky, L., Barton, S., & Luborsky, L. (1975). Comparative studies of psychotherapies: Is it true that "everyone has won and all must have prizes"? *Archives of General Psychiatry, 32,* 995–1008.

Luborsky, L., Diguer, L., Seligman, D. A., Rosenthal, R., Krause, E. D., Johnson, S., et al. (1999). The researcher's own therapy allegiances: A "wild card" in comparisons of treatment efficacy. *Clinical Psychology: Science and Practice, 6,* 95–106.

Luborsky, L., McLellan, A. T., Diguer, L., Woody, G., & Seligman, D. A. (1997). The psychotherapist matters: Comparison of outcomes across twenty-two therapists and seven patient samples. *Clinical Psychology: Science and Practice, 4,* 53–65.

McDermut, W., Miller, I. W., & Brown, R. A. (2001). The efficacy of group psychotherapy for depression: A meta-analysis and review of the empirical research. *Clinical Psychology: Science and Practice, 8,* 98–116.

McFall, R. (1991). Manifesto for a science of clinical psychology. *The Clinical Psychologist, 44*(6), 75–88.

Meehl, P. E. (1954). *Clinical vs. statistical prediction.* Minneapolis: University of Minnesota Press.

Messer, S. (2001). Empirically supported treatments: What's a nonbehaviorist to do? In B. D. Slife, R. N. Williams, & D. Barlow (Eds.), *Critical issues in psychotherapy: Translating new ideas into practice* (pp. 3–19). Thousand Oaks, CA: Sage.

Mineka, S., Watson, D., & Clark, L. A. (1998). Comorbidity of anxiety and unipolar mood disorders. *Annual Review of Psychology, 49,* 377–412.

Mitchell, J. E., Maki, D. D., Adson, D. E., Ruskin, B. S., & Crow, S. J. (1997). The selectivity of inclusion and exclusion criteria in bulimia nervosa treatment studies. *International Journal of Eating Disorders, 22,* 243–252.

Morrison, C., Bradley, R. & Westen, D. (2003). The external validity of efficacy trials for depression and anxiety: A naturalistic study. *Psychology and Psychotherapy: Theory, Research and Practice, 76,* 109–132.

Mueller, T. I., Leon, A. C., Keller, M. B., Solomon, D. A., Endicott, J., Coryell, W., et al. (1999). Recurrence after recovery from major depressive disorder during 15 years of observational follow-up. *American Journal of Psychiatry, 156,* 1000–1006.

Nakash-Eisikovits, O., Dierberger, A., & Westen, D. (2002). A multidimensional meta-analysis of pharmacotherapy for bulimia nervosa: Summarizing the range of outcomes in controlled clinical trials. *Harvard Review of Psychiatry, 10,* 193–211.

Nathan, P. E. (1998). Practice guidelines: Not yet ideal. *American Psychologist, 53,* 290–299.

Nathan, P. E., Stuart, S. P., & Dolan, S. L. (2000). Research on psychotherapy efficacy and effectiveness: Between Scylla and Charybdis? *Psychological Bulletin, 126,* 964–981.

Newman, D. L., Moffitt, T., Caspi, A., & Silva, P. A. (1998). Comorbid mental disorders: Implications for treatment and sample selection. *Journal of Abnormal Psychology, 107,* 305–311.

Oldham, J. M., Skodol, A. E., Kellman, H. D., Hyler, S. E., Doidge, N., Rosnick, L., et al. (1995). Comorbidity of Axis I and Axis II disorders. *American Journal of Psychiatry, 152,* 571–578.

Ost, L., & Westling, B. E. (1995). Applied relaxation vs. cognitive behavior therapy in the treatment of panic disorder. *Behaviour Research and Therapy, 33,* 145–158.

Persons, J. B. (1991). Psychotherapy outcome studies do not accurately represent current models of psychotherapy: A proposed remedy. *American Psychologist, 46,* 99–106.

Persons, J. B., & Silberschatz, G. (1998). Are results of randomized controlled trials useful to psychotherapists? *Journal of Consulting and Clinical Psychology, 66,* 126–135.

Persons, J., & Tompkins, M. (1997). Cognitive-behavioral case formulation. In T. D. Ells (Ed.), *Handbook of psychotherapy case formulation* (pp. 314–339). Oakland, CA: Center for Cognitive Therapy.

Popper, K. (1959). *The logic of scientific discovery.* London: Hutchinson.

Rosenthal, R. (1991). *Meta-analytic procedures for social research* (Revised ed.). Thousand Oaks, CA: Sage.

Rosenthal, R. (1995). Writing meta-analytic reviews. *Psychological Bulletin, 118,* 183–192.

Rosenthal, R., & DiMatteo, M. R. (2000). Meta analysis: Recent developments in quantitative methods for literature reviews. *Annual Review of Psychology, 52,* 59–82.

Roth, A., & Fonagy, P. (1996). *What works for whom? A critical review of psychotherapy research.* New York: Guilford Press.

Scheel, K. R. (2000). The empirical basis of dialectical behavior therapy: Summary, critique, and implications. *Clinical Psychology: Science and Practice, 7,* 68–86.

Segal, Z. V., Gemar, M., & Williams, S. (1999). Differential cognitive response to a mood challenge following successful cognitive therapy pharmacotherapy for unipolar depression. *Journal of Abnormal Psychology, 108,* 3–10.

Seligman, M. E. P. (1995). The effectiveness of psychotherapy. *American Psychologist, 50,* 965–974.

Shea, M., Elkin, I., Imber, S., Sotsky, S., Watkins, J., Collins, J., et al. (1992). Course of depressive symptoms over follow-up: Findings from the National Institute of Mental Health Treatment of Depression Collaborative Research Program. *Archives of General Psychiatry, 49,* 782–787.

Shea, M., Widiger, T., & Klein, M. (1992). Comorbidity of personality disorders and depression: Implications for treatment. *Journal of Clinical and Consulting Psychology, 60,* 857–868.

Shear, M. K., Pilkonis, P. A., Cloitre, M., & Leon, A. C. (1994). Cognitive behavioral treatment compared with nonprescriptive treatment of panic disorder. *Archives of General Psychiatry, 51,* 395–402.

Skinner, B. F. (1953). *Science and human behavior.* New York: Macmillan.

Smith, M., & Glass, G. (1977). Meta-analysis of psychotherapy outcome studies. *American Psychologist, 32,* 752–760.

Snyder, D. K., Wills, R. M., & Grady, F. A. (1991). Long-term effectiveness of behavioral versus insight-oriented marital therapy: A 4-year follow-up study. *Journal of Consulting and Clinical Psychology, 59,* 138–141.

Steiger, H., & Stotland, S. (1996). Prospective study of outcome in bulimics as a function of Axis-II comorbidity: Long-term responses on eating and psychiatric symptoms. *International Journal of Eating Disorders, 20,* 149–161.

Stiles, W. B., & Shapiro, D. A. (1989). Abuse of the drug metaphor in psychotherapy process-outcome research. *Clinical Psychology Review, 9,* 521–543.

Strupp, H. H., Horowitz, L. M., & Lambert, M. J. (Eds.). (1997). *Measuring patient changes in mood, anxiety, and personality disorders: Toward a core battery.* Washington, DC: American Psychological Association.

Stuart, G. L., Treat, T. A., & Wade, W. A. (2000). Effectiveness of an empirically based treatment for panic disorder delivered in a service clinic setting: 1-year follow-up. *Journal of Consulting and Clinical Psychology, 68,* 506–512.

Sullivan, H. S. (1953). *The interpersonal theory of psychiatry.* New York: Norton.

Tang, T., & DeRubeis, R. J. (1999). Sudden gains and critical sessions in cognitive–behavioral therapy for depression. *Journal of Consulting and Clinical Psychology, 67,* 894–904.

Task Force on Psychological Intervention Guidelines. (1995). *Template for developing guidelines: Interventions for mental disorders and psychosocial aspects of physical disorders.* Washington, DC: American Psychological Association.

Thase, M. E., Simons, A. D., McGeary, J., Cahalane, J., Hughes, C., Harden, T., et al. (1992). Relapse after cognitive behavior therapy of depression: Potential implications for longer courses of treatment. *American Journal of Psychiatry, 149,* 1046–1052.

Thompson-Brenner, H., Glass, S., & Westen, D. (2003). A multidimensional meta-analysis of psychotherapy for bulimia nervosa. *Clinical Psychology: Science and Practice, 10,* 269–287.

Thompson-Brenner, H., & Westen, D. (2004a). *Accumulating evidence for personality subtypes in eating disorders: Differences in comorbidity, adaptive functioning, treatment response, and treatment interventions in a naturalistic sample.* Unpublished manuscript. Boston University, Boston.

Thompson-Brenner, H., & Westen, D. (2004b). *A naturalistic study of psychotherapy for bulimia nervosa: Comorbidity, outcome, and therapeutic interventions in the community.* Unpublished manuscript. Boston University, Boston.

van Blakom, A. J. L. M., van Oppen, P., Vermeulen, A. W. A., van Dyck, R., & Harne, C. M. V. (1994). A meta-analysis on the treatment of obsessive compulsive disorder: A comparison of antidepressants, behavior, and cognitive therapy. *Clinical Psychology Review, 14,* 359–381.

Wampold, B., Mondin, G., Moody, M., Stich, F., Benson, K., & Ahn, H. (1997). Methodological problems in identifying efficacious psychotherapies. *Psychotherapy Research, 7,* 21–43.

Watson, D., & Clark, L. A. (1992). Affects separable and inseparable: On the hierarchical arrangement of the negative affects. *Journal of Personality and Social Psychology, 62,* 489–505.

Watson, D., Clark, L. A., Weber, K., Assenheimer, J. S., Strauss, M. E., & McCormick, R. A. (1994). Testing a tripartite model: II. Exploring the symptom structure of anxiety and depression in student, adult, and patient samples. *Journal of Abnormal Psychology, 104,* 15–25.

Weersing, V. R., & Weisz, J. R. (2002). Community clinic treatment of depressed youth: Benchmarking usual care against CBT clinical trials. *Journal of Consulting and Clinical Psychology, 70,* 299–310.

Weinberger, J. (1995). Common factors aren't so common: The common factors dilemma. *Clinical Psychology: Science and Practice, 2,* 45–69.

Weinberger, J. (2000). *Why can't psychotherapists and psychotherapy researchers get along? Underlying causes of the EST–effectiveness controversy.* Unpublished manuscript. Adelphi University, Garden City, NY.

Weiss, B., Catron, T., & Harris, V. (2000). A 2-year follow-up of the effectiveness of traditional child psychotherapy. *Journal of Consulting and Clinical Psychology, 68,* 1094–1101.

Wenzlaff, R. M., & Eisenberg, A. R. (2001). Mental control after dysphoria: Evidence of a suppressed, depressive bias. *Behavior Therapy, 32,* 27–45.

West, J. C., Zarin, D. A., Peterson, B. D., & Pincus, H. A. (1998). Assessing the feasibility of recruiting a randomly selected sample of psychiatrists to participate in a national practice-based research network. *Social Psychiatry and Psychiatric Epidemiology, 33*(12), 620–623.

Westen, D. (1998a). Case formulation and personality diagnosis: Two processes or one? In J. Barron (Ed.), *Making diagnosis meaningful* (pp. 111–138). Washington, DC: American Psychological Association.

Westen, D. (1998b). The scientific legacy of Sigmund Freud: Toward a psychodynamically informed psychological science. *Psychological Bulletin, 124,* 333–371.

Westen, D. (1999). Psychodynamic theory and technique in relation to research on cognition and emotion: Mutual implications. In T. Dalgleish & M. J. Power (Eds.), *Handbook of cognition and emotion* (pp. 727– 746). New York: Wiley.

Westen, D. (2000). Integrative psychotherapy: Integrating psychodynamic and cognitive-behavioral theory and technique. In C. R. Snyder & R. Ingram (Eds.), *Handbook of psychological change: Psychotherapy processes and practices for the 21st century* (pp. 217–242). New York: Wiley.

Westen, D. (2002). Manualizing manual development. *Clinical Psychology: Science and Practice, 9,* 416–418.

Westen, D., & Arkowitz-Westen, L. (1998). Limitations of Axis II in diagnosing personality pathology in clinical practice. *American Journal of Psychiatry, 155,* 1767–1771.

Westen, D., & Harnden-Fischer, J. (2001). Personality profiles in eating disorders: Rethinking the distinction between Axis I and Axis II. *American Journal of Psychiatry, 165,* 547–562.

Westen, D., Heim, A. K., Morrison, K., Patterson, M., & Campbell, L. (2002). Simplifying diagnosis using a prototype-matching approach: Implications for the next edition of the DSM. In L. Efeutler & M. L. Malik (Eds.), *Rethinking the DSM: A psychological perspective* (pp. 221–250). Washington, DC: American Psychological Association.

Westen, D., & Morrison, K. (2001). A multidimensional meta-analysis of treatments for depression, panic, and generalized anxiety disorder: An empirical examination of the status of empirically supported therapies. *Journal of Consulting and Clinical Psychology, 69,* 875–899.

Westen, D., Moses, M. J., Silk, K. R., Lohr, N. E., Cohen, R., & Segal, H. (1992). Quality of depressive experience in borderline personality disorder and major depression: When depression is not just depression. *Journal of Personality Disorders, 6,* 382–393.

Westen, D., Muderrisoglu, S., Fowler, C., Shedler, J., & Koren, D. (1997). Affect regulation and affective experience: Individual differences, group differences, and measurement using a Q-sort procedure. *Journal of Consulting and Clinical Psychology, 65,* 429–439.

Westen, D., & Shedler, J. (1999a). Revising and assessing Axis II, Part 1: Developing a clinically and empirically valid assessment method. *American Journal of Psychiatry, 156,* 258–272.

Westen, D., & Shedler, J. (1999b). Revising and assessing Axis II, Part 2: Toward an empirically based and clinically useful classification of personality disorders. *American Journal of Psychiatry, 156,* 273–285.

Westen, D., Shedler, J., Durrett, C., Glass, S., & Martens, A. (2003). Personality diagnosis in adolescence: DSM-IV Axis II diagnoses and an empirically derived alternative. *American Journal of Psychiatry, 160,* 952–966.

Westen, D., & Weinberger, J. (2003). *When clinical description becomes statistical prediction.* Unpublished manuscript. Emory University, Atlanta, GA.

Wiers, R. W., van Woerden, N., Smulders, F. T. Y., & De Jong, P. J. (2002). Implicit and explicit alcohol-related cognitions in heavy and light drinkers. *Journal of Abnormal Psychology, 111,* 648–658.

Williams, J. M., Mathews, A., & MacLeod, C. (1996). The emotional Stroop task and psychopathology. *Psychological Bulletin, 120,* 3–24.

Wilson, G. T. (1998). Manual-based treatment and clinical practice. *Clinical Psychology: Science and Practice, 5,* 363–375.

Wilson, G. T. (1999). Rapid response to cognitive behavior therapy. *Clinical Psychology: Science and Practice, 6,* 289–292.

Wilson, G. T., Fairburn, C. G., & Agras, W. S. (1997). Cognitive-behavioral therapy for bulimia nervosa. In D. M. Garner & P. E. Garfinkel (Eds.), *Handbook of treatment for eating disorders* (2nd ed., pp. 67–93). New York: Guilford Press.

Wixom, J., Ludolph, P., & Westen, D. (1993). Quality of depression in borderline adolescents. *Journal of the American Academy of Child & Adolescent Psychiatry, 32,* 1172–1177.

Wolf, E. M., & Crowther, J. H. (1992). An evaluation of behavioral and cognitive-behavioral group interventions for the treatment of bulimia nervosa in women. *International Journal of Eating Disorders, 11,* 3–15.

Zimmerman, M., McDermut, W., & Mattia, J. (2000). Frequency of anxiety disorders in psychiatric outpatients with major depressive disorder. *American Journal of Psychiatry, 157,* 1337–1340.

Zinbarg, R. E., & Barlow, D. H. (1996). Structure of anxiety and the anxiety disorders: A hierarchical model. *Journal of Abnormal Psychology, 105,* 181–193.

Evidence-Based Psychodynamic Psychotherapies

Peter Fonagy, PhD[1]

Editor's Note: This article essays to cover the same ground as the preceding chapter by Westen and his collaborators, but with an even larger reference list that more comprehensively covers the wider psychotherapy research world outside the United States, with Fonagy's own arena of work centrally in the United Kingdom. Fonagy's meta-analysis of evidence-based outcome research studies is centered more on (research) efficacy rather than (naturalistic) effectiveness studies, and progresses systematically through the assessment of diagnosis-specific disorders, starting with major depressions, and going through varieties of anxiety disorders, eating disorders, substance abuse disorders, and personality disorders.

In proceeding in this manner, Fonagy uses the traditional DSM conceptions of the categorization of discrete mental illnesses which this entire volume is an effort to transcend, both diagnostically and therapy assessment-wise, and is of course in contrast with the earlier papers in this section by Blatt, et al. and by Shedler and Westen, which propose more complex psychoanalytically based understandings of mental functioning and the therapeutic process as the basis for diagnostic and treatment assessments. Fonagy shows, however, that even when using DSM symptom clusters, there is considerable evidence of efficacy for psychodynamically based therapies for a variety of disorders and shares with Westen, et al. a meta-analytic portrayal of how much can be learned about treatment results from within the more limited DSM framework, but without the important focus by Westen et al. upon the limitations simultaneously operative within that frame.

INTRODUCTION

This review is based on an exhaustive review of the psychotherapy outcome literature, undertaken originally at the instigation of the UK Department of Health by Roth and Fonagy (Department of Health, 1995). We have recently updated this review (Fonagy, Target, Cottrell, Phillips, & Kurtz, 2002; Roth & Fonagy, in press) and extended it to identify all studies of psychoanalytic psychotherapy. The usual methods for identifying studies were employed (Fonagy, Target, et al., 2002; Roth & Fonagy, in press). The key questions that should be

---

[1] Freud Memorial Professor of Psychoanalysis, University College, London, England

asked of this literature given the current state of research in this area (also see Westen, Morrison, & Thompson-Brenner, 2004) are: (1) are there any disorders for which short-term psychodynamic psychotherapy (STPP) can be considered evidence-based; (2) are there any disorders for which STPP is uniquely effective as either the only evidence-based treatment or as a treatment that is more effective than alternatives, and (3) is there any evidence base for long-term psychodynamic psychotherapy (LTPP) either in terms of achieving effects not normally associated with short-term treatment, or addressing problems which have not been addressed by STPP? In this context, short-term therapy is conceived of as a treatment of around 20 sessions carried out usually once weekly.

From the standpoint of psychodynamic psychotherapy, the database of research studies has significant limitations. Westen and colleagues (Westen, et al., 2004) recently offered a powerful critique of the research methods used to assign the status of "empirically supported or unsupported therapies." Research that is considered empirically supported tends to have three characteristics: (1) studies address a single disorder (usually Axis I) with diagnostic assessments to ensure homogeneity of samples, (2) treatments are manualized and are of brief and fixed duration to ensure the integrity of the "experimental manipulation," and (3) outcome assessments focus on the symptom(s) that represent the declared priority of the study (and often the intervention). The underlying aim is the maximization of internal validity by random assignment, controlling confounding variables, and standardising procedures. Westen, et al. (2004) identify four poorly supported assumptions underpinning the application of randomized controlled trial (RCT) methodology to psychotherapy research: (1) that psychopathology is so malleable that a brief intervention is likely to change it permanently, (2) that most patients can be treated for a single disorder or problem, (3) that psychiatric disorders can be treated with psychosocial interventions without regard to personality factors that are less likely to change with brief treatments, and (4) that experimental methods provide a helpful "gold standard" for evaluating these packages. In reality, most forms of psychopathology encountered in specialist centers are treatment resistant (Kopta, Howard, Lowry, & Beutler, 1994) and comorbid with other disorders (Kessler, Stang, Wittchen, Stein, & Walters, 1999) which need to be tackled in the broader context of the patient's personality structure (e.g., Thompson-Brenner, Glass, & Westen, 2003) and experimental methods need to be supplemented by correlational analysis to ascertain the effective components of treatment (Ablon & Jones, 2002).

METHODOLOGICAL CONSIDERATIONS

Evidence for Evidence-Based Practice

This review is based on what funders and researchers currently regard as appropriate evidence (Clarke & Oxman, 1999). The criteria, which are used to determine what counts as evidence based practice, must themselves be empirically tested. Their specificity (the likelihood of falsely identifying a treatment as effective) and sensitivity (the chance of misclassifying an effective treatment as ineffective) should be established against a variety of other public health criteria. The same empirical standards should be applied to these criteria as would be expected in association with other clinical decision making tasks. Face validity, which is what we currently have, is clearly insufficient. Treatments designated as "evidence based" by some criteria must be distinguishable from treatments that do not meet these criteria on several concurrent independent but relevant indicators such as theoretical coherence, public health impact, user/consumer acceptability, etc.

The Absence of Evidence or Evidence for Ineffectiveness

Current categorization in evidence-based psychotherapies conflates two radically different groups of treatments: Those that have been adequately tested and found ineffective for a patient group, and those that have not been tested at all. It is important to make this distinction, since the reason that a treatment has not been subjected to empirical scrutiny may have little to do with its likely effectiveness. It may have far more to do with the intellectual culture within which researchers operate, the availability of treatment manuals, and peer or third party payer perceptions of the value of the treatment (which can be critical for both research funding and publication). The British psychodynamically oriented psychiatrist, Jeremy Holmes (2002), has eloquently argued in the *British Medical Journal* that the absence of evidence for psychoanalytic treatment should not be confused with evidence of ineffectiveness. In particular, his concern was that cognitive therapy would be adopted by default because of its research and marketing strategy rather than its intrinsic superiority. He argued that: (1) the foundations of cognitive therapy were less secure than often believed; (2) the impact of Cognitive Behavioral Therapy (CBT) on long term course of psychiatric illness was not well demonstrated; (3) in one "real life trial," at least the CBT arm had to be discontinued because of poor compliance from a problematic group of patients who, nevertheless, accepted and benefited from couples therapy (Leff, et al., 2000); (4) the effect size of CBT is exaggerated by comparisons with wait-list controls; and (5) the emergence of a post-cognitive behavior therapy approach (e.g., Teasdale, et al., 2000; Young, 1999) that leans increasingly on psychodynamic ideas.

While I am entirely in sympathy with Jeremy Holmes' perspective, even if my work with Tony Roth was part of the target of his criticism, it is only fair to expose the shortcomings of his communication. Nick Tarrier (2002), in a commentary on Holmes' piece, writes with passion:

> Holmes relies on the specious old adage that absence of evidence is not evidence of absence [of effectiveness] .... I would have more enthusiasm for this argument if traditional psychotherapy were new. It has been around for 100 years or so. The argument, therefore, becomes a little less compelling when psychotherapy's late arrival at the table of science has been triggered by a threat to pull the plug on public funding because of the absence of evidence. (p. 292)

Tom Sensky and Jan Scott (Sensky & Scott, 2002) were similarly distressed, both by Holmes' selective review of evidence and his allegations that some cognitive therapists are starting to question aspects of their discipline. The message from the CBT camp is this: If psychodynamic clinicians are going to address the issue of evidence-based practice, they will have to do more than gripe and join in the general endeavor to acquire data.

Of course, psychodynamic clinicians are at a disadvantage and not simply because they are late starters (after all, many new treatments find a place at the table of evidence-based practice). There are profound incompatibilities between psychoanalysis and modern natural science. Paul Whittle (2000) has drawn attention to the fundamental incompatibility of an approach that aims to fill in gaps in self-narrative with cognitive psychology's commitment to minimal elaboration of observations, a kind of Wittgensteinian cognitive asceticism. The making of meaning around a life narrative is fundamental to human nature. It is, therefore, inconceivable that psychoanalysis (or any process very much like it) will ever not be part of the range of approaches that people with mental health problems desire. However, in this context, success is measured as eloquence (or meaningfulness) which is not reducible to either symptom or suffering. Moreover, psychoanalytic explanations invoke personal history, but behavior genetics has brought environmental accounts into disrepute. While cognitive behavioral therapy also has environmentalist social learning theory at its foundations, it has been more effective in moving away from a naïve environmentalist position. To make matters worse, within psychoanalysis there has been a tradition of regarding the uninitiated with contempt, scaring off most open-minded researchers. The engagement of psychoanalytic clinicians in research programs is a desirable goal.

Psychoanalysts are more than ever before, but not yet fully, committed to systematically collecting data with the potential to challenge and contradict as well as to confirm cherished ideas. The danger that must be avoided at all costs is that research is embraced selectively only when it confirms previously held views. This may be a worse outcome than the wholesale rejection of the entire enterprise of seeking evidence since it immunizes against being affected by findings at the same time as creating an illusion of participation in the virtuous cycle of exploring, testing, modifying, and re-exploring ideas.

The Scope of the Task

Most United Kingdom evidence-based treatment reviews have been uniquely based on RCTs. In psychosocial treatments, RCTs are often regarded as inadequate because of their low external validity or generalizability (Anon, 1992). In brief, it is claimed that they are not relevant to clinical practice—a hotly debated issue in the field of psychotherapy (Hoagwood, Hibbs, Brent, & Jensen, 1995) and psychiatric research (Olfson, 1999). There are a number of well publicized reasons, which I have not the space to go into here, as to why randomized trials in many areas of health care may have low external validity: (1) the unrepresentativeness of health care professionals participating, (2) the unrepresentativeness of participants screened for inclusion (in order to maximize homogeneity), (3) the possible use of atypical treatments designed for a single disorder, and (4) limiting the measurement of outcome to the symptom that is the focus of the study and is easily measurable but far from the only relevant dimension (Fonagy, 1999a).

RCTs cover only a limited number of treatments, and many treatments remain unevaluated in relation to many conditions. Because there are at least 200 disorders of child and adult mental health (by DMS criteria) and many hundreds of different forms of intervention, most of which have many components and many characteristic patterns of delivery, it is inconceivable that a matrix of types of therapy by types of disorder could ever be populated by appropriate studies (Goldfried & Wolfe, 1996). This is no trivial issue. Studies that attempt to identify which component of a treatment program is essential to its success frequently find that apparently, most of the layers of the onion can be removed and the effect is still there. Because outcome studies rarely help identify either the effective elements of treatments or the process of change that leads to improvement, many traditional influential supporters of outcome investigations are calling for fewer rather than more outcome studies. Alan Kazdin (1998), for example, recommended a so-called "dismantling" strategy that one by one removes potential components of change until the genuinely effective component is identified. Some have suggested that meta-analyses might offer a direct solution to this problem (e.g., Borkovec & Ruscio, 2001), but this is by no means a straightforward task.

A recent meta-analysis by Wilson McDermut and colleagues (McDermut, Miller, & Brown, 2001) identified group therapy as efficacious for depression with average ES of 1.06. However, the group treatments involved teaching a wide range of different strategies in different studies (self-control techniques, problem-solving skills, relaxation skills, disputation of negative thinking). So was teaching a skill truly addressing a depression-related deficit? Matching patients to treatments that emphasized the specific deficits they presented with did not increase the effect size, and even attention-control groups resulted in a reduction of symptoms. Yalom (1995) outlined 11 therapeutic factors in group therapy but none of the studies reviewed by McDermut, et al. discussed any one of these. We simply do not know what aspects of group treatments for depression make them so effective.

Beyond these fairly well-publicized issues, the question arises of whether manualized treatments or treatment packages are the appropriate level of analysis in our search for effective interventions. For example, a study by Olfson and colleagues (Olfson, Mechanic, Boyer, & Hansell, 1998) followed up schizophrenic patients discharged from hospital, and found that patients who had contact with the outpatient clinician prior to discharge were better off in terms of symptom reduction than those who had no communication with outpatient staff. Similar, apparently minor, process parameters of care may be far more important in determining outcome than entire treatment packages. It is hard to imagine that a sufficient number of RCTs could ever be performed to assess all such, potentially key, parameters of care. Evidence-based practice needs to look beyond the current database and look at practice-based evidence in order to comprehensively establish evidence based practice.

The Ideal Outcome Research Program

This was proposed by Alan Kazdin a number of years ago, but as it would require us to rethink our entire approach to outcome studies and evidence-based practice it is unlikely ever to be implemented. Basically, he suggests that:

- Treatment research should begin with the identification of key dysfunctions associated with a disorder and the empirical demonstration of these dysfunctions in a sizeable proportion of the clinical group.
- A conceptual link must be established between a proposed treatment method and the dysfunctional mechanism hypothesized to underpin the disorder.
- Only when the conceptual link has been established can manualization commence.
- This is followed by the collection of the hierarchy of evidence that forms the body of systematic reviews.
- Process-outcome studies can then be implemented to establish key treatment components and necessary treatment length.

Experimental studies of hypothesized processes and mechanisms need to confirm the correlational findings from process-outcome investigations. Finally, the boundary conditions for the treatment need establishing, in terms of patient and environmental characteristics that promote or undermine the effectiveness of the therapy. You will notice that this is a radically different approach to the one normally undertaken where the starting point is the evaluation of a designated treatment. Currently, the identification of key psychological processes is at best post hoc. No wonder there are too many different treatment modalities. No wonder that we know so little about why any of them work. Reversing this process would be a remarkable achievement of scientific enterprise.

Pragmatic Trials

The answer to the controversy between efficacy and effectiveness studies of psychotherapy may lie in so called pragmatic or "real-world" trials. These minimal effort trials require experimentation in addition to ongoing outcome measurement. The experimental component of pragmatic trials includes randomization to alternative methods of care. Importantly, non-specific aspects of care are controlled under these circumstances, yet questions of direct relevance to the clinicians may be asked and answered. Patients who participate naturally reflect the clinical population and exclusion criteria are kept to a minimum. Comparison treatments are with routine practice, which usually involves combination treatments, and treatments titrated according to the client's response. The pragmatic trial imposes minimal constraints on management. The only major sacrifice to internal validity is the loss of blindness in assessment. Blindness, which is likely to be imperfect in psychosocial treatments, in any case, may offer little advantage as regards objectivity of outcome assessment. Double blindness imposes unrealistic restrictions even upon routine pharmacological care, and deviations from normal practice threaten the validity and generalizability of any cost data used in the estimation of cost effectiveness. Concealment of allocation (the prevention of foreknowledge about the group to which the patient will be allocated if recruited) that is an important source of selection bias, is readily achievable in this context. The unique feature of such trials lies in the relevance of the questions that clinicians may ask of their routine practice. Ideally, clinical equipoise (genuine uncertainty concerning outcome) should drive the search for evidence. In evidence-based practice, clinical curiosity is sadly, rarely the motivator.

Pragmatic trials could be a key additional line of information for evidence based practice. In combination with more rigorous RCTs (particularly relevant to new treatments) and the judicious use of observational data, they will provide evidence of sufficient richness to significantly advance standards of mental health care. The establishment and support of a profession-wide methodology for pragmatic trials should be considered an important additional task of evidence based practice psychotherapy initiatives.

Clinical Guidelines

Closing the gap between practice and evidence brings us to another quantum leap in the sophistication with which evidence for psychotherapeutic clinical psychological services is considered. It is increasingly recognized that evidence does not speak for itself and to be usefully applied it needs to be reviewed and integrated by a group of unbiased experts, including individuals whose expertise is as users and caregivers. Clinical guidelines that integrate evidence and front-line experience drawn up by multi-disciplinary panels, which as a collection of individuals have full awareness of the limitations of everyday clinical practice, is a key step that has all too often been omitted in the past when the sole experience applied to the interpretation of evidence was one of management.

Research, with its focus on selected patient populations, cannot, of course, tell clinicians what to do with specific individuals. Clinicians have to ask the research database specific questions with an individual patient in mind. How to pose this massive accumulation of such questions and, even more challengingly, how to obtain meaningful answers? These are far more complex skills than that of generating a systematic review. Many hope that clinical guidelines can and will perform the role of translation of research into practice increasingly well. The controversy that surrounds this issue is beyond the scope of this paper. It is, perhaps, sufficient for us to say that we cannot see guidelines, however sophisticated, ever substituting for clinical skill and experience any more than the Highway Code can substitute for skilled driving. Future research should perhaps look at the skill with which clinicians implement particular treatments and the relationship of that to patient outcome.

In addressing the failure of translation of guidelines into clinical behavior (Chilvers, Harrison, Sipos, & Barley, 2002; Higgitt & Fonagy, 2002), it is useful to differentiate between "diffusion," "dissemination," and "implementation" (Palmer & Fenner, 1999). These are inter-related and increasingly active phases of a process. Publication in a journal article (diffusion) is a passive form of communication, haphazard, untargeted, and uncontrolled (seemingly insufficient to achieve much in the way of change in clinical practice). The development of practice guidelines, overviews, etc. are more active and targeted to an intended audience. Implementation is yet more active, with sanctions and incentives, monitoring, and adjustment to local needs. The methods for translating guidelines into practice include the use of written materials, educational efforts, product champions, financial incentives, patient-mediated interventions, and reminder systems. Notwithstanding problems of the currency of guidance, there is a very real question about the extent to which guidance is utilized. At a recent Australian meeting to review the fate of 14 guidelines, none was found to have fared well. The shorter they were, the more likely they were to have had a noticeable impact. Successful implementation was most likely if it was initiated at a local level.

The Brain and the Mind

The question is not whether psychotherapy is still relevant in the days of Prozac, but how can we make it really count against a background increasingly fragmented social support systems and how can we use it efficiently where current medication is not enough? Drugs and psychotherapy both work to the extent that they do because they both impact on the functioning of the brain. How else could it be, since the brain is the organ of the mind and diseases of the mind are unequivocally diseases of the brain? The outcome of psychotherapy, therefore, should be as easy (or easier) to measure in terms of brain function as in terms of behavior or subjective reports.

But the brain is not the final frontier of our knowledge about the mind. Emotions may be crudely changed by drugs, but without giving any meaning to the experience of mental disorder or to the drug-induced change. Psychotherapy is the crystallization of the principle of psychological causation—that mental disorder, in many instances, may be most usefully seen in psychological terms, as the product of specific beliefs, desires, and emotions. Without understanding mental disorder psychologically, it would be impossible to understand the self-evident social pathways to mental disorder: Poverty, unemployment, incest, homelessness, spiritual despair at the violence and heartlessness of abusive parenting, the almost limitless methods that people can find of inflicting human misery—all these ignominies influence people's expectations about others, the trust that they may be capable of feeling, their anger about their treatment, the complex ways we all find to learn to live in the social context that the fortunes or misfortunes of our birth have presented for us. Turning away from therapy could mean shutting our ears to such anguish. Psychotherapists blew the whistle on the prevalence and long term impact of child maltreatment. It is the feelings, wishes, beliefs, thoughts, and desires in the wake of despair that psychotherapy must be retained to address.

Severe social disadvantage increases the risk of mental disorder by orders of magnitude. That this is a psychological rather than a merely physical process is borne out by the predictive power of relative rather than absolute destitution. The further down the social pile the greater the misery, regardless of the actual material wealth of the individual. It is felt disadvantage that is psychologically toxic. Of course, in this and every other case, it can be argued that experience of deprivation is a brain state, but the logical conclusion from that argument was foreshadowed in Huxley's *Brave New World* (Huxley, 1932). No one would seriously suggest that the most appropriate ethical way of addressing the gigantic issues raised by social disadvantage might be the suppression by medication of the misery of social exclusion.

But the native land of psychotherapy, the mental world of beliefs, desires, and emotions—central for a while in 20th Century psychiatry—is a fragile creature. Maintaining the causal significance of meaning runs the gauntlet of a powerful human need for concreteness and simplicity, which the physics and biology of brain research represent. Only a psychological Luddite would ignore the immense benefit we have drawn from brain research. But we would be equally deluded were we to deny its cost. Brain research has impacted our culture. The answers it has provided, when translated into exuberant media sound bites, have undermined the ethos of seeking for psychological meaning in the way therapists work with patients. The natural human desire to create a narrative, a story, around one's experience has given way under economic as well as political pressures to a profound disrespect for the mental, born less of disillusionment with the efficacy of psychotherapy than of the reductionism of certain biological psychiatrists. Over the last 15 years, the United States has witnessed a devastation of concern with the psyche. Many HMOs (protectors of insurance company profit margins) will fund either no psychotherapy or, at most, a half a dozen sessions. Not surprisingly, and coincidental with the biological revolution in psychiatry, spending on mental health care in the U.S. has decreased in real terms by a factor of 50%.

Psychotherapy is essential to whole-person mental health care. We cannot afford to abandon it, if we are to offer meaningful and respectful care to those in distress. My concern here is with the risk of irreparable, even if unintended, damage to a perspective which enshrines in psychiatry what is unique about our species—that we recognize in each other the presence of a mind, the presence of emotions, wishes, and beliefs as the motivators of behavior, adaptive or maladaptive. Turning away from psychological therapy, from the truth of the importance of mind, risks apocalyptic cultural and social changes, inevitable if we mock personal experience and start to deride the feelings, thoughts, and desires of our fellow humans.

Science and Scientism

Finally, a word about science and scientism in psychotherapy research. We all have a need for certainty and experience discomfort with not knowing, and risk anxious retreat from ignorance into pseudo knowledge (so characteristic of the early years of medicine). A scientific approach has obviously been incredibly helpful and has saved many millions of lives. To argue against it is not just churlish, it is clearly unethical and destructive. But to argue for a mechanical reading of evidence, as some clinical psychologists have done (Chambless & Hollon, 1998; Chambless, et al., 1996), equally skirts the risk of doing harm.

Research evidence collected as part of the present initiative will need to be carefully weighed. Multiple channels of evaluation are needed and they need to be kept open and actively maintained. No self-respecting clinicians will change their practice overnight. They would be unwise to do so. Evidence has to be read, evaluated, and placed into the context of what is possible, desirable, and fits with existing opportunities. It should be remembered that in mental health, at least, but also probably in most areas of clinical treatment method, accounts can be given for a relatively small proportion of the variance in outcome relative to the nature of the patient's problem (Weisz, Weiss, Han, Granger, & Morton, 1995; Weisz, Weiss, Morton, Granger, & Han, 1992), which may well interact with the skills of the attending clinician. This latter form of variance is to be cherished, because not only that is where the art of medicine lies, but also because it is in the study of that variability that future major advances in health care may be made, as long as we can submit these to empirical scrutiny.

MAJOR DEPRESSION

About 20 psychodynamic psychotherapy trials have been published dealing with the treatment of depressive and anxiety disorders or symptoms (Crits-Christoph, 1992; Leichsenring, 2001). Along with other therapies, it has been shown to have better effectiveness in open trials or compared to wait-list (Shefler, Dasberg, & Ben-Shakhar, 1995) or outpatient treatment in general (Guthrie, Moorey, Margison, et al., 1999). In the light of relatively readily available alternative treatments, the critical demonstrations concern that of an equivalence, or perhaps even superiority, to alternative treatment approaches.

Reviews

There have been two recent relevant reviews of the literature (Churchill, et al., 2001; Leichsenring, 2001). In addition, the National (England and Wales) Institute for Clinical Excellence (NICE) is conducting a systematic review in order to produce guidelines for treatment of depression within the National Health Service. The Churchill review concerned treatments for depression of 20 sessions or less published up to 1998. Of the studies suitable to include in meta-analysis, six involved psychodynamic therapy. Improvement was found to be over twice as likely with cognitive behavior therapy (CBT) as it was with psychodynamic therapy. However, to conclude from this that CBT is superior to psychoanalytic psychotherapy in the treatment of depression may be premature in the light of the following considerations:

- There was no superiority of CBT over other therapies where follow-up was available.
- Differences between CBT and other therapies were limited in severely depressed groups.
- A number of therapies identified in the review as "psychodynamic" were not "bona fide" therapies (Wampold, 1997).

This last point is very important. An earlier meta-analysis by Gloaguen (1998) similarly concluded that CBT was superior to other therapies. However, once interventions that were not theoretically-based and had no scientific base were removed from these comparisons, the superiority of CBT over other therapies could no longer be demonstrated (Wampold, Minami, Baskin, & Callen-Tierney, 2002). Meta-analytic reviews should not confound estimates of the effectiveness of STPP with those of "non-bona fide" therapies.

A more positive picture apparently emerges from the review by Leichsenring (2001). This review identified six RCTs of at least 13 sessions in length studies that contrasted manualized STPP and CBT (Barkham, Rees, Shapiro, et al., 1996; Elkin, 1994; Gallagher-Thompson & Steffen, 1994; Hersen, Bellack, Himmelhoch, & Thase, 1984; Shapiro, et al., 1994; Shapiro, et al., 1995; Shea, et al., 1992; Thompson, Gallagher, & Breckenridge, 1987). The review concludes that the two forms of therapy are not substantially different as only one of the studies reviewed suggests a possible superiority of CBT. We calculate the overall Risk Ratio (RR) for the comparison to be 0.91 (95% Confidence Interval [CI]: 0.77 to 1.06) indicating that CBT is only 9% more likely to generate remission than STPP. Although not reported by Leichsenring, meta-analytic comparison of follow-up data available for these studies actually reveals a slight superiority for CBT (RR = 0.82, 95% CI: 0.70, 0.96). This indicates that CBT increases the chance of continued remission by 20% more than STPP.

We should consider the possibility of selection bias in this review. Leichsenring includes the NIMH Collaborative Depression Trial in the meta-analysis, which is, to say the least, controversial, as IPT was included as an STPP merely because the therapist was psychodynamically trained (Elkin, 1994; Shea, et al., 1992). As neither the developers nor other reviewers consider IPT to be a psychodynamic therapy, it seems wiser not to include it in reviews of STPP. However, even if this study is excluded, the superiority of CBT over STPP remains (RR=0.82, 95% CI: 0.70, 0.96). However, the remaining four studies include a trial of social skills training relative to STPP (Hersen, et al., 1984) and a study of CBT offered to caregivers (Gallagher-Thompson & Steffen, 1994), neither of which seems relevant to the assessment of the relative effects of CBT for depression. Of the two studies remaining, one was group rather than individual therapy carried out with an older adult population (Thompson, et al., 1987). The most appropriate conclusion at this stage might be that a meta-analysis of this literature is premature.

Consideration of Individual Studies Contrasting Psychodynamic Therapy with Other Psychotherapies

This conclusion reflects the regrettable fact that there are fewer controlled studies of psychodynamic therapy for depression than one might expect given the wide use of this treatment for this problem. In fact, most investigators employ STPP as a contrast to an alternative therapy to which they have an allegiance. Not surprisingly, dynamic therapy is usually found to be significantly less effective (Covi & Lipman, 1987; Kornblith, Rehm, O'Hara, & Lamparski, 1983; McLean & Hakstian, 1979; Steuer, et al., 1984). Given that the researchers' lack of investment in the "control" treatment reflects a lack of equipoise, findings from these investigations should be treated with great caution. Consistent with this formulation, better designed and implemented studies report no difference between CBT and STPP (Bellack, Hersen, & Himmelhoch, 1981; Thompson, et al., 1987). Nevertheless, small sample size and design weaknesses argue against basing conclusions concerning psychodynamic therapy for depression on these investigations. Two major studies stand out as sound comparisons of a cognitive behavioral and a psychodynamic approach to the treatment of depression because of their size, the quality of randomization, the care of implementation, baseline assessment, and outcome measurement, and clarity of the therapeutic interventions assessed. These are The Sheffield Psychotherapy Project and The Helsinki Psychotherapy Study.

The Sheffield Psychotherapy Project

The Sheffield Psychotherapy Project (Barkham, Rees, Stiles, et al., 1996; Shapiro, et al., 1994; Shapiro, et al., 1995) randomized 169 patients meeting criteria for Manic-Depressive Disorder (MDD) to CBT or STPP. Of the 117 who completed the study; 103 were followed up at one year. Treatment was brief (8 or 16 sessions). Most would agree that eight sessions represents a "sub-clinical dose" of STPP. In line with this, those who received only 8 sessions of psychodynamic therapy were doing less well at one year than those with 8 sessions of CBT. At 16 sessions, the two treatments appeared to be equally effective (RR= 0.93, 95% CI: 0.68, 1.27). A further important finding was that those with more severe depression at the start of treatment were less likely to maintain gains in both arms of the trial. Patients with severe depression (Beck Depression Index [BDI] score > 27) appeared to require longer treatment regardless of treatment type. About 30% of patients remained asymptomatic from post-treatment to one year follow-up. This interaction, however, was not found in a small-scale, community-based attempt at replication (Barkham, Rees, Shapiro, et al., 1996). Overall, neither of these short-term treatments (CBT or STPP) appeared to be strikingly effective in the medium term, but STPP performed broadly comparably to CBT.

The Helsinki Psychotherapy Study

The fullest assessment of psychodynamic psychotherapy for mood disorder thus far comes from the initial report of the Helsinki Psychotherapy Study (Knekt & Lindfors, 2004). In many ways, this exemplary randomized study compared a problem-solving, solution-focused therapy (SFT) to short- and long-term psychodynamic psychotherapy. The study also had an arm for full psychoanalysis, to which subjects were self-selected and additionally screened for suitability. So far, only findings related to the two short-term arms of the trial are available.

SFT is a relatively novel approach (Lambert, Okiishi, Finch, & Johnson, 1998) that emphasizes the collaborative efforts of patient and therapist to identify a problem and find solutions to it. It is conducted once every second or third week up to a maximum of 12 sessions (the actual number of sessions in the trial was 10 over about 7.5 months). STPP, following Malan's approach (Malan, 1976), was scheduled over 20 once-weekly sessions over a period of 5 to 6 months (actual number of sessions in the trial was 15 over a period of about 6 months). Data was collected on auxiliary treatments, such as psychotropic medication and the additional use of psychotherapy services. An unusually wide range of assessments are administered at various time points (5 assessment points in the first year) up to 60 months after baseline measurement, in order to pick up the long term and "meta-symptomatic" changes believed to be associated with STPP.

Six-hundred thirty-eight patients were referred from clinical services (not recruited for the study by advertisement or the like) of whom 381 were eligible and willing to participate in the study. Ninety-seven patients were allocated to SFT, 101 to STPP and 128 to LTPP. Over 82% of the sample met DSM criteria for depressive disorder and 43% for some type of anxiety disorder. Fifty-seven percent had mood disorder alone and 14% had anxiety disorder alone. The sample appears moderately severe (average Global Assessment of Functioning [GAF] score was 55, and SCL-90 GSI 1.29) slightly less severe than the Sheffield sample. The average Hamilton Depression (HAM-D) score was 15.7. Surprisingly, only about 25% were on any kind of psychotropic medication.

Given the careful design and implementation of the complex methodology and the exceptionally large sample size (adequate power to detect a 20% difference), the observation of an absence of significant differences between the two groups is impressive. At 12 months, the reduction in depression and anxiety scores was relatively large, e.g., the BDI decreased by almost 50% (from 18 to 10) and the Hamilton decreased by almost 30% (from 15 to 11). The average Global Assessment of Functioning (GAF) increased to about 65. On most of the measures the gains were apparent by 7 months and remained stable thereafter. About one-third of the 82% of patients who were suffering from a mood disorder lost the diagnosis by 7 months and changes after that were no longer statistically significant. Both forms of therapy showed about 20% of recovery from personality disorders by 7 months. This increased to 46% in the STPP group by 12 months, but in SFT the percentage recovered from Personality Disorder (PD) diagnosis did not increase (RR = 2.1, 95% CI: 1.36, 3.25). However, we cannot make too much of this difference, given the absence of adjustments for Type I error and the great number of comparisons carried out. Measuring recovery in terms of achieving below clinical cut-point scores on the BDI and Hamilton ratings, SFT appeared to achieve somewhat more change faster, although there were, again, no significant differences after the 9 months time point ($RR_{BDI@3months} = 0.49$, 95% CI: 0.27, 0.88). Work ability index improved for both groups, but only by about 10%, and this was achieved by 7 months with little change thereafter. Interestingly, days of sick leave was reduced significantly for both groups. Similarly, a range of measures on social functioning improved over the first 7 months, but produced no notable change later and no differences were seen between the treatment groups.

In summary, the trial demonstrated rapid and generally similar decreases on self-reported and observer-rated depressive symptoms during the first months of therapy and less prominent reductions in symptoms later. Remission was somewhat more rapid with SFT, and continued recovery from a PD diagnosis was more marked for STPP. The rate of recovery reported here is comparable to those found in other studies involving CBT. Broadly, the study demonstrates that a fairly generic form of brief psychoanalytic psychotherapy is as effective in the treatment of depression as a less generic, but previously established as empirically-supported, form of CBT (Mynors-Wallis, Davies, Gray, Barbour, & Gath, 1997; Mynors-Wallis, Gath, Day, & Baker, 2000; Mynors-Wallis, Gath, Lloyd-Thomas, & Tomlinson, 1995). The study was unusual in the breadth of outcomes covered. It permitted the observation that recovery of work ability, social functioning, and personality functioning appears to be far smaller than reductions of acute psychiatric symptoms (e.g., Pre-Post Standardized Mean Difference$_{BDI}$ (SMD) = 9.65, 95% CI: 8.66, 10.64; Pre-Post SMD$_{SAS(work)}$ = 3.33, 95% CI: 3.79, 12.84). Measurement in social adjustment domains does not appear to advantage the less symptom-focused STPP. This is important in the interpretation of other trials. The limited gain observed in social adjustment is consistent with current models of change in psychotherapy (Howard, Lueger, Maling, & Martinovitch, 1993).

The absence of a no-treatment control group in this study makes it hard to estimate the proportion of observed reductions in symptoms that were not due to psychotherapy. However, since effective treatments for depression exist, randomization of patients to a purely placebo arm for a 12 months period would be unethical—adequately designed studies will inevitably lack a no-treatment control arm. The treatments were well described, but not fully manualized. Adherence is not reported.

Consideration of Individual Studies Contrasting Psychodynamic Therapy with Pharmacotherapy

When offered alone, psychotherapy and medication are of equivalent efficacy and psychotherapy is rarely superior (Roth & Fonagy, in press). There is evidence of "added value" when psychotherapy is added to medication, but most of this evidence is from IPT and CBT studies. Two recent studies assessed adding STPP to an antidepressant regimen. A Dutch study (de Jonghe, Kool, van Aalst, Dekker, & Peen, 2001) assigned 84 patients to antidepressant and 83 to combined therapy. The pharmacotherapy protocol started with fluoxetine and allowed a switch to amitryptyline, if participants were non-responsive, and finally to moclobemide. The psychotherapy was a psychoanalytically-oriented, brief supportive therapy associated with the work of the first author (de Jonghe, Rijnierse, & Janssen, 1994). An unexpectedly large number of patients refused pharmacotherapy alone, so of the 167 patients randomized, 57 started in pharmacotherapy and 72 in combined therapy. Intent-to-treat remission rate in the combined psychodynamic psychotherapy and pharmacotherapy on the Hamilton Depression Rating Scale (HDRS) was 37%, while it was only 15% in the pharmacotherapy sample ($RR_{HDRS<7} = 2.36$, 95% CI: 1.33, 4.18). The findings indicate that not only is combined STPP and pharmacotherapy accepted better, but symptomatic indicators of success rate, both clinician- and self-rated, suggest high levels of success. The success rate of 37%, defined by HDRS less than 7, for the combined group is not impressive. Across a range of measures, however, by 24 months the success rate of the combined therapy is nearly 60% and that of pharmacotherapy alone rises to 40% ($RR_{HDRS<7} = 1.5$, 95% CI: 1.09, 2.06). The superiority of the combined treatment is maintained, but does not appear to increase. It is not clear how combined treatment would compare with a psychotherapy alone condition. In some analyses, this has been a difficult difference to demonstrate (Thase, et al., 1997).

A second comparison study (Burnand, Andreoli, Kolatte, Venturini, & Rosset, 2002) randomly assigned 95 patients to a combination (clomipramine and STTP) or a clomipramine alone condition. Despite an attrition rate of 22%, the intent to treat analysis revealed somewhat fewer treatment failures for the combined treatment, as well as better work adjustment scores. No group differences were noted on the HDRS, however. There were more frequent instances of hospitalization and more days spent in hospital for the clomipramine alone treatment. Combined therapy was also associated with fewer days lost from work. This, together with saving on hospitalization costs, led to an estimated cost saving per episode of $2,300. It should be noted that the benefits of STPP were detectable, even though the pharmacotherapy group had some non-specific psychological input (attention placebo) and the psychotherapy was delivered by nurses rather than certified psychotherapists. This latter finding echoes the success of other psychodynamic interventions where the therapist is supervised by, but is not a fully trained psychoanalytic psychotherapist (Bateman & Fonagy, 2001).

Process Factors and Moderating Variables

Support for a psychodynamic approach to the treatment of depression may also accrue from the demonstration that the inclusion of interventions specific to a psychoanalytic approach is associated with good outcome even in therapies for depression born of a different orientation. For example, in a study of CBT, the extent of focus on "parental issues" turned out to be positively associated with outcome (Hayes, Castonguay, & Goldfried, 1996). In another study, of CBT and STPP, the differences between the success of either intervention appeared to be correlated with the use of interventions prototypically considered "psychoanalytic" (Ablon & Jones, 1998). However, similar evidence can be readily mustered to support CBT. Using the same instrument (Enrico Jones's Psychotherapy Q-sort) on tapes of the NIMH treatment of depression trial, Ablon and Jones demonstrated the superiority of therapies where process codings of both IPT and CBT more closely resembled the CBT prototype (Ablon & Jones, 1999; 2002). Thus far, studies of psychodynamic psychotherapy process and outcome have not demonstrated powerful associations between change and putative mechanism of action. For example, a negative association has been reported between the number of transference interpretations and therapy outcome, indicating that the overuse of this technique frequently regarded by clinicians as essential to therapeutic success, may even be iatrogenic (Connolly, et al., 1999).

Summary

The current evidence base of psychodynamic therapy for depression is weak, relative to the number of psychoanalytic therapists and the rate at which evidence is accumulating for other approaches. The psychodynamic approach may be marginalized, not by its relative lack of effectiveness, but by the sparseness of compelling demonstrations of its comparability to "empirically supported" alternatives. There is some evidence relating to brief psychodynamic therapy (up to 24 sessions), but no evidence for long-term therapy or psychoanalysis, despite the fact that data from trials of depression indicate the need for more intensive treatment. As Westen and Morrison (2001) observe, the evidence for the effectiveness of CBT for depression in the medium term is not sound. However, none of the therapies appear to differ markedly from each other. In the two cases where brief psychodynamic therapy was compared with CBT or problem-solving therapy, the observed size of the effects were similar in the groups contrasted and, in turn, similar to results reported in other studies of CBT, IPT, and couples therapy.

Broadly speaking, in 4 to 6 months of therapy, about half of those treated are likely to remit; about half of these will experience a remission in the succeeding 12 months. As Roth and Fonagy (Roth & Fonagy, in press) observe, the data are consistent with the assumption that a proportion of patients in any research sample will respond to therapeutic intervention of any kind. An appropriate future strategy for psychodynamic psychotherapy research on depression might be to compare the effectiveness of relatively long-term psychodynamic psychotherapy with alternative forms of intervention in patients who are non-responders in trials of CBT, IPT, or pharmacotherapy. A further weakness of the evidence base for psychodynamic treatment studies of depression is that no STPP was tested twice by independent research groups (Chambless & Hollon, 1998), most manuals subjected to systematic inquiry are idiosyncratic, and their testing is restricted to the location in which they were developed.

ANXIETY DISORDERS

Research on anxiety disorders is normally subdivided into research on phobia, generalized anxiety disorder, panic disorder (with and without agoraphobia), post-traumatic stress disorder (PTSD), and obsessive-compulsive disorder (OCD). These, often comorbid with depression (Brown, Campbell, Lehman, Grisham, & Mancill, 2001), are the most commonly encountered disorders either in community surveys or in primary mental health services. Anxiety disorders are central to psychoanalytic theory (Milrod, Cooper, & Shear, 2001) and are probably the most common presenting complaints in psychodynamic therapeutic practice. Disappointingly, for at least two of the most common anxiety problems (social phobias and specific phobias), there are no diagnosis-specific controlled trials of psychodynamic therapy. The field is dominated by CBT packages that combine a range of approaches with almost no studies of non-behavioral approaches, except for a small trial of interpersonal therapy (Lipsitz, Markowitz, Cherry, & Fyer, 1999).

Generalized Anxiety Disorder

Treatments developed for generalized anxiety disorder are dominated by anxiety management (relaxation, positive self talk) and cognitive therapy focusing on identifying and modifying worrying thoughts. Because of the sparsity of the literature, meta-analytic and systematic reviews are not very informative. Westen and Morrison's meta-analysis (Westen & Morrison, 2001) identifies a study of psychodynamic therapy (supportive expressive therapy) (Crits-Christoph, Connolly, Azarian, Crits-Christoph, & Shappell, 1996), but does not address differences in efficacy across the four types of therapy examined. Another meta-analysis (Fisher & Durham, 1999) establishes a clinical cut-off on the Spielberger Trait Anxiety Scale, to identify the proportion of participants who recover at post-therapy, remain in remission at 6 months, as well as those who recover in the 6 months post-therapy period. By these criteria, overall, at 6 months 36% are unchanged, 24% are improved and 38% are recovered. Only 4% of patients are considered as recovered following psychodynamic therapy; however, this is based on just one study (Durham, et al., 1994). This contrasts with 60% for individual applied relaxation therapy and 51% for CBT. Notably, non-directive therapy was shown to have recovery rates of 38%, suggesting that neither relaxation nor restructuring of worrying thoughts are necessary for substantial improvement. However, the review includes too few trials to be a definitive statement about the relative effectiveness of these therapies in anxiety.

A number of individual studies of psychodynamic psychotherapy have provided some relevant data. Two open trials have been reported. Crits-Christoph and colleagues (Crits-Christoph, et al., 1996) followed 26 patients for a year. The patients had 16 once-weekly sessions followed by booster sessions once every 3 months. At post-therapy, 79% no longer met diagnostic criteria for Generalized Anxiety Disorder (GAD).

A second study by Durham and colleagues (Durham, et al., 1999) contrasted analytically-based psychotherapy with CBT and anxiety management training in an RCT. Ninety-nine patients with a GAD diagnosis for at least 6 months (mean duration 30 months) were randomly assigned to either high frequency or low frequency (weekly or fortnightly) CBT or analytic psychotherapy. Unfortunately, the groups ended up poorly matched with the CBT patients in the low frequency condition significantly less severely affected. Importantly, the gains from psychoanalytic psychotherapy were less than those for cognitive therapy and were also less likely to be maintained at one-year follow-up. Thus, while 60% of patients treated by CBT met clinically significant change criteria at one-year follow-up, only 14% of those in analytic psychotherapy did so ($RR_{HARS} = 0.11$, 95% CI: 0.03, 0.37). At this stage, higher frequency was associated with better maintenance of gains for both CBT and analytic psychotherapy. However, when the sample was followed up almost a decade after the end of treatment (Durham, Chambers, MacDonald, Power, & Major, 2003), only about half of those who had achieved recovery at 6 months maintained their gains in the very long term. By this stage, there was no difference in outcome between CBT and non-CBT treated participants.

A major limitation of this trial, but also a helpful pointer, was the nature of the psychoanalytic therapy offered. The two therapists, although both experienced psychiatrists, were training in psychoanalysis, are not reported to have had special training in brief therapeutic methods, and had no manual to follow. Under these circumstances, it is highly likely that the therapy delivered was not an effective version of STPP. If the effectiveness of cognitive therapy were assessed on the basis of two individuals trained in generic CBT, without further training specific to the trial, this would generally be considered unacceptable. It is possible, as the techniques used are not specified in the report, that these therapists used inappropriate techniques borrowed from the long-term therapy in which they were currently training and unhelpfully applied these in a time-limited context.

Panic Disorder

As with GAD, non-directive psychodynamic therapies have been used as control treatments in a number of CBT trials (e.g., Beck, Sokol, Clark, Berchick, &

Wright, 1992; Craske, Maidenberg, & Bystritsky, 1995). The relative absence of therapeutic equipoise makes these trials suspect and evidence from them can have few implications for the effectiveness of short-term psychodynamic treatments. When more effort is made to create a credible placebo, differences between treatment and control groups are reduced or disappear completely. For example, one study randomized 45 patients with panic disorder to 15 sessions of CBT or a therapy described as "non-prescriptive" where the therapist was encouraged to offer reflective listening (Shear, Pilkonis, Cloitre, & Leon, 1994). No significant differences were found at either post-therapy or at 6 months follow-up. In a partial replication, the same group (Shear, Houck, Greeno, & Masters, 2001) did find a difference between CBT and this non-prescriptive form of therapy, but the difference is small relative to less credible control interventions. In the meta-analysis by Nordhus and Pallesen (2003) of psychological treatments for later life anxiety, a number of studies are noted where the effectiveness of CBT is reduced or even reversed when the control condition is a highly credible psychotherapeutic placebo (e.g., Wetherell, Gatz, & Craske, 2003).

There are few trials of brief psychodynamic therapy for panic and none unequivocally addresses the effectiveness of this approach. Milrod and her colleagues have worked over a number of years to establish the evidence base for a manualized, panic-focused psychodynamic psychotherapy (Busch, Milrod, Cooper, & Shapiro, 1996; Busch, Milrod, & Singer, 2000; Milrod, Busch, Cooper, & Shapiro, 1997). This team reports an open trial of psychoanalytic psychotherapy with 21 patients seen twice weekly over 12 weeks and with a 6 month follow-up (Milrod, Busch, et al., 2001; Milrod, et al., 2000). Sixteen of the 21 participants showed remission (defined as a reduction from baseline of more than 50% on the panic disorder severity scale). The results proved stable at an unusually long follow-up period of 40 weeks. Of those completing treatment, 93% were considered remitted at the end of treatment and 90% at follow-up.

The study is, in many ways, exemplary. In particular, there was careful attention to measurement issues, careful training of therapists, and attention to treatment integrity. It is also remarkable for the involvement of senior psychoanalysts in the design and delivery of this structured and symptom-focused, but unequivocally psychoanalytic treatment. Although the effect sizes are comparable to those observed in the best trials of cognitive behavioral therapy (e.g., Barlow, Gorman, Shear, & Woods, 2000), the absence of a control group and relatively small sample size limits the generalizability of the conclusions.

Wiborg and Dahl (Wiborg & Dahl, 1996) reported a controlled study that examined the effect of adding psychodynamic therapy to treatment with clomipramine. Thirty patients were randomized to clomipramine or clomipramine with 15 weeks of manualized dynamic psychotherapy based on the work of Davanloo (1978), Malan (1976), and Strupp and Binder (1984). There was a follow-up at 6, 12, and 18 months of treatment. At the end of treatment, all patients in the combined treatment group were free of panic attacks ($RR_{HRSD} = 1.33$, 95% CI: 1.04, 1.72), but at 6 months follow-up, all clomipramine-treated subjects were panic-free. By 18 months, 75% of the drug-only group had relapsed, but only 20% of the group who had received psychotherapy ($RR_{HRSD} = 3.2$, 95% CI: 1.45, 7.05). The differences were apparent, even when adjustments were made for initial severity of symptoms and social adjustment. Further advantages were observed in terms of the psychotherapy group reporting fewer side effects from the medication. This study provides evidence that STPP is an effective adjunct to pharmacotherapy in panic disorder, but, of course, cannot speak to the effectiveness of this treatment in the absence of clomipramine. It is also important to note that clomipramine was administered by the treating psychotherapist in the experimental arm of the trial, but by a non-psychiatrically trained general physician in the control group. The findings confirm the results of an early trial (Klein, Zitrin, Woerner, & Ross, 1983) where the effect of imipramine for phobic problems was (to the authors' surprise) as strongly enhanced by STPP as by behavior therapy ($RR = 0.97$, 95% CI: 0.66, 1.43).

As described above, the Helsinki Psychotherapy Study (Knekt & Lindfors, 2004) included a significant number of individuals diagnosed with panic disorder ($n = 34$) and generalized anxiety disorder ($n = 37$). In addition, the authors observed that practically all the patients (more than 95%) had Hamilton Anxiety scores higher than 7 at baseline. There was a slight, but not statistically significant, difference between the groups in terms of the impact of the treatment on anxiety problems: 56% of those with anxiety disorders lost their diagnosis by 7 months of STTP, compared with 42% of those in SFT ($RR_{HARS} = 1.34$, 95% CI: 1.0, 1.78). By 12 months, the difference had narrowed to 62% and 52% respectively ($RR_{HARS} = 1.19$, 95% CI: 0.93, 1.51). While this difference is not significant, it underscores the potential for STPP to rapidly assist in the problems of anxiety as well as depression. There was a 34% decrease in the Hamilton Anxiety Rating Scale for STPP, and a 28% decrease for SFT at 12 months, but almost all of this had been achieved by 7 months.

Stress Related Conditions: Post-Traumatic Stress Disorder (PTSD) and Complex Grief Reaction

Psychodynamic approaches to PTSD focus on the meaning of the traumatic event for the person's sense of self and their place in the outside world (Horowitz, Marmar, Weiss, DeWitt, & Rosenbaum, 1984). Studies supporting this approach are either case reports or open trials. Open trials of the psychodynamic treatment of female victims of sexual assault have tended to be positive, but methodologically problematic (Cryer & Beutler, 1980; Perl, Westlin, & Peterson, 1985; Roth, Dye, & Lebowitz, 1988). Scarvalone and colleagues (Scarvalone,

Cloitre, & Difede, 1995) contrasted a psychodynamic group therapy with a wait-list control group. All participants (N = 40) had histories of sexual abuse although not all had current symptoms of PTSD. After treatment, 39% of those in the psychodynamic group, as opposed to 83% of those in the control group, met diagnostic criteria. ($RR_{DPTSD} = 0.47$, 95% CI: 0.27, 0.83).

A relatively large randomized controlled trial (RCT) from Holland (Brom, Kleber, & Defares, 1989) contrasted psychodynamic therapy, hypnotherapy, and trauma desensitization in the treatment of 114 individuals with PTSD diagnosis. Many were bereaved, and only about 20% reported experiencing a traumatic event. There was also a wait-list control group. Mean length of treatment varied somewhat between conditions (trauma desensitization = 15 weeks, hypnotherapy = 14.4 weeks, STPP = 18.8 weeks). The study reports all treatments to be superior to the wait-list control group with clinically significant improvements in about 60% of treated patients and 26% of the untreated ($RR_{DPTSD} = 2.28$, 95% CI: 1.12, 4.64). At post-treatment, psychodynamic therapy seemed to have the weakest effects, but therapeutic changes continued in this group and by follow-up they matched or exceeded those of other therapies. Interestingly, trauma desensitization had stronger influence on intrusions and psychodynamic therapy had more influence on avoidance.

Complex grief reaction was the focus of a further RCT of brief individual psychotherapy, contrasted with a group therapy run by non-clinician volunteers who were experts by experience (Marmar, Horowitz, Weiss, Wilner, & Kaltreider, 1988). The therapy was based on Horowitz's model of pathological bereavement and was delivered by experienced therapists. Sixty-one patients were randomized and outcomes were assessed at the end of treatment and at four-month and one-year follow-ups. Patients received 12 sessions of therapy in each group. The superiority of the psychotherapy group was principally in terms of reducing attrition in the early and late phases of the treatment. Nearly a third of those in group treatment terminated in the first third of the treatment ($RR_{DROPOUT} = 0.42$, 95% CI: 0.24, 0.73). Self-report results provided evidence of the superiority of psychotherapy at four months and one year on the general severity index of the SCL-90 ($SMD_{SCL90} = -0.6$, 95% CI: -1.1, -0.8). Other than the GSI, observer ratings and self-report differences favored the psychotherapy group, but were not statistically significant. This was most likely because the self-help group was surprisingly effective, at least for those who attended them. This trial was designed before the wider recognition of the value of self-help groups; otherwise, perhaps the investigators might have chosen a less challenging comparison.

An impressive program of work by William Piper and colleagues (Piper, et al., 1991; Piper, Joyce, McCallum, & Azim, 1998) examined the effects of time-limited interpretive therapy, in both an individual and in a partial hospitalization context (Piper, Rosie, Joyce, & Azim, 1996). However, these studies were conducted with heterogeneous samples of psychiatric outpatients and, therefore, are not relevant to a diagnosis-based review. An important trial explored the value of interpretive versus supportive group therapy for individuals with complicated grief reactions (Ogrodniczuk, Piper, McCallum, Joyce, & Rosie, 2002; Piper, McCallum, Joyce, Rosie, & Ogrodniczuk, 2001). Both therapies were modified to be appropriate for group treatment of grief, but, while interpretive therapy was aimed to enhance insight about repetitive conflicts associated with the losses, supportive therapy included praise and gratification. The treatments were manualized, sessions were videotaped, and the groups met for one 90-minute session per week for 12 weeks. Both treatments were effective in terms of an exceptionally broad range of outcome measures, covering general symptoms, grief symptoms, and target problems. The most informative finding to emerge from this study was the interaction between type of therapy and a measure of object relatedness. Psychological-mindedness was associated with improvement in both interpretive and supportive therapy. An intriguing and complex interview-based measure of the quality of object relations (QOR) (Piper, et al., 1991) was found to interact with these modes of therapy in a fashion meaningfully related to psychodynamic formulations. High quality or mature object relations on the QOR appear to predict greater benefit from interpretive therapy, while those whose relationships are judged to be more primitive, searching, or controlling were more likely to benefit from supportive therapy. Subsequent investigation (Piper, Ogrodniczuk, McCallum, Joyce, & Rosie, 2003) suggested that the balance of positive and negative affect expressions during therapy was the important mediator of this association. This well-conducted program suggests that STPP may be a relatively effective treatment for complex grief reactions and that individuals with more mature representations of interpersonal relationships are most likely to benefit.

Summary

Anxiety treatment research represents the "home base" of cognitive behavioral approaches. GAD represents its most significant challenge. One uncontrolled trial suggested that STPP might have something to offer these patients. A controlled trial comparing an unspecified form of STPP to cognitive therapy showed the latter to be substantially more effective in the short and medium term. The disappointing results from the psychodynamic arm of the trial may relate to the non-specificity and unstructured nature of this therapy.

Panic attacks appear to be relatively well treated by 15 to 20 sessions of CBT. There is a promising psychodynamic therapeutic approach to panic that might match CBT in efficacy that requires extension and replication in multi-center controlled trials. The superiority of CBT over other approaches is probably limited, as shown by reduced effect sizes in controlled trials that have active placebo treatments. The challenge for a psychodynamic approach is to identify a way to address limitations in CBT, either in terms of long-term efficacy (Milrod & Busch, 1996) or a more pervasive impact on social functioning. Interestingly, evidence from the Helsinki trial, where this was a focus of investigation, did not support the view that short-term psychodynamic therapy had a wider impact on social functioning than problem-focused treatments. Evidence on the treatment of PTSD is also sparse, notwithstanding the central involvement of psychoanalytic clinicians in mapping the consequences of childhood and later trauma. Available controlled studies concern complicated grief and bereavement reactions, and not exposure to trauma. Nonetheless, findings from such trials are generally positive although by no means uniquely effective.

It is striking that little research has been done to establish the pertinence of psychodynamic approaches to anxiety, which is so central to both psychoanalytic theory and practice. Possibly, psychodynamic therapists do not consider anxiety symptoms important enough, as Freud's term "signal anxiety" might suggest. Bypassing the surface problem of the anxiety symptoms, they attempt to achieve change in the underlying structures, even in brief therapies. Losing focus, they find change relatively difficult to bring about. It requires an approach such as Milrod's, which retains focus on the symptom at the same time as exploring unconscious determinants, to achieve rapid change. The importance of anxiety-related problems demands that further studies should be initiated.

EATING DISORDERS

Anorexia Nervosa

Most current treatment approaches for anorexia nervosa (behavior therapy [BT], CBT, family therapy, psychodynamic psychotherapy) recognize the importance of establishing an appropriate dietary regime, which is common to all treatments. An early study (Hall & Crisp, 1987), assigned 30 anorexic patients to either dietary advice or psychotherapy. The psychotherapy was psychodynamic, either delivered individually or involving the whole family for 12 sessions at two-week intervals. The dietary advice group entailed 15 one-hour sessions with a dietician at weekly or fortnightly intervals. There was no difference between the groups on body weight at post-treatment or at one-year follow-up. Those receiving psychotherapy showed better social and sexual adjustment scores. The sample sizes made it difficult to interpret these results, as the majority of the participants in the anorexic arm showed substantial weight gain and the inferior mean relative to the control groups was due to three individuals who showed a substantial weight loss. Needless to say, in this early study the psychotherapy (STPP) was not manualized.

An influential study by Russell and colleagues (Russell, Szmukler, Dare, & Eisler, 1987) contrasted family and individual therapy for 80 inpatients, the majority of whom (57) were anorexic. The therapy was not strictly psychodynamic, as it included cognitive and strategic techniques. Broadly, the majority of patients in both groups had poor outcome at one year (61%), with just under a quarter having good outcomes. While indicating the general difficulty of treating this group of patients, this study also suggested that late-onset patients (onset after age 19) did better with individual therapy. This finding was partially confirmed in a 5-year follow-up (Eisler, et al., 1997). The superiority of family therapy is restricted to anorexics with early onset and relatively short history.

The largest trial involving STPP is that of Dare and colleagues (Dare, Eisler, Russell, Treasure, & Dodge, 2001). Eighty-four patients were recruited to STPP based on Malan's approach (Malan, 1976). All therapeutic interventions were conducted by experienced therapists (family therapy [Dare & Eisler, 1997] and cognitive analytic therapy [Ryle, 1990]). The control group received standard psychiatric care (from trainee psychiatrists). This trial was carried out in a tertiary care setting; most patients had had one or more treatment failures. Not surprisingly, outcomes were poor (mean weight gains were small and left patients with under-nutrition), but provided evidence for all three treatment approaches. After one year of treatment, about a third of the patients in the three specialist psychotherapies no longer met DSM criteria for anorexia nervosa as compared with only 5% of those in routine treatment ($RR_{DAN} = 7.0$, 95% CI: 1.0, 48.9). It was not possible to differentiate clearly between the three specialized psychotherapies in terms of an improvement based on weight gain, regularity of menstruation and bulimic symptoms although the odds ratio for improvement in STPP and family therapy was better and significantly different from routine treatment ($RR_{FOCAL} = 1.99$, 95% CI: 0.85, 4.68) ($RR_{FAMTHER} = 1.55$, 95% CI: 0.63, 3.84). The study was, however, under-powered and follow-up was only partial.

Crisp and colleagues (Crisp, et al., 1991) report an RCT with 20 patients allocated to each of four treatment arms: inpatient treatment, outpatient individual and family psychotherapy (12 sessions over 10 months), 10 group therapy sessions, and initial assessment along with treatment as usual in the community. The individual therapy group was significantly better than both the inpatient and the minimal treatment group at the end of treatment. The individual psychotherapy was structured, somewhat eclectic in orientation, and delivered by experienced psychotherapists. The inpatient group received a range of treatments based on behavioral techniques coupled with milieu treatment and individual and family therapy. Gowers and colleagues (Gowers, Norton, Halek, & Crisp, 1994) reported on the outcome of the outpatient group compared with the minimal treatment group two years after the end of treatment. The outpatient group maintained, and further improved, their weight gain, which was more than twice that of the control group. While 60% of the psychotherapy group were judged to be well (within 15% of Mean Matched Population Weight [MMPW], normal menstruation and eating habits) or nearly well (within 15% of MMPW, nearly normal menstruation and/or abnormal eating habits), only 20% of the control group were judged to be so ($RR_{DAN} = 3.0$, 95% CI: 1.16, 7.73). Despite the small sample size, the study suggests that substantial benefits accrue to anorexic patients from psychodynamic therapy supported by family therapy. However, the form of therapy offered was eclectic rather than a pure form of STPP; therefore, effective elements may actually be associated with the strategic or directive elements.

Bulimia Nervosa

The majority of trials in the literature (around 30) employed either behavioral or cognitive-behavioral techniques (Hay & Bacaltchuk, 2001; Thompson-Brenner, et al., 2003). Intent-to-treat recovery rates are only around 33%, with an advantage to individual therapies and no clear superiority to CBT over alternative active psychological interventions. No non-CBT studies report long term follow-up, and meta-analytic studies show a tendency towards deterioration in effect size of follow-up samples relative to post therapy observations. The meta-analyses do not speak to the specific efficacy of psychodynamic therapies.

Garner and colleagues (Garner, Rockert, Davis, & Garner, 1993) reported a study contrasting STPP based on Luborsky's supportive expressive model (Luborsky, 1984) with CBT. Sixty patients were randomized to 19 individual treatment sessions over an 18-week period. Five patients withdrew from each treatment arm. The two treatments were equally effective in their impact for binge frequency. CBT was somewhat more effective (but not statistically significantly) in reducing vomiting frequency and significantly more effective in reducing depression. Both treatments are considered by the authors to be effective, but where differences emerged these favored CBT. No follow up is reported for the study, which would be critical in this context.

A different psychodynamic approach was taken in a study of 33 bulimic patients (Bachar, Latzer, Kreitler, & Berry, 1999) assigned to either nutritional counseling alone or in conjunction with a form of cognitive therapy or a form of self-psychological dynamic therapy. A range of measures was used including measures of symptomatology, attitudes to food, self structure, and general psychiatric symptoms. The groups were inappropriately small and preclude comments on relative efficacy. However, pre-post effects appear to be substantial for psychodynamic treatment, less notable for cognitive therapy, and almost negligible for nutritional guidance. The study is further weakened by the mixture of anorexic and bulimic patients identified and the non-standard cognitive approach applied. Nevertheless, it suggests psychodynamic treatment may have significantly better outcomes compared to an almost untreated group.

Walsh (Walsh, et al., 1997) reported an impressive investigation that contrasted psychodynamically oriented supportive psychotherapy with CBT and antidepressant medication (desipramine followed by fluoxetine). One-hundred-twenty women with bulimia were randomized to five treatment arms. In this trial, CBT was superior to psychodynamic psychotherapy in reducing bulimic symptoms. Supportive psychotherapy appeared to offer little additional benefit to medication alone, but CBT and medication combined produced greater improvement than medication alone. The results suggest that supportive psychotherapy is not particularly helpful for bulimia.

Obesity

Beutel and colleagues (Beutel, Thiede, Wiltlink, & Sobez, 2001) reported an unusual trial involving inpatient treatment of obesity (Body Mass Index [BMI] > 35kg/m2) . Ninety-eight consecutive patients were randomly allocated to 6 weeks of either inpatient behavioral (n = 46) or psychodynamic (n = 52) treatments entailing individual and group work in both approaches. They measured weight loss, eating behavior, body image, and life satisfaction. While both interventions were associated with substantial gains, there were no differences between the two programs in terms of weight loss or eating behavior changes.

Summary

There have been four trials of psychodynamic psychotherapy for anorexia nervosa, all of which found it to be as effective as other treatments, including intensive behavioral and strategic family therapy. None of the trials were powered adequately to distinguish conclusively between alternative treatments. Taking the results together, it seems that relative to TAU, psychodynamic therapy for anorexia nervosa holds its own. The trials were performed in two London specialist units, but the particular brands of psychoanalytic psychotherapy practiced were not comparable, so they cannot be considered replications.

STPP fares less well in the treatment of bulimia. One trial indicated that STPP was somewhat less effective than CBT, while in another study the superiority of STPP is based on a small sample size and an unusual implementation of cognitive therapy. In a trial exploring combined pharmacological and psychosocial treatments, non-specific supportive STPP turned out to be less effective than CBT in enhancing the effect of medication.

Overall, as in other contexts, when STPP is modified for a specific clinical problem it is far more likely to be effective; it is comparable to a similarly refined cognitive behavioral approach. As a generic supportive treatment, it is unlikely to be an appropriate recommendation for any of the eating disorders considered, but as a specific approach it is perhaps more likely to be of benefit.

SUBSTANCE MISUSE

Psychoanalytic therapies do not have a strong tradition in the treatment of substance misuse. There have been theoretical and clinical investigations of the problems, but few substantive case series studies (Hopper, 1995; Johnson, 1999; Radford, Wiseberg, & Yorke, 1972). However, in the light of emerging data concerning the prevalence rates of alcohol and drug dependence—perhaps in excess of 7% (Hickman, et al., 1999; Kessler, et al., 1994; Kraus, et al., 2003)—it seems important to establish whether psychoanalytic psychotherapy has something to contribute to this major public health problem.

Alcohol Misuse

A research group led by William Miller has produced an exhaustive, and periodically updated, report concerning the relative effectiveness of a range of psychosocial treatments for alcohol dependence (Miller & Wilbourne, 2002; Miller, Wilbourne, & Hettema, 2003). Using a simple, but relatively robust method of identifying empirical support (Finney & Monahan, 1996), in terms of the number of studies in the literature yielding positive outcomes, they identified brief interventions and motivational enhancement as best supported, followed by community reinforcement and bibliotherapy, then various behavioral interventions (contracting, self control, etc.), followed by social skills. Psychotherapy is placed last in a long line.

Indeed, evidence for the efficacy of psychotherapy and counseling is very limited. An early study (Levinson & Sereny, 1969) described assigning inpatients to a generic insight-oriented therapy, with additional educational sessions or treatment as usual, which at the time included recreational therapy and occupational therapy. At one-year follow-up, no differences were observed in terms of drinking behavior, with somewhat greater improvements being reported from the control group. Miller's database contains other similar examples (e.g., Pattison, Brissenden, & Wohl, 1967; Tomsovic, 1970).

Looking at more specific dynamic psychotherapies, there are some studies of dynamic therapy, which show superiority to a no-treatment control group (Brandsma, Maultsby, & Welsh, 1980; Kissin & Gross, 1968). However, when the contrast is with minimal intervention approaches, there appears to be little demonstrable benefit from dynamic psychotherapeutic treatment (Crumbach & Carr, 1979; Zimberg, 1974). Studies which do suggest differences (e.g., Pomerleau, Pertshuk, Adkins, & d'Aquili, 1978) are characterized by poor methodology (Miller & Hester, 1986). There is only one trial (amongst the 381 trials listed in the Miller database) that supports a psychodynamic approach (Sandahl, Herlitz, Ahlin, & Rönnberg, 1998). Investigators randomized 49 patients meeting criteria for alcohol dependence to group psychodynamic or group cognitive-behavioral therapy. All patients had already completed inpatient treatment. There were no statistically significant differences between the groups, but at post-therapy and, more importantly, at 15 months follow-up, both groups improved. While not statistically significant, the tendency was for the psychodynamic psychotherapy group to show better maintenance of gains.

Even with the most effective treatment, the prognosis for alcohol dependence is not good, particularly for patients with greater chronicity. There is insufficient evidence in the literature to support psychodynamic psychotherapy as an adequate first-line therapy for patients with alcohol dependency problems. Given the comorbidity of alcohol dependence with other psychiatric problems, STPP may possibly be helpful in dealing with residual psychiatric disorder after alcohol dependence has been addressed. This suggestion will need to be subjected to empirical tests.

Cocaine Dependency

The outcome of cocaine abuse from naturalistic studies is similar to alcohol. A study of the effectiveness of community treatment (Simpson, Joe, Fletcher, Hubbard, & Anglin, 1999) revealed that 90-day relapse rates for long-term residential treatment were 15%; for short-term in-patient treatment, 38%; and outpatient programs, 29%. Given the under-reporting of cocaine use, the rates of relapse are likely 10 to 20% higher (Simpson, Joe, & Broome, 2002).

Kang and colleagues (Kang, et al., 1991) reported a major trial to study the efficacy of once-weekly psychotherapy or family therapy contrasted with group therapy led by a para-professional among patients with cocaine use disorders. Participants were recruited from those seeking outpatient treatment and 168 consented to be randomized to one of three arms in the trial. One-hundred twenty-two of those in the trial were interviewed 6 and 12 months later and addiction severity indices were compared. Attrition was extremely high with only about 50% attending more than one session and 22% more than six sessions. Nineteen percent of those who attended more than three sessions reported abstinence at six months. There was a significant impact for the cohort as a whole. This reflected the 19% of the 122 subjects who were no longer using cocaine at follow-up. There was a strong relationship between achieving abstinence and improvements in psychiatric symptoms and family problems. There was no relationship between attendance at therapy sessions and outcome. The results of the trial were considered by the author to indicate that outpatient once weekly psychotherapy is an insufficient treatment for cocaine use disorder. The results indicate that inpatient treatment or more intensive outpatient treatment may be required.

A second trial, the National Institute for Drug Abuse Collaborative Cocaine Study (Crits-Christoph, et al., 1997; Crits-Christoph, et al., 1999; Crits-Christoph, et al., 2001) randomized 487 severely cocaine-dependent patients who met criteria for cocaine misuse, with 75% smoking crack cocaine and 33% also meeting criteria for alcohol dependence, to one of four treatments: (1) group drug counseling (GDC) following the 12 steps model, (2) GDC combined with individual drug counseling (IDC), (3) GDC combined with CBT, or (4) GDC combined with STPP. Treatments were offered over six months during which participants had 24 group sessions and a maximum of 36 individual sessions. The treatment lacked acceptability. By the third month, 50% of the participants had left treatment and, overall, only 28% completed. All treatments showed significant improvements from baseline to post-baseline in cocaine use (past 30 days). The greatest improvement was with IDC. By the sixth month, an estimated 40% of available patients in the IDC group reported cocaine use, compared with 58% in CBT, 50% in STPP, and 52% in GDC alone ($RR_{IDCvsSTPP@6months}$ = 1.24, 95% CI: 0.94, 1.64) ($RR_{IDCvsCBT@6months}$ = 1.35, 95% CI: 1.03, 1.77). At 12 months follow-up, these percentages were 40%, 46%, 48%, and 47%, respectively. The difference between IDC and other treatments was statistically significant. CBT and STPP retained patients better, but IDC produced more improvement in terms of abstinence. Interestingly, higher levels of alliance were associated with better retention in IDC and STPP, but with worse retention in CBT (Crits-Christoph, et al., 2001). There was no difference between the treatments in terms of associated psychological, social, and interpersonal measures (Crits-Christoph, et al., 2001). It should be noted that, while this is one of the most sophisticated tests of the value of STPP, there are some crucial flaws in the design. In the extended (2 weeks) assessment, 46% of the initial participants (those with the highest level of dependency needs) were lost to the trial, and patients on psychotropic medication who might have benefited most from STPP or CBT were excluded.

Opiate Dependency

Meta-analyses of the treatment of opiate dependency (Brewer, Catalano, Haggerty, Gainey, & Fleming, 1998; Prendergast, Podus, Chang, & Urada, 2002) identified short treatment length, low treatment integrity, and low levels of staff training to be associated with relatively poor outcome. Meta-analyses reveal effect sizes to be relatively low (0.3) and, unusually, fail to identify a particular treatment type as especially beneficial.

Woody and colleagues (Woody, McLellan, Luborsky, & O'Brien, 1987; Woody, et al., 1983; Woody, McLellan, Luborsky, & O'Brien, 1990; Woody, McLellan, Luborsky, & O'Brien, 1995) performed a crucial randomized study of supportive expressive therapy contrasted with CBT in opiate dependent individuals on methadone. These two forms of therapy were compared with 24 weeks of drug counseling alone. The numbers of sessions for the three conditions were not equal: 17 for drug counseling alone, 12 for STPP, and 10 for CBT. Of 305 patients who met criteria, 185 of these agreed to take part, but only 110 engaged in the trial. Patients in all three groups showed improvements in lessened drug use, criminal behavior, and psychological function at 7 months follow-up. There were advantages to the STPP group in psychological problems, days worked, money legally earned, and advantages to CBT in dealing with legal problems. Both therapy groups did better than drug counseling only group. At 12 months follow-up, data were available from 93 participants, with the two psychotherapy groups showing more improvement. CBT showed the same kind of advantages on most measures as STPP. However, 44% of STPP vs. 26% in CBT and 18% in drug counseling alone were off methadone at 12 months ($RR_{STPPVSCBTMETHADONE} = 1.71$, 95% CI: 0.88, 3.31) ($RR_{STPPVSCONTROLMETHADONE} = 2.44$, 95% CI: 1.12, 5.3) (Woody, et al., 1987).

A partial replication of this study (Woody, et al., 1995) in a community setting addressed a limitation of the previous study that psychotherapy participants had both a drug counselor and a psychotherapist. In the replication study, the clients randomized to drug counseling alone (n = 41) had access to two drug counselors, matching the psychotherapy group (n = 82). The number of sessions between the arms were also equated in the community replication. There were no differences between the groups in positive opiate urine samples, but there was a difference as far as cocaine urine analysis was concerned (22% in STPP and 36% in DC) ($RR_{COCAINESTPPVSDC} = 0.6$, 95% CI: 0.34, 1.06). The pattern of results across time consistently indicated that while the groups were equivalent at the end of treatment, the drug counseling alone group worsened during follow-up, while the STPP group improved over the same period. The study, however, encountered the problems that face effectiveness as opposed to efficacy (rapid staff changes, sub-optimal clinical protocols, lack of co-operation from clinical sites). Thus, the degree of change observed is even more impressive.

Summary

Many studies considered the efficacy of brief interventions for alcohol dependence. For alcohol problems of low severity, brief interventions seem to be the interventions of choice. Psychodynamic psychotherapy, along with other formal psychological therapies, appears not to be particularly helpful when offered as a stand-alone treatment. On the whole, successful interventions appear to be targeted at drinking behavior and testable psychodynamic protocols of this kind have not yet been developed.

Again, for low levels of cocaine dependency, briefer treatments appear to be appropriate. But for individuals with more severe problems, both engaging with treatment and maintaining commitment to formal psychotherapy appears problematic. Supportive expressive psychotherapy appears of almost no value in the context of cocaine misuse. In fact, treatments that do not engage with clients in the community context appear to be of limited relevance. It is an obvious question as to whether STPP could be modified to incorporate community involvement.

A different picture emerges in the context of opiate abuse where psychodynamic treatment was shown to be efficacious in two trials, unfortunately (from the standpoint of EST criteria) carried out by the same team. However, in this context, there is a prima facie case for the unique effectiveness of supportive expressive therapy, as neither IPT (Rounsaville, Glazer, Wilber, Weissman, & Kleber, 1983) nor certain cognitive therapies (Dawe, et al., 1993; Kasvikis, Bradley, Powell, Marks, & Gray, 1991) appear to have quite the same impact. Nevertheless, generic counseling or certain types of family-based interventions may enhance the effectiveness of methadone treatment, just as STPP appears to. In this area, there is urgent need for replication by an independent group of workers willing to implement the supportive-expressive therapeutic strategy.

If a place is to be found for psychodynamic psychotherapy in substance abuse protocols, it is unlikely to be in offering formal therapy as a primary treatment. Rather, taking the lead from the opiate work, a niche needs to be found where psychodynamic intervention provides appropriate support for what is ultimately a physical dependency requiring physical treatment rather than hoping that a psychological intervention by itself is capable of resolving a physical dependency. There is urgent need to identify protocols that sequence traditional forms of psychosocial treatments with interventions for physical dependence within a single integrated package.

PERSONALITY DISORDERS

Personality disorders (PD) represent a special challenge for outcome research because of the high level of comorbidity between Axis I and Axis II diagnoses and within Axis II diagnoses (Swartz, Blazer, & Winfield, 1990; Zimmerman & Coryell, 1990). Treatment research is somewhat limited, powerfully enhanced by recent activity in new approaches to cognitive behavioral therapy (Blum, Pfohl, John, Monahan, & Black, 2002; Koons, et al., 2001; Linehan, et al., 1999), as well as psychodynamic treatments (Bateman & Fonagy, 2004; Clarkin, et al., 2001; Clarkin, Levy, Lenzenweger, & Kernberg, 2004b; Ryle & Golynkina, 2000).

There have been two meta-analyses of psychological therapies. Perry and colleagues (Perry, Banon, & Ianni, 1999) identified 15 studies, including six randomized trials. Substantial effect sizes (ES) were identified pre- to post-treatment (ES = 1.1-1.3), which reduced to around 0.7 in studies where active control treatments were used. A more focused meta-analysis (Leichsenring & Leibing, 2003) considered only trials that used either CBT or psychodynamic therapy and identified 22 studies, 11 of which were RCTs. Pre-post effect size for psychodynamic therapy was 1.31, based on 8 studies, and for CBT was 0.95, based on 4 studies. There was an insignificant correlation between treatment length and outcome.

The limited number of studies, compounded by heterogeneity of clinical populations and methods applied, suggests that meta-analysis at this stage may be premature. Further, many of the studies included in these meta-analyses did not have the aim of treating Axis II disorders. Notwithstanding these limitations, the broad conclusion from these aggregated figures would be that CBT and psychodynamic therapy are equally effective.

Borderline Personality Disorder

There are more studies of borderline personality disorder (BPD) than of other PDs. There have been a number of uncontrolled open trials of the psychodynamic treatment of BPD. The Menninger Study of 42 patients carried out in the 1950s is historically important as the first serious, relatively methodologically sound attempt to evaluate the outcome of any type of psychological therapy (Wallerstein, 1986, 1989). It was a study of psychoanalysis and expressive or supportive psychodynamic psychotherapy. One may well ask what happened to this pioneering spirit. The study's findings are complex, but broadly imply that more mature personalities with better interpersonal relationships responded well to expressive interpretive therapy, whereas those with low ego strength responded better to supportive interventions. There have been a number of other naturalistic studies (Antikainen, Hintikka, Lehtonen, Koponen, & Arstila, 1995; Karterud, et al., 1992; Monsen, Odland, Faugli, Daae, & Eilertsen, 1995; Tucker, Bauer, Wagner, Harlam, & Sher, 1987; Waldinger & Gunderson, 1984; Wilberg, et al., 1998). These studies, with varied sample sizes, speak to the relative efficacy of various forms of psychodynamic therapy, but had too little in common in terms of treatment protocols to permit conclusions concerning the effectiveness of this approach.

An Australian uncontrolled trial stands out in terms of methodological rigor (Meares, Stevenson, & Comerford, 1999; Stevenson & Meares, 1992; 1999). In this open trial, 48 patients received twice-weekly interpersonal self-psychological psychodynamic outpatient therapy over 12 months. The contrast was with patients on a waiting list for 12 months. Unfortunately, allocation was not random and severity in the wait-list group was slightly less. Thirty percent of the treatment group no longer met criteria for BPD at the end of one year. There was little indication of change in the control group. However, intent-to-treat calculations would only estimate a 19% remission rate, which is comparable to the spontaneous change in follow-along studies. A wait-list control group is problematic and sometimes referred to as a "nocebo" group, as the implicit contingencies of being on a waiting list imply no change.

A further large-scale uncontrolled trial of psychodynamic psychotherapy is worth singling out. Dolan and colleagues (Dolan, Warren, & Norton, 1997) reported on the outcome of a therapeutic community run on strictly democratic principles, for example patients having a veto on the appropriateness of an admission. Of 598 patients referred, 239 were admitted and 137 (23%) returned assessment questionnaires at the one-year follow-up. About equal numbers of admitted and non-admitted patients returned the questionnaires, about 80% of whom met diagnostic criteria for BPD. Clinically significant change on self-reported borderline symptomatology was seen in 43% of the treated and 18% of the untreated patients (30 versus 12) ($RR_{STPPVSCONTROL} = 2.39$, 95% CI: 1.34, 4.27). Length of stay was associated with improvement. The comparison group places profound limitations on the study, not just because of the absence of randomization and the varied reasons for being in the no treatment group, but also because the pre-post time period covered in the treatment group was significantly longer (19 versus 12 months). Nevertheless, the study provides data concerning the likely change to be observed in a specialist, but routine, service context.

The Cornell group (Clarkin, et al., 2001) reported the outcomes of 23 female patients treated in transference-focused psychotherapy. The trial, which was a pilot for the Personality Disorders Institute Borderline Personality Disorder Research Foundation RCT (Clarkin, et al., 2004b), was a carefully conducted follow-along study of 23 female patients. After one year of treatment, suicidal behavior substantially decreased and the pre-post comparison of inpatient days suggested significant cost savings.

Gabbard, et al. (2000) reported a prospective, naturalistic, and uncontrolled study of consecutive patients admitted to the Menninger Hospital. Only 35% of the 216 completed in the sample were diagnosed with BPD. About half the patients had mixed PD or PD Not Otherwise Specified. An important feature of the study was the telephone follow-up at one year. GAF scores increased: only 3.7% had GAF scores above 50 on admission, which increased to 55% at discharge and 66% at follow-up. Other measures reflected a similar pattern. The study suggests that inpatient treatment can initiate improvement even in relatively severely dysfunctional patients. But the absence of a comparison group, and the unknown selection bias introduced by limited participation, reduces the generalizability of the data. Further the treatment package offered, while relatively consistent across patients, was not monitored in relation to each discipline. Given the wide diversity of length of stay, it is hard to link progress to psychotherapeutic experience.

Chiesa and colleagues (Chiesa & Fonagy, 2000, 2003; Chiesa, Fonagy, Holmes, & Drahorad, 2004; Chiesa, Fonagy, Holmes, Drahorad, & Harrison-Hall, 2002) reported a further controlled, but not randomized, trial of inpatient psychodynamic treatment. Two forms of hospital-based treatment were contrasted with a general community-based psychiatric treatment model. In the first protocol, patients were admitted for approximately 12 months with no aftercare. In the second, patients were admitted for only 6 months but this was followed by 12 months of outpatient therapy with community support. The third arm received community psychiatric care (medication and brief hospital admissions as necessary). Two-hundred ten patients with at least one diagnosis of personality disorder were allocated according to geographical criteria into the three groups. Outcome was evaluated at 6, 12, and 24 months on self-harm and suicide attempts, and self-reports of symptom severity and social adaptation. At 24 months, only the phased or step-down condition showed improvements, while patients in the long-term residential model showed no improvements in self-harm, attempted suicide, and number of readmissions. There were significant reductions in symptom severity, improvements in social adaptation, and global functioning. Patients in the general psychiatric group showed no improvement in these variables, except for self-harm. Forty-seven percent of the inpatient group, 73% of the step-down group, and 71% of the general psychiatric group reported no self-harm in the previous 12 months ($RR_{INPVSTAU@24MONTHS} = 0.66$, 95% CI: 0.47, 0.93; $RR_{SDPVSTAU@24MONTHS} = 1.03$, 95% CI: 0.81, 1.32). At 24 months, more of the inpatient group had hospital admissions in the previous 12 months (49% for inpatient group compared to 11% for the step-down and 33% for the general psychiatric care groups ($RR_{INPVSTAU@24MONTHS} = 1.5$, 95% CI: 0.92, 2.45; $RR_{SDPVSTAU@24MONTHS} = 0.34$, 95% CI: 0.14, 0.85).

Thus, in terms of clinical outcome the general psychiatric treatment group were somewhat inferior to the step-down group and superior to the inpatient group. The findings indicate that long-term inpatient therapy may be iatrogenic and may undermine some of the effective components of a treatment mode, which results in substantial positive outcomes in more moderate doses. Only about 10 to 12% of the general psychiatric group showed clinically significant change in symptomatology and social adjustment compared to over half of the step-down group and about a quarter of the inpatient group. Mean Global Security Index (GSI) scores were more or less unchanged in the general psychiatry group. They were reduced by half a standard deviation in the inpatient group and by a whole standard deviation in the step-down group.

Only one randomized controlled study is available. Bateman and Fonagy (1999; 2001; 2003) reported on a study of 38 patients assigned to specialist partial hospitalization or to routine care. Over 18 months, partial hospitalization showed significant gains over controls on measures of suicidality, self-harm, and inpatient stay. These became apparent at 6 to 12 months of treatment and increased over time. Follow-up at 18 months, which included an intent-to-treat analysis, demonstrated that not only did patients in the program maintain their gains, but further improvements were observed. At the end of treatment, 84% of the treatment-as-usual (TAU) and 36% of the partial hospital patients had showed self-harming behaviors in the previous 6 months ($RR_{SH@18MOS} = 0.43$, 95% CI: 0.24, 0.75). At 36 months, 58% of the controls and 8% of the partial hospital patients had harmed themselves in the previous 6 months ($RR_{SH@36MONTHS} = 0.14$, 95% CI: 0.03, 0.55). A cost-benefit analysis suggested that in the course of the treatment, additional costs of the program are offset by reductions in inpatient and emergency room care costs, as well as in reduced medication. The difference in costs per patient became apparent in the follow-up period. The mean annual cost-of-service utilization was $15,500 for the TAU group and $3,200 for the partial hospitalization group. This is an enormous discrepancy.

The second controlled trial carried out by Clarkin and colleagues (2004a) is the most ambitious and comprehensive trial of psychodynamic psychotherapy in any context. It contrasts transference-focused psychotherapy (TFP) (Clarkin, Kernberg, & Yeomans, 1999) with dialectical behavior therapy (DBT) (Linehan, 1993) and psychoanalytic supportive psychotherapy (SPT) (Rockland, 1987). TFP is based on Kernberg's object relations model and is a twice-weekly outpatient therapy using clarification, confrontation, and transference interpretation. Psychodynamic supportive psychotherapy eschews transference interpretation, focuses on the strengthening of adaptive defenses, forming an alliance, and providing reassurance. All therapists were experienced in the conduct of their modality. Of 207 patients interviewed for the trial, 109 met the criteria; 19 refused randomization, but the remaining 90 were randomized to TFP, DBT, or SPT. The baseline GAF score was about 50, quite severe for an outpatient sample. Results are available to 12 months. In all therapies, GAF scores increased by about 10 points. Beck Depression Index (BDI) scores decreased significantly and social adjustment scores increased. There was no significant change in anxiety scores. The majority of patients showed improvement in their suicidality; only a minority appeared to be getting worse. Hierarchical linear modeling showed that TFP and DBT improved significantly on suicidality, but that patients in SPT treatment did not, and that all three treatment groups improved significantly in terms of global functioning and depression. On the Adult Attachment Interview (AAI) (Main & Goldwyn, 1998), ratings of coherence (closely related to attachment security) improved for all three groups. The improvement was most marked for the TFP group, but this difference was not statistically significant. Reflective function scores (Fonagy, Target, Steele, & Steele, 1998), based on the AAI and related to mentalization, showed slight improvements in the other two treatments, but was only significant for the transference-focused psychotherapy group (Levy & Clarkin, in press). Other than this significant interaction, there were no differences between the treatment groups, except for a significantly higher early termination rate from DBT that could reflect more rapid improvement or lower acceptability of this treatment within this group.

Antisocial Personality Disorder

There are no trials of psychodynamic treatment of antisocial personality disorder (ASPD), and only a small number of observational studies of individuals detained in high security settings (e.g., Reiss, Grubin, & Meux, 1996). These studies were reviewed by Warren, et al. (2003) and, while it is likely that at least some of these individuals would meet criteria for ASPD, this cannot be assumed. In general, improvements are noted, but the methodology is too weak to permit generalization.

More recently, Saunders (1996) contrasted CBT and STPP. The treatment was offered to men who were violent with their partners and, of the 136 participants, 40% met criteria for ASPD. No differences are reported between the groups in terms of recidivism and, in the absence of a no-treatment control group, it is difficult to judge if either treatment was effective. A prison service in the UK (Grendon) is currently run along relatively coherent psychodynamic principles. Taylor (2000) describes outcomes from a 7 year follow-up of 700 individuals who participated in this therapeutic community. The comparison groups in the report consist of demographically matched individuals who were never admitted to Grendon from the wait list group and 1,400 individuals treated from a general prison population. Attendance at the psychodynamic therapeutic community at Grendon was associated with a reduced rate of re-offending. Further, there was a link between length of stay at Grendon and outcome. However, when prior criminal histories are controlled for, the apparent impact of Grendon is reduced. Thornton and colleagues (Thornton, Mann , Bowers, Sheriff, & White, 1996) looked at a subgroup who were sex offenders. When matched with a group with similar forensic histories, those at the chronic end of the severity spectrum (at least two previous convictions for sex offenses) had better outcomes.

Cluster C (Anxious-Fearful) Personality Disorder

Cluster-C personality disorders include avoidant PD (social discomfort, timidity), dependent PD (dependent on reassurance), and obsessive-compulsive PD. These are the most prevalent personality disorders in the general population (10%) (Torgersen, Kringlen, & Cramer, 2001).

We know of only one open trial of psychodynamic therapy that explicitly focuses on avoidant PD (Barber, Morse, Krakauer, Chittams, & Crits-Christoph, 1997). They used supportive expressive psychotherapy in the treatment of 38 individuals—two-thirds with avoidant and one-third with obsessive-compulsive PD. Attrition was high, with 50% of the avoidant PDs leaving therapy prematurely; 40% of those with avoidant PD who stayed with therapy retained their diagnosis. Those with obsessive-compulsive PD had better retention rates and better outcomes.

A small Norwegian trial (Svartberg, Stiles, & Seltzer, 2004) compared STPP with cognitive therapy for outpatients with cluster C personality disorder. Fifty-one patients were randomly allocated to receive 40 weekly sessions of dynamic therapy (Malan's approach) or cognitive therapy (Beck's approach). Sessions were videotaped and adherence and integrity checks were performed with both therapies. Only two patients did not attend follow-up assessments at 6, 12, and 24 months. Both groups improved and continued to improve after treatment, both symptomatologically and in terms of personality profile (Millon's Clinical Multiaxial Inventory). On the SCL-90, 38% and 17% for STPP and CBT, respectively, were recovered, with asymptomatic status (below the clinical cut-point) at the end of treatment ($RR_{SCL90@12MONTHS} = 2.6$, 95% CI: 0.94, 7.22). However, at 2-year follow-up these had increased to 54% and 42%, respectively ($RR_{SCL90@24MONTHS} = 1.46$, 95% CI: 0.8, 2.65). These figures were somewhat lower for personality change on the Millon—63% of the STPP group and 48% of the CBT group changed on this measure ($RR_{MILLON@24MONTHS} = 1.39$, 95% CI: 0.83, 2.31). The results of the clinical equivalence test (within interval of 20% of a zero difference) suggests that the group differences on the Millon are probably trivial, but the differences on the SCL-90 may be of clinical significance. Sadly, the study is underpowered to detect more than a large effect size, which is unlikely to be observed in this kind of context.

A randomized trial compared STPP for predominantly cluster C personality disordered individuals (n = 31), along the lines developed by Malan (1976) and Davanloo (1978), with brief adaptive psychotherapy (BAP) developed by the authors (n = 32) (Winston, et al., 1994). There was also a wait-list control group (n = 26). The former form of STPP is believed by the authors to be more confrontational, but both appear to address defensive behavior and elicit affect in interpersonal contexts. Thirty-two patients were randomly allocated to BAP and 31 to more traditional STPP. Twenty-five completed STPP and 30, BAP. Mean treatment length was 40 sessions, but the wait-list control group lasted only 15 weeks. A large number of therapists participated. Treatment manuals and video-taping were employed for adherence checks. A variable-length follow-up reached about two-thirds of the treated groups. The two treated groups both showed significant change on the GSI of the SCL-90 of approximately one standard deviation and some change on the Social Adjustment Scale (SAS). There were no significant differences between the two treated groups—not surprising, given the similarity of the approaches. There were some differences between the groups in terms of gender and Axis I diagnoses and heterogeneity as to Axis II diagnoses. The study was under-powered to look at specific benefits of each therapy in relation to particular PD types. An earlier study by the same group (Winston, et al., 1991) contrasted the same therapies and reported essentially the same results with similar effect sizes on the GSI and the SAS. This study had a more robust follow-up at 18 months (Winston, et al., 1994) and indicated that the gains were maintained.

LONG TERM PSYCHOTHERAPY

In the previous sections, we considered evidence available to support thera-peutic interventions, which are derivatives of psychoanalysis. However, there is a certain degree of disingenuity in psychoanalysis embracing these investigations. Most analysts would consider that the aims and methods of short-term, once-a-week psychotherapy are not comparable to "full analysis." What do we know about the value of intensive and long-term psychodynamic treatment? Here, the evidence base becomes even more patchy and we cannot restrict the review to ran-domized controlled trials.

The Boston Psychotherapy Study (Stanton, et al., 1984) compared long-term psychoanalytic therapy (two or more times a week) with supportive therapy for clients with schizophrenia in a randomized controlled design. On the whole, clients who received psychoanalytic therapy fared no better than those who received supportive treatment. The partial-hospital RCT (Bateman & Fonagy, 1999) included in the psychoanalytic arm of the treatment, included therapy groups three times a week, as well as individual therapy once or twice a week, over an 18-month period. A further controlled trial of intensive psychoanalytic treatment of children with chronically poorly-controlled diabetes reported signifi-cant gains in diabetic control in the treated group, which was maintained at one-year follow-up (Moran, Fonagy, Kurtz, Bolton, & Brook, 1991). Experimental sin-gle case studies carried out with the same population supported the causal rela-tionship between interpretive work and improvement in diabetic control and physical growth (Fonagy & Moran, 1991). The work of Chris Heinicke also sug-gests that four or five times weekly sessions may generate more marked improve-ments in children with specific learning difficulties than a less intensive psychoanalytic intervention (Heinicke & Ramsey-Klee, 1986).

One of the most interesting studies to emerge recently was the Stockholm Outcome of Psychotherapy and Psychoanalysis Project (Blomberg, Lazar, & San-dell, 2001; Grant & Sandell, 2004; Sandell, et al., 2000). The study followed 756 persons who received national insurance-funded treatment for up to three years in psychoanalysis or psychoanalytic psychotherapy. The groups were matched on many clinical variables. Four or five times weekly analysis had similar outcomes at termination, when compared with one to two sessions per week psychother-apy. During the follow-up period, psychotherapy patients did not change, but those who had had psychoanalysis continued to improve, almost to a point where their scores were indistinguishable from those obtained from a non-clinical Swedish sample. While the results of the study are positive for psycho-analysis, certain findings are quite challenging. For example, therapists whose atti-tude to clinical process most closely resembled that of a so-called "classical analyst" (neutrality, exclusive orientation to insight) had psychotherapy clients with the worst, commonly negative, outcomes.

The German Psychoanalytic Association undertook a major follow-up study of psychoanalytic treatments undertaken in that country between 1990 and 1993 (Leuzinger-Bohleber, Stuhr, Ruger, & Beutel, 2003; Leuzinger-Bohleber & Target, 2002). A representative sample (n = 401) of all the patients who had terminated their psychoanalytic treatments with members of the German Psychoanalytical Association (DPV) were followed up. Between 70 and 80% of the patients achieved good and stable psychic changes (average 6.5 years after the end of treatment), according to the evaluations of the patients themselves, their analysts, independent psychoanalytic and non-psychoanalytic experts, and questionnaires commonly applied in psychotherapy research. The evaluation of mental health costs showed a cost reduction through fewer days of sick leave during the 7 years following the end of long-term psychoanalytic treatments. Qualitative analysis of the data also pointed to the value that patients continued to attach to their analytic experience. In the absence of pre-treatment measures, it is impossible to estimate the size of the treatment effect.

Another large pre-post study of psychoanalytic treatments has examined the clinical records of 763 children who were evaluated and treated at the Anna Freud Centre, under the close supervision of Anna Freud (Fonagy & Target, 1994, 1996; Target & Fonagy, 1994a, 1994b). Children with certain disorders (e.g., depression, autism, conduct disorder) appeared to benefit only marginally from psychoanalysis or psychoanalytic psychotherapy. Interestingly, children with severe emotional disorders (three or more Axis I diagnoses) did surprisingly well in psychoanalysis, although they did poorly in once or twice a week psychoanalytic psychotherapy. Younger children derived greatest benefit from intensive treatment. Adolescents appeared not to benefit from the increased frequency of sessions. The importance of the study is, perhaps, less in demonstrating that psychoanalysis is effective, although some of the effects on very severely disturbed children were quite remarkable, but more in identifying groups for whom the additional effort involved in intensive treatment appeared not to be warranted.

The Research Committee of the International Psychoanalytic Association has recently prepared a comprehensive review of North American and European outcome studies of psychoanalytic treatment (Fonagy, et al., 2002). The committee concluded that existing studies failed to unequivocally demonstrate that psychoanalysis is efficacious relative to either an alternative treatment or an active placebo. A range of methodological and design problems was identified, including absence of intent to treat controls, heterogeneous patient groups, lack of random assignments, the failure to use independently-administered standardized measures of outcome, etc. Nevertheless, the report, which ran to several hundred pages and briefly describes more than fifty studies, is encouraging to psychoanalysts. Another overview (Gabbard, Gunderson, & Fonagy, 2002) suggested that psychoanalytic treatments may be necessary when other treatments prove to be ineffective. The authors concluded that psychoanalysis appears to be consistently helpful to patients with milder disorders and somewhat helpful to those with more severe disturbances. More controlled studies are necessary to confirm these impressions. A number of studies testing psychoanalysis with "state of the art" methodology are ongoing and are likely to produce more compelling evidence over the next years. Despite the limitations of the completed studies, evidence across a significant number of pre and post investigations suggests that psychoanalysis appears to be consistently helpful to patients with milder (neurotic) disorders and somewhat less consistently so for other, more severe, groups. Across a range of uncontrolled or poorly controlled cohort studies, mostly carried out in Europe, longer intensive treatments tended to have better outcomes than shorter, non-intensive treatments (demonstration of a dose-effect relationship). The impact of psychoanalysis was apparent beyond symptomatology in measures of work functioning and reductions in health care costs.

CONCLUSIONS

Considerable evidence has accumulated for the efficacy of psychoanalytic approaches for a range of diagnostic conditions. The strength of the evidence varies across clinical groups and, in the case of some groups, there is little current evidence supporting the approach. In no area is the evidence compelling, but in most areas where systematic investigation has been carried out, outcomes are comparable to those obtained by other therapeutic methods. There are disorders where the outcome of psychoanalytic therapy is, in certain respects, better than alternative treatments (e.g., borderline personality disorder). In other areas (e.g., depression), there are opportunities for the psychodynamic approach created by the known limitations of rival orientations. In relation to treatment-resistant conditions, technical innovation is called for and this has been a significant barrier to psychoanalytically-oriented investigations. Even where original and effective approaches have been developed, replication of findings by groups other than those responsible for the development of the program are hard to find.

There can be few valid excuses for the currently thin evidence base of psychoanalytic treatment. In the same breath that we, as psychoanalysts, often claim to be at the intellectual origin of other talking cures (e.g., systemic therapy, cognitive behavior therapy), we also seek to shelter behind the relative immaturity of the discipline as an account for the absence of research evidence for its efficacy. Yet the evidence base of these "derivatives" of psychoanalytic therapy has been far more firmly established than evidence for the approach at the root of the psychotherapy movement (Holmes, 2002).

Of course, there are reasons for this, such as the long-term nature of the therapy, the subtlety and complexity of its procedures, the elusiveness of its self-declared outcome goals, and the incompatibility of direct observation and the need for absolute confidentiality. None of these reasons can stand up to careful scrutiny. The scientific method has been, in recent years, extended to a wide range of highly complex phenomena, and our understanding of the psychological processes that are at work in mental disorders and their psychosocial therapy is a focus of intense inquiry from a range of perspectives. Neither the subject matter nor the difficulties inherent to its systematic investigation account for the relative lack of support for empirical and systematic qualitative studies of the process and outcome of psychoanalytic therapies. Currently, political considerations make funded research in this field difficult, but, historically, this has not always been the case. A more likely reason for the absence of psychoanalytic outcome research lies in the fundamental incompatibilities in the world view espoused by psychoanalysis and most of current social science (Whittle, 2000) that will require a shift in epistemology on the part of psychoanalytic psychotherapists.

There are several components to this attitude change:

1. The incorporation of data gathering methods beyond the anecdotal, methods that are now widely available in social and biological science.

2. Moving psychoanalytic constructs from the global to the specific, which will facilitate cumulative data gathering and identifying the psychological mechanisms which account for change in psychodynamic therapy.

3. Routine consideration of alternative accounts for behavioral observations of change.

4. Increasing psychoanalytic sophistication concerning social and contextual influences on pathological behavior and its response to treatment.

5. Ending the "splendid isolation" of psychoanalysis by undertaking active collaboration with other scientific and clinical disciplines.

6. Using the knowledge-base of psychoanalysis to generate innovative treatment approaches to currently treatment-resistant conditions.

7. Integrating successful psychotherapeutic manipulations from other disciplines into a psychodynamic approach.

8. Identifying clinical groups for whom the psychodynamic method is particularly effective.

9. Adopting a scientific attitude that celebrates the value of the replication of observations rather than their uniqueness.

Rather than fearing that fields adjacent to psychoanalysis might destroy the unique insights offered by long-term intensive individual therapy, psychoanalysts must embrace the rapidly evolving "knowledge chain," focused at different levels of the study of brain-behavior relationships. As Kandel (1998; 1999) has pointed out, this may be the major route to the preservation of the hard-won insights of psychoanalysis.

REFERENCES

Ablon, J. S., & Jones, E. E. (1998). How expert clinicians' prototypes of an ideal treatment correlate with outcome in psychodynamic and cognitive-behavioural therapy. *Psychotherapy Research, 8,* 71-83.

Ablon, J. S., & Jones, E. E. (1999). Psychotherapy process in the National Institute of Mental Health Treatment of Depression Collaborative Research Program. *Journal of Consulting & Clinical Psychology, 67(1),* 64-75.

Ablon, J. S., & Jones, E. E. (2002). Validity of controlled clinical trials of psychotherapy: findings from the NIMH Treatment of Depression Collaborative Research Program. *American Journal of Psychiatry, 159(5),* 775–783.

Anon. (1992). Cross design synthesis: A new strategy for studying medical outcomes. *Lancet, 340,* 944-946.

Antikainen, R., Hintikka, J., Lehtonen, J., Koponen, H., & Arstila, A. (1995). A prospective three-year follow-up study of borderline personality disorder inpatients. *Acta Psychiatr Scand, 92(5),* 327-335.

Bachar, E., Latzer, Y., Kreitler, S., & Berry, E. M. (1999). Empirical comparison of two psychological therapies. Self psychology and cognitive orientation in the treatment of anorexia and bulimia. *Journal of Psychotherapy Practice and Research, 8(2),* 115-128.

Barber, J. P., Morse, J. Q., Krakauer, I. D., Chittams, J., & Crits-Christoph, K. (1997). Change in obsessive-compulsive and avoidant personality disorders following time-limited supportive-expressive therapy. *Psychotherapy, 34(2),* 133-143.

Barkham, M., Rees, A., Shapiro, D. A., Stiles, W. B., Agnew, R. M., Halstead, J., et al. (1996). Outcomes of time-limited psychotherapy in applied settings: replicating the Second Sheffield Psychotherapy Project. *Journal of Consulting and Clinical Psychology, 64(5),* 1079-1085.

Barkham, M., Rees, A., Stiles, W. B., Shapiro, D. A., Hardy, G. E., & Reynolds, S. (1996). Dose-effect relations in time-limited psychotherapy for depression. *Journal of Consulting and Clinical Psychology, 64(5),* 927-935.

Barlow, D. H., Gorman, J. M., Shear, M. K., & Woods, S. W. (2000). Cognitive-behavioral therapy, imipramine, or their combination for panic disorder: A randomized controlled trial. *Journal of the American Medical Association, 283(19),* 2529-2536.

Bateman, A., & Fonagy, P. (1999). The effectiveness of partial hospitalization in the treatment of borderline personality disorder: A randomised controlled trial. *American Journal of Psychiatry, 156,* 1563-1569.

Bateman, A., & Fonagy, P. (2001). Treatment of borderline personality disorder with psychoanalytically oriented partial hospitalization: an 18-month follow-up. *American Journal of Psychiatry, 158(1),* 36-42.

Bateman, A., & Fonagy, P. (2003). Health service utilization costs for borderline personality disorder patients treated with psychoanalytically oriented partial hospitalization versus general psychiatric care. *American Journal of Psychiatry, 160(1),* 169-171.

Bateman, A. W., & Fonagy, P. (2004). *Psychotherapy for borderline personality disorder: Mentalization based treatment.* Oxford: Oxford University Press.

Beck, A., Sokol, L., Clark, D., Berchick, R., & Wright, F. (1992). A crossover study of focused cognitive therapy for panic disorder. *American Journal of Psychiatry, 149,* 778-783.

Bellack, A., Hersen, M., & Himmelhoch, J. (1981). Social skills training compared with pharmacotherapy and psychotherapy for depression. *American Journal of Psychiatry, 138,* 1562-1567.

Beutel, M., Thiede, R., Wiltlink, J., & Sobez, I. (2001). Effectiveness of behavioral and psychodynamic in-patient treatment of severe obesity: First results from a randomized study. *International Journal of Obesity, 25,* 96-98.

Blomberg, J., Lazar, A., & Sandell, R. (2001). Outcome of patients in long-term psychoanalytical treatments: First findings of the Stockholm Outcome of Psychotherapy and Psychoanalysis (STOPP) study. *Psychotherapy Research, 11,* 361-382.

Blum, N., Pfohl, B., John, D. S., Monahan, P., & Black, D. W. (2002). STEPPS: A cognitive-behavioral systems-based group treatment for outpatients with borderline personality disorder. A preliminary report. *Comprehensive Psychiatry, 43(4),* 301-310.

Borkovec, T. D., & Ruscio, A. M. (2001). Psychotherapy for generalized anxiety disorder. *Journal of Clinical Psychiatry, 62(Suppl 11),* 37-42; discussion 43-35.

Brandsma, J., Maultsby, M., & Welsh, R. (1980). *The outpatient treatment of alcoholism: A review and a comparative study.* Baltimore: University Park Press.

Brewer, D. D., Catalano, R. F., Haggerty, K., Gainey, R. R., & Fleming, C. B. (1998). A meta-analysis of predictors of continued drug use during and after treatment for opiate addiction. *Addiction, 93(1),* 73-92.

Brom, D., Kleber, R., & Defares, P. (1989). Brief psychotherapy for PTSD. *Journal of Consulting and Clinical Psychology, 57,* 607-612.

Brown, T. A., Campbell, L. A., Lehman, C. L., Grisham, J. R., & Mancill, R. B. (2001). Current and lifetime comorbidity of the DSM-IV anxiety and mood disorders in a large clinical sample. *Journal of Abnormal Psychology, 110(4),* 585-599.

Burnand, Y., Andreoli, A., Kolatte, E., Venturini, A., & Rosset, N. (2002). Psychodynamic psychotherapy and clomipramine in the treatment of major depression. *Psychiatric Services, 53(5),* 585-590.

Busch, F., Milrod, B., Cooper, A., & Shapiro, T. (1996). Grand rounds: Panic focused psychodynamic psychotherapy. *Journal of Psychotherapy Research and Practice, 5,* 72-83.

Busch, F., Milrod, B., & Singer, M. (2000). Theory and technique in the psychodynamic treatment of panic disorder. *Review Theories of Psychiatry, 4100,* 16-17.

Chambless, D. L., & Hollon, S. (1998). Defining empirically supported therapies. *Journal of Consulting and Clinical Psychology, 66,* 7-18.

Chambless, D. L., Sanderson, W. C., Shoham, V., Johnson, S. B., Pope, K. S., Crits-Christoph, P., et al. (1996). An update on clinically validated therapies. *The Clinical Psychologist, 49,* 5-18.

Chiesa, M., & Fonagy, P. (2000). Cassel Personality Disorder Study: Methodology and treatment effects. *British Journal of Psychiatry, 176,* 485-491.

Chiesa, M., & Fonagy, P. (2003). Psychosocial treatment for severe personality disorder: 36-month follow-up. *British Journal of Psychiatry, 183,* 356-362.

Chiesa, M., Fonagy, P., Holmes, J., & Drahorad, C. (2004). Residential versus community treatment of personality disorder: A comparative study of three treatment programs. *American Journal of Psychiatry, 162,* 1463-1470.

Chiesa, M., Fonagy, P., Holmes, J., Drahorad, C., & Harrison-Hall, A. (2002). Health service use costs by personality disorder following specialist and nonspecialist treatment: A comparative study. *Journal of Personal Disorders, 16(2),* 160-173.

Chilvers, R., Harrison, G., Sipos, A., & Barley, M. (2002). Evidence into practice: Application of psychological models of change in evidence-based implementation. *British Journal of Psychiatry, 181(2),* 99-101.

Churchill, R., Hunot, V., Corney, R., Knapp, M., McGuire, H., Tylee, A., et al. (2001). A systematic review of controlled trials of the effectiveness and cost-effectiveness of brief psychological treatments for depression. *Health Technology Assessment, 5(35).*

Clarke, M., & Oxman, A. D. (1999). *Cochrane Reviewers' Handbook 4.0* [updated July 1999]. In Review Manager [Computer Program]: Version 4.0. Oxford: The Cochrane Collaboration.

Clarkin, J. F., Foelsch, P. A., Levy, K. N., Hull, J. W., Delaney, J. C., & Kernberg, O. F. (2001). The development of a psychodynamic treatment for patients with borderline personality disorder: A preliminary study of behavioral change. *Journal of Personal Disorders, 15(6)*, 487-495.

Clarkin, J. F., Kernberg, O. F., & Yeomans, F. (1999). *Transference-focused psychotherapy for borderline personality disorder patients*. New York, NY: Guilford Press.

Clarkin, J. F., Levy, K. N., Lenzenweger, M. F., & Kernberg, O. F. (2004a). *The Personality Disorders Institute/Borderline Personality Disorder Research Foundation randomized control trial for borderline personality disorder: Progress report*. Paper presented at the Annual Meeting of the Society for Psychotherapy Research, Rome, Italy.

Clarkin, J. F., Levy, K. N., Lenzenweger, M. F., & Kernberg, O. F. (2004b). The Personality Disorders Institute/Borderline Personality Disorder Research Foundation randomized control trial for borderline personality disorder: rationale, methods, and patient characteristics. *Journal of Personality Disorders, 18(1)*, 52-72.

Connolly, M. B., Crits-Christoph, P., Shappell, S., Barber, J. P., Luborsky, L., & Shaffer, C. (1999). Relation of transference interpretations to outcome in the early sessions of brief supportive-expressive psychotherapy. *Psychotherapy Research, 9*, 485-495.

Covi, L., & Lipman, R. S. (1987). Cognitive-behavioral group psychotherapy combined with imipramine in major depression. *Psychopharmacology Bulletin, 23*, 173-176.

Craske, M. G., Maidenberg, E., & Bystritsky, A. (1995). Brief cognitive-behavioral versus nondirective therapy for panic disorder. *Journal of Behavior Therapy and Experimental Psychiatry, 26(2)*, 113-120.

Crisp, A. H., Norton, K., Gowers, S., Halek, C., Bowyer, C., Yeldham, D., et al. (1991). A controlled study of the effect of therapies aimed at adolescent and family psychopathology in anorexia nervosa. *British Journal of Psychiatry, 159*, 325-333.

Crits-Christoph, P. (1992). The efficacy of brief dynamic psychotherapy: A meta-analysis. *American Journal of Psychiatry, 159*, 325-333.

Crits-Christoph, P., Connolly, M. B., Azarian, K., Crits-Christoph, K., & Shappell, S. (1996). An open trial of brief supportive-expressive psychotherapy in the treatment of generalized anxiety disorder. *Psychotherapy, 33*, 418-430.

Crits-Christoph, P., Siqueland, L., Blaine, J., Frank, A., Luborsky, L., Onken, L. S., et al. (1997). The National Institute on Drug Abuse Collaborative Cocaine Treatment Study. Rationale and methods. *Archives of General Psychiatry, 54(8)*, 721-726.

Crits-Christoph, P., Siqueland, L., Blaine, J., Frank, A., Luborsky, L., Onken, L. S., et al. (1999). Psychosocial treatments for cocaine dependence: National Institute on Drug Abuse Collaborative Cocaine Treatment Study. *Archives of General Psychiatry, 56(6)*, 493-502.

Crits-Christoph, P., Siqueland, L., McCalmont, E., Weiss, R. D., Gastfriend, D. R., Frank, A., et al. (2001). Impact of psychosocial treatments on associated problems of cocaine-dependent patients. *Journal of Consulting & Clinical Psychology, 69(5)*, 825-830.

Crumbach, J. C., & Carr, G. L. (1979). Treatment of alcoholics with logotherapy. *International Journal of the Addictions, 14*, 847-853.

Cryer, L., & Beutler, L. (1980). Group therapy: An alternative approach for rape victims. *Journal of Sex and Marital Therapy, 6*, 40-46.

Dare, C., & Eisler, E. (1997). Family therapy for anorexia nervosa. In D. G. Garner & P. E. Garfinkel (Eds.), *Handbook of Treatment for Eating Disorders* (2nd ed.). New York: Guilford.

Dare, C., Eisler, I., Russell, G., Treasure, J., & Dodge, L. (2001). Psychological therapies for adults with anorexia nervosa: randomised controlled trial of out-patient treatments. *British Journal of Psychiatry, 178*, 216-221.

Davanloo, H. (1978). *Basic principles and techniques in short-term dynamic psychotherapy*. New York: Spectrum.

Dawe, S., Powell, J., Richards, D., Gossop, M., Marks, I., Strang, J., et al. (1993). Does post-withdrawal cue exposure improve outcome in opiate addiction? A controlled trial. *Addiction, 88(9)*, 1233-1245.

de Jonghe, F., Kool, S., van Aalst, G., Dekker, J., & Peen, J. (2001). Combining psychotherapy and antidepressants in the treatment of depression. *Journal of Affect. Disorders, 64(2-3)*, 217-229.

de Jonghe, F., Rijnierse, P., & Janssen, R. (1994). Psychoanalytic supportive psychotherapy. *Journal of the American Psychoanalytic Association, 42*, 421–446.

Department of Health (1995). *Strategic Report on the Psychotherapies*. London: HMSO.

Dolan, B., Warren, F., & Norton, K. (1997). Change in borderline symptoms one year after therapeutic community treatment for severe personality disorder. *British Journal of Psychiatry, 171*, 274-279.

Durham, R. C., Chambers, J. A., MacDonald, R. R., Power, K. G., & Major, K. (2003). Does cognitive-behavioural therapy influence the long-term outcome of generalized anxiety disorder? An 8-14 year follow-up of two clinical trials. *Psychological Medicine, 33(3)*, 499-509.

Durham, R. C., Fisher, P. L., Treliving, L. R., Hau, C. M., Richard, K., & Stewart, J. B. (1999). One year follow-up of cognitive therapy, analytic psychotherapy and anxiety management training for generalized anxiety disorder: Symptom change, medication usage and attitudes to treatment. *Behavioural and Cognitive Psychotherapy, 27*, 19-35.

Durham, R. C., Murphy, T., Allan, T., Richard, K., Treliving, L. R., & Fenton, G. W. (1994). Cognitive therapy, analytic psychotherapy and anxiety management training for generalized anxiety disorder. *British Journal of Psychiatry, 165*, 315-323.

Eisler, I., Dare, C., Russell, G. F., Szmukler, G., le Grange, D., & Dodge, E. (1997). Family and individual therapy in anorexia nervosa. A 5-year follow-up. *Archives of General Psychiatry, 54(11)*, 1025-1030.

Elkin, I. (1994). The NIMH treatment of depression collaborative research program: Where we began and where we are. In A. E. Bergin & S. L. Garfield (Eds.), *Handbook of psychotherapy and behavior change* (4th ed.). New York: Wiley.

Finney, J. W., & Monahan, S. C. (1996). The cost-effectiveness of treatment for alcoholism: A second approximation. *Journal of Studies on Alcohol, 57(3)*, 229-243.

Fisher, P. L., & Durham, R. C. (1999). Recovery rates in generalized anxiety disorder following psychological therapy: an analysis of clinically significant change in the STAI-T across outcome studies since 1990. *Psychological Medicine, 29(6)*, 1425-1434.

Fonagy, P. (1999a). Process and outcome in mental health care delivery: A model approach to treatment evaluation. *Bulletin of the Menninger Clinic, 63(3)*, 288-304.

Fonagy, P., Kachele, H., Krause, R., Jones, E., Perron, R., Clarkin, J., et al. (2002). *An open door review of outcome studies in psychoanalysis* (2nd ed.). London: International Psychoanalytical Association.

Fonagy, P., & Moran, G. S. (1991). Studies of the efficacy of child psychoanalysis. *Journal of Consulting and Clinical Psychology, 58*, 684-695.

Fonagy, P., & Target, M. (1994). The efficacy of psychoanalysis for children with disruptive disorders. *Journal of the American Academy of Child and Adolescent Psychiatry, 33*, 45-55.

Fonagy, P., & Target, M. (1996). Predictors of outcome in child psychoanalysis: A retrospective study of 763 cases at the Anna Freud Centre. *Journal of the American Psychoanalytic Association, 44*, 27-77.

Fonagy, P., Target, M., Cottrell, D., Phillips, J., & Kurtz, Z. (2002). *What works for whom? A critical review of treatments for children and adolescents*. New York: Guilford.

Fonagy, P., Target, M., Steele, H., & Steele, M. (1998). *Reflective functioning manual, version 5.0, for application to adult attachment interviews*. London: University College London.

Gabbard, G. O., Coyne, L., Allen, J. G., Spohn, H., Colson, D. B., & Vary, M. (2000). Evaluation of intensive inpatient treatment of patients with severe personality disorders. *Psychiatric Services, 51(7)*, 893-898.

Gabbard, G. O., Gunderson, J. G., & Fonagy, P. (2002). The place of psychoanalytic treatments within psychiatry. *Archives of General Psychiatry, 59,* 505-510.

Gallagher-Thompson, D., & Steffen, A. M. (1994). Comparative effects of cognitive-behavioral and brief psychodynamic psychotherapies for depressed family caregivers. *Journal of Consulting and Clinical Psychology, 62,* 543-549.

Garner, D. M., Rockert, W., Davis, R., & Garner, M. D. (1993). A comparison between CBT and supportive expressive therapy for bulimia nervosa. *American Journal of Psychiatry, 150,* 37-46.

Gloaguen, V., Cottraux, J., Cucherat, M., & Blackburn, I. (1998). A meta-analysis of the effects of cognitive therapy in depressed patients. *Journal of Affective Disorders, 49(1),* 59-72.

Goldfried, M. R., & Wolfe, B. E. (1996). Psychotherapy practice and research: Repairing a strained alliance. *American Psychologist, 51,* 1007-1016.

Gowers, S., Norton, K., Halek, C., & Crisp, A. H. (1994). Outcome of outpatient psychotherapy in a random allocation treatment study of anorexia nervosa. *International Journal of Eating Disorders, 15,* 165-177.

Grant, J., & Sandell, R. (2004). Close family or mere neighbours? Some empirical data on the differences between psychoanalysis and psychotherapy. In P. Richardson, H. Kächele, & C. Renlund (Eds.), *Research on psychoanalytic psychotherapy with adults* (pp. 81-108). London: Karnac.

Guthrie, E., Moorey, J., Margison, F., Barker, H., Palmer, S., McGrath, G., et al. (1999). Cost-effectiveness of brief psychodynamic-interpersonal therapy in high utilizers of psychiatric services. *Archives of General Psychiatry, 56(6),* 519-526.

Hall, A., & Crisp, A. N. (1987). Brief psychotherapy in the treatment of anorexia nervosa. *British Journal of Psychiatry, 151,* 185-191.

Hay, P. J., & Bacaltchuk, J. (2001). *Psychotherapy for bulimia nervosa and binging* (Cochrane Review). In The Cochrane Library, Issue 4, 2002. Oxford: Update Software.

Hayes, A. M., Castonguay, L. G., & Goldfried, M. R. (1996). Effectiveness of targeting the vulnerability factors of depression in cognitive therapy. *Journal of Consulting and Clinical Psychology, 64(3),* 623-627.

Heinicke, C. M., & Ramsey-Klee, D. M. (1986). Outcome of child psychotherapy as a function of frequency of sessions. *Journal of the American Academy of Child Psychiatry, 25,* 247-253.

Hersen, M., Bellack, A. S., Himmelhoch, J. M., & Thase, M. E. (1984). Effects of social skills training, amitriptyline and psychotherapy in unipolar depressed women. *Behavior Therapy, 15,* 21-40.

Hickman, M., Cox, S., Harvey, J., Howes, S., Farrell, M., Frischer, M., et al. (1999). Estimating the prevalence of problem drug use in inner London: A discussion of three capture-recapture studies. *Addiction, 94(11),* 1653–1662.

Higgitt, A., & Fonagy, P. (2002). Clinical effectiveness. *British Journal of Psychiatry, 181(2),* 170-174.

Hoagwood, K., Hibbs, E., Brent, D., & Jensen, P. (1995). Introduction to the special section: Efficacy and effectiveness in studies of child and adolescent psychotherapy. *Journal of Consulting and Clinical Psychology, 63,* 683-687.

Holmes, J. (2002). All you need is cognitive behaviour therapy? *British Medical Journal, 324* (7332), 288-290; discussion 290-294.

Hopper, E. (1995). A psychoanalytical theory of "drug addiction:" Unconscious fantasies of homosexuality, compulsions and masturbation within the context of traumatogenic processes. *International Journal of Psychoanalysis, 76,* 1121-1142.

Horowitz, M. J., Marmar, C., Weiss, D. S., DeWitt, K. N., & Rosenbaum, R. (1984). Brief psychotherapy of bereavement reactions: The relationship of process to outcome. *Archives of General Psychiatry, 41,* 438-448.

Howard, K., Lueger, R., Maling, M., & Martinovitch, Z. (1993). A phase model of psychotherapy: Causal mediation of outcome. *Journal of Consulting & Clinical Psychology, 61,* 678-685.

Huxley, A. (1932). *Brave new world.* London/Garden City, NY: Chatto and Windus/Harper and Brothers.

Johnson, B. (1999). Three perspectives on addiction. *Journal of the American Psychoanalytic Association, 47,* 791-815.

Kandel, E. R. (1998). A new intellectual framework for psychiatry. *American Journal of Psychiatry, 155,* 457–469.

Kandel, E. R. (1999). Biology and the future of psychoanalysis: A new intellectual framework for psychiatry revisited. *American Journal of Psychiatry, 156,* 505-524.

Kang, S. Y., Kleinman, P. H., Woody, G. E., Millman, R. B., Todd, T. C., Kemp, J., et al. (1991). Outcomes for cocaine abusers after once-a-week psychosocial therapy. *American Journal of Psychiatry, 148(5),* 630-635.

Karterud, S., Vaglum, S., Friis, S., Irion, T., Johns, S., & Vaglum, P. (1992). Day hospital therapeutic community treatment for patients with personality disorders: An empirical evaluation of the containment function. *Journal of Nervous Mental Disorders, 180(4),* 238-243.

Kasvikis, Y., Bradley, B., Powell, J., Marks, I., & Gray, J. A. (1991). Postwithdrawal exposure treatment to prevent relapse in opiate addicts: A pilot study. *International Journal of Addiction, 26(11),* 1187-1195.

Kazdin, A. E. (1998). *Research design in clinical psychology.* Needham Heights, MA: Allyn and Bacon.

Kessler, R. C., McGonagle, K. A., Zhao, S., Nelson, C. B., Hughes, M., Eshleman, S., et al. (1994). Lifetime and 12-month prevalence of DSM-III-R psychiatric disorders in the United States. *Archives of General Psychiatry, 51,* 8-19.

Kessler, R. C., Stang, P., Wittchen, H. U., Stein, M., & Walters, E. E. (1999). Lifetime comorbidities between social phobia and mood disorders in the US National Comorbidity Survey. *Psychological Medicine, 29(3),* 555–567.

Kissin, B., & Gross, M. M. (1968). Drug therapy in alcoholism. *American Journal of Psychiatry, 125,* 31-41.

Klein, D. F., Zitrin, C. M., Woerner, M. G., & Ross, D. C. (1983). Treatment of phobias: II. Behavior therapy and supportive psychotherapy: Are there any specific ingredients? *Archives of General Psychiatry, 40(2),* 139–145.

Knekt, P., & Lindfors, O. (Eds.). (2004). *A randomized trial of the effects of four forms of psychotherapy on depressive and anxiety disorders: Design methods and results on the effectiveness of short term psychodynamic psychotherapy and solution focused therapy during a 1-year follow-up* (Vol. 77). Helsinki: Social Insurance Institution.

Koons, C. R., Robins, C. J., Tweed, J. L., Lynch, T. R., Gonzalez, A. M., Morse, J. Q., et al. (2001). Efficacy of dialectical behavior therapy in women veterans with borderline personality disorder. *Behavior Therapy, 32,* 371-390.

Kopta, S., Howard, K., Lowry, J., & Beutler, L. (1994). Patterns of symptomatic recovery in psychotherapy. *Journal of Consulting and Clinical Psychology, 62,* 1009-1016.

Kornblith, S. J., Rehm, L. P., O'Hara, M. W., & Lamparski, D. M. (1983). The contribution of self-reinforcement training and behavioral assignments to the efficacy of self-control therapy for depression. *Cognitive Therapy and Research, 7,* 499-528.

Kraus, L., Augustin, R., Frischer, M., Kummler, P., Uhl, A., & Wiessing, L. (2003). Estimating prevalence of problem drug use at national level in countries of the European Union and Norway. *Addiction, 98(4),* 471-485.

Lambert, M.J., Okiishi, J.C., Finch, A.E., & Johnson,L.D. (1998). Outcome assessment: From conceptualization to implementation. *Professional Psychology: Research and Practice 29*: 63-70.

Leff, J., Vearnals, S., Brewin, C. R., Wolff, G., Alexander, B., Asen, E., et al. (2000). The London Depression Intervention Trial: Randomised controlled trial of antidepressants v. couple therapy in the treatment and maintenance of people with depression living with a partner. Clinical outcome and costs. *British Journal of Psychiatry, 177,* 95-100.

Leichsenring, F. (2001). Comparative effects of short-term psychodynamic psychotherapy and cognitive-behavioral therapy in depression: A meta-analytic approach. *Clinical Psychological Review, 21(3),* 401-419.

Leichsenring, F., & Leibing, E. (2003). The effectiveness of psychodynamic therapy and cognitive behavior therapy in the treatment of personality disorders: A meta-analysis. *American Journal of Psychiatry, 160(7),* 1223-1232.

Leuzinger-Bohleber, M., Stuhr, U., Ruger, B., & Beutel, M. (2003). How to study the quality of psychoanalytic treatments and their long-term effects on patients' well-being: A representative, multi-perspective follow-up study. *International Journal of Psychoanalysis, 84,* 263-290.

Leuzinger-Bohleber, M., & Target, M. (Eds.). (2002). *The outcomes of psychoanalytic treatment.* London: Whurr.

Levinson, T., & Sereny, G. (1969). An experimental evaluation of insight therapy for the chronic alcoholic. *Canadian Psychiatric Association Journal, 14,* 143-146.

Levy, K. N., & Clarkin, J. F. (in press). To examine the mechanisms of change in the treatment of borderline personality disorder. *Journal of Clinical Psychology.*

Linehan, M. M. (1993). *Cognitive-behavioural treatment of borderline personality disorder.* New York: Guilford.

Linehan, M. M., Schmidt, H., Dimeff, L. A., Craft, J. C., Kanter, J., & Comtois, K. A. (1999). Dialectical behavior therapy for patients with borderline personality disorder and drug dependence. *American Journal on Addictions, 8,* 279-292.

Lipsitz, J. D., Markowitz, J. C., Cherry, S., & Fyer, A. J. (1999). Open trial of interpersonal psychotherapy for the treatment of social phobia. *American Journal of Psychiatry, 156(11),* 1814-1816.

Luborsky, L. (1984). *Principles of psychoanalytic psychotherapy: A manual for supportive-expressive treatment.* New York: Basic Books.

Main, M., & Goldwyn, R. (1998). *Adult attachment scoring and classification systems.* Unpublished manuscript. University of California at Berkeley.

Malan, D. H. (1976). *Toward the validation of dynamic psychotherapy.* New York: Plenum Press.

Marmar, C. R., Horowitz, M. J., Weiss, D. S., Wilner, N. R., & Kaltreider, N. B. (1988). A controlled trial of brief psychotherapy and mutual-help group treatment of conjugal bereavement. *American Journal of Psychiatry, 145(2),* 203-209.

McDermut, W., Miller, I., & Brown, R. (2001). The efficacy of group psychotherapy for depression: A meta-analysis and review of the empirical research. *Clinical Psychology: Science and Practice, 8(1),* 98-116.

McLean, P. D., & Hakstian, A. R. (1979). Clinical depression: Comparative efficacy of outpatient treatments. *Journal of Consulting and Clinical Psychology, 47,* 818-836.

Meares, R., Stevenson, J., & Comerford, A. (1999). Psychotherapy with borderline patients: I. A comparison between treated and untreated cohorts. *Australian and New Zealand Journal of Psychiatry, 33(4),* 467-472.

Miller, W. R., & Hester, R. K. (1986). The effectiveness of alcoholism treatment: What research reveals. In W. R. Miller & N. Heather (Eds.), *Treating addictive behaviors: The process of change.* New York: Plenum Press.

Miller, W. R., & Wilbourne, P. L. (2002). Mesa Grande: A methodological analysis of clinical trials of treatments for alcohol use disorders. *Addiction, 97,* 265-277.

Miller, W. R., Wilbourne, P. L., & Hettema, J. E. (2003). What works? A summary of alcohol treatment outcome research. In R. K. Hester & W. R. Miller (Eds.), *Handbook of alcoholism treatment approaches: Effective alternatives* (3rd ed., pp. 13-63). Boston, MA: Allyn and Bacon.

Milrod, B., & Busch, F. (1996). Long-term outcome of panic disorder treatment: A review of the literature. *Journal of Nervous and Mental Disorders, 184(12)*, 723-730.

Milrod, B., Busch, F., Cooper, A., & Shapiro, T. (1997). *Manual of panic: Focused psychodynamic psychotherapy.* Washington, DC: APA Press.

Milrod, B., Busch, F., Leon, A. C., Aronson, A., Roiphe, J., Rudden, M., et al. (2001). A pilot open trial of brief psychodynamic psychotherapy for panic disorder. *Journal of Psychotherapy Practice Research, 10,* 239–245.

Milrod, B., Busch, F., Leon, A. C., Shapiro, T., Aronson, A., Roiphe, J., et al. (2000). Open trial of psychodynamic psychotherapy for panic disorder: A pilot study. *American Journal of Psychiatry, 157(11),* 1878–1880.

Milrod, B., Cooper, A., & Shear, M. (2001). Psychodynamic concepts of anxiety. In D. Stein & E. Hollander (Eds.), *Textbook of anxiety disorders* (pp. 89-103). Washington, DC: American Psychiatric Press.

Monsen, J. T., Odland, T., Faugli, A., Daae, E., & Eilertsen, D. E. (1995). Personality disorders: Changes and stability after intensive psychotherapy focusing on affect consciousness. *Psychotherapy Research, 5,* 33-48.

Moran, G., Fonagy, P., Kurtz, A., Bolton, A., & Brook, C. (1991). A controlled study of psychoanalytic treatment of brittle diabetes [see comments]. *Journal of The American Academy of Child And Adolescent Psychiatry, 30(6),* 926-935.

Mynors-Wallis, L., Davies, I., Gray, A., Barbour, F., & Gath, D. (1997). A randomised controlled trial and cost analysis of problem-solving treatment for emotional disorders given by community nurses in primary care. *British Journal of Psychiatry, 170,* 113-119.

Mynors-Wallis, L. M., Gath, D. H., Day, A., & Baker, F. (2000). Randomised controlled trial of problem solving treatment, antidepressant medication, and combined treatment for major depression in primary care. *British Medical Journal, 320(7226),* 26-30.

Mynors-Wallis, L. M., Gath, D. H., Lloyd-Thomas, A. R., & Tomlinson, D. (1995). Randomised controlled trial comparing problem solving treatment with amitriptyline and placebo for major depression in primary care. *British Medical Journal, 310(6977),* 441-445.

Nordhus, I. H., & Pallesen, S. (2003). Psychological treatment of late-life anxiety: An empirical review. *Journal of Consulting and Clinical Psychology, 71(4),* 643-651.

Ogrodniczuk, J. S., Piper, W. E., McCallum, M., Joyce, A. S., & Rosie, J. S. (2002). Interpersonal predictors of group therapy outcome for complicated grief. *International Journal of Group Psychotherapy, 52,* 511-535.

Olfson, M. (1999). Emerging methods in mental health outcomes research. *Journal of Practical Psychiatry and Behavioural Health, 5,* 20-24.

Olfson, M., Mechanic, D., Boyer, C. A., & Hansell, S. (1998). Linking inpatients with schizophrenia to outpatient care. *Psychiatric Services, 49,* 911-917.

Palmer, C., & Fenner, J. (1999). *Getting the message across: Review of research and theory about disseminating information within the NHS.* London: Gaskell.

Pattison, E. M., Brissenden, A., & Wohl, T. (1967). Assessing specific aspects of in-patient group psychotherapy. *International Journal of Group Psychotherapy, 17,* 283-297.

Perl, M., Westlin, A. B., & Peterson, L. G. (1985). The female rape survivor: Time limited therapy with female/male co-therapists. *Journal of Psychosomatic Obstetrics and Gynaecology, 4,* 197-205.

Perry, J. C., Banon, E., & Ianni, F. (1999). Effectiveness of psychotherapy for personality disorders. *American Journal of Psychiatry, 156(9),* 1312-1321.

Piper, W. E., Rosie, J. S., Joyce, A. S., & Azim, H. F. A. (1996). Psychiatric partial hospitalization: A review of the research. In W. E. Piper, J. S. Rosie, A. S. Joyce, & H. F. A. Azim (Authors), *Time-limited day treatment for personality disorders: Integration of research and practice in a group program.* Washington, DC: American Psychological Association

Piper, W. E., Azim, H. F. A., Joyce, A. S., McCallum, M., Nixon, G. W. H., & Segal, P. S. (1991). Quality of object relations vs interpersonal functioning as a predictor of the therapeutic alliance and psychotherapy outcome. *Journal of Nervous and Mental Disease, 179*, 432-438.

Piper, W. E., Joyce, A. S., McCallum, M., & Azim, H. F. (1998). Interpretive and supportive forms of psychotherapy and patient personality variables. *Journal of Consulting and Clinical Psychology, 66(3)*, 558–567.

Piper, W. E., McCallum, M., Joyce, A. S., Rosie, J. S., & Ogrodniczuk, J. (2001). Patient personality and time-limited group psychotherapy for complicated grief. *International Journal of Group Psychotherapy, 51*, 525–552.

Piper, W. E., Ogrodniczuk, J. S., McCallum, M., Joyce, A. S., & Rosie, J. S. (2003). Expression of affect as a mediator of the relationship between quality of object relations and group therapy outcome for patients with complicated grief. *Journal of Consulting and Clinical Psychology, 71(4)*, 664-671.

Pomerleau, O., Pertshuk, M., Adkins, D., & d'Aquili, E. (1978). Treatment for middle-income problem drinkers. In P. E. Nathan, G. A. Marlatt, & T. Loberg (Eds.), *Alcoholism: New directions in behavioral research and treatment*. New York: Plenum Press.

Prendergast, M. L., Podus, D., Chang, E., & Urada, D. (2002). The effectiveness of drug abuse treatment: a meta-analysis of comparison group studies. *Drug Alcohol Dependency, 67(1)*, 53-72.

Radford, P., Wiseberg, S., & Yorke, C. S. B. (1972). A study of "main-line" heroin addiction: A preliminary report. *Psychoanalytic Study of the Child, 27*, 156-180.

Reiss, D., Grubin, D., & Meux, C. (1996). Young psychopaths in special hospital: Treatment and outcome. *British Journal of Psychiatry, 168*, 99-104.

Rockland, L. H. (1987). A supportive approach: Psychodynamically oriented supportive therapy. Treatment of borderline patients who self-mutilate. *Journal of Personality Disorders, 1*, 350-353.

Roth, A., & Fonagy, P. (in press). *What works for whom? A critical review of psychotherapy research. 2nd edition*. New York: Guilford Press.

Roth, S., Dye, E., & Lebowitz, L. (1988). Group therapy for sexual-assault victims. *Psychotherapy, 25*, 82–93.

Rounsaville, B. J., Glazer, W., Wilber, C. H., Weissman, M. M., & Kleber, H. D. (1983). Short-term interpersonal psychotherapy in methadone-maintained opiate addicts. *Archives of General Psychiatry, 40(6)*, 629-636.

Russell, G. F. M., Szmukler, G. I., Dare, C., & Eisler, I. (1987). An evaluation of family therapy in anorexia nervosa and bulimia nervosa. *Archives of General Psychiatry, 44*, 1047-1056.

Ryle, A. (1990). *Cognitive analytic therapy: Active participation in change*. Chichester: Wiley.

Ryle, A., & Golynkina, K. (2000). Effectiveness of time-limited cognitive analytic therapy of borderline personality disorder: factors associated with outcome. *British Journal of Medical Psychology, 73(Pt. 2)*, 197–210.

Sandahl, C., Herlitz, K., Ahlin, G., & Rönnberg, S. (1998). Time-limited group therapy for moderately alcohol dependent patients: A randomised controlled trial. *Psychotherapy Research, 8*, 361-378.

Sandell, R., Blomberg, J., Lazar, A., Carlsson, J., Broberg, J., & Rand, H. (2000). Varieties of long-term outcome among patients in psychoanalysis and long-term psychotherapy: A review of findings in the Stockholm Outcome of Psychoanalysis and Psychotherapy Project (STOPP). *International Journal of Psychoanalysis, 81(5)*, 921-943.

Saunders, D. G. (1996). Feminist cognitive-behavioral and process-psychodynamic treatments for men who batter: Interaction of abuser traits and treatment models. *Violence and Victims, 11*, 393-414.

Scarvalone, P., Cloitre, M., & Difede, J. (1995). *Interpersonal process therapy for incest survivors: Preliminary outcome data.* Paper presented at the Society for Psychotherapy Research Conference, Vancouver.

Sensky, T., & Scott, J. (2002). All you need is cognitive behaviour therapy? Critical appraisal of evidence base must be understood and respected. *British Medical Journal, 324(7352),* 1522.

Shapiro, D. A., Barkham, M., Rees, A., Hardy, G. E., Reynolds, S., & Startup, M. (1994). Effects of treatment duration and severity of depression on the effectiveness of cognitive-behavioral and psychodynamic-interpersonal psychotherapy. *Journal of Consulting and Clinical Psychology, 62(3),* 522-534.

Shapiro, D. A., Rees, A., Barkham, M., Hardy, G., Reynolds, S., & Startup, M. (1995). Effects of treatment duration and severity of depression on the maintenance of gains following cognitive behavioral and psychodynamic interpersonal psychotherapy. *Journal of Consulting and Clinical Psychology, 63,* 378-387.

Shea, M. T., Pilkonis, P. A., Beckham, E., Collins, J. F., Elkin, I., Sotsky, S. M., et al. (1992). Personality disorders and treatment outcome in the NIMH treatment of depression collaborative research program. *American Journal of Psychiatry, 147,* 711-718.

Shear, M. K., Houck, P., Greeno, C., & Masters, S. (2001). Emotion-focused psychotherapy for patients with panic disorder. *American Journal of Psychiatry, 158(12),* 1993-1998.

Shear, M. K., Pilkonis, P. A., Cloitre, M., & Leon, A. C. (1994). Cognitive behavioral treatment compared with non-prescriptive treatment of panic disorder. *Archives of General Psychiatry, 51,* 395-401.

Shefler, G., Dasberg, H., & Ben-Shakhar, G. (1995). A randomised controlled outcome and follow-up study of Mann's time-limited psychotherapy. *Journal of Consulting and Clinical Psychology, 63,* 585-593.

Simpson, D. D., Joe, G. W., & Broome, K. M. (2002). A national 5-year follow-up of treatment outcomes for cocaine dependence. *Archives of General Psychiatry, 59(6),* 538-544.

Simpson, D. D., Joe, G. W., Fletcher, B. W., Hubbard, R. L., & Anglin, M. D. (1999). A national evaluation of treatment outcomes for cocaine dependence. *Archives of General Psychiatry, 56(6),* 507-514.

Stanton, A. H., Gunderson, J. G., Knapp, P. H., Vancelli, M. L., Schnitzer, R., & Rosenthal, R. (1984). Effects of psychotherapy in schizophrenia: I. Design and implementation of a controlled study. *Schizophrenia Bulletin, 10,* 520-563.

Steuer, J., Mintz, J., Hammen, C., Hill, M. A., Jarvik, L. F., McCarley, T., et al. (1984). Cognitive-behavioral and psychodynamic group psychotherapy in treatment of geriatric depression. *Journal of Consulting and Clinical Psychology, 52,* 180-192.

Stevenson, J., & Meares, R. (1992). An outcome study of psychotherapy for patients with borderline personality disorder. *American Journal of Psychiatry, 149,* 358-362.

Stevenson, J., & Meares, R. (1999). Psychotherapy with borderline patients: II. A preliminary cost benefit study. *Australian and New Zealand Journal of Psychiatry, 33(4),* 473-477.

Strupp, H. H., & Binder, J. L. (1984). *Psychotherapy in a new key: A guide to time-limited dynamic psychotherapy.* New York: Basic Books.

Svartberg, M., Stiles, T. C., & Seltzer, M. H. (2004). Randomized, controlled trial of the effectiveness of short-term dynamic psychotherapy and cognitive therapy for cluster C personality disorders. *American Journal of Psychiatry, 161(5),* 810-817.

Swartz, M., Blazer, D., & Winfield, I. (1990). Estimating the prevalence of borderline personality disorder in the community. *Journal of Personality Disorders, 4,* 257.

Target, M., & Fonagy, P. (1994a). The efficacy of psychoanalysis for children with emotional disorders. *Journal of the American Academy of Child and Adolescent Psychiatry, 33,* 361-371.

Target, M., & Fonagy, P. (1994b). The efficacy of psychoanalysis for children: Developmental considerations. *Journal of the American Academy of Child and Adolescent Psychiatry, 33,* 1134-1144.

Tarrier, N. (2002). Commentary: Yes, cognitive behaviour therapy may well be all you need. *British Medical Journal, 324*, 288-294.

Taylor, R. (2000). A seven year reconviction study of HMP Grendon Therapeutic Community. Home Office.

Teasdale, J. D., Segal, Z. V., Williams, J. M., Ridgeway, V. A., Soulsby, J. M., & Lau, M. A. (2000). Prevention of relapse/recurrence in major depression by mindfulness-based cognitive therapy. *Journal of Consulting and Clinical Psychology, 68(4)*, 615-623.

Thase, M. E., Greenhouse, J. B., Frank, E., Reynolds, C. F., Pilkonis, P. A., Hurley, K., et al. (1997). Treatment of major depression with psychotherapy or psychotherapy-pharmacotherapy combinations. *Archives of General Psychiatry, 54*, 1009-1015.

Thompson, L. W., Gallagher, D., & Breckenridge, J. S. (1987). Comparative effectiveness of psychotherapies for depressed elders. *Journal of Consulting and Clinical Psychology, 55*, 385-390.

Thompson-Brenner, H., Glass, S., & Westen, D. (2003). A multidimensional meta-analysis of psychotherapy for bulimia nervosa. *Clinical Psychology: Science and Practice, 10*, 269-287.

Thornton, D., Mann , R., Bowers, L., Sheriff, N., & White, T. (1996). Sex offenders in a therapeutic community. In J. Shine (Ed.), *Grendon: A compilation of Grendon research.*

Tomsovic, M. (1970). A follow-up study of discharged alcoholics. *Hospital and Community Psychiatry, 21*, 94–97.

Torgersen, S., Kringlen, E., & Cramer, V. (2001). The prevalence of personality disorders in a community sample. *Archives of General Psychiatry, 58*, 590-596.

Tucker, L., Bauer, S. F., Wagner, S., Harlam, D., & Sher, I. (1987). Long-term hospital treatment of borderline patients: A descriptive outcome study. *American Journal of Psychiatry, 144*, 1443-1448.

Waldinger, R. J., & Gunderson, J. G. (1984). Completed therapies with borderline patients. *American Journal of Psychotherapy, 38*, 190-202.

Wallerstein, R. S. (1986). *Forty-two lives in treatment: A study of psychoanalysis and psychotherapy.* New York: Guilford Press.

Wallerstein, R. S. (1989). The psychotherapy research project of the Menninger Foundation: An overview. *Journal of Consulting and Clinical Psychology, 57*, 195-205.

Walsh, B. T., Wilson, G. T., Loeb, K. L., Devlin, M. J., Pike, K. M., Roose, S. P., et al. (1997). Medication and psychotherapy in the treatment of bulimia nervosa. *American Journal of Psychiatry, 154(4)*, 523-531.

Wampold, B. E. (1997). Methodological problems in identifying efficacious psychotherapies. *Psychotherapy Research, 7*, 21-43.

Wampold, B.E., Minami, T., Baskin, T., & Callen-Tierney, S. (2002). A meta-(re)analysis of the effects of cognitive therapy versus 'other therapies' for depression. *Journal of Affective Disorders, 68(2-3)*, 159-165.

Warren, F., Preedy-Fayers, K., McGauley, G., Pickering, A., Norton, K., Geddes, J. R., et al. (2003). *Review of treatments for severe personality disorder.* Home Office Online Report 30/03 (http://www.homeoffice.gov.uk/rds/pdfs2/rdsolr3003.pdf). (Accessed 1/30/06.)

Weisz, J. R., Weiss, B., Han, S. S., Granger, D. A., & Morton, T. (1995). Effects of psychotherapy with children and adolescents revisited: A meta-analysis of treatment outcome studies. *Psychological Bulletin, 117(3)*, 450–468.

Weisz, J. R., Weiss, B., Morton, T., Granger, D., & Han, S. (1992). *Meta-analysis of psychotherapy outcome research with children and adolescents.* Los Angeles: University of California.

Westen, D., & Morrison, K. (2001). A multidimensional meta-analysis of treatments for depression, panic, and generalized anxiety disorder: An empirical examination of the status of empirically supported therapies. *Journal of Consulting and Clinical Psychology, 69*, 875-899.

Westen, D., Morrison, K., & Thompson-Brenner, H. (2004). The empirical status of empirically supported psychotherapies: Assumptions, findings, and reporting in controlled clinical trials. *Psychological Bulletin, 130,* 631-663.

Wetherell, J. L., Gatz, M., & Craske, M. G. (2003). Treatment of generalized anxiety disorder in older adults. *Journal of Consulting and Clinical Psychology, 71(1),* 31-40.

Whittle, P. (2000). Experimental psychology and psychoanalysis: What we can learn from a century of misunderstanding. *Neuro-Psychoanalysis, 1,* 233-245.

Wiborg, I. M., & Dahl, A. A. (1996). Does brief dynamic psychotherapy reduce the relapse rate of panic disorder? *Archives of General Psychiatry, 53(8),* 689-694.

Wilberg, T., Friis, S., Karterud, S., Mehlum, L., Urnes, O., & Vaglum, P. (1998). Outpatient group psychotherapy: A valuable continuation treatment for patients with borderline personality disorder treated in a day hospital. A three year follow-up study. *Nordic Journal of Psychiatry, 52,* 213-221.

Winston, A., Laikin, M., Pollack, J., Samstag, L. W., McCullough, L., & Muran, J. C. (1994). Short-term psychotherapy of personality disorders. *American Journal of Psychiatry, 151,* 190-194.

Winston, A., Pollack, J., McCullough, L., Flegenheimer, W., Kestenbaum, R., & Trujillo, M. (1991). Brief psychotherapy of personality disorders. *Journal of Nervous and Mental Disease, 179,* 188-193.

Woody, G. E., Luborsky, L., McLellan, A. T., O'Brien, C. P., Beck, A. T., Blaine, J., et al. (1983). Psychotherapy for opiate addicts. Does it help? *Archives of General Psychiatry, 40(6),* 639-645.

Woody, G. E., McLellan, A. T., Luborsky, L., & O'Brien, C. P. (1987). Twelve-month follow-up of psychotherapy for opiate dependence. *American Journal of Psychiatry, 144(5),* 590-596.

Woody, G. E., McLellan, A. T., Luborsky, L., & O'Brien, C. P. (1990). Psychotherapy and counseling for methadone-maintained opiate addicts: Results of research studies. In L. S. Onken & J. D. Blaine (Eds.), *Psychotherapy and counseling in the treatment of drug abuse.* NIDA Research Monograph 104.

Woody, G. E., McLellan, A. T., Luborsky, L., & O'Brien, C. P. (1995). Psychotherapy in community methadone programs: a validation study. *American Journal of Psychiatry, 152(9),* 1302-1308.

Yalom, I. D. (1995). *The Theory and Practice of Group Psychotherapy* (4th ed.). New York: Basic Books.

Young, J. E. (1999). *Cognitive therapy for personality disorder: A schema-focused approach (3rd ed.).* Sarasota, FL: Professional Resource Press/Professional Resource Exchange, Inc.

Zimberg, S. (1974). Evaluation of alcoholism treatment in Harlem. *Quarterly Journal of Studies on Alcohol, 35,* 550-557.

Zimmerman, M., & Coryell, W. H. (1990). Diagnosing personality disorders within the community: A comparison of self-report and interview measures. *Archives of General Psychiatry, 47,* 527.

Review of Meta-Analyses of Outcome Studies of Psychodynamic Therapy

Falk Leichsenring, DSc[1]

Editor's Note: The last article provides a third overview, this one from Germany, rather than the UK (Fonagy) or the USA (Westen, et al.). It is overall a shorter list of studies but with a much stronger focus on the German literature, some published in German, but much of it in English in general psychiatric and psychoanalytic journals, and also in empirical research-oriented journals.

Leichsenring, like Fonagy, presents his meta-analyses in relation to the study of outcome in specific illness disorders, depressive disorders, personality disorders, borderline disorders, etc., and again within the stipulations of DSM diagnostic categories, and the constraints of efficacy studies within the random clinical trial (RCT) model. But he also cautions that the findings that emerge within the strictures of these efficacy studies cannot be directly transferred to routine naturalistic clinical practice. In a number of places he takes issue with some of Fonagy's assessments of his own (Leichsenring's) conclusions in his articles that Fonagy reviews. The reader here can go back and forth between these views as expressed in both articles.

Overall, this entire array of 12 chapters in Part III of this volume is intended to indicate both the considerations and the issues and problems in response to which this Psychodynamic Diagnostic Manual (PDM) has been brought into being, and also to demonstrate some of the major conceptual and empirical supports for a psychodynamic construction.

In times of evidence-based medicine and empirically supported treatments, there is a need for empirical outcome research in psychodynamic and psychoanalytic therapy (Gunderson & Gabbard, 1999). However, what criteria are appropriate to demonstrate that a treatment works is the subject of controversial discussions. A major aspect of this controversy is the question whether randomized controlled trials (RCTs) truly represent the "gold standard" of outcome research (Beutler, 1998; Chambless & Hollon, 1998; Chambless & Ollendick, 2001; Henry, 1998; Persons & Silberschatz, 1998; Seligman, 1995; Westen, Novotny, & Thompson-Brenner, 2004, p. 691 of this volume). RCTs are carried out in an experimental research setting (efficacy studies), whereas effectiveness studies are carried out under the usual conditions of clinical practice. Recently, a proposal has been made to resolve this controversy by clarifying and

---

[1] Clinic of Tiefenbrunn and Department of Psychosomatics and Psychotherapy, University of Goettingen, Germany

differentiating what research questions can be adequately addressed by RCTs, and what questions, rather, require research effectiveness studies (Leichsenring, 2004). The two types of study designs lead to different intended applications. For this reason, they are not in a competitive relationship (Leichsenring, 2004). Recent reviews of efficacy studies of psychodynamic therapy in specific psychiatric disorders have been given by Peter Fonagy in this book (p. 765), and also by Fonagy, Roth and Higgitt (2005), Leichsenring (2005), and Roth and Fonagy (2005).

In this section, results of recent meta-analyses of psychodynamic therapy are presented. Various meta-analyses have addressed the efficacy of short-term psychodynamic psychotherapy (STPP). Svartberg and Stiles (1991) found STPP to be superior to no-treatment controls, but to be inferior to alternative psychotherapies. Crits-Christoph (1992) reported that STPP achieved large effect sizes compared with untreated waiting-list control patients and was found to be equally effective compared with other forms of therapy such as cognitive behavioral therapy (CBT) or psychopharmacological treatment. Although the effect sizes assessed by Anderson and Lambert (1995) were a bit lower than those reported by Crits-Christoph, their results corroborated his findings. Unlike Svartberg and Stiles, Crits-Christoph and Anderson and Lambert included studies of interpersonal therapy (IPT) as representatives of STPP—a subject of controversial discussion that is discussed later in this paper.

The outcome of a meta-analysis is heavily influenced by the selection and the quality of the studies included in the evaluation (e.g., Chambless & Hollon, 1998). As Messer and Warren (1995) have pointed out, many of the studies included in the meta-analysis of Svartberg and Stiles (1991) had severe conceptual and methodological flaws. This is also true for the meta-analysis of Grawe, Donati, and Bernauer (1994) comparing STPP and CBT (Leichsenring, 1996; Tschuschke & Kächele, 1996; Tschuschke, et al., 1998). However, Crits-Christoph (1992) included in his meta-analysis only studies that fulfilled rigorous methodological criteria (e.g., use of therapy manuals, experienced therapists, minimum of sessions, etc.). Wampold, et al. (2002) assessed the efficacy of all bona fide treatments and did not find differences between different methods of psychotherapy. At present, two disorder-specific reviews or meta-analyses of STPP are available: One deals with the effects of STPP in depressive disorders (Leichsenring, 2001), the other one with the effects of psychodynamic psychotherapy in personality disorders (Leichsenring & Leibing, 2003).

META-ANALYSES OF DEPRESSIVE DISORDERS

At present, two disorder-specific reviews or meta-analyses of STPP are available—the review of Leichsenring (2001) studied the efficacy of STPP compared to CBT in the treatment of depression. In fact, it is more a review than a meta-analysis. Because of the small number of studies that could be included, the results were discussed separately for each study. Some meta-analytic evaluations were made when it seemed appropriate. This review used inclusion criteria similar to Crits-Christoph's meta-analysis (1992). In addition, taking the results reported by Howard, et al. (1986) into account, studies were only included in which at least 13 sessions of therapy had taken place. After 13 sessions, 60% of the depressed patients had improved according to Howard, et al. (1986, p. 163). However, "improvement" does not mean that these patients had achieved maximum benefit (Howard, et al., 1986, p. 163) or had returned to fully normal functioning (Kopta, Howard, Lowry, & Beutler, 1994). Thus, the criterion of 13 sessions of STPP was a minimum rather than an optimal threshold. In order to ensure both an acceptable statistical power and also that randomization was effective (Hsu, 1989), studies were only included in which at least 20 patients were treated in each condition. Only six studies could finally be included in the review (Barkham, et al., 1996; Elkin, et al., 1989; Gallagher-Thompson & Steffen, 1994; Hersen, Himmelhoch, & Thase, 1984; Shapiro, et al., 1994; Thompson, Gallagher, & Breckenridge, 1987). Additional data from these studies were reported by Shapiro, et al. (1995) and Shea, et al. (1990). Like Crits-Christoph (1992) and Anderson and Lambert (1995), I included studies of interpersonal therapy (IPT) as representative of STPP. However, of the studies finally included, this only refers to the study of Elkin, et al. (1989). Outcome was assessed separately for depressive symptoms, general psychiatric symptoms, and social functioning. In the studies included, between 16 and 20 treatment sessions were held. Different forms of STPP were applied. However, this was also true for the (comparative) studies of CBT included in this review. Three studies provided the data necessary to calculate effect sizes in the form of Cohen's statistic (Cohen, 1988; Hersen, Himmelhoch, & Thase, 1984; Shapiro, et al., 1994; Shapiro, Rees, Barkham, & Hardy, 1995; Thompson, Gallagher, & Breckenridge, 1987).

According to the results, STPP achieved large effect sizes ($d \geq 0.80$) with regard to depressive symptoms, general psychiatric symptoms, and social functioning (Leichsenring, 2001). With the exception of the NIMH follow-up (Shea, et al., 1990), a stable reduction of the depressive symptoms after STPP was reported (Barkham, et al., 1996; Gallagher-Thompson, & Steffen, 1994; Hersen, Himmelhoch, & Thase, 1984; Shapiro, Barkham, & Hardy, 1995). In order to compare the efficacy of STPP and CBT, the between-group tests of significance performed by the authors of the six studies were reviewed. In total, 60 comparisons applying tests of significance were carried out. In 58 of the 60 comparisons (i.e., 97%) performed in the six studies and their follow-ups, no significant difference could be detected between STPP and CBT concerning the effects in depressive symptoms, general psychiatric symptoms, and social functioning. Furthermore, STPP and CBT were compared with regard to the number of patients that were reported as remitted or improved. Five studies provided the necessary data (Elkin, et al., 1989; Gallagher-Thompson & Steffen, 1994; Hersen, Himmelhoch, & Thase, 1984; Shapiro, et al., 1994; Shapiro, Barkham, & Hardy, 1995; Thompson, Gallagher, & Breckenridge, 1987). I evaluated the data separately for the end of treatment and the follow-up assessments. Here again, no significant differences were found between STPP and CBT with regard to the number of patients regarded as remitted or improved, either on the level of the single studies or in a meta-analytic evaluation of all five studies. The mean difference between STPP and CBT concerning the number of patients that were judged as remitted or improved corresponded to a small effect size (post assessment: $\phi = 0.08$, follow-up assessment: $\phi = 0.12$). In this case, the ϕ-correlation is the appropriate statistic to assess the effect size (Cohen, 1988). A value of $\phi = w \leq 0.10$ is regarded as a small effect (Cohen, 1988). As the ϕ-correlation is equivalent to the difference in success rates (Rosenthal, 1995; Rosenthal & Rubin, 1982), the (non-significant) difference in success rates between STPP and CBT was 8% ($\phi = 0.08$) at the end of therapy and 12% ($\phi = 0.12$) at follow-up in favor of CBT. According to the meta-analytic evaluation of these five studies, STPP and CBT were equally effective methods in the treatment of depression.

This review had some limitations. Above all, the number of studies which met the inclusion criteria was small. Thus, the results can only be preliminary. Furthermore, the results only apply to the specific forms of STPP that were examined in the selected studies (e.g., Horowitz, 1976; Mann, 1973; Rose & Del Maestro, 1990; Shapiro & Fith, 1985). They cannot be generalized to other forms of STPP. Further studies are needed to examine the effects of specific forms of STPP in depression in both controlled and natural settings. The NIMH study of depression (Shea, et al., 1990) has shown that only 24% of the total sample was free of symptoms for both eight weeks after the end of therapy and during the 18-month follow-up period. CBT, interpersonal therapy, and pharmacotherapy did not differ significantly in this regard (Shea, et al., 1990, p. 784). According to the latter results, 16 to 20 sessions of interpersonal therapy, CBT and pharmacotherapy of a comparable duration, are insufficient for most patients to achieve lasting remission. Future studies and meta-analyses should address the effects of longer treatments of depression.

In a re-evaluation of the data in my 2001 review, Fonagy (research included in this book, p. 765) found a superiority of CBT over STPP that I, he asserts, had not reported (Leichsenring, 2001). According to the inclusion criteria that I had applied in that review, studies of fewer than 13 sessions were excluded. This also applies to studies including fewer than 20 patients per condition. For this reason, I had neither included the 8-session condition of the Shapiro, et al. (1994, 1995) study nor the data of the maintenance treatment of the Hersen, et al. (1984) study. The superiority of CBT reported by Fonagy may be due to his inclusion of these data. At least the inclusion of an eight-session treatment of depression seems to be questionable, taking the data on dose-effect relationship reported by Howard, et al. (1986) into account.

The inclusion of interpersonal therapy (IPT) as representative of STPP is controversial. This critique refers to the meta-analyses and reviews of Crits-Christoph (1992), Anderson and Lambert (1995), and Leichsenring (2001). However, as indicated in my 2001 paper (Leichsenring, 2001, p. 413), it can be shown that the results of my review do not change substantially if the study of Elkin, et al. (1989) is excluded. I included the interpersonal therapy of Klerman, et al. (1984) applied in the NIMH study of depression (Elkin, et al., 1989) in my 2001 review as a form of psychodynamic therapy, because the NIMH Treatment of Depression Collaborative Research Program (Elkin, et al., 1985, p. 307) identified the interpersonal therapy as within the psychodynamic domain and contrasted it to CBT. Furthermore, only therapists who had had psychodynamic training were selected to perform the interpersonal therapies in that study. Also, Elkin, et al. (1989, p. 978) had concluded: "... it is impossible in this study to separate treatments from the therapists carrying out these treatments." For this reason Crits-Christoph (1992) included IPT in his meta-analysis of STPP as well. Today, however, arguments and data are available that suggest that IPT not be included as a form of STPP (Ablon & Jones, 2002; Markowitz, Svartberg, & Swartz, 1998). For this reason, studies of IPT were not included in the later meta-analyses of psychodynamic therapy we have made (Leichsenring & Leibing, 2003; Leichsenring, Rabung & Leibing, 2004).

Fonagy (p. 765) discusses a possible selection bias in my 2001 review. As the problem of including IPT has already been discussed, I shall only briefly address his other points of critique. Fonagy states that two studies I included do not seem "relevant to the assessment of the relative effects of CBT for depression." He refers to the study of Hersen, et al. (1984) using social skills training as a behavioral treatment of depression, and to the study of Gallagher-Thompson and Steffen (1994) who examined CBT treatment of depressive caregivers. Fonagy does not give an explanation for his point of view, and I do not see why these studies are not relevant to the study of the effects of CBT in depression.[2] This applies also to Fonagy's judgment of the study of Thompson, et al. (1987) which he described as "group rather than individual therapy carried out with an older adult population." In that study, individual therapy was used (Thompson, Gallagher, & Breckenridge, 1987, p. 385) and, therefore, I do not see why there is such a problem in treating and studying elderly depressed patients.

META-ANALYSES OF PERSONALITY DISORDERS

In another meta-analysis for specific psychiatric disorders, the effects of STPP and CBT in the treatment of personality disorders were assessed (Leichsenring &

---

[2] In the study of Gallagher-Thompson and Steffen (1994), 68% of the depressive caregivers suffered from a major depression, and 30% from a minor depression. Hersen, et al. (1984) used social skills training for depression according to a treatment manual in patients with a major depressive disorder.

Leibing, 2003). This meta-analysis included only studies that used standardized methods to make personality disorder diagnoses, applied reliable and valid instruments for the assessment of outcome, and reported data that allowed calculation of within group effect sizes or assessment of percentages of recovery from personality disorders. Fourteen studies of psychodynamic therapy and eleven studies of cognitive-behavioral therapy were included. Of these 25 studies, 14 applied a randomized controlled design. For psychodynamic psychotherapy, six RCTs and eight CBT were available. We assessed effect sizes for the overall treatment effect, for self-report and observer-rated measures, as well as for measures more specific to the personality disorder psychopathology (e.g., DSM criteria personality disorders, measures of interpersonal problems, or self esteem). Data of the longest follow-up period were used for the meta-analytic evaluation, in order to assess long-term rather than short-term changes which seem to be more appropriate for the study of personality disorders. The main results were as follows.

In most of the studies, psychodynamic psychotherapy was time-limited. Psychoanalysis was not employed. For psychodynamic psychotherapy, the mean treatment duration was 37.18 weeks (SD = 26.80). The number of sessions ranged from 12 to 40 (mean = 23.17, SD = 11.63). For CBT, the mean treatment duration was 16.36 weeks (SD = 16.63) and the number of sessions ranged from 6 to 32 (mean = 13.19, SD = 8.59). For psychodynamic psychotherapy, the mean follow-up period was 78.13 weeks (SD = 60.39). For CBT, the mean follow-up period was 12.50 weeks (SD = 17.82).

In these studies, the following forms of personality disorders were treated with psychodynamic psychotherapy: (1) borderline personality disorder (BPD), (2) mixed samples of the three clusters of DSM-III personality disorders, and (3) patients with an Axis I disorder and a concomitant diagnosis of a personality disorder. In the CBT studies, (1) patients with BPD, avoidant personality disorder, (2) bulimia nervosa and a comorbid personality disorder, and (3) patients with an Axis I disorder and a concomitant diagnosis of a personality disorder were treated.

According to the results, psychodynamic therapy yielded an overall mean pre-post effect size within treatment of 1.46, which represents a large effect (Cohen, 1988; Kazis, et al., 1989). For self-report measures, the mean effect size was 1.08, for observer-rated measures it was 1.79. For CBT, the corresponding effect sizes were 1.00, 1.20, and 0.87. For more specific measures of personality disorder pathology (e.g., DSM criteria of personality disorder, interpersonal problems, self esteem), psychodynamic therapy yielded a large mean pre-post (within treatment) effect size of 1.56. As the data of the longest follow-up period were used for the meta-analytic evaluation, the effect sizes indicate long-term rather than short-term change in personality disorders. This is particularly true for psychodynamic psychotherapy with a mean follow-up period of 1.5 years (78 weeks), whereas the mean follow-up period for CBT was considerably shorter (13 weeks).

EFFECTS OF PSYCHODYNAMIC PSYCHOTHERAPY IN PATIENTS WITH BORDERLINE PERSONALITY DISORDER

In eight studies included in our 2003 meta-analysis, the effects of psychodynamic therapy in patients with borderline personality disorder (BPD) were reported (Antikainen, et al., 1995; Bateman & Fonagy, 1999; Karterud, et al., 1992; Lieberman & Eckman, 1981; Munroe-Blum & Marziali, 1995; Stevenson and Mears, 1992; Tucker, et al., 1987; Wilberg, et al., 1998). The mean overall effect size achieved by psychodynamic psychotherapy in patients with BPD was 1.31 (SD = 0.71). The mean effect size for self-rated measures was 1.00 (SD = 0.25), and 1.45 (SD = 1.09) for observer-rated measures. These effect sizes were significantly different from zero (Leichsenring & Leibing, 2003). The mean treatment duration was 33 weeks (SD = 26.85). Four studies reported the effects of CBT in patients with borderline personality disorder (Bohus, et al., 2000; Liberman & Ekman 1981; Linehan, Tutek, Heard, & Amstrong, 1994; Linehan, et al., 1999). The mean overall effect size for CBT was 0.95 (SD = 0.31). The mean effect size for self-rated measures was 0.97 (SD = 0.24), and 0.81 (SD = 0.54) for observer-rated measures. The mean treatment duration was 22 weeks (SD = 26.84).

According to these results, there is evidence that both psychodynamic therapy and cognitive-behavioral therapy are effective treatments of personality disorders. The effect sizes we reported for CBT and psychodynamic psychotherapy cannot be compared directly between the two methods of therapy, because the data did not come from same experiment comparisons. The studies differed with respect to various aspects of therapy, patient samples, outcome assessment and other variables. For this reason, the conclusion cannot be drawn that "CBT and psychodynamic therapy are equally effective," (Fonagy, p. 765). However, a more recent RCT found CBT and short-term psychodynamic psychotherapy equally effective in the treatment of cluster C personality disorders (Svartberg, Stiles & Seltzer, 2004).

Certainly, our meta-analysis of psychodynamic psychotherapy and CBT in personality disorders has some limitations as well. First of all, the number of studies that could be included is again limited. This applies to both CBT (11 studies) and psychodynamic psychotherapy (14 studies). The small number of studies reduces both the results' potential generalization and their statistical power (Cohen, 1988). Thus, the conclusions that can be drawn are again only preliminary. Furthermore, most of the studies included focused on outcome measures that referred to Axis I pathology associated with personality disorders (e.g., symptoms of depression or anxiety). However, this seems to be justified as most of the personality disorder patients included had a comorbid Axis I pathology. This is especially true of severe personality disorders such as BPD. Studies that included patients with both Axis I and Axis II pathology (Diguer, Barber, & Luborsky, 1993; Hardy, et al., 1995; Karterud, et al., 1992) reported more pathological pretreatment scores in the outcome measures applied for patients with personality disorders compared with patients with Axis I pathology only. Thus, to study Axis I pathology seems to be of some relevance for personality disorders as well. Furthermore, seven studies of psychodynamic psychotherapy used measures that referred to aspects of core personality pathology. We found a large effect size of 1.56 for these measures.

With regard to limitations, within-group effect sizes may be an overestimate of the true change on account of unspecific therapeutic factors, spontaneous remission or regression to the mean. However, in two randomized controlled studies of psychodynamic psychotherapy (Bateman & Fonagy, 1999; Winston, et al., 1994), the mean effect sizes for psychodynamic psychotherapy exceeded that of the control condition. This was true as well for the patients of the Bateman and Fonagy study in an 18-month follow-up (Bateman & Fonagy, 2001).

Referring to the meta-analyses of Perry, et al. (1999) and to our meta-analysis (Leichsenring & Leibing, 2003), Fonagy (p. 765) asserts that "many of the studies included in these meta-analyses did not have the aim of treating Axis II disorders." However, as far as our meta-analysis is concerned (Leichsenring & Leibing, 2003), this is true only for 3 of 14 studies (21%) of psychodynamic psychotherapy (Diguer, Barber, & Luborsky, 1993; Hardy, et al., 1995). Most of the studies did aim at treating personality disorders. In a second step of evaluation, the authors of the three original studies had analyzed their data with regard to effects in comorbid Axis II pathology (Diguer, Barber, & Luborsky, 1993; Hardy, et al., 1995). I do agree with Fonagy regarding the heterogeneity of clinical populations and of methods applied as a problem for a meta-analytic evaluation. In order to take this problem into account, we assessed changes both in measures more specific to personality disorders and in effects for specific diagnostic groups. Further studies which examined specific forms of psychotherapy with specific types of personality disorders using measures of core personality psychopathology are required. Both longer treatments and follow-up studies should be included.

META-ANALYSIS OF PSYCHODYNAMIC PSYCHOTHERAPY WITH SPECIFIC PSYCHIATRIC DISORDERS

Since the publication of the meta-analyses of Svartberg and Stiles (1991), Crits-Christoph (1992), and Anderson and Lambert (1995), several studies of STPP have been published that have not yet been included in meta-analyses. The most recent study, which was included by Anderson and Lambert was published in 1993; that is now more than 10 years ago. For this reason, we conducted a new meta-analysis which included the more recent studies of STPP (Leichsenring, Rabung, & Leibing, 2004). As the results of a meta-analysis depend on the quality of the studies included, we applied rigorous inclusion criteria. Studies were only included that fulfilled the following methodological requirements:

- a randomized controlled design was applied;

- a specific form of STPP as represented in a treatment manual or manual-like guide was applied and treatment integrity was ensured;

- therapists were specifically trained and /or experienced in STPP techniques;

- only patients with specific psychiatric disorders were treated (no mixed samples, no analogue studies);

- the patient sample was clearly described;

- only diagnostic procedures and outcome measures for which reliability and validity have been demonstrated were used; and

- data were reported that were necessary to calculate pre-post effect sizes.

Contrary to the meta-analyses of Anderson and Lambert (1995), Crits-Christoph (1992), and Leichsenring (2001), studies of IPT were not included (e.g., Elkin, et al., 1989) for the reasons already discussed. Thus, this review includes only studies for which there is a general agreement that they represent proper models of STPP.

As it is questionable to aggregate the results of very different outcome measures which refer to different areas of psychological functioning (Rosenthal & Rubin, 1986), we assessed the efficacy of STPP separately for target symptoms, general psychiatric symptoms (i.e., comorbid symptoms), and social functioning. This procedure is analogous to Crits-Christoph's (1991) meta-analysis. As outcome measures of target problems, we included both patient ratings of target problems and measures referring to symptoms that are specific to the patient group under study, e.g., measures of anxiety for studies investigating treatments of anxiety disorders. For the efficacy of STPP with general (concomitant) psychiatric symptoms, both broad measures of psychiatric symptoms, such as the Symptom-Check List (SCL-90) (Derogais, 1977) and specific measures that did not refer specifically to the disorder under study were included, e.g., the Beck Depression Inventory (BDI) applied in patients with personality disorders (Beck, et al., 1961). For the assessment of social functioning, the Social Adjustment Scale (SAS) and similar measures were included (Weissman & Bothwell, 1976).

Results

Seventeen studies of STPP met the inclusion criteria. Of the 17 studies that were identified, 13 (76%) had not yet been included in other meta-analyses of STPP. Only two of the 19 studies that Svartberg and Stiles (1991) included in their meta-analysis met our inclusion criteria (Fairburn, Kirk, O'Connor, & Cooper, 1986; Thompson, Gallagher, & Breckenridge, 1987). Of the 26 studies of the Anderson and Lambert meta-analysis (1995), only four studies were included (Brom, Kleber, & Defares, 1989, Thompson, Gallagher, & Breckenridge, 1987,

Winston, et al., 1994; Woody, Luborsky, McLellan, & O'Brien, 1990). Of the eleven studies included by Crits-Christoph (1991), we included only four (Brom, Kleber, & Defares, 1989, Thompson, Gallagher, & Breckenridge, 1987, Winston, et al., 1994; Woody, Luborsky, McLellan, & O'Brien, 1990). As reported above, Crits-Christoph and Anderson and Lambert included studies of IPT, which we excluded. Only two studies of the meta-analysis of Leichsenring were included (Shapiro, et al., 1994, Thompson, Gallagher, & Breckenridge, 1987) and only one study (Munroe-Blum & Marziali, 1995) of Leichsenring and Leibing's meta-analysis (2003).[3] Accordingly, only a limited portion of the studies that were included in previous meta-analyses of STPP was included in our 2004 meta-analysis.

Models of STPP

In the 17 studies included in our meta-analysis, different models of STPP were applied (Leichsenring, Rabung, & Leibing, 2004). The most frequently applied concepts of STPP were the methods developed by Davanloo (1980), Horowitz (1976), Luborsky (1984), and Shapiro and Firth (1985).

Therapy Duration

In the 17 studies of STPP, between 7 and 40 sessions were conducted. Short therapies of seven sessions were carried out in the study of Hamilton, et al. (2000); longer therapies were carried out in the studies of Winston, et al. (1994) and Svartberg, et al. (2004), who studied the treatment of personality disorders. The mean number of sessions of STPP was 20.97 (SD = 10.90).

Duration of Follow-Up

The mean length of the follow-up period was about one year (M = 61.42 weeks, SD = 71.26).

Effect Sizes of STPP

Target Problems

For target problems, STPP yielded an effect size of 1.39 post therapy and of 1.57 at follow-up. Both effect sizes differ significantly from zero (Leichsenring, Rabung, & Leibing, 2004). The limits of a 95% confidence interval were 0.97 and 1.82 (post assessment) and, respectively, 1.10 and 2.04 (follow-up assessment).

---

[3] The study of Bateman and Fonagy (1999) was not included in our 2004 meta-analysis as we only examined studies of short-term psychodynamic psychotherapy.

General Psychiatric Symptoms

For general psychiatric symptoms, STPP yielded an effect size of 0.90 post therapy and of 0.95 at follow-up. Both effect sizes differ significantly from zero (Leichsenring, Rabung, & Leibing, 2004). The limits of a 95% confidence interval were 0.64 and 1.17 (post assessment) and, respectively, 0.65 and 1.25 (follow-up assessment).

Social Functioning

For social functioning, STPP yielded an effect size of 0.80 post therapy and of 1.19 at follow-up. Both effect sizes differ significantly from zero (Leichsenring, Rabung, & Leibing, 2004). The limits of a 95% confidence interval were 0.56 and 1.05 (post assessment) and, respectively, 0.58 and 1.79 (follow-up assessment).

Stability of Effect Sizes

In order to assess the stability of effects, we compared the pre-post effect sizes with the pre-follow-up effect sizes for only those studies that included follow-up assessments. For STPP the pre-follow-up effect sizes were stable and tended to increase (target problems: 1.44. vs. 1.57; general psychiatric symptoms: 0.91 vs. 0.95; and social functioning: 0.89 vs. 1.19). For CBT, the effect sizes were stable as well (target problems: 1.37. vs. 1.33; general psychiatric symptoms: 1.01 vs. 0.97; and social functioning: 0.97 vs. 1.05).

STPP vs. No Treatment and Treatment as Usual

In order to compare STPP with no treatment and with treatment as usual (TAU), we tested if the between-group effect sizes between STPP, on the one hand, and no treatment, and TAU, on the other hand, were significantly different from zero. According to the results, STPP was significantly superior to no treatment and TAU with regard to target problems, general psychiatric symptoms and social functioning (Leichsenring, Rabung, & Leibing, 2004). Because of the small number of studies, these tests were only performed for the post-therapy effect sizes. The between-group effect sizes were large for target problems (post: 1.17); that is, STPP was superior to control conditions by more than one standard deviation (Leichsenring, Rabung, & Leibing, 2004). For general psychiatric symptoms and social functioning the between-group effect sizes were of a medium to large size (Leichsenring, Rabung, & Leibing, 2004).

STPP vs. Other Forms of Psychotherapy

Fifteen studies included a comparison of STPP with other forms of psychotherapy, e.g., CBT (Leichsenring, Rabung, & Leibing, 2004). For these studies, no significant differences were found between STPP and other forms of psychotherapy in target symptoms, general psychiatric symptoms, and social functioning. This was true for both the pre-post effect sizes and the pre-follow-up effect sizes.

Therapy Duration and Effect Sizes

We tested whether the effect sizes of STPP correlate with the duration of therapy (number of sessions). For STPP, all (Spearman) correlations with any outcome measure were insignificant (rs $\leq$ 0.21, p = 0.64).

DISCUSSION

The available meta-analyses provided some evidence that psychodynamic psychotherapy is an efficacious treatment of psychiatric disorders which is superior to TAU or wait list conditions and as effective as other forms of psychotherapy such as CBT. However, further studies of STPP with specific psychiatric disorders are urgently needed. This applies, for example, to anxiety disorders. Although anxiety is such an important concept in psychodynamic theory and therapy (Zerbe, 1990), randomized controlled studies of psychodynamic therapy with anxiety disorders are widely lacking (Leichsenring, 2005). Furthermore, it is an interesting question for future research to find out if there are areas of psychological functioning in which STPP is superior to other forms of psychotherapy.

STPP was judged as "probably efficacious" by the Task Force on Promotion and Dissemination of Psychological Procedures of the Division 12 (Clinical Psychology) of the American Psychological Association (1995). The evaluation problem with STPP was that no two studies of independent research groups were found demonstrating efficacy of the same form of STPP with the same psychiatric disorder. At present, this judgment still seems to hold (Fonagy, Roth, & Higgitt, 2005; Leichsenring, 2005). The Task Force concluded that further evidence for STPP with specific psychiatric disorders is required if this clinically validated form of treatment is to survive in the present market.

In the studies reviewed here, different models of STPP were applied. Whether and how they "really," that is, empirically, differ is an interesting question: "Relying on brand names of therapy can be misleading" (Ablon & Jones, 2002, p. 775). Studies addressing this problem are relevant for considering whether some of the different models of STPP are similar enough to be lumped together. If this turns out to be the case, empirical evidence for one model of psychodynamic psychotherapy would also be valid for another model that has proved to be similar enough.

Ablon and Jones (2002) compared CBT and IPT as they were performed in the NIMH treatment of depression study. According to the results, both forms of therapy adhered most strongly to the ideal prototype of CBT. In addition, adherence to the CBT prototype yielded more positive correlations with outcome measures across both types of treatment. However, STPP was not included in this comparison. Thus, it is not clear how STPP, CBT, and IPT differ empirically with regard to therapist behavior. In the NIMH treatment of depression study, IPT was close to CBT. However, IPT could be even closer to STPP than to CBT. In an earlier study (Luborsky, 1984), therapists' behavior was compared between the Penn-VA study (Luborsky, Woody, McLellan, & Rosenzweig, 1982), the Yale study (Rounsaville, et al., 1983), and the Temple study (Sloane, et al., 1975). The profiles of types of therapists' statements were compared across the different treatments. According to the results, IPT fell between the profiles of supportive expressive therapy and CBT (Luborsky, 1984, p. 37). However, the results differ depending on the category of therapists' statements that are compared. For example, with regard to both interpretation/clarification and directive statements, IPT was very close to CBT. In contrast, nondirective statements were most frequently used both by supportive expressive therapy and IPT. In another study, CBT and IPT could be successfully discriminated (DeRubeis, Hollon, Evans, & Bemis, 1982). Thus, the results reported by Ablon and Jones (2002) may be quite specific to the NIMH treatment of depression study, and not generalizable to IPT and CBT in general. Goldsamt, et al. (1992) compared a demonstration session carried out by Beck, Meichenbaum, and Strupp with the same patient. They found as many significant differences between Beck and Meichenbaum as between Meichenbaum and Strupp. Most differences were found between Beck and Strupp. Meichenbaum was somewhere between Beck and Strupp, and raters could not differentiate between Meichenbaum and Strupp, although they represent different therapeutical approaches, i.e., CBT vs. psychodynamic therapy.

The question of whether the "different" models of psychodynamic psychotherapy differ among themselves empirically is importantly open to further research. This question cannot be answered by inspection comparing the manuals with regard to the included interventions. Empirical studies of actual therapy sessions are required. In a review of empirical studies, Blagys and Hilsenroth (2000) identified seven features that were significantly more frequently observed in psychodynamic, psychodynamic-interpersonal or interpersonal psychotherapy than in CBT.[4] However, the review of Blagys and Hilsenroth did not address the question of whether different models of STPP differ among themselves and from IPT. The features that were found to discriminate IPT from CBT were distinctive of STPP as well (see Tables 1-7 of Blagys & Hilsenroth, 2000, pp. 170-184). Comparing prototypic sessions of different variants of STPP empirically would be a very

---

[4] However, whether two or more methods of therapy can be reliably discriminated or identified on the basis of these features is open to further research. Significant mean differences are a necessary, but not a sufficient, condition for this purpose.

interesting and promising project of research. Other forms of therapy (e.g., CBT, IPT) should also be included.

However, adherence to a treatment manual can be achieved with considerable differences in the underlying interpersonal processes, and it is these processes which may be most significantly related to outcome (Henry, Schacht, & Strupp, 1990; Henry, et al., 1993;). Differences between therapists should also be studied. Crits-Cristoph and Mintz (1991), for example, have shown that individual therapists applying the same form of therapy differed in regard to their efficacy. Thus, in a second step, the factors that may be identified to characterize specific forms of psychodynamic psychotherapy should be related to outcome.

The evidence reported here came from randomized controlled trials carried out under experimental conditions. These results cannot be directly transferred to routine clinical practice, as patients, treatments, and therapists may differ significantly from those in research settings. For this reason, studies are required that test whether a treatment that had worked under experimental conditions works equally well in routine clinical practice. The National Institute of Mental Health in the United States has specifically called for more effectiveness research (Krupnick, et al., 1996), i.e., research under conditions of routine clinical practice. According to recent studies from the general realm of evidence-based medicine, observational studies are reported not to systematically overestimate treatment effects (Benson & Hartz, 2000; Concato, Shah, & Horwitz, 2000). This seems to be true for psychotherapy as well (Shadish, Matt, Navarro, & Phillips, 2000). Quasi-experimental designs can be used to improve the internal validity of observational studies (Shadish, Cook, & Campbell, 2002; Leichsenring, 2004). This is especially relevant for long-term psychodynamic psychotherapy, for which randomized controlled designs are hardly appropriate (Leichsenring, 2004, 2005).

REFERENCES

Ablon, J. S., & Jones, E. E. (2002). Validity of controlled clinical trials of psychotherapy, findings from the NIMH Treatment of Depression Collaborative Research Program. *American Journal of Psychiatry, 159,* 775-783.

Anderson, E. M., & Lambert, M. J. (1995). Short-term dynamically oriented psychotherapy. A review and meta-analysis. *Clinical Psychology Review, 15,* 503–514.

Antikainen, R., Hintikka, J., Lehtonen, J., Koponen, H., & Arstil, A. (1995). A prospective follow-up study of borderline personality disorder inpatients. *Acta Psychiatrica Scandinavica, 92,* 327-335.

Barkham, M., Rees, A., Shapiro, D. A., Stiles, W. B., Agnew, R. M., Halstead, J., et al. (1996). Outcomes of time-limited psychotherapy in applied settings. Replication of the second Sheffield Psychotherapy Project. *Journal of Consulting and Clinical Psychology, 64,* 1079-1085.

Bateman, A., & Fonagy, P. (1999). The effectiveness of partial hospitalization in the treatment of borderline personality disorder, a randomized controlled trial. *American Journal of Psychiatry, 156,* 1563-1569.

Bateman, A., & Fonagy, P. (2001). Treatment of borderline personality disorder with psycho-analytically oriented partial hospitalization: An 18-month follow-up. *American Journal of Psychiatry, 158,* 36-42.

Beck, A. T., Ward, C. H., Mendelson, M., Mock, J., & Erbaugh, J. (1961). An inventory for measuring depression. *Archives of General Psychiatry, 4,* 561-571.

Benson, K., & Hartz, A. J. (2000). A comparison of observational studies and randomized, controlled trials. *New England Journal of Medicine, 342,* 1878-1886.

Beutler, L. E. (1998). Identifying empirically supported treatments: What if we didn't? *Journal of Consulting and Clinical Psychology, 66,* 113-120.

Blagys, M. D., & Hilsenroth, M. J. (2000). Distinctive features of short-term psychodynamic-interpersonal psychotherapy: A review of the comparative psychotherapy process literature. *Clinical Psychology, Science and Practice, 7,* 167-188.

Bohus, M., Haaf, B., Stiglmayr, C., Phl, U., Böhme, R., & Linehan, M. (2000). Evaluation of inpatient Dialectical-Behavioral Therapy for borderline personality disorder: A prospective study. *Behavior, Research and Therapy, 38,* 875-887.

Brom, D., Kleber, R. J., & Defares, P. B. (1989). Brief psychotherapy for posttraumatic stress disorders. *Journal of Consulting and Clinical Psychology, 57,* 607-612.

Chambless, D. L., & Hollon, S. D. (1998). Defining empirically supported treatments. *Journal of Consulting and Clinical Psychology, 66,* 7-18.

Chambless, D. L., & Ollendick, T. H. (2001). Empirically supported psychological interventions: Controversies and evidence. *Annual Review of Psychology, 52,* 685-716.

Cohen, J. (1988). *Statistical power analysis for the behavioral sciences.* Hillsdale, NJ: Lawrence Erlbaum.

Concato, J., Shah, N., & Horwitz, R. I. (2000). Randomized, controlled trials, observational studies, and the hierarchy of research designs. *New England Journal of Medicine, 342,* 1887-1892.

Crits-Christoph, P. (1992). The efficacy of brief dynamic psychotherapy: A meta-analysis. *American Journal of Psychiatry, 149,* 151-158.

Crits-Christoph, P., & Mintz, J. (1991). Implications of therapist effects for the design and analysis of comparative studies of psychotherapies. *Journal of Consulting and Clinical Psychology, 59,* 20-26.

Davenloo, H. (1980). *Short-term dynamic psychotherapy.* New York: Jason Aronson.

Derogais, L. (1977). *The SCL-90 Manual I: Scoring, administration and procedures for the SCL-90-R.* Baltimore: Clinical Psychometric Research.

DeRubeis, R. J., Hollon, S. D., Evans, M. D., & Bemis, K. M. (1982). Can psychotherapies for depression be discriminated? A systematic investigation of cognitive therapy and interpersonal therapy. *Journal of Consulting and Clinical Psychology, 50,* 744-756.

Diguer, L., Barber, J. P., & Luborsky, L. (1993). Three concomitants: Personality disorders, psychiatric severity, and outcome of psychodynamic therapy of major depression. *American Journal of Psychiatry, 150,* 1146-1248.

Elkin, I., Parloff, M. B., Hadley, S. W., & Autry, J. H. (1985). NIMH Treatment of Depression Collaborative Research Program. *Archives of General Psychiatry, 42,* 305-316.

Elkin, I., Shea, T., Watkins, J. T., Imber, S. D., Sotsky, S. M., Collins, J. F., et al. (1989). National Institute of Mental Health Treatment of Depression Collaborative Research Program. *Archives of General Psychiatry, 46,* 971-982.

Fairburn, C. G., Kirk, J., O'Connor, M., & Cooper, P. J. (1986). A comparison of two psychological treatments for bulimia nervosa. *Behavioral Research Therapy, 24,* 629-643.

Fonagy, P., Roth, A., & Higgitt, A. (2005). Psychodynamic psychotherapies: Evidence-based practice and clinical wisdom. *Bulletin of the Menninger Clinic, 69,* 1-58.

Gallagher-Thompson, D. E., & Steffen, A. M. (1994). Comparative effects of cognitive-behavioral and brief psychodynamic psychotherapies for depressed family caregivers. *Journal of Consulting and Clinical Psychology, 62,* 543-549.

Goldsamt, L. A., Goldfried, M. R., Hayes, A. M., & Jerr, S. (1992). Beck, Meichenbaum, and Strupp: A comparison of three therapists on the dimension of therapist feedback. *Psychotherapy, 29,* 167-176.

Grawe, K., Donati, R., & Bernauer, F. (1994). *Psychotherapie im Wandel.* Von der Konfession zur Profession. Göttingen: Hogrefe.

Hamilton J., Guthrie E., Creed, F., et al. (2000). A randomized controlled trial of psychotherapy in patients with chronic functional dyspepsia. *Gastroenterology, 119,* 661-669.

Hardy, G. E., Barkham, M., Shapiro, D. A., Stiles, W. B., Rees, A., & Reynolds, S. (1995). Impact of cluster C personality disorders on outcomes of contrasting brief psychotherapies for depression. *Journal of Consulting and Clinical Psychology, 63,* 997-1004.

Henry, W. P. (1998). Science, politics, and the politics of science, the use and misuse of empirically validated treatment research. *Psychotherapy Research, 8,* 126-140.

Henry, W. P., Schacht, T. E., & Strupp, H. H. (1990). Patient and therapist introject, interpersonal process and differential psychotherapy outcome. *Journal of Consulting and Clinical Psychology, 58,* 768-774.

Henry, W. P., Strupp, H. H., Butler, S. F., Schacht, T. E., & Binder, J. L. (1993). The effects of training in time-limited dynamic psychotherapy. Changes in therapist behavior. *Journal of Consulting and Clinical Psychology, 58,* 768-774.

Hersen, M., Himmelhoch, J. M., & Thase, M. E. (1984). Effects of social skill training, Amitriptyline and psychotherapy in unipolar depressed women. *Behavior Therapy, 15,* 21-40.

Horowitz, M. (1976). *Stress response syndromes.* New York: Aronson.

Howard, K. I., Kopta, S. M., Krause, M. S., & Orlinsky, D. E. (1986). The dose-effect relationship in psychotherapy. *American Psychologist, 41,* 159-164.

Hsu, L. M. (1989). Random sampling, randomization and equivalence of contrasted groups in psychotherapy outcome research. *Journal of Consulting and Clinical Psychology, 57,* 132-137.

Karterud, S., Vaglum, S., Friis, S., Irion, T., Johns, S., & Vaglum, P. (1992). Day hospital therapeutic community treatment for patients with personality disorders. *Journal of Nervous Mental Disorders, 180,* 238-243.

Kazis, L. E., Anderson, J. J., & Meenan, R. F. (1989). Effect sizes for interpreting changes in health status. *Medical Care, 27,* (3 Suppl.), S178-189.

Klerman, G. L., Weissman, M. M., Rounsaville, B. J., & Chevron, E. S. (1984). *Interpersonal psychotherapy of depression.* New York: Basic Books.

Kopta, S. M., Howard, K. I., Lowry, J. L., & Beutler, L. E. (1994). Patterns of symptomatic recovery in psychotherapy. *Journal of Consulting and Clinical Psychology, 62,* 1009-1016.

Krupnick, J. L., Sotsky, S. M., Simmens, S., Moyer, J., Elkin, I., Watkins, J., et al. (1996). The role of the therapeutic alliance in psychotherapy and pharmacotherapy outcome: Findings in the National Institute of Mental Health Treatment of Depression Collaborative Research Program. *Journal of Consulting and Clinical Psychology, 64,* 532-539.

Leichsenring, F. (1996). Zur meta-analyse von Grawe, Bernauer und Donati. (The meta-analysis of Grawe, Bernauer und Donati) *Gruppenpsychotherapie und Gruppendynamik, 32,* 205-234.

Leichsenring, F. (2001). Comparative effects of short-term psychodynamic therapy and cognitive-behavioral therapy in depression: A meta-analysis. *Clinical Psychology Review, 21,* 401-419.

Leichsenring, F. (2004). Randomized controlled vs. naturalistic studies: A new research agenda. *Bulletin of the Menninger Clinic, 68,* 115-129.

Leichsenring, F. (2005). Are psychoanalytic and psychodynamic psychotherapies effective: A review. *International Journal of Psychoanalysis, 86,* 1-26.

Leichsenring, F., & Leibing, E. (2003). The effectiveness of psychodynamic psycho-therapy and cognitive–behavioral therapy in personality disorders. A meta-analysis. *American Journal of Psychiatry, 160,* 1223-1232.

Leichsenring, F., Rabung, S., & Leibing, E. (2004). The efficacy of short-term psychodynamic therapy in specific psychiatric disorders: A meta-analysis. *Archives of General Psychiatry, 61,* 1208-1216.

Libermann, R. P., & Eckman, T. (1981). Behavior therapy vs. insight-oriented therapy for repeated suicide attempters. *Archives of General Psychiatry, 38,* 1126-1130.

Linehan, M. M., Schmidt, H., Dimeff, L. A., Craft, J. C., Kanter, J., & Comtois, K. A. (1999). Dialectical behavior therapy for patients with borderline personality disorder and drug-dependence. *American Journal of Addition, 8,* 279-292.

Linehan, M. M., Tutek, D. A., Heard, H. L., & Armstrong, H. E. (1994). Interpersonal outcome of cognitive behavioral treatment for chronically suicidal borderline patients. *American Journal of Psychiatry, 151,* 1771–1776.

Luborsky, L. (1984). *Principles of psychoanalytic psychotherapy.* Manual for supportive-expressive treatment. New York: Basic Books.

Luborsky, L., Woody, G. E., McLellan, A. T., & Rosenzweig, J. (1982). Can independent judges recognize different psychotherapies? An experiment with manual-guided therapies. *Journal of Consulting and Clinical Psychology, 30,* 49-62.

Mann, J. (1973). *Time-limited psychotherapy.* Cambridge MA: Harvard University Press.

Markowitz, J. C., Svartberg, M., & Swartz, H.A. (1998). Is IPT time-limited psychodynamic psychotherapy? *Journal of Psychotherapy Practice and Research, 7,* 185-195.

Messer, S. B., & Warren, C. S. (1995). *Models of brief psychodynamic therapy: A comparative approach.* New York: Guilford Press.

Munroe-Blum, H., & Marziali, E. (1995). A controlled trial of short-term group treatment for borderline personality disorder. *Journal of Personality Disorders, 9,* 190-198.

Perry, J. C., Banon, E., & Floriana, I. (1999). Effectiveness of psychotherapy for personality disorders. *American Journal of Psychiatry, 156,* 1312-1321.

Persons, J. B., & Silberschatz, G. (1998). Are results of randomized trials useful to psychotherapists? *Journal of Consulting and Clinical Psychology, 66,* 126-135.

Rose, J., & Del Maestro, S. (1990). Separation-individuation conflict as a model for understanding distressed caregivers. Psychodynamic and cognitive case studies. *The Gerontologist, 30,* 693-697.

Rosenthal, R. (1995). Progress in clinical psychology, is there any? *Clinical Psychology, Science and Practice, 2,* 133-149.

Rosenthal, R., & Rubin, D. B. (1982). A simple, general purpose display of magnitude of experimental effect. *Journal of Educational Psychology, 74,* 166-169.

Rosenthal, R., & Rubin, D. B. (1986). Meta-analytic procedures for combining studies with multiple effect sizes. *Psychological Bulletin, 99,* 400-406.

Roth, A., & Fonagy, P. (2005). *What works for whom? A critical review of psychotherapy research.* 2nd ed. New York: Guilford Press.

Rounsaville, B. J., Glazer, W., Wilber, C. H., Weissman, M. M., Kleber, H. D. (1983). Short-term interpersonal psychotherapy in methadone-maintained opiate addicts. *Archives of General Psychiatry, 140,* 629-636.

Seligman, M. E. P. (1995). The effectiveness of psychotherapy. The Consumer Reports study. *American Psychologist, 50,* 965-974.

Shadish, W. R., Matt, G., Navarro, A., & Phillips, G. (2000). The effects of psychological therapies under clinically representative conditions: A meta-analysis. *Journal of Consulting and Clinical Psychology, 126,* 512–529.

Shadish, W. R., Cook, T. D., & Campbell, D. T. (2002). *Experimental and quasi-experimental designs for generalized causal inference.* Boston: Houghton Mifflin Company.

Shapiro, D. A., Barkham, M., Rees, A., Hardy, G. E., Reynolds, S., & Startup, M. (1994). Effects of treatment duration and severity of depression on the effectiveness of cognitive-behavioral and psychodynamic-interpersonal psychotherapy. *Journal of Consulting and Clinical Psychology, 62,* 522-534.

Shapiro, D. A., & Firth, J. A. (1985). *Exploratory therapy manual for the Sheffield Psychotherapy Project (SAPU Memo 733).* University of Sheffield: Sheffield, England.

Shapiro, D. A., Rees, A., Barkham, M., & Hardy, G. E. (1995). Effects of treatment duration and severity of depression on the maintenance of gains after cognitive-behavioral and psychodynamic-interpersonal psychotherapy. *Journal of Consulting and Clinical Psychology, 63,* 378-387.

Shea, T., Pilkonis, P. A., Backham, E., Collins, J. F., Elkin, I., Stuart, M., et al. (1990). Personality disorders and treatment outcome in the NIMH Treatment of Depression Collaborative Research Program. *American Journal of Psychiatry, 147,* 711-718.

Sloane, R. B., Staples, F. R., Cristol, A. H., Yorkston, N. J., & Whipple, K. (1975). Short-term analytically oriented psychotherapy versus behavior therapy. *American Journal of Psychiatry, 132,* 373-377.

Stevenson, J., & Meares, R. (1992). An outcome study of psychotherapy for patients with borderline personality disorder. *American Journal of Psychiatry, 149,* 358-362.

Svartberg, M., & Stiles, T. C. (1991). Comparative effects of short-term psychodynamic psychotherapy: A meta-analysis. *Journal of Consulting and Clinical Psychology, 59,* 704-714.

Svartberg, M., Stiles, T., & Seltzer, M. H. (2004). Randomized, controlled trial of the effectiveness of short-term dynamic psychotherapy and cognitive therapy for Cluster C personality disorders. *American Journal of Psychiatry, 161,* 810-817.

Task Force on Promotion and Dissemination of Psychological Procedures. (1995). Training and dissemination of empirically-validated psychological treatments. Report and recommendations. *Clinical Psychologist, 48,* 3-23.

Thompson, L. W., Gallagher, D., & Breckenridge, J. S. (1987). Comparative effectiveness of psychotherapies for depressed elders. *Journal of Consulting and Clinical Psychology, 55,* 385-390.

Tschuschke, V., Bänninger-Huber, E., Faller, H., Fikentscher, E., Fischer, G., Frohburg, I., et al. (1998). Psychotherapieforschung—Wie man es (nicht) machen sollte. Eine Experten/innen-Reanalyse von Vergleichsstudien bei Grawe, et al. (1994). [Psychotherapie research—How it should not be done. An expert re-analysis of the comparative outcome studies of Grawe, et al. (1994)]. *Psychotherapie, Psychosomatik, Medizinische Psychologie, 48,* 430-444.

Tschuschke, V., & Kächele, H. (1996). What do psychotherapies achieve? A contribution to the debate centered around differential effects of different treatment concepts. In U. Esser, W. Pabst, & G. W. Speierer (Eds.), *The power of the person-centered approach—new challenges, perspectives, answers.* Köln: Gesellschaft für wissenschaftliche Gesprächspsychotherapie (GwG).

Tucker, L., Bauer, S. F., Wagner, S., Harlam, D., & Sher, I. (1987). Long-term hospital treatment of borderline patients: A descriptive outcome study. *American Psychiatrist, 144,* 1443-1448.

Wampold, B., Minami, T., Baskin, T. W., & Tierney, S. C. (2002). A meta-(re)analysis of the effects of cognitive therapy versus 'other therapies' for depression. *Journal of Affective Disorders, 68,* 159-165.

Weissman, M. M., & Bothwell, S. (1976). Assessment of social adjustment by patient self-report. *Archives of General Psychiatry, 33,* 1111-1115.

Westen, D., Novotny, C. M., & Thompson-Brenner, H. (2004). The empirical status of empirically supported psychotherapies, assumptions, findings, and reporting in controlled clinical trials. *Psychological Bulletin, 130,* 631-663.

Wilberg, T., Friis, S., Karterud, D., Mehlum, L., Urnes, O., & Vaglum, P. (1998). Outpatient group psychotherapy. A valuable continuation treatment for patients with borderline personality disorder treated in a day hospital. *Nord Journal of Psychiatry, 52,* 213-221.

Winston, A., Laikin, M., Pollack, J., Samstag, L. W., McCullough, L., & Muran, J. C. (1994). Short-term psychotherapy of personality disorders. *American Journal of Psychiatry, 151,* 190-194.

Woody, G. E., Luborsky, L., McLellan, A. T., & O'Brien, C. P. (1990). Corrections and revised analyses for psychotherapy in methadone maintenance patients. *Archives of General Psychiatry, 47,* 788-789.

Zerbe, K. J. (1990). Through the storm, psychoanalytic theory in the psychotherapy of the anxiety disorders. *Bulletin of the Menninger Clinic, 54,* 171-183.

Index